IMPROVING THE COMMON WEAL

IMPROVING THE COMMON WEAL

Aspects of Scottish Health Services
1900–1984

Edited by Gordon McLachlan

Published by
Edinburgh University Press
for
The Nuffield Provincial Hospitals Trust

© 1987
The Nuffield Provincial Hospitals Trust

Published for the Trust by
Edinburgh University Press
22 George Square, Edinburgh

Printed in Great Britain by
Eyre & Spottiswoode Ltd
The Thanet Press, Margate

British Library Cataloguing
  in Publication Data
Improving the common weal:
    aspects of Scottish health
    services 1900–1984;
    a collection in honour of the late
    Sir John Brotherston.
1. Medical care—Scotland—
    History—20th century
  I. Brotherston, *Sir* John
  II. Nuffield Provincial Hospitals Trust
362.1'09411   RA305.G6
ISBN 0 85224 551 3

CONTENTS

PROLOGUE

A 'Complaint of the Common Weill of Scotland'?[1]

The Concept

When John Brotherston in 1982 approached me asking whether the Trustees would be interested in financing a history of Scottish Health Services since 1900, neither of us was under any illusion that to incorporate in one volume an integrated account of the period to encompass the complex range of services and interests which are involved, would be a difficult task. At the same time he felt the time was appropriate, and was confident that he could rely on the help of a number of colleagues who had been concerned with health development in Scotland in the major sectors in the run-up to the Second World War and its immediate aftermath. Above all because of their active participation in the changes which had taken place, together they would be capable of providing a background to his own observations, by producing appreciations and analyses of such changes, and their effects, as direct consequences of the National Health Service (Scotland) Act 1947.

In the belief that 'time future (is) contained in time past'[2] and because Scotland has an identifiable *persona* separate from England and its Regions, the Trustees approved the study in the hope in time, of having for comparative purposes, an analysis and review of developments and improvements of health services in a unique area of the United Kingdom furth of London, which is in the geographical area served by the Trust, the provinces referred to in the Trust's title being that part of the UK outside the Metropolitan Police District of London. This was not so much in pursuit of one of the Scottish mythologies fostered by the observation of Queen Victoria's Consort 'England does not know what she owes to Scotland,'[3] as an attempt to glean some truths about health arrangements 'within a political and social system which history has differentiated at many key points from that of England'[4]. The Trust's experience is that many of the current problems which are associated with the NHS in the UK as a whole, are best studied in a more localised context to which people can more confidently relate, than from the inevitably less personalized, more corporate, national point of view. In these days of instant media coverage and comment, many issues are obscured by the transfer of isolated, sometimes dramatic if minor incidents, to the national stage, which for a better appreciation of the implications need deeper analysis. This is important in order to chart the way to the kind of improvement which is the prime purpose of the Trust. Significantly, in a Scottish connection, the purpose of improvement was fundamental to the Age of Scottish Enlightenment, a period of intellectual activity in Scotland currently being remembered with pride when 'A concept of improvement meant an interest in history and change...'[5]. The outline of the study promised much in this respect and with the appointment of a research assistant, Dr John Brims, John Brotherston proceeded to the task of commissioning a number of papers and assessing the formidable amount of rich primary source material accumulated over the years, which is a special feature of the health care sector.

Sir John Brotherston

It is not to exaggerate, that John Brotherston's death in May 1985[6] was a tragedy in that it robbed him of the opportunity of completing the ambitious task he had set himself and for which he was particularly fitted. He was unfortunately unable to see certain essays at all, and some only in penultimate draft, and he had thus, no opportunity of revising and completing the draft of his own review of the crucial period from 1948.

In order to pursue its policies a body such as the Trust has to depend mainly on those prominent and influential in its field of action, and the Trust had been helped considerably by John over the years. Archie Duncan in his moving funeral tribute reproduced as the Epilogue to this volume[7] spoke for all who knew John and appreciated his immense talents and humanity. He had an outstanding record in the Public Health movement in its purest sense, not only on the Scottish but also on the world scene. For the last thirty years of his life Scotland was his base, and the influential appointments he held there in academic and government fields make the ideal foundation for a comprehensive view of the health field related to the needs of individuals as members of communities. Indeed, the award to him of the prestigious Bronfman Prize by the American Public Health Association recognised this. His contributions to Trust publications such as 'Medical History and Medical Care' (OUP for NPHT, 1971)[9] and 'Medical Education and Medical Care' (OUP for NPHT, 1977)[10] and 'Basic Medical Education in the British Isles' (NPHT 1977)[11] reveal his grasp of the problems and the implications for the future, of this most complex of services for humanity.

In addition to his outstanding academic career at Edinburgh University where for a considerable time he was Dean of the Medical School while Professor of Public Health and Social Medicine (and later Community Medicine), an important period in John Brotherston's career was as Chief Medical Officer. There he played a very important part in helping to forge the links necessary for good practice between the key individuals and institutions in central government, academic and clinical circles, and local government, as well as voluntary bodies. This role gave him an exceptional opportunity to observe and gauge the elements promoting growth and change in this important period of social history. Even if death may have prevented him from putting the final touches to the Introduction to this collation in his own distinctive way, what he did produce and what he so impressively commissioned is unrivalled as primary source material and as a corpus and distillation of knowledge about health services in a country, which through its graduates in Public Health, has contributed much to the advancement of the application of medical knowledge throughout the world. The references alone are likely to be a goldmine for historians and scholars of medical care. It is also possible to distinguish important contemporary lines of discourse, illuminating possibly as never before, a number of major issues of our time, particularly relevant to Scotland but not exclusively so.

The Trust and Research

As General Editor of the Nuffield Provincial Hospitals Trust's publications, an old friend of John's and a Scot, it has fallen to me to try and follow the scheme of attack drawn up by John, and as faithfully as I can, *not* to attempt to complete what he set out to do in the Introduction, for that was intended as a personal review, but to edit and present on my own responsibility what was available of his own work, and the commissions.

This has been a daunting assignment even though I knew John for most of the thirty years that I was Secretary of the Nuffield Provincial Hospitals Trust and the nature of my job has ensured I have had a close interest in Scottish affairs. Scotland has always been an important example in the geographical area of the UK in which the NPHT operates, and for obvious reasons, particularly because it is a nation and not a Region of the UK, with its own institutions and history, the record of its arrangements for medical care are of special interest to all concerned with how to promote improvement. Notably the perspective of Scotland and many of the aspects of its medical care history, provide a useful comparison against which the approach to some of the major problems which bedevil medical care in the UK can be judged. The structure in England is essentially based on Regions, each with special environmental characteristics but without the benefit of a national character, and as current health policies seem to point to a greater role for Regional Authorities there, the Scottish experience is important as a guide. To many observers the services have in the past, seemed better in Scotland. The close relations which all professions in the health service even at the periphery have had with Ministers and with the civil servants in St Andrew's House, do not exist elsewhere, and Scotland has seemed a model for mutual understanding between different layers and professions in a public service, with potentially rich dividends if the lessons could be applied elsewhere.

Scottish Health Services – a sub-system of the NHS?

One of the many difficulties of considering solutions to the problems of current developments in services, is the way in which health services have been shaped since 1948 by governments of all complexions, endeavouring to fit Scotland's peculiar social economic and political status and problems to UK policies, which tend to be composite and rarely allow for other than relatively trivial local initiatives. The concept of a National Health Service, even if it required *de jure* three different enactments for England and Wales, for Scotland and for Northern Ireland, is essentially of universal *political* application in the United Kingdom, irrespective of geographical and environmental differences. It is impossible to escape the strong impression from this volume that, although Scotland has its special problems as well as traditions, these cannot be tackled appropriately by blanket decisions on a UK corporate model, however cosmetically applied. It does not require much in the way of imagination to see that since 1948, those at the centre of administration in St Andrews' House have striven in many ways not to be diverted from native Scottish tradition and principle; but because of the precedence any specially Scottish arrangements might create to upset philosophies and policies emanating from London and applied to the UK as a whole, the battle for separate policies is doomed to be lost. This has been specially so in recent years in which many government enquiries have been initiated, sometimes ending in 'reforms' designed for a UK 'system' possessing a uniformity for North, South, East and West which does not really exist at all. As a result, there have been notable restraints in the direction and scope of developments which those more directly concerned with Health Service policies in Scotland, would doubtless like to have taken to meet peculiarly Scottish needs. In the search for understanding and improvement involving individuals and institutions with their own traditions, historical perspectives can only be ignored at some peril, especially where in the case of Scotland, there is the consciousness of a separate identity as a nation. Medicine is essentially a conservative sector of the social fabric of any country and while this collation unfolds accounts of how services have developed since the turn of the century, it is evident that the roots of many of the arrangements peculiarly related to the Scots were embedded in the Scottish social and political fabric, long before the 1939–45 World War and the NHS (Scotland) Act of 1947, and actions which disturb these put healthy growth at risk. Indeed it is clear from this collation that building on a tradition given boosts in the Victorian period in the efforts to counter environmental conditions, Scottish concern for the 'Public Health' became a special feature in this century giving rise to social and political considerations which could not be ignored by people claiming to be civilised. It is specially notable in this connection that as far back as the 1930s, the Cathcart Committee Report[12] recommended a Scottish health service, with a key position for the general practitioner, thirty years and more before the General Practitioner Charter!

Health Services as Part of Social History

The accounts and comments in the whole volume are indeed an important part of the social history of this century and are thrown into striking relief by the background provided by some of the observations on social conditions and their effects, made in T.C. Smout's lively 'A Century of the Scottish People, 1830–1950'[13]. In the recent history of medical care, the growth and strengthening of health services since the 1939–45 War are universal phenomena and an important part of the social history of any country, the shape of services in each differing according to local and ethnic circumstances, even if a common characteristic is increased government participation. This is especially so in the history of social welfare in Scotland[14] which has its intellectual origins in the Scottish Enlightenment[15] which begat the pressures for social justice in the Victorian era, after the lull occasioned by the Napoleonic Wars. The development of such services has been the resultant of many forces – social, economic and political – all of which had their effects on the complex web and the woof of personal services which make up health care as we know it now, and to the way in which they were provided as a result of the stimulation and the reactions to many events, and often by the way in which opinions were introduced, moulded and disseminated in the circumstances of the times.

Natural and Local Pressures

Thus, while the successive steps towards the ideal of a comprehensive national health service are accelerated by such eventful happenings as the accidents of war, when society tends to be mobilised nationally on many fronts in the face of national dangers, in efforts to support the morale of the civilian population as well as the armed forces, the concept of social reforms of which health care is a prime, perhaps the most complex example, has much deeper roots. These lie in the political realisation that Government intervention is sometimes imperative to achieve the social stability and social and economic advancement which is the life blood of a nation. It seems quite clear from this collation of essays, which adds a special dimension to the chronicle of the development of the various services and the professional groups, that forces had been at work to that end, some way even before the Boer War. In particular in Scotland, the social susceptibilities reacting to the growing public sense of need, and in the face of the relative failure of private charitable action to meet the needs of the more deprived among the population, ensured that public services were slowly but surely being evolved. These were mainly at local levels in order to provide essential services for all classes of the population, in the light of accumulating scientific knowledge about the origins of many of the problems, and what medicine could do about these. Indeed, the Scottish experience would seem to highlight the need for a reconciliation between national and local initiatives, and between public and personal attitudes and responsibilities, in order to achieve full mobilisation of all kinds of resources for the common weal.

Professor Smout, in his 'Century of the Scottish People' has drawn attention to the local nature of public endeavour through the observation made by a writer in the 'Fortnightly Review' in 1903 about the way things were going in Scotland:

"[In Glasgow a citizen] may live in a municipal house; he may walk along the municipal street, or ride on the municipal tramcar and watch the municipal dust cart collecting the refuse which is to be used to fertilise the municipal farm. Then he may turn into the municipal market, buy a steak from an animal killed in the municipal slaughterhouse, and cook it by the municipal gas stove. For his recreation he can choose amongst municipal libraries, municipal art galleries and municipal music in municipal parks. Should he fall ill, he can ring up his doctor on the municipal telephone, or he may be taken to the municipal hospital in the municipal ambulance by a municipal policeman. Should he be so unfortunate as to get on fire, he will be put out by a municipal fireman, using municipal water; after which he will, perhaps, forego the enjoyment of a municipal bath, though he may find it necessary to get a new suit in the municipal old clothes market."[16].

This reminds us starkly, of the extent 80 years ago, of the public services of Glasgow, then at its prime as a centre of private enterprise in industry and commerce. The Glasgow public enterprises were indeed a classical application of the often ignored part of the *dicta* of its celebrated (adopted) son, Adam Smith, concerning the role of government[17] –

albeit at a local level, which complements the observation of his friend and leading figure in the Scottish Enlightenment, the philosopher David Hume, that 'Public utility is the sole origin of justice'[18]. Such public ventures were not intended to make a profit or subsidise the rates, but were designed as the best way of making specific services cheaper and better for the citizens. This point is also made by Tom Ferguson in his tandem of books on Scottish Welfare up to 1914[19], in particular, the significance to public welfare of the change which took place in public attitudes to social problems, and the pressures to try and ameliorate these through public action.

The Objection to London Supervision

It is noteworthy too, that above all, there was a marked reluctance in matters of public welfare on the part of the Scots to have their own institutions supervised from London[20], for it was widely recognised that apart from natural pride in these, the accompanying bureaucratic tendencies accentuated by distance, had several drawbacks. Many of these constraints, arising from distance and centralisation, unfortunately still remain in the 1980s. One fact relevant to the present scene, is that perhaps all too frequently, official 'quangos' set up to assess current problems as seen from London implying the recognition of a need for change, assume common problems within a supposedly unitary UK system which however is not always coherent. The resulting reports are definitely more bland than those which dealt with the problems in earlier times. Their anonymity, bred from the cautious professionalism of a *corps d'elite* of civil servants fails to hide the fact they tend to see the UK as a consistent whole (which it certainly is not) from the base of London. That they are professionally written and scrupulously if selectively researched, is beyond question, but it is inevitable that the unique characteristics and the problems arising for example from the different morbidities and traditional practices in different parts of the country (e.g. the North and South-East), far less a nation such as Scotland, are ignored, because they deal cautiously with lowest common factors, to accommodate the discrepancies between different parts of the Kingdom. There was no such anonymity nor restraint about Chadwick[21], a much revered figure, and much quoted in treatises on the foundations of public health, yet it is doubtful in the face of the kind of overwhelming professional bureaucracy which obtains now to support UK policies, if he could have wielded as much influence as he did in the nineteenth century with his largely personal report: and it has to be remembered that while Chadwick included Scotland in his review, the principles enunciated were carefully checked with the Scots and applied to suit the Scottish circumstances of the time[22].

Official Reports and Lowest Common Factors

The NHS of our era with its deployment of enormous resources presents of course a much more complicated picture than that evidenced by the lack of health care policies in the nineteenth century, or even those in the changing scene up to 1948. It is however questionable whether the succession of inevitably bland, anonymous, frequently anodyne comments from committees and commissions, inevitably originating from London, with which we have been assailed in recent years and which are faithfully accounted for with exhaustive references in this volume, have contained sustained attempts to understand the present through the past. Many of these deal in essence with general issues important to the wellbeing of man, but unfortunately because official 'quangos' tend to be brought into being to fight forest fires which flare up, and are usually doused without too close analyses of their causation, most of their reports have tended to end in actions designed to deal with the most obvious of the lowest common factorial problems, if not in the event consigned to libraries, or lie forgotten in dead files. Indeed, it is tempting to speculate how the need for many reforms is obscured by the lowest common factor syndrome, because the logical argument for this or that action, is not based on an appreciation of history to which succeeding phases of intellectual and political action should be keyed.

A Scottish System and the UK Model

This volume is rich in matters which illuminate the operation of health services which are there to be mined by social historians and commentators. Yet, these issues are also of more than interest to those concerned with policy; and although of the very stuff of effective management, they are rarely touched upon in the reports of official enquiries, since they are often obscured because they fail to conform to a UK 'National' model. They thus often tend to be ignored when priorities for action for improvement are considered.

Especially notable in the Scottish experience, are the functions and effect of Ministers actually on the spot: the close relationship which exists between the Civil Servants in St Andrew's House, and not only with members of the health authorities throughout Scotland but their officials and their professional staffs: the special links in Scotland because of the dominance of the medical schools, between academic and clinical medicine: the evident potential which requires to be encouraged and indeed exploited, in actions of the Royal Medical Corporations in Scotland on the quality of care, and in exploring such an important issue as the interaction of medical and nursing practice: the successes and failures of such experimental ventures as the Planning Council and the Common Services Agency: the particular experience of the latter on information gathering and the use of (and failure to use) the resulting intelligence, both for improving medical practice and for management: the generally accepted success of the experience of Scotland in health services research: the special arrangements in the practice of community medicine: the public/private mix of health care which is quite different from that in England, and perhaps reflects the order of relative resources employed.

This is not to suggest that the inbuilt inertia of the current bureaucracy operating a UK model can be easily overcome by the presentation of private comments and authoritative analyses as are contained in this volume; but it has been designed to, and does serve to illuminate as never before, a welter of important issues concerned with crucial matters. The Scottish experience portrayed in these papers is invaluable and should be assessed for its lessons.

A Gloomy Assessment of the Future?

It is difficult in reading the Introduction to avoid the conclusion that John Brotherston had begun to believe that however great the concept of the NHS is – (and no one can doubt it is here to stay as a 'public utility purveying justice') – something is going fundamentally wrong in Scotland[23]. It seems all too evident, (and it is becoming increasingly paralleled in the English Regions) that a great deal is being lost in the failure to mobilise local institutions and the wealth of individual talents which can be deployed there, to ensure overall improvement in this most human and personal of services. It is clear that there is a need in the case of the NHS in Scotland, for an effective reconciliation to be made between a UK 'national' model and a political system which does not easily fit well with the ruling UK system. Indeed, the problems of the NHS in Scotland add weight to Professor Kellas' contention that there is indeed a definite Scottish political system[24], made critical now with the current political make-up of Scottish members in Parliament, which is at odds with the political realities of the concept of democracy; and it is important to consider the effects. A major problem has been the inability of what was pre- National Health Service, a unique Scottish health system to be allowed to evolve naturally from its own thriving institutions, and indeed to shake itself free on health matters from what seems to be accepted as broad English practice in a UK 'system' and 'model' within the special perspective of a quite separate nation, and not a British Provincial Region similar to Trent or the West Midlands.

Pointers to Future Policies

There are indeed interesting points, both for public and private action concerning future policies, to be distilled from this volume. It is also useful to separate those relevant to the UK government, and those relevant to Scottish interests.

(a) The United Kingdom

It cannot be denied that Scotland has been enabled to deploy relatively greater resources in the health field than England. Yet for all that, and although there have been advances in the range and quality of services over the last thirty years, Scotland is not exactly doing too well in the league tables of achievement in morbidity and mortality statistics and a Golden Age has not yet been assured. Does this therefore go some way to confirm that greater resources are likely to do no more than assuage a more fundamental disfunction? Should not the policy makers at every level in health (if they exist other than occasionally) take a closer look at the structure and operation of services in Scotlard to see why with relatively greater resources 'all is not well'?

(b) The challenge to Scotland

But for the Scots themselves there are lessons from this collation. The record of achievement is impressive enough, even if it adds to the feeling that as in the UK as a whole, we should have had greater dividends in terms of medical advances from the kind of 'intelligence' which clinicians and managers ought to be able to derive from a National Health Service. But if Scotland is indeed in future to be regarded as little more than another Region of the United Kingdom and trail along as a peculiar British region, as appears to be John Brotherston's sober conclusion, it is surely time for the Scots themselves to take stock of their history. It is just not a microcosm of the UK 'system', but it is an example richer in evidence of where health services succeed and fail, and what improvements can be achieved, than in any other part of the UK, or for that matter any other country of comparable size. This is not to plead the case for such a sweeping political change in the machinery of government as a complete devolution for Scottish affairs, which would still leave the fundamental questions to be addressed, so much as for seeking improvements by attempting to work out how to achieve the development of a public utility structure based on Scottish institutions, which will allow for local and private initiative within an enlightened central administration. Even if the population of Scotland is of similar order to some of the larger Regional Health Authorities in England[25], the special characteristics and traditions of its institutions and people give it a unique base with a potentiality for development more promising than exists in any of the English Regions and indeed in most other countries.

At a time when there is uneasiness not only about the economic state but about the troubled state and future of the more cherished Scottish institutions and professions in education, in the law and in medicine, which interacting should provide the intellectual ferment essential for improvement in the common weal, should there not be a strenuous attempt to mobilise private, apolitical effort to examine the likely future of health services against their history and contemporary philosophical, political, economic and social considerations?

It is a challenge for a renaissance of national character, and for a new Age of Scottish Enlightenment which should not await a central government initiative, for the thinking will have to be done in any case; and against the kind of authoritative, intellectual and professional weight which could be deployed in the effort, the results could not be easily ignored. Any untoward delay would be unfortunate and to the detriment to the cause of public health and the common weal.

Gordon McLachlan

References

(1)   Sir David Lyndsay of the Mount. '*The Complaint of the Common Weill of Scotland.*' Poems by Sir David of the Mount (Maurice Lindsay, Ed.) Oliver and Boyd for Saltire Society, Edinburgh 1948.

(2)   T.S. Eliot, '*Four Quartets, Burnt Norton, 1.*' Collected Poems 1909-62. Faber and Faber, London 1963.

(3)   Quotation from the Royal Archives Z.491/13v. in the Introduction by Delia Miller to '*The Highlanders of Scotland.*' Haggerston Press, London 1986.

(4)   James G. Kellas, '*The Scottish Political System*'. C.U.P., Cambridge 1984.

(5)   David Daiches, '*The Scottish Enlightenment*' in '*A Hotbed of Genius*'. (Daiches, Jones and Jones (Eds.)), E.U.P., Edinburgh 1986.

(6)   Sir John Brotherston died on 12 May 1985.

(7)   Professor Duncan's funeral oration is reproduced as the Epilogue to this volume, pp.613-16.

(8)   The Bronfman Prize was awarded to Sir John Brotherston by the American Public Health Association in 1971 for his outstanding contribution to Public Health.

(9)   '*Medical History and Medical Care*'. McLachlan and McKeown (Eds.), O.U.P. for N.P.H.T.; London 1971.

(10) '*Medical Education and Medical Care*'. McLachlan (Ed.) O.U.P. for N.P.H.T., London 1977.

(11) '*Basic Medical Education in the British Isles*', with a preface by Sir John Brotherston, N.P.H.T.; London 1977.

(12) The Cathcart Committee's report was entitled "Department of Health for Scotland '*Committee on Scottish Health Services Report*'. Cmnd.5204, (Edinburgh, 1936)".

(13) Smout, T.C., '*A Century of the Scottish People, 1830–1950*'. Collins, London 1986.

(14) Thomas Ferguson (i) '*The Dawn of Scottish Social Welfare*'. Nelson, London 1948; and (ii) '*Scottish Social Welfare 1864–1914*', Livingstone, Edinburgh 1958.

(15) The essays in '*A Hotbed of Genius*', (Daiches Jones and Jones (Eds)). Edinburgh University Press, Edinburgh 1986, afford stimulating reading about the Scottish Enlightenment.

(16) Smout, T.C., *op. cit.*, p.45: Quotation from '*The Fortnightly Review*', January 1903. Acknowledged as provided by Dr W.H. Fraser.

(17) Raphael, D.D., 'Adam Smith' in '*A Hotbed of Genius*', *op. cit.*

(18) Peter Jones, 'David Hume' in '*A Hotbed of Genius*', *op. cit.*

(19) Thomas Ferguson, *op. cit.*

(20) Flinn, M.W., in Introduction p.62 in "Chadwick, Edwin, '*Report on the Sanitary Condition of the Labouring Population of Great Britain (1842)*', (Edited with an Introduction by Flinn M.W.), E.U.P., 1965".

(21) *Ibid.*, Introduction.
(22) *Ibid.*, Introduction pp.72-3.
(23) See Introduction to this volume (Section 3) p.150.
(24) Kellas, *op. cit.*, Particularly Chapters 1 and 14.

Aspects of Scottish Health Services 1900–1984

PART I:
Introduction

Sir John Brotherston
(Research Assistant: John Brims)

CONTENTS

1. *Scottish Health Services in the Nineteenth Century*

CONTENTS

About the Authors

SIR JOHN BROTHERSTON whose career is sketched out in the Epilogue by Professor Duncan was assisted in the vast research required for the period 1900–1984 by **DR JOHN BRIMS** whom he wished to recognise as co-author of the essay 'The Development of Public Medical Care 1900–1948'. Although Sir John died before proofs were available, he had approved essays 1. and 2., and essay 3. is substantially the same as his last draft. (Ed.)

Scottish Health Services in the Nineteenth Century

The background

In the history of the health services in modern Scotland the end of the 19th century might be said to have marked the end of the beginning. By 1900, after a protracted struggle, Scotland had come to accept the need for publicly run and funded systems of public health surveillance, drainage, water supply, and medical care both for paupers and for those suffering from certain highly infectious diseases. The growing involvement of the state in public health and its entry, on however limited a scale, into the field of medical care were major developments, the importance of which it is perhaps difficult for us who are accustomed to paying for the complex apparatus of modern central and local government to appreciate fully. Yet the importance of these developments cannot be overestimated. In retrospect it seems reasonably clear that what was at stake in the 19th century was the survival of modern industrial, urban civilisation in this country.

Scottish social legislation in the 19th century was generally tardy and cautious, following well behind developments in England. Why was this so? In attempting to answer this complex question four things must be borne in mind: Scotland's constitutional relationship with England; the structure of politics in both Scotland and Britain as a whole; the inability of Parliament to find sufficient time for the discussion of Scottish business; and perhaps most importantly, the doggedly individualistic outlook of most 19th century Scots. Since 1707 all Scottish legislation had had to pass through a Parliament largely composed of men who knew little of Scotland. The natural consequence of this was that much needed reforms were often considerably delayed. Where Scots and English agreed on the solution to a particular problem, the legislative delay was minimal. But there was always likely to be some delay, for legislation had to be adapted to suit Scottish conditions. Where there was no all-British agreement, the prospects were generally bleak. The parliamentary union safeguarded certain distinctively Scottish institutions, but it did not encourage the adoption of distinctively Scottish solutions to new problems. Thus the parliamentary union, by provincialising Scottish political life, virtually ensured that important Scottish legislation would follow on an English initiative and would either be closely modelled on that initiative or stick close to previous Scottish legislation. The inbuilt conservatism of this constitutional arrangement naturally suited conservative interests in Scotland. Until the 1880s the political system was dominated by property owners who were slow to appreciate the need for radical social legislation and slower to agree to finance the required reforms. However, it is important to add that there is little evidence to suggest that prior to the 1880s there was any great popular demand for radical social reforms, and much to suggest that the community as a whole largely shared the individualistic ethos of the property owners.

The second half of the 18th century had seen a gradual improvement in the welfare of the country. The movement was uneven and slow, and the condition of the people at the end of it left much to be desired; nevertheless the improvement was real. The 19th century opened with a period of relative prosperity assisted by wartime spending. It is therefore surprising at first glance to read the critical accounts of the conditions of the country which began to appear after 1820. The comments became steadily more gloomy and increased in volume during the 'Condition of the People' controversies of the 1830s, culminating about 1840 in the writings of the Scottish Poor Law and sanitary reformers which revealed the extent of destitution in the country and the deplorable state of sanitation. An atmosphere of crisis is deliberately created in the mind of the reader by these tracts. Was there some sudden deterioration in the state of the people, or were the terrible conditions revealed by the reformers the result of some long continued decline? Was the state of affairs first discovered at this late date by minds recently devoted to the problem, or had it long been appreciated and understood?

To both questions the answer lies midway. The improvements of the 18th century were mainly in the rural population. The nutritional level of the people was generally raised, but the special problems of the towns remained untouched. The towns were notoriously more unhealthy places than the rural areas, and their population was steadily increasing with the growth of industry. For a short period, at the end of the 18th century and the beginning of the 19th century, there was some expansion in the area and housing space of the towns as the better-off citizens moved out to suburbs, but the good effects were short-lived, for the growth of the towns failed to keep pace with the much more rapid growth of urban population by immigration. Gross overcrowding became inevitable. A situation developed analogous to that in the 'shanty towns' in contemporary Third World cities. The new urban populations were largely supplied from the rural areas, and the rustics who came to the towns were particularly susceptible to the diseases prevalent there. Moreover the growing industrial sector of the economy, which created these problems was liable to frequent break-downs. Each setback to industry threw large numbers into unemployment and poverty, and increased their susceptibility to disease.

These events took place in a country which had no social or administrative machinery adapted to deal adequately with these new stresses and strains. Nor was public opinion sufficiently educated to see the relationship of cause and effect between industrial and urban growth on the one hand and the prevalent distress on the other. The country had a long history of dearth and distress behind it, and it was excited by the prospect of the new wealth and power created by the Industrial Revolution. It was inevitably a considerable time before the more prosperous citizens were prepared to accept new responsibilities.

It was during the period of readjustment following on the end of the French wars in 1815 that the consequences were first felt in their full force. Destitution increased in the towns. Poverty and overcrowding brought epidemics of increasing severity, and the death rate, which had been falling during the previous 50 years, began to rise again. Moreover, as the pace of urbanisation increased, so the high urban death rates began to operate on a steadily rising proportion of the total population. As the wealth and power of the nation began to shift from the countryside to the towns, so urban conditions became a major concern and a subject worthy of increasing study. When disease and destitution began to interfere with the workings of industry and threaten future prosperity, then it was time for at least some men to question whether they represented something other than a visitation from a wrathful God upon a sinful nation. The attention devoted to endemic and epidemic typhus fever, for example, was no coincidence, for the major killing disease of that time specialised in killing the wage-earner, thereby injuring the industrial machine and leaving widows and orphans to swell the ranks of paupers for whom provision of some sort had to be made.

The cholera epidemic of 1831–2 helped to concentrate attention on health problems. There was something dreadful and dramatic about the sharp onslaught of Asiatic cholera after its slow and well publicised approach across the continents. Moreover, unlike typhus, which concentrated its attack in the poorest and most overcrowded areas, cholera attacked more widely, and even the well-to-do were not exempt. The advent of cholera produced a flurry of activity, with temporary Boards of Health being created, but, when the danger had passed, the country returned to its normal state of inactivity. However, eventually the voice of reform was heard, and wide agreement was reached that something must be done to combat the scourge of epidemic disease. In England the miasmatists, led by Sir Edwin Chadwick (1800–1890), succeeded in concentrating attention upon 'sanitary' reform, but in Scotland, where expert medical opinion, led by Professor William Pulteney Alison (1790–1859) of Edinburgh University, favoured the contagion theory of disease, attention was focused on the problem of destitution as the chief cause of increasing misery, overcrowding, and disease.

The Care of the Poor

Poor relief in Scotland, as it was before 1845, had grown to meet the simple needs of a basically agrarian community. It was later said that 'outside the principal centres of population the old Scottish Poor Law may best be described as a regulated and legalized scheme of begging, supplemented by voluntary assessments and the charities of the Church'[1]. By 1845 the community had long outgrown the stage where its poverty could be dealt with by such a system of licensed begging and church alms.

An adequate system of poor relief was a first necessity in preventing disease and lowering mortality rates, according to the Association for obtaining an Official Inquiry into Pauperism in Scotland, of which Professor W.P. Alison was a leading member. In 1840 he came to the forefront with the publication of his closely argued pamphlet *Observations on the Management of the Poor in Scotland and its effects on the Health of the Great Towns*, which had considerable influence on opinion. The movement for reform became unstoppable after 1843, when the Disruption in the Church of Scotland rendered the old poor law unworkable, and in 1845 the Poor Law (Scotland) Amendment Act was passed. The Act was a very cautious development of the previous law, and it maintained most of the characteristics of the Scottish system. The parish remained as the unit of administration, but parochial relief was henceforth managed by Parochial Boards consisting of elected representatives, with the chief magistrate as *ex officio* member. A central Board of Supervision was established, but its powers were limited to supervision and investigation of the work of the Parochial Boards, with the right to remonstrate. It is noteworthy that it was still left to the Parochial Boards to decide whether or not assessment, a tax similar to modern local rates, was required to provide adequate funds for the relief of the poor. Moreover relief was still limited to the aged and infirm poor, the Poor Law Commissioners having recommended that it was neither necessary nor expedient to give funds raised by assessment to the able-bodied poor in times of depression. The system of outdoor relief was to be maintained where possible, and although the provision of poor-houses by parishes over a certain size, or by unions of parishes, was recommended, it was not made compulsory.

Altogether no great change could be expected in the social scene from a measure of this kind. None the less it made clear the duty of the parish to provide relief. The Parochial Board had to appoint an Inspector of Poor, and to him was entrusted the direct control of relief, subject to the supervision of the Board. He was liable at law for the death of any person whose application for relief had been refused; and his tenure of office was secured against local pressures, for he could be dismissed only by the Board of Supervision. Although assessment had not been made compulsory, it became almost a necessity if the other conditions of the Act were to be carried out. The number of assessed parishes increased rapidly. In

1845 there were 230 assessed parishes, but within one year that number had risen to 420. By 1894 840 parishes were assessed, and by 1909 all of Scotland's 870 parishes had accepted the need for assessment.

The medical provisions of the Act are perhaps the most interesting part of it, for they created a statutory obligation to provide for the sick poor. Thus Section 66 of the Act laid down that 'In cases in which poorhouses shall be erected, or enlarged, or altered, under the provisions of this Act there shall be proper and sufficient arrangements for dispensing and supplying medicines to the sick poor and there shall be provided by the Parochial Board proper medical attendance for the inmates of every such poorhouse, and for that purpose it shall be lawful for the Parochial Board to nominate and appoint a properly qualified medical man, who shall give regular attendance at such poorhouses, and to fix a reasonable remuneration to be paid to him'. Section 69 stated that 'the Parochial Board are required ... to provide for medicines, medical attendance, nutritious diet, and clothing' for the poor.

Thus, for the first time, statutory provision was made for the treatment of ill health within part of the community and a duty was laid upon newly created statutory bodies to arrange this provision out of public funds. The Board of Supervision seems to have worked from the start to make the medical service as efficient as possible. It was satisfied with the medical provision in the poorhouses, but the discretionary arrangements for outdoor medical relief continued to be unsatisfactory, especially in rural and remote parishes. To remedy this, Parliament in 1848 voted a grant of £10,000 to provide part of the cost of an improved medical service. The Board used this grant as a lever to raise efficiency. It was laid down as a condition of receiving a subsidy that a Parochial Board must appoint a Medical Officer with a fixed salary to attend sick paupers. In the meantime the Poor Law reform movement had perhaps one unfortunate result: by concentrating attention on one aspect of reform it may have served to slow down other necessary improvements. It was to be another twenty years before Scotland started to tackle in earnest the problems of sanitation and the control of epidemic disease.

Sanitary Reform

As early as the late eighteenth century the principles of medical police, or public health as it was later called, were understood by leading medical men. In 1769 William Buchan (1729–1805) had disseminated a summary of these principles in his popular book *Domestic Medicine*. Andrew Duncan (Senior) (1744–1828) had delivered lectures on medical police in Edinburgh in 1791, the contents of which reveal an appreciation of the principles formulated by the German Johann Peter Frank, whose *Complete System of Medical Police* (1784) was the first comprehensive statement of the problems pertaining to the health of a nation, and of the measures thought necessary to deal with them. A chair of Medical Jurisprudence was founded in Edinburgh University in 1807, with Andrew Duncan (Junior) (1773–1832), its first occupant, devoting part of his time to lecturing on medical police, while in 1809 John Roberton (1776–1840) published in Edinburgh his important *Treatise on Medical Police*. In 1819 Professor W.P. Alison succeeded Duncan in the chair of Medical Jurisprudence, and his lectures reveal the close attention which was being paid by the Scottish medical men of the period to the work of the great armed services doctors such as Pringle, Lind, and Blane. That such developments had succeeded in creating a body of medical opinion informed in the essentials of sanitation is shown by the flood of medical pamphlets which poured forth in the 1820s and 1830s urging the need for such essential sanitary measures as enforcement of cleanliness within and without the house, suppression of overcrowding, regulation of lodging houses, demolition of unhealthy tenements, and the opening up of densely populated districts. However half a century passed before effective steps were taken to implement these measures.

There was obviously still some hope that the necessary reforms could be accomplished by the kind of communal voluntary action the earlier English medical reformers such as Percival, Ferrier and Haysgarth had attempted. Alison, in his lectures on medical police in 1820, outlined the provisions which had been made in Edinburgh during the typhus epidemic in 1817, as a model for his students to note. He discussed the importance of getting all cases into hospital quickly, and the methods of overcoming the general reluctance to go into hospital, which arose because of the popular fear of hospitals and because the infected wage earner knew that by going to hospital he left his family destitute. Alison explained that since the recent opening of Queensberry House as a temporary fever hospital to supplement the accommodation available in Edinburgh Royal Infirmary

> "no instance has occurred of a Patient being refused admittance for want of room – or of delay in his removal. A Fever Committee has been established, and this Committee has an officer always at the Infirmary who receives the recommendation of the admissions of the Fever Patients – the removal and the burial if the case terminates fatally takes place at the expense of the Committee. The support of the family of the Patient is undertaken by the Destitute Sick Society, ... Persons are employed by the Committee, on the recommendation of a medical man, to fumigate the rooms with oxymuriatic acid gas, and (what is of more importance) to thoroughly wash the bed furniture, to scour other articles of furniture, to white-wash the walls of the house, and to ventilate the place completely; and sometimes, where there is much poverty, a bed or two are lent for the time to the Family

by the Destitute Sick Society... The Destitute Sick Society, for their own benevolent purposes, have divided the city into districts and each district is visited weekly by two of their body, in order that the medical man belonging to the district (there being one appointed to each) may know at once of any case of the disease there existing... I say that even in large towns there is no necessity that the establishment for the reception of Fever Patients should be permanent; thus two wards of the Royal Infirmary were found sufficient for the accommodation of such patients for many years, and when the fever is more prevalent than usual, it is easy to provide some additional temporary establishment. It is quite necessary, however, that the Society or Association with which the management of the preventive measures rests should be permanent and one or two officers should always be employed in its service; and then, if the disease should become prevalent, it will be easy to obtain more subscriptions, and to take more persons into employment. But if the whole thing has to be started from the beginning each time much valuable time will be lost"[2].

Such measures probably prevailed in early 19th century Edinburgh, but were inadequate to deal with the greater health problems posed by the more populous, overcrowded, and unsanitary cities of the mid 19th century. Later Alison commented ruefully that the capacity to cope with such problems 'was in great measure in the power of the community, although at present beyond the powers of many of its individuals'. In other words, the time had come to abandon the purely voluntary system and move to some more radical solution.

In mid 19th century Scotland the fevers causing the greatest problems were still typhus and relapsing fever, louse-borne diseases notoriously associated with times of war, famine, and destitution, which cause overcrowding of individuals in conditions of squalor promoting infestation with lice. Although typhoid fever is shown separately in vital statistics for the first time in 1866 and was already beginning to be identified clinically separate from typhus in the mid 19th century, the indigenous epidemic fevers were still thought to be spread by contagion. Hence among Scottish medical opinion there was considerable opposition to the argument promoted by the English sanitary reformers that all problems would be solved by banishing 'filth' from the city slums.

The movement for sanitary reform had obtained impetus from the cholera epidemics, which stimulated great official activity on the part of the Central Board of Health in London and led to the establishment of many local Boards of Health. It appeared that the disease sought out the places most befouled with excrement and other filth. From that time onwards filth was raised from the level of private disgust to the important status of a public enemy in the propaganda of the sanitarians. This development was especially apparent in England where the sequelae of the English Poor Law reform gave influence for a time to a body of men centred round Sir Edwin Chadwick (1800–1890) who were whole-hearted in their belief in the miasmatic theory, which stated that epidemic fevers were caused by miasmatic or poisonous vapours arising from rotting organic matter. Large-scale investigations were organised into the conditions of urban areas of England which were aimed at demonstrating the truth of this theory so clearly that a convinced public opinion would banish dirt from the towns for ever. In 1839 the English Poor Law Commissioners obtained permission to turn their attention to Scotland. In that country they appealed for information to the Provosts of burghs, and, through them, to officers of medical charities and other medical practitioners.

The results of these investigations were published in 1842 in the *Reports on the Sanitary Conditions of the Labouring Populations of Great Britain 1842: Local Reports relating to Scotland*. Although these reports revealed much dirt and squalor, the conclusion drawn from these conditions by the Scottish reporters did not meet with the approval of the epidemiologists who advised the English Commissioners. The reports throw some useful light on the difficulties in the way of Chadwickian sanitary reform in Scotland. It was difficult to persuade medical men trained and brought up on the treatment of 'fever' (i.e. typhus and relapsing fever) that these diseases were caused by miasmata. It was only too apparent to them that contagion was the means of spread of infection, and that poverty and misery were the underlying causes. They quoted various efforts which had been made to reduce pollution but which had had no effect on the prevalence of fevers. Therefore the reports urged the primary necessity for an attack upon the causes of destitution, and placed the sanitary reforms beloved of the English Commissioners in a secondary position, without by any means dismissing them as of no importance.

This was to have significant effect in keeping Scotland out of the scope of the Public Health Act of 1848. The application of this Act to Scotland was opposed largely because of widespread resistance to the ideas of Chadwick and his disciples in the English Board of Health who were the main proponents of the legislation. A Committee of the Royal College of Physicians of Edinburgh gave evidence to the Commissioners, stating that:

> "The Committee will take the liberty of adding that although they had a high respect for individual members of the General Board of Health in London, the confident expression of opinion which those gentlemen have made on several important questions touching the diffusion of epidemic diseases, which the Committee regard as very difficult and doubtful, and on which they know that some of the most experienced

practitioners in Scotland hold a very definite opinion, have by no means tended to increase their expectations of the efficiency of measures applicable to Scotland, for restraining the diffusion of epidemics, which may proceed from that source"[3].

This evidence indicates the resistance in Scotland to being treated as an undifferentiated part of the United Kingdom.

Despite resistance to the Chadwickian solution, the reports by no means condemned the idea of sanitary reform. On the contrary the need was clearly realised, but the need for new institutions and laws was stressed if these reforms were to be effective. Burgh Police Acts had aimed at reforms in the past, but they were ineffective because of the lack of proper authorities to enforce them and because of the inadequate state of the law governing nuisances. For Edinburgh an organisation of medical police with stipendiary medical officers was recommended, while the recommendations for Glasgow went so far as to propose the setting up of a Sanitary Commission with power to appoint a medical or other officer, inspectors, clerks, and servants. However, there were in the Victorian community certain economic interest groups which could mobilise to obstruct reform, and which account for some of the delay in implementing effective solutions despite strong support for them. For example, we can note the fate of a Sanitary Improvement Bill sponsored by the Edinburgh Town Council in 1846. This measure would have enabled considerable public health reforms to be carried out, but would have materially affected the commercial interests of the owners of the irrigated lands to the east of the city, the mill owners on the Water of Leith, the spirit trade, the owners of private slaughterhouses, the pawnbrokers, the dealers in second-hand goods, the proprietors of the houses to which sanitary measures were to be applied, and others. These groups either actively or passively opposed the Bill and, in the event, it was withdrawn.

With the passage of time the situation if anything deteriorated. A major typhus epidemic in 1847 and two cholera epidemics in 1848–49 and 1853–54 occurred before the problem was tackled. The first initiative was taken in Glasgow, where demands for the municipal provision of a pure water supply had been rising since the early 1830s. In 1852 Loch Katrine was proposed as the source of water supply for the city, but the private water companies (one of which had been supplying polluted water from the river Clyde) and ratepayers' organisations combined to oppose the scheme. Further opposition, this time from the Admiralty, which claimed that the removal of water from Loch Katrine would lead to the silting up of the Firth of Forth, the Navy's only anchorage north of the Humber, led to greater delay, and it was 1855 before the Glasgow Corporation Water Works Act was passed. This Act authorised Glasgow Corporation to take over the private water companies supplying the city and establish a municipal water supply based on Loch Katrine, which was to give Glasgow the finest water supply in the United Kingdom.

In 1857 a 'Committee of Nuisances' was appointed in Glasgow, and for the first time public health was differentiated as a special function of local government. This was done under powers given by the Nuisance Removal (Scotland) Act of 1856. In 1859 John Ure, the chairman of the committee, submitted a scheme for the sanitary reform of Glasgow. He recommended the creation of a special department under a medical officer with a staff of inspectors charged with discovering nuisances and controlling disease. The Town Council sent Ure, another Councillor, the Chief Constable, and the Master of Works to visit the chief towns of the United Kingdom and report on their sanitary government and powers. They reported that while the sanitary condition of Glasgow might not be excelled in Scotland or Ireland, it was greatly surpassed in England; a situation which, allowing for 'the more cleanly habits of the English Working Classes' and the different style of building, they thought was 'undoubtedly also attributable to the extensive powers possessed by the local authorities, the thorough organization of their sanitary departments, and the enforcement of their sanitary regulations'[4].

The local powers in Glasgow were considered to be inadequate. Ure's scheme for a sanitary department was adopted, along with his recommendation for increased powers. The necessary powers were obtained in the Glasgow Police Act of 1862, and in 1863 Professor W.T. Gairdner (1824–1907) was appointed as the first Medical Officer of Health of the City. This Act marks the start of the modern public health movement in Scotland, but all was not yet plain sailing. The situation was summed up in 1870 by Gairdner. Speaking of medical reformers, he said,

> "our difficulty has been all along the fear that our own position is not sufficiently secure – the fear and the certainty, indeed, that we could not propose, with any chance of carrying public opinion with us, measures of the extremely strong and radical order that are absolutely necessary to cope with the immense evils we have to deal with. Till we have public opinion with us and this is not only having the arm of the law, as represented by the authorities, with us, but the large concurring force of public opinion – till then, I believe we shall be too weak to cope successfully with the evil"[5].

Improvement throughout the 19th century was limited by the unwillingness of the better off to accept additional taxes, an unwillingness based upon the argument that high local taxes damaged the ability of the locality to generate jobs and incomes.

In Edinburgh it required the fall of an old building in the High Street in 1861 to awaken the inhabitants to the needs of the situation. This accident, in which 35 people were killed, seems to have caused more stir than had any of the epidemics. Dr Henry Littlejohn (1828–1914) was appointed Medical Officer in 1862, and his detailed *Report on the Sanitary*

Conditions of Edinburgh, published in 1865, led to the Edinburgh Improvement Act of 1867. The work of the reformers over the half-century had at last educated public opinion to the point where it was prepared to do something about the problems of the town.

The central Government was slow to show interest in public health administration, and local communities faced the increasingly complex problems of epidemic control and sanitation for many years before the central authorities came to their aid in 1867 with the passing of the Public Health (Scotland) Act. Prior to this Act, central government had only intervened in public health matters in a spasmodic and intermittent fashion. The half century or more during which there was no central Government policy whatsoever was interrupted for only a brief period during the cholera epidemic of 1831–32, when the Privy Council was forced to set up a Central Board of Health in London to deal with that particular emergency. It was logical that the next step should be the establishment of machinery to deal with future emergencies, such machinery to operate only after a state of emergency had been declared, and only for such time as the emergency was officially considered to last. This change of policy from spasmodic to intermittent interference was introduced by the Nuisance Removal Acts, of which the first was passed in 1846. Dr J.B. Russell, who succeeded Professor Gairdner as Medical Officer of Health of Glasgow in 1870, summed up the cause and effect of this policy:

> "Having been taught all that was known of sanitary practice, its method, and the occasion for its use, under the lash of epidemic disease, it is not surprising that the legislature should have, in such a school, learned a system of spasmodic sanitation. Such was the method of applying Privy Council orders – legal instruments, under the authority of which affrighted authorities proceeded to administer, in drastic doses, that which they ought to have, from day to day, exhibited as a mild tonic to keep the body of the community in constant health. This evil method was introduced into Scotland in the Nuisance Removal Acts, various editions of which were passed from 1846 to 1856. They conferred no effective powers for ordinary times, no medical officer, and only in extremity of epidemic pressure, by Orders in Council, duly published in the *Gazette*, and for specified devoted localities, brought into operation house-to-house visitation, suppression of overcrowding, special cleansing, power to dispense medicine, and provide medical attendance and hospital accommodation"[6].

It was not until 1867 that the passing of Scotland's first Public Health Act marked the long overdue change of government policy from intermittent interference to an admission of responsibility for constant supervision of public health affairs.

It was the passing of the Poor Law Act of 1845 which made possible the policy introduced under the Nuisance Removal Acts, for the 1845 Act established both a statutorily constituted body in every parish, known as the Parochial Board, and a Board of Supervision capable of exerting control from the centre. The administrative structure was streamlined with the passage of the Nuisance Removal Act of 1856. Prior to this Act the Board of Health in London had acted as intermediary between the Privy Council and the Board of Supervision. From 1856, however, the Board of Supervision was the unique central authority in Scotland, and it was vested with certain important powers in order to carry out orders that might be issued by the Privy Council. It could appoint a medical officer at a salary not exceeding £200 per annum, and issue regulations providing for the speedy interment of the dead, for house to house visitations, for dispensing of medicines, and for affording medical aid to persons afflicted by epidemic diseases. It was also allowed to regulate overcrowding of houses.

However, the Board of Supervision and its successor, the Local Government Board for Scotland, were primarily responsible for supervising the Poor Law, and for a long time their approach to their health responsibilities was influenced by the parsimony derived from their primary responsibility. Along with its Annual Report of 1869 the Board of Supervision printed a copy of an 'instructional letter' to the Poor Law Officers in relation to the Public Health Act of 1867. This letter stated that:

> "The Board do not wish you at present to make such regular and minute inspections of your district with reference to its sanitary condition as would seriously interfere with your ordinary duties as General Superintendents of the Poor . . . You will understand that the Board do not expect that the whole of the provisions of the Public Health Act can be immediately and substantially put in force in all places . . . It is the desire of the Board you should keep in view, and as closely as may be carry out, the general principles upon which you have been instituted to carry out your duties as an officer under the Poor Law"[7].

Surveillance by medical officers of health and sanitary inspectors was one of the key elements of public health reform. However, the Public Health Act of 1867 did not require local authorities to appoint medical officers of health, and, in the event, relatively few authorities made appointments. Only with the passing of the Local Government (Scotland) Act of 1889 did it become compulsory for local authorities to appoint medical officers of health, and in response to increasing demand for medical officers of health a number of universities developed post graduate programmes in public health. Some of the early medical officers of health were clinicians of eminence like Professor Gairdner, Dr Roger

McNeill, Medical Officer of Health of Argyll, and Dr John C. McVail (1849–1926), Medical Officer of Health of Stirlingshire. The Board of Supervision was more active in promoting the appointment of sanitary inspectors, although, as with the medical officers of health in the early days, it was often difficult to obtain suitably trained sanitary inspectors. A sanitary inspector in a country district was often Inspector of Poor and schoolmaster as well. It had been said that, outside large towns, any person who could be persuaded to accept the smallest possible salary would be appointed as sanitary inspector. By 1872 the Board required 62 local authorities, with an urban population of over 2,000, to appoint sanitary inspectors, fix proper salaries for such inspectors, and report to the Board the name, address, and salary of the inspector appointed. However, the remuneration of the sanitary inspector often remained inadequate despite the efforts of the Board of Supervision. The Sanitary Inspectors' Association (later to become the Royal Sanitary Association of Scotland) was formed in 1874 in order to raise standards, and, by the end of the century, it had helped to produce a generation of reasonably well informed sanitary inspectors – an essential element of any improvement in basic public health practice.

Public works to improve water supplies and drainage came slowly and spasmodically. Despite the magnificent lead given by Glasgow in creating the Loch Katrine scheme, which involved piping water 50 miles to the city, many authorities remained reluctant to take effective action which necessarily involved incurring expenditure. There was also opposition from those who had vested interests in private water schemes. Even as late as 1905 the Local Government Board was having to apply steady pressure on some of the smaller urban local authorities who seemed to be making little effort to improve the water supply of their districts, even when epidemic disease had drawn attention to the dangers of their present supply.

A necessary consequence of improved water supplies, as well as a necessity on other public health grounds, was a corresponding improvement of drainage systems. In 1872 the Board of Supervision lamented that a considerable number of towns and larger villages were still without sewerage, and noted that they had encountered a good deal of opposition to their requests for improvement. The Board stated that in the future, resistance to their remonstrances would lead to legal proceedings. However, work proceeded, if slowly. For example Glasgow increased its mileage of sewers from 40 in 1850 to 100 in 1890.

A big issue was whether or not it was appropriate to connect the house sinks and water-closets to the main drainage system. On the whole the experts seemed to be of the view that there was too much ignorance of these contraptions in poor areas to risk such connections. Dr J.B. Russell, in a paper presented to the Philosophical Society of Glasgow in 1877, produced figures to show that the inhabitants of 1 and 2 apartment houses ran an increased risk of contamination with germs when sinks and water-closets were introduced into their houses[8].

The housing of the people has long been one of the most unsatisfactory features of the Scottish scene. Early in the nineteenth century Scottish housing already compared unfavourably with that south of the Border, particularly in respect of overcrowding. Reform made slow progress, due more to the magnitude of the problem and the willingness of the people to tolerate low standards than to the lack of legislation, for there were many Acts of Parliament on the subject, both general and local, between 1866 and 1914. Various simple lessons had to be learnt before legislation could be effective. For example, slum clearance without provision of alternative accommodation simply led to the creation of new slums as those displaced sought refuge elsewhere. First introduced in Glasgow, 'ticketing', i.e. the public definition of the permitted numbers of persons in a given room or apartment, was a useful weapon. Long after he became Medical Officer of Health of Glasgow in 1870, Dr J.B. Russell spent much of his time attempting to persuade the artisans of that city, including the decent and well-doing, that money spent on a good house was money well spent.

Much legislation was required to meet the requirements of public health reform, but only the most significant statutes can be noted here. In 1878, Greenock obtained a local Police Act requiring householders to notify cases of infectious disease to the sanitary inspector and not, it should be noted, to the Medical Officer of Health. The Medical Officer of Health remarked that the original intention had been to get doctors to notify such cases for a fee of 2s6d (12.5p) but the doctors had refused, regarding this as a breach of confidentiality. The Act proved less than successful, for many householders failed to notify. Edinburgh also tried to get agreement to a Police Bill requiring notification by doctors, but they voiced strong opposition. Nevertheless, Edinburgh went ahead in 1879, offering the participating doctors a fee of 2s6d for each case notified. Dr Henry Littlejohn, the Edinburgh Medical Officer of Health, stated that the clause was a great success, in that it enabled the local authority to gauge from day to day the health of the community and to make preparations for epidemics. Unfortunately the Infectious Diseases (Notification) Act of 1889 was adoptive rather than mandatory. The Board of Supervision urged local authorities to use a measure which applied to smallpox, cholera, diphtheria, membranous croup, erysipelas, scarlet fever, typhus, typhoid, relapsing and puerperal fever. In 1891 the Board reported that the Act had been adopted by the local authorities with jurisdiction over 60 *per cent* of the population, and by 1894 88 *per cent* of the population was covered.

The Local Government Act of 1889 promoted the creation within counties of special drainage and water supply districts which were much more likely to be effective than the Parochial Boards. By these means the larger villages and populous places were led to install drainage systems along the same lines as those in towns. With the passing of the Burgh Police Act of 1892, and the Public Health Act of 1897, local authorities directed their attention increasingly to requiring the introduction of sinks and water-closets into houses. The notice served on owners usually specified that a sink was to be fitted in a window recess or other well lighted and ventilated place with suitable connections to the sewers. The extent of provision required of water-closets was usually on the basis of at least one convenience for every three tenants.

Under the Local Government Act of 1889 and the Public Health Act of 1897 each County and District Committee was also required to appoint a medical officer of health and a sanitary inspector. It was to be a condition of appointment that the medical officer of health should have no private practice, and the later statute required him to have a qualification in sanitary science. After the 1889 Local Government Act county medical officers of health were appointed, and were soon able to report improvements, for the Act granted the Board of Supervision new powers to issue obligatory regulations governing the duties of medical officers of health. Each medical officer of health and sanitary inspector was required to write an annual report, while the medical officer of health was also required to report epidemics and every case of smallpox to the Board of Supervision. The Act produced a significant improvement in the structure of public health administration. Before 1889 1,046 local authorities were involved in the administration of public health; but subsequently the number was reduced to 305. Not all the authorities were zealous, but in the main the Act promoted a considerable advance. The Board of Supervision reported in 1893 that, with few exceptions, complaints about sanitary defects were promptly dealt with when transmitted by the Board to the relevant local authority. Only on rare occasions was the Board obliged to take legal action.

The Public Health Act of 1897 confirmed the local authorities responsible for public health as the town councils of burghs, and in rural areas the district committees or, in their absence, the county councils. It obliged local authorities to provide hospitals for infectious diseases when required to do so by the central authority. Local authorities were empowered by the Act to provide and maintain mortuaries, and they could also make bye-laws related to new building in their areas.

The central authority, the 1897 Public Health Act confirmed, was the Local Government Board for Scotland. It now prepared draft regulations on the duties of medical officers of health and sanitary inspectors. As some small local authorities had difficulty in obtaining a medical officer of health with the required statutory qualifications in public health, they were allowed to make arrangements to secure the services of the county medical officer of health.

The central authority had changed its name in 1894, but it still possessed some of the less admirable traits and Poor Law predilections of its predecessor. Much remained to be done. Writing a good deal later, Mr David Ronald, Chief Engineer of the Department of Health for Scotland, observed that at the turn of the century,

"the outstanding feature of almost every town and village in the industrial areas was their filthy condition from a sanitary point of view, although the people thought a great improvement had been effected by the cessation of throwing household refuse out of the windows and doors into the streets. The introduction of the ashpit and privy midden were no doubt a great advance, but in the light of today's knowledge they were little short of abominations. These were usually built in the court or yard behind the houses, and every form of waste and putrescible matter was thrown into them and the contents of the privies adjoining were also emptied into them and removed with the household waste. In towns this material was removed at regular intervals, probably weekly or fortnightly, depending on the district. The procedure was that the scavenger wheeled the material from the ashpit to the street, where it was dumped in a heap and thereafter removed by horse and cart. The cleansing might or might not be done by the local authority. In some cases it was, in others it was let out on contract, generally to a farmer. The farmer's interest was not always the removal of town refuse but the working of his farm, and he only removed the refuse at times when it was not possible to do other work on the farm".

On the supply of water, Ronald remarked:

"It is probably inconceivable to the present generation that prior to the general introduction of gravitation water supplies to a house the householder had to carry water from a tap, or, in some instances, a well, and store it in the house as required. In villages – and no doubt in many towns – vessels for carrying the water were known as 'stoups'. In many instances this water carried from wells was far from pure, and what its condition might be after it had been stored in a wooden vessel for probably a day in a sleeping apartment can be conjectured. It should be remembered that this water was not kept in a separate apartment but generally in the kitchen, which is now known as the living-room, and was exposed to dust and other sources of contamination. Local authorities embarked on what were then considered water schemes of great magnitude, and almost every local paper about this time was filled with debates of town councils proposing to embark on water schemes, which were described by the pessimistic members as something which would ruin the town. In spite of this opposition, the schemes progressed, and much to the delight of everyone, instead of towns and districts being ruined it was the first thing that brought prosperity and health to their areas"[9].

Hospital Care

Since their foundation the great city infirmaries have been the basis of hospital provision for the main populations of the country. No understanding of subsequent development, e.g. the structure of the National Health Service in Scotland, is possible without taking account of this.

At the beginning of the 18th century there had been only rudimentary hospital provision for the sick and infirm. At the end of the 17th century a plan was formed in the College of Physicians of Edinburgh to found a complete medical school in the city along the lines of that in Leyden in the Netherlands, to which many young Scots had gone for training. This necessitated the provision of a hospital. In 1729 the Edinburgh Infirmary was opened, with accommodation for six patients. In 1738 building was begun on a new hospital to provide room for 228 patients, which was opened in 1741. All Edinburgh and the surrounding country joined in a remarkable response to the project. Lord Provost George Drummond (1687–1766) gave a lead for the Town Council. The General Assembly of the Church of Scotland, the only representative national body of the time, ordered collections to be made at all church doors. Societies in Edinburgh contributed money; merchants gave building materials; farmers and carriers supplied carts; and mechanics and labourers gave many days work for nothing.

In Glasgow the interest of the civic leaders was also apparent. A Town's Hospital with a small infirmary was founded in 1733, being maintained by the Town Council, the Merchants House, the Trades House, and the general Kirk Session, all of which contributed to its upkeep in definite proportions. The members of the Faculty of Physicians and Surgeons gave their services free. The Glasgow Royal Infirmary was opened in 1794 when the Town's Hospital became inadequate for the city's growing needs. In 1874 the Western Infirmary was opened to provide a teaching hospital adjacent to the University's new site on Gilmorehill, and in 1890 the Victoria Infirmary was founded to provide for the south side of the ever growing city.

In Aberdeen a public meeting of citizens was convened in 1739 by the Town Council to moot the idea of building an infirmary. The plan was approved and a civic dignitary, the Convenor of Trades, was sent to Edinburgh and Glasgow to study the hospitals there. He prepared plans and the Infirmary was opened in 1742 with six beds, which were increased shortly after the middle of the century to 80. Arrangements made by some parishes to ensure treatment for their sick foreshadow more modern schemes. An Aberdeenshire reporter in the Old Statistical Account stated,

> "There is an excellent Infirmary at Aberdeen, which is of great service to the poor of all neighbouring parishes. An annual collection is made at the church doors for that Infirmary, which entitles the poor to medical advice and assistance, when they labour under any bodily distress; and likewise to proper accommodation, while their cure is in progress"[10].

Other towns in Scotland followed the lead. The Dumfries and Galloway Infirmary was founded in 1776. The Montrose Royal Infirmary and Dispensary was founded in 1782. Dundee Infirmary was opened in 1798. Houses of recovery were added to existing dispensaries in Paisley and Greenock in 1805 and 1807 respectively. The Northern Infirmary at Inverness was opened in 1804, serving the whole of the north of Scotland for more than a century. In Elgin, Gray's Hospital was opened in 1819. In Perth the Infirmary was opened in 1838, and by 1845 there were infirmaries at Ayr and Kelso. By 1845 there were 270 beds in the Aberdeen Infirmary, 120 in Dundee, 100 in Greenock, 84 in Perth, and 80 in Dumfries, while Elgin and Montrose each had 60 and Ayr 40. Some of the infirmaries provided remuneration, usually between £20 and £60 *per per annum*, for their medical staff, but in others there had never been any remuneration or it had been abandoned.

These hospitals were supported not by taxes, but rather by voluntary subscriptions, donations, and legacies. Nevertheless, they should be considered as community rather than private institutions. Citizens of all ranks took both an interest and a pride in the establishment and maintenance of these charitable foundations which symbolised the Christian virtues, civic responsibility, and status of their communities. Financial support was forthcoming not only from within the burghs in which the hospitals were located, but also from the rural hinterlands beyond, and in the case of the Edinburgh Royal Infirmary support was almost national, with monies being received from as far away as Shetland.

Provision for special categories of patient came later. For example, Sick Children's Hospitals were opened in 1860 in Edinburgh, in 1877 in Aberdeen, and in 1883 in Glasgow. The Lock Hospital in Glasgow was founded in 1805 to treat sufferers from venereal disease. The Edinburgh Institution for the Deaf and Dumb was founded in 1810. In Glasgow the Deaf and Dumb Institute was opened in 1831, while in the same city the Blind Asylum and Eye Infirmary was opened in 1827. Maternity hospitals had been founded in Edinburgh, Glasgow, Aberdeen, and Dundee (where the maternity unit was part of the Royal Infirmary) by the late 19th century.

The second half of the 19th century witnessed the establishment in many Scottish towns of small, unpretentious cottage hospitals. Aberfeldy Cottage Hospital, which opened in 1879, was a typical example, having developed from an earlier philanthropic venture which provided, among other things, a home for the sick and poor of the parish. Many of these new hospital ventures, which started in a humble way, developed a bias to surgical treatment as distinct from medical, as surgery developed at the end of the 19th century. One notable example of this trend was Falkirk cottage hospital, which developed into the Falkirk Infirmary.

In fact, by the end of the 19th century, the revolution in surgery was transforming large hospitals as well as small, and changing attitudes to hospital care, although it is important to note that even in the 1830s, before anaesthesia and antisepsis, surgical techniques were being advanced. Anaesthesia had been practised since the identification of the use of nitrous oxide in 1844, of ether by Morton in 1846, and especially since Sir James Y. Simpson (1811–1870) reported the properties of chloroform in 1847. Anaesthetics alone did nothing to improve the safety of surgery, although it reduced its agonies, and it may in fact have increased risks for a short while by tempting the surgeon to take greater risks and thus increase the hazards of infection. For example, the operative mortality reported in the Glasgow Royal Infirmary increased from 10.8 *per cent* in the period 1851–60 to 12.4 *per cent* in the decade 1861–70. It did not fall till the next decade 1871–80, when it fell to 8.6 *per cent*. Joseph Lister (1827–1912) published the first accounts of his work on antisepsis in 1867. This breakthrough was followed later by Sir William Macewen's (1848–1924) development of aseptic surgical techniques. By 1900 the number of operations in the Glasgow Infirmary had increased from 2,014 in 1860 to 16,749, while the case mortality had fallen to 7.2 *per cent* even though many more radical procedures were attempted. The period of surgical supremacy, which was to continue into the 1930s, was now beginning with its surgical 'princes', such as Sir William Macewen, and active general practitioner surgeons in every cottage hospital. About this time the advantages of hospital treatment, even for the well-to-do, were in sight, although it was not until the early years of the 20th century that these advantages were fully established. Until then hospitals, if not 'houses of death' as William Farr called them, were regarded as appropriate refuges only for the sick poor, or at any rate for those without decent housing of their own. The preferred place for the care of the better off was the home, even when surgery was required. The development of radiology at the end of the 19th century was another reason for change. The hospital was soon to begin its great technological advance as the success story of 20th century medical care, although it was only from the 1930s onwards that the pharmaceutical revolution enabled physicians to compete with surgeons for pride of place in the public mind.

Nursing

Improvements in nursing standards in late 19th century hospitals increased the attractiveness of hospital care. According to Florence Nightingale (1820–1910), nursing in earlier times had been left to those 'who were too old, too weak, too drunken, too dirty, too stupid or too bad to do anything else'[11]. Obstacles to change were the indelicacy of the tasks and the fact that the hospital was a refuge for the poor. The better off stayed at home and were nursed by relatives. But Florence Nightingale was not the only force for change, nor was the previous situation always as bad as she made out. Middle-class conversion to the hospital was a cause as well as a result of the nursing reform which changed nursing during the period 1860–1900. The daughters of the Victorian middle class were ready to fill a new professional career structure. The improvement in nursing began about 1870. Previously the Governess of the Royal Infirmary in Edinburgh hired a cook, chambermaids, and one ordinary nurse for each ward. The nurse had to clean the ward, make the beds, attend on the patients, and carry the medicine bottles to and from the apothecary shop. Supernumerary nurses were engaged for those patients who required constant and special attention. There were no ordinary nurses on night duty, and when a patient required watching after a serious operation, the student dressers were called upon to take four-hourly watches and to see that the patient was properly looked after. The nurses had no training beyond the practical expertise that they had picked up in the course of their work. In the 1860s the Nightingale School, the first training school for nurses in Britain, had been established in London, and in 1866 the Governess of the Edinburgh Infirmary was relieved of the duty of superintending nurses. In 1870 Miss Elizabeth Anne Barclay from St Thomas's Hospital was appointed the first Lady Superintendent, bringing with her a party of nurses, popularly known as 'the Nightingales'. Nurses of the old type were gradually ousted, and women of better education and ability underwent a three year training programme. Other Scottish towns followed Edinburgh's initiative, and improved nursing was introduced in less prestigious hospitals. Dr J.B. Russell, who had been the Medical Superintendent of Glasgow's new fever hospital before he became Medical Officer of Health, commented that,

> "nurses have no organisation as a class, no *morale*. The popular idea ... resembles that of a washerwoman – drinking is inseparable from both ... For all this we have ourselves to blame'.

Good nurses, he added, would only be obtained when education, organisation, supervision, good pay, and superannuation were provided[12]. Russell introduced training into the local authority hospitals. Even in the Poor Law infirmaries improvements were taking place. In 1878 the Board of Supervision referred for the first time to defective arrangements in poorhouses for nursing sick and bedridden inmates. Malcolm McNeil (1839–1919), one of their visiting officers, wrote regarding the need for better nursing:

> "I am informed that any woman of activity and moderate intelligence, if a sufficient number of patients are available for purposes of tuition, can be taught to be of some service as a nurse in 3 to 6 months, i.e. she can be drilled in regular habits, promptitude, tidiness, obedience to medical orders, the modes of moving helpless persons, simple bandaging etc."[13].

The daily average of the sick and bedridden in Scottish poorhouses at that time was 2,942, while only three sick nurses, and not a single probationer, were employed. In 1880, the Board of Supervision drew up Rules and Regulations for the management of hospitals and infirmaries in poorhouses where a trained head nurse or lady superintendent was employed. These rules laid down that when a superintendent nurse was appointed, the matron of the poorhouse would have no jurisdiction within the hospital. The superintendent nurse was to conform to the instructions of the medical officer as to the treatment, diet, and hygiene of the hospital. By 1897 nearly half of the poorhouses had trained nurses. In that year the English Local Government Board issued an order prohibiting nursing by pauper inmates in workhouses, but the Scottish Local Government Board doubted if they had powers to issue such an order, and in any case they said it was not expedient because of the number of small poorhouses where it was not practical. They advised the removal of acute cases to the infirmaries. Pauper nursing was still prevalent in Scotland at the time of the visits by the Royal Commission on the Poor Laws 12 years later but some progress had been made since the 1890s. By 1902 four poorhouse hospitals had training schools for nurses, while in 1907 the Local Government Board introduced written, oral and practical examinations for nurses.

Nursing standards outside the hospital were also progressing. Many localities took steps to provide themselves with a resident nurse. Sometimes the laird installed a nurse at his own expense. Sometimes local associations were formed to employ a nurse. Parish Councils were authorised and encouraged to subscribe to the funds of these associations if they undertook the treatment of paupers. The Local Government Act of 1889, which instituted County Councils and District Committees as health authorities, made possible the great developments in nursing services which took place subsequently in rural areas.

Care of the mentally ill is another strand in the story of institutional provision. The first institution dedicated to the purpose was the Montrose Asylum, opened in 1782. The Aberdeen Asylum was opened in 1800. The Royal Edinburgh Asylum was granted its Royal Charter in 1807. The Glasgow Asylum was opened in 1814, while that in Dundee was founded in 1812. The Royal Asylum in Perth and the Crichton

Royal Institution at Dumfries were opened in 1827 and 1838 respectively. Provision for the mentally handicapped came later. Baldovan Asylum was opened in 1855, in Edinburgh an Institution was founded in 1855, and the Royal Scottish National Institution in Larbert was opened in 1863. In 1855 Dorothea Dix (1802–1887), the American reformer in the field of mental illness, visited Scotland on invitation and, having investigated conditions for treating the insane, reported adversely. Following her report a Royal Commission was appointed to investigate the situation. It found much to criticise, and its recommendations led to the Lunacy (Scotland) Act of 1857 which established a Central Board of Commissioners in Lunacy and District Boards of Lunacy. It laid down conditions for certification, and contained two important provisions not found in English Lunacy Acts which were to be responsible for the relative freedom from complaints in Scotland. These were the power to keep a patient under observation for six months in doubtful cases without certificate and the power to board out harmless lunatics with private persons. As from 1858 jurisdiction regarding the insane or feeble-minded poor was transferred from the aggrieved Board of Supervision to the Central Board of Commissioners in Lunacy for Scotland.

The main burden of caring for the sick and infirm paupers, however, continued to rest with the Board of Supervision and the Parochial Boards, and the result was an unsatisfactory compromise between a rigid attempt to control costs and a sense of responsibility towards the sick and infirm. The Poor Law Amendment Act of 1845 had laid down clearly the duty of maintaining proper and sufficient arrangements for the sick poor, including proper medical attendance. On the other hand, the Board was determined to keep the poorhouse as a severe test of genuine poverty, explaining in a circular that the 'poorhouse will be literally useless as a test unless it is conducted under rules and regulations as to discipline and restraint so strict as to render it more irksome than labour'. As a result Poor Law hospitals lagged far behind voluntary hospitals. For example, in 1884 the Barony poorhouse medical officers in Glasgow noted the difficulties of surgery conducted in the wards amidst other patients because there was no surgical theatre available. Backward even by the standards of the times as these institutions were, they came to play an ever increasing role in the provision of medical care. Prior to 1845 there had been hardly any poorhouses in Scotland, but by 1895 there were 62 of these establishments catering in some fashion for the needs of 15,392 inmates, almost one-third of whom were sick and infirm. With the democratisation of the political process in the 1880s the Poor Law authorities became more responsive to the demands for improved care for the sick poor. Glasgow led the way in gradually upgrading the hospital part of its poorhouses, and in providing purpose built Poor Law hospitals separate from the poorhouses. The Royal Commission on the Poor Law in its 1909 report exempted Glasgow 'with its 3 new Poor Law Hospitals' from its cutting criticism of Scottish Poor Law hospitals. The slow metamorphosis had begun which turned Poor Law hospitals into modern institutions for the care of the sick.

In the meantime deep seated prejudices against the Poor Law infirmaries were engrained in the public consciousness. The responsibility of Poor Law authorities for the sick and infirm created by the Poor Law Amendment Act of 1845 included the provision of 'outdoor' medical relief. The 1886 rules of the Board of Supervision stated that 'all poor persons in need of medical relief must be duly and punctually attended by a competent Medical Practitioner'. No practitioner was to be regarded as competent unless he had a medical degree or diploma from a University or other approved body in Great Britain. The medical officer was to report in writing to the Inspector of the Poor the relief necessary for treatment, and the practitioner was to attend personally, at the house of the patient if necessary.

The Poor Law created many new posts for doctors. It encouraged all parishes to appoint a doctor, but many were slow to do so. Parliament in 1847–48 voted an extra sum of £10,000 to be spent on medical relief for the poor in Scotland. This grant acted as an incentive, and by 1902 only 79 out of 874 parishes were still outside the scheme. There were, however, special difficulties in finding practitioners for outlying, poverty stricken areas where private practice was unremunerative. Nevertheless, it was the Poor Law, supported by Treasury grants, which brought a doctor for the first time to many parishes in the Highlands and Islands.

Poor law medical practice had few admirers within the medical profession. The cheeseparing of Poor Law authorities created disillusionment and a dislike of public service among doctors which was to cloud later discussions between the profession and the government. The terms of service were the cause of much heated controversy regarding methods of appointment, duties and pay. Usually the appointment was permanent, but some parishes tried to keep it subject to annual review. It was sometimes put out to tender, with the doctor who was willing to carry out the duties of the post for the smallest salary being given the appointment. Usually the service was to be comprehensive and included the supply of all necessary medicines. The Parochial Board decided on the amount to be paid. A negotiating committee of the profession sought to obtain acceptable terms, especially for rural medical officers who found it difficult to press their claims.

There was another form of public hospital at that time – the fever hospital. Traditionally the main work of dealing with fevers had been left to the great infirmaries, and it was only when a particularly severe epidemic threatened to overwhelm the entire life of the town that the public authorities were stirred to action, and then the action was short lived. This situation was well described by Dr J.B. Russell, who won his

spurs in the struggle to establish municipal fever hospitals. Describing the
history of epidemic fever management in Glasgow, he wrote that:
> "Each epidemic was a tragedy. When it was played out all
> the properties were dispersed and the stage left
> unfurnished . . . From its opening in 1794 for seventy years the
> [Glasgow] Royal Infirmary was the centre of every provision
> for isolation. At one time indeed the managers even disin-
> fected the houses from which they removed fever patients.
> The usual course of events was the rapid extension of the
> epidemic until the Infirmary Fever House was overflowing:
> then public excitement, public meetings, the appointment of
> a 'Fever Committee', or a 'Board of Health', as in 1832 and
> 1837, the collection of funds, a rushing about for sites for
> temporary hospitals, attendance at home, the organisation of
> a staff of fumigators, etc. Then the disease in due time began
> to decline: it shrank within the capacity of the Royal
> Infirmary: the hospitals were pulled down, the doctors,
> nurses and fumigators who had not been buried were paid
> off; a report of the receipts and disbursements was submitted
> and the Board of Committee ceased to be. The play was over;
> the old properties were not even stowed away, they were
> burned"[14].

In Edinburgh, Queensberry House was used as the fever overflow
hospital from the Infirmary.

Eventually the voluntary infirmaries rebelled against this system.
Glasgow was the first to act. An isolation hospital was opened in Parliamentary Road in 1865, in 1870 Belvidere Hospital was founded, and in
1900 Ruchhill Hospital opened its wards for the first time. In Edinburgh,
the managers of the Royal Infirmary announced in 1885 that they could
no longer provide for fever patients, and for some years the old surgical
house of the old infirmary was used as a fever hospital. It was 1903 before
a purpose built municipal fever hospital, the City Hospital, was opened
in Edinburgh. Dundee provided a permanent fever hospital at King's
Cross in 1889. The Board of Supervision applied pressure to local authorities to provide fever hospitals, as they were empowered to do under the
Public Health Act of 1867, and a good many small hospitals were opened
as a result. The larger fever hospitals developed their own nurse training
schemes, and a standard of patient care superior to that in the Poor Law
hospitals. Important as the development of municipal fever hospitals
undoubtedly was, we may question whether separation of hospital responsibility for infections from the main stream of clinical development
has been a good thing for Scottish medicine in the long run. In the
U.S.A., where this separation never took place, there has been more
research and development devoted to the ever-present hazards of infection than in this country.

The high prevalence of infectious disease, and the epoch-making advances in bacteriology in the late nineteenth century, began to persuade the administrative authorities that it would be valuable to have the resources of bacteriological laboratories available to practitioners within their districts, particularly in connection with the diagnosis of cases of diphtheria, typhoid fever, tuberculosis, and the examination of water supplies. In his report for 1896 the Medical Officer of Health of Aberdeen suggested a combination of local authorities and an arrangement with Professor David J. Hamilton (1849–1909) of the University, whereby necessary bacteriological examinations could be carried out either on behalf of the local authorities themselves or any practitioner within their districts. Within two years Dr Watt was able to report that 31 local authorities, covering a population of 350,000, were participating in the scheme. At about the same time the city of Glasgow set up a bacteriological laboratory, and in 1902 the county of Lanark decided to follow suit.

Tuberculosis was a special form of infection which was creating increasing anxiety at the end of the 19th century. In the five years from 1866 to 1870 there were nearly 12,000 deaths from tuberculosis in Scotland – 17 *per cent* of all deaths. This was the high point in death rates from tuberculosis, and from then on mortality fell steadily. In the meantime Dr Robert W. Philip (1859–1939) was developing his pioneer system of care for tuberculosis which was to be a pattern for medical care organisations in many countries and was to win him a knighthood in 1913. The central point of his system was a dispensary, the threefold object of which was to diagnose and treat tuberculosis, and prevent the spread of infection to contacts. Philip's system also included a sanatorium which aimed to effectively arrest early cases of tuberculosis; a hospital for patients in advanced stages of the disease which sought chiefly to limit the spread of infection; and a colony for the aftercare of patients who would probably relapse if not under supervision. Tuberculosis control, he maintained, should be a separate and well defined department of the medical officer of health.

The Medical Profession

The greatest strength of the Scottish health service to this day probably lies in the size and strength of its medical schools. The story begins effectively with the foundation of the Edinburgh University Medical Faculty in 1726. The early success of the Edinburgh medical school owed everything to a conjunction of circumstances: the coming together of a group of young, ambitious and talented men; the willingness of the City's Town Council and farsighted Lord Provost to support the development; the decay of Leyden from its earlier pre-eminence among European medical schools; and the recondite and impractical state of medical education in the old English universities. The closure of Oxford and Cambridge to denominations other than the Church of England, and the demand for doctors for the armed services during a period of almost continuous war, led to the rapid ascendancy of an Edinburgh school which was ably supported for a century or so by individual teachers and scientists of great talent who attracted large numbers of students to Edinburgh, both to the University and to the expanding extra-mural schools, from all over the English-speaking world. The development of the Glasgow Medical School, however, was hindered by the hostility of the Faculty of Physicians and Surgeons and by the absence of a sizeable teaching hospital, until the opening of Glasgow Royal Infirmary in 1794, and consequently the Glasgow school was unable to compete with its eastern rival until the early nineteenth century. Aberdeen medical school, despite the early existence of its 'mediciner' or professor of medicine, did not really prosper until the union of Marischal and King's Colleges in 1860, while the development of the St Andrews school was crippled by the lack of clinical teaching facilities until 1899 when these were made available in Dundee.

By the mid 19th century Scotland had lost her true international ascendancy in the scientific forefront of medicine and medical education to France and Germany, where the great advances in physiology and pathology were being made, although the outlay on medical education remained relatively large for such a small country. In 1858 two Acts of the greatest importance came on to the statute books; the first, an Act regulating the qualifications of practitioners in medicine and surgery, and the second an Act creating the General Medical Council to establish and supervise a register of medical practitioners. These Acts, which had long been delayed by the struggles between the universities and the medical corporations for supremacy, removed various anomalies and difficulties interfering with the freedom of qualified practitioners to practise anywhere within the British Empire. At the time when these Acts were passed some 50 *per cent* of registered practitioners in the United Kingdom had received their qualifications from one of the Scottish universities or one of the Scottish Colleges. Since that date the total output of the Scottish schools has diminished relatively, as has the proportion of Scottish-trained doctors, which is now around 17 *per cent*. Nevertheless the production of doctors is such that it has been possible to maintain a more numerous establishment of doctors relative to population in Scotland than in other parts of the United Kingdom, and the great teaching hospitals on which the medical schools are based are the vital power-houses driving the machinery of medical care, and in no sense ivory towers withdrawn from the main battle front.

It is not easy to trace the origins of the hard and fast lines which differentiate categories in the modern medical profession, and in particular the separation of the general practitioner from the specialist. The forefather of the general practitioner in Scotland seems to have been the surgeon-apothecary. By the end of the 17th century the surgeon-apothecaries, who were firmly based on the College of Surgeons in Edinburgh and the Faculty of Physicians and Surgeons in Glasgow, had seen off the apothecaries, who unlike their brothers in England were henceforth limited to the roles of prescribing chemists. To the extent that the surgeon-apothecaries came out of similar processes of recruitment and education as the physicians and surgeons, the profession in Scotland thereby largely avoided the 'class' division between the tradesmen apothecary trained by apprenticeship and the gentleman university-educated physicians which prevailed in England. The distinction should not, however, be too finely drawn. The Scottish surgeon-apothecaries did not all hold a University or College qualification. Even into the mid 19th century many, particularly in rural areas, were trained by apprenticeship, and were consequently regarded by their colleagues as of distinctly lower status. In Glasgow, surgeon-apothecaries who operated a dispensing 'shop' were ineligible for Fellowship of the Faculty of Physicians and Surgeons.

Medical practice was still frequently ineffective, and was sometimes positively dangerous. There was therefore a good deal of justified public suspicion of doctors, although the distribution of doctors depended very much on the financial resources of the area. The Highlands and Islands remained in parts a medical desert until well on in to the 20th century. Even the existence of Poor Law posts offered scant pickings, and in some of the poorer areas doctors were few and far between. Although there was some notable exceptions, doctors tended to be of low quality; they had huge distances to travel and there was often no fee for them at the end. The Royal College of Physicians of Edinburgh had carried out a survey of practice in the Highlands in 1852. Letters were sent to ministers and doctors in 155 parishes. It was found that 62 parishes had adequate services, 52 were partially supplied, and 41 were rarely if ever visited by a doctor. The report's findings anticipated those of the Dewar Committee in 1912 which were to lead to the establishment of the Highlands and Islands Medical Service. This dearth was not only found in the Highlands. In Aberdeenshire there was only one doctor for 50 miles north of Aberdeen at the beginning of the 18th century. In these rural areas, in the absence of practitioners, it was necessary that clergymen and lairds should know something about medicine, and if after 1769 they possessed a copy of William Buchan's best selling *Domestic Medicine* their clients were probably no worse off than if they had found a medical practitioner. By contrast, McCracken[15] has shown that in the wealthy county of Roxburgh there was one doctor for 1,840 patients in 1760, and that by 1795 it was one to 1,390, possibly the most favourable ratio ever found in that area. In the cities, the population and the number of doctors more or less kept pace with each other. In Glasgow, by the end of the 19th century, there were in fact proportionately more doctors to total population than there had been at the beginning of the century, partly as a result of the increased number of paid appointments available to doctors, which had multiplied by more than a factor of ten. Another factor creating additional income for the profession was the large scale intervention into the field of medical insurance of the Friendly Societies. By the late 19th century industrial growth had provided a large class of skilled working men who could afford to pay for medical insurance. This need was met by the Friendly Societies and, to a lesser extent, by commercial organisations. The Friendly Societies became a strong enough force to be a factor in medical politics in the early 20th century. Such was the growth of the Friendly Society movement that by 1892 there were 1,320 societies in Scotland with 280,000 members and £1.25 million funds. The Friendly Societies were hard faced and tight-fisted employers, and the medical profession was as resentful of what it regarded as their exploitation of 'contract practitioners' as it was of the treatment meted out to parochial medical officers by the Poor Law authorities.

Hospital specialisation, as we know it today, was in its infancy, being generally resisted by the grandees of the profession, although obstetrics, ophthalmology, and ENT were well established specialisms by the 1820s and 1830s. There was already some evidence in the cities of demarcation between the doctors with and without hospital affiliations, from which the separation of specialist from general practitioner later developed, but it should be noted that most of the prestigious hospital physicians carried on high class general practice well into the 20th century. There was also some tension between the two categories, for the doctors without hospital jobs were apt to blame the hospitals for attending free of charge in out-patient departments to patients who could afford a fee. To some extent this grievance was abated after the National Insurance Act of 1911.

Maternity and Child Welfare

The history of the Maternity and Child Welfare movement more properly belongs to the 20th century, but towards the end of the 19th century some premonitory developments can be identified. The higher child death rates of children of low social groups had attracted the notice of early Victorians. Professor Robert Cowan (1796–1841) of Glasgow wrote in 1840 that 'the contrast between the labouring classes and those in easy circumstances is in no part so strongly marked as the relative number of births and deaths of their children'[16]. At an earlier stage smallpox and measles had been regarded by some as the poor man's friend because they were apt to decimate his overly numerous family. Smallpox vaccination was not made compulsory in Scotland until 1864, 10 years after England. According to the Registrar General, diphtheria first showed itself in

Scotland in 1857. There was a great reduction of mortality from diphtheria following the introduction of antitoxin in 1894, but measles and whooping cough were rarely absent from large centres.

Anxiety created by baby-farming scandals led to the Infant Life Protection Acts of 1872 and 1897. It became compulsory for anybody earning money from caring for a child over one and under five to notify the local authority. Prevention of Cruelty to Children Acts for Glasgow were passed in 1884, for Edinburgh in 1885, and for the whole of Scotland in 1890. Dr J.B. Russell, the Medical Officer of Health of Glasgow, was concerned about uncertified deaths and their relationship to illegitimacy long before the official maternity and child welfare movement. In 1874 he wrote 'the more dependent and helpless of itself the life is, the less attention it receives'[17]. Russell conducted Glasgow's first enquiry into its high infant mortality rates, publishing his results in 1876.

Resources were beginning to be made available. The Royal Edinburgh Hospital for Sick Children was founded in 1858. Dr John Thomson (1856–1926) was a Scottish pioneer in paediatrics, who published a textbook on his specialism in 1898. Dr John W. Ballantyne (1861–1923) of Edinburgh was the first doctor in the United Kingdom to establish an antenatal clinic which provided supervision for expectant women. In 1901 a bed for this purpose was endowed in the Simpson Maternity Hospital in Edinburgh, and in 1915 an ante-natal department was created.

The 19th Century Legacy

It had been widely expected that as a result of the development of public health services during the 19th century the death rate would fall. It did, but the infant mortality rate and the maternal rate did not. With the fall in the birth rate which aroused fears of depopulation, a clamour began to arise for greater action in child welfare.

As we know that the effects of adverse environmental change are likely to show themselves firstly and most acutely among the child population, it seems beyond doubt that the century of industrialisation, overcrowding, and slum dwelling must have had adverse effects on Scottish urban populations. The nutrition experts of the later 19th century were clear that there had been marked deterioration in the urban diet compared with the traditional oatmeal and milk diet of rural populations. Poor diet, chronic and dire overcrowding, and the generally polluted urban environment must have scathed our population. How many generations will it take for the Scots to free themselves from the physical and cultural stunting which have resulted?

References

(1)   *Report of the Royal Commission on the Poor Laws. Report on Scotland.* (1909) Parliamentary Papers XXXVIII, p.192.

(2)   Brotherston, J.H.F. *Observations on the Early Public Health Movement in Scotland.* (London, 1952), pp.65–66.

(3)   Ferguson, T. *The Dawn of Scottish Social Welfare. A survey from medieval times to 1863.* (Edinburgh, 1948), pp.147–148.

(4)   Brotherston, J.H.F. *op.cit.*, p.87.

(5)   Russell, J.B. *Public Health Administration in Glasgow.* (Glasgow, 1905), pp.32–33.

(6)   *Ibid*, pp.82–83.

(7)   Ferguson, T. *Scottish Social Welfare 1864–1914.* (Edinburgh, London, 1958), p.11.

(8)   *Ibid*, pp.193–194.

(9)   *Committee on Scottish Health Services Report.* Cmd.5204 (Edinburgh, 1936), pp.40–41.

(10) *The Statistical Account of Scotland, drawn up from the communications of the ministers of the different parishes* (Ed. Sir John Sinclair) (Edinburgh, 1791–1799), XV, p.223.

(11) Gaffney, R. 'Women as doctors and nurses', in Checkland, O., and Lamb, M., *Health Care as Social History*: The Glasgow Case. (Aberdeen University Press, 1982), p.139.

(12) *Ibid*, pp.140–141.

(13) Ferguson, T. *Scottish Social Welfare 1864–1914.* (Edinburgh & London, 1958), p.304.

(14) Russell, J.B. *Public Health Administration in Glasgow.* (Glasgow, 1905), pp.15–16.

(15) McCracken, I.E. 'Eighteenth Century Medical Care: a study of Roxburghshire', *Proc. Roy. Soc. Med.* 1949, 42, pp.410–6.

(16) Ferguson, T. *The Dawn of Scottish Social Welfare. A survey from medieval times to 1863.* (Edinburgh, 1948), p.285.

(17) Checkland, O. 'Maternal and Child Welfare', in Checkland, O., and Lamb, M., *Health Care as Social History: The Glasgow Case.* (Aberdeen University Press, 1982), p.119.

2. The Development of Public Medical Care: 1900–1948

CONTENTS

The Development of Public Medical Care 1900–1948

The opening of the century

Victorian society was based on the twin foundations of self-help and Christian philanthropy, and, at the beginning of this century, the State played a limited role in the provision of health care. Local authorities could be required, under the Public Health (Scotland) Act of 1897, to provide hospital treatment for those suffering from infectious diseases, and were, under the influence of the pioneer Sir Robert Philip, coming increasingly to recognise the need for concerted action in alliance with voluntary agencies against the scourge of pulmonary tuberculosis. The State, however, accepted responsibility only for the treatment of sick paupers. Many people of limited financial means therefore subscribed a small weekly sum to a Friendly Society or similar organisation which provided a medical practitioner to attend them when they were sick. Others who were too poor or too improvident to make such arrangements relied in time of ill-health upon the services provided by dispensaries, the outpatient departments of voluntary hospitals, or general practitioners, whose fees were adjusted according to the economic circumstances of their patients and were frequently waived entirely. Others again turned to folk remedies or patent medicines. In certain remote areas of the country, and in the poverty-stricken western Highlands and Islands in particular, health care was totally inadequate. There were too few doctors living too far away from patients who, in any case, were generally unable to afford medical services. In many rural areas hospital provision was hopelessly insufficient for the needs of the population. Many medical practitioners, public health officials, and interested laymen realised that health care services were far from satisfactory, but there is little evidence of widespread public disquiet and none of any determined effort to secure radical reform.

It has long been accepted that, like the first and second world wars in later periods, the Boer War played a significant part in transforming British attitudes towards health policy. The military embarrassments experienced in South Africa created profound anxieties in a Britain which was already becoming worried by its recent economic difficulties and by the threat posed by the increasing economic and military might of the United States and Germany. In 1902 a Royal Commission was appointed to ascertain what opportunities existed in the Scottish education system for the physical training of children and adolescents, and to suggest 'how such opportunities may be increased' so as 'to contribute towards the sources of national strength'[1]. It is important to emphasise that the Royal Commission was not appointed to inquire into the health of children, and that, as Dr W. Leslie Mackenzie later pointed out, its terms of reference assumed 'that, given adequate opportunity and organisation of physical training at all stages of school life and afterwards, the fitness of children and adolescents could be secured'[2]. The lack of essential scientific data relating to the physique of Scottish school children led the Royal Commission to set up its own inquiry to provide the requisite information. This inquiry, which was conducted by Professor Matthew Hay in Aberdeen and Leslie Mackenzie in Edinburgh, revealed an alarming picture of widespread ill-health among Scottish children, and demonstrated the close link between poverty and ill-health. The inquiry's findings made a great impact on the Royal Commission, and in its report, which was published in March 1903, it not only recommended improvements in the Scottish physical education system, but also advocated the establishment of a scheme of medical inspection for school children, and pointed out the importance of nutritious diet to the satisfactory physical and mental development of children[3].

The publication of the Royal Commission's report created no stir, and aroused no immediate demand for fundamental changes in health policy. The *Glasgow Herald* welcomed the recommendations in favour of more emphasis on physical education in Scottish schools, but ignored the wider recommendations on the importance of a nutritious diet and the provision of a system of medical inspection for Scottish school children[4]. The correspondence subsequently published in that newspaper strongly suggests that its readership did not disagree with the views of its leader writers. The *Scotsman* showed some interest in the Royal Commission's findings regarding the relationship between poor housing and physical unfitness, commenting that they seem 'to make good the rule that "the poorer the house the thinner the child"', but it too displayed no enthusiasm for any scheme of medical inspection for school children, and offered no solution to the old Scottish problem of bad housing[5].

The publication of the Royal Commission's report stimulated only one of the *Scotsman's* readers to take pen to paper, and significantly the concerned reader in question was a public health official rather than a layman. Dr William Robertson, Medical Officer of Health for Leith, wrote that 'everyone interested in public health will hail with immense satisfaction the lucid and enlightened report of the Commission on Physical Culture in Schools'. He congratulated the Commission on grasping the importance of the provision of food in school, and claimed that the recommendation in favour of 'a systematic medical inspection of schools and scholars... will strongly appeal to the medical officers of health of every large district'[6]. Robertson's claim was soundly based. In 1904 Dr W. Leslie Mackenzie, Medical Inspector to the Local Government Board for Scotland, pointed out that 'for many years medical officers of health [and others] have suggested the desirability of instituting a medical inspection of schools'[7]. Indeed, Dr William Robertson had himself drawn up a scheme of medical inspection for Paisley school children in 1900, which he persuaded the local authority and School Board to adopt. However, when the Scottish Education Department informed the School Board that rate monies could not legally be applied for such a purpose the project had been reluctantly dropped[8].

The frustration experienced by enlightened public health officials and progressive local authorities at the lack of response to the Royal Commission's report was probably compounded by the reception given by the leaders of 'informed' Scottish opinion to the Interdepartmental Committee's report on Physical Deterioration. Over sixteen months had elapsed since the publication of the report of the Royal Commission on Physical Training, but the mature reflection thus afforded did nothing to alter Scottish views. Scottish members of Parliament greeted the Committee's report with the seeming indifference that had characterised their response to its predecessor in 1903. On matters of health policy at least, they were, with few exceptions, strangely silent indeed. The local authorities were apparently equally unmoved. The Convention of Royal Burghs, the collective voice of Scottish urban local government, regarded the subject of medical inspection of school children as undeserving of debate. A similar indifference was displayed by the *Glasgow Herald*, which considered the Interdepartmental Committee's report unworthy of editorial comment. In assessing the report's findings the *Scotsman* refused to be ruffled by alarmist talk of national degeneracy, and argued complacently that there is 'a mean physical standard which is the inheritance of the nation as a whole, and the tendency of the race is to maintain this inherited mean.' Moreover the same newspaper dismissively labelled as 'wastrels' those who had been rejected for military service on medical grounds. It would appear that, in the view of the *Scotsman* at least, the health problems of the sub-class of casual unskilled workers (from which the army usually drew its recruits) were largely of their own making[9].

A somewhat different view of the cause of ill-health among the poorer sections of society was taken by the Liberal *Dundee Advertiser*. The *Advertiser* found much in the report to support its strong temperance opinions, commenting that 'chief among the principal causes of physical deterioration the Committee places alcoholism'. This was a serious misrepresentation of the report's findings, but it enabled the leader writer to claim that 'if we could only deal with this root-matter [i.e., the overconsumption of alcohol] the things referred to in the other recommendations of the Committee would either come of themselves or be rendered superfluous'[10]. The prominent place held by drink in the demonology of both the skilled working class and the lower middle class in Scotland was such that there can be no doubt that the *Dundee Advertiser*'s views on the primary cause of poverty and its associated ill-health reflected those of a great number of ordinary Scots of differing political persuasions. It was pressure from the popular and politically influential temperance movement which led to the so-called Local Veto Act of 1913, a measure which permitted ballots to be held on whether or not licensed premises would be allowed to operate in specified areas. In 1920 the Independent Labour Party and its mouthpiece *Forward* (whose editor, Tom Johnston, a staunch prohibitionist, refused to accept advertisements for alcoholic drinks) championed a massive 'No Licence Campaign' in Scotland. The campaign was less than successful, with only 41 areas voting to prohibit the sale of alcohol, but temperance was to remain an important part of the increasingly powerful Labour movement's political creed in Scotland into the period after the second world war. Indeed, the Glasgow Labour Party only abandoned its policy of maintaining 'dry' council estates in 1965, and it was 1982 before the Party did anything to implement its decision[11].

Important as temperance was to many Scots, an increasing number of people came to accept that it could not be a panacea for all the ills of the poor. Slowly but surely old opinions came to be re-examined in the light of the findings of the Royal Commission on Physical Training and the Interdepartmental Committee on Physical Deterioration. By 1906, for example, both the Unionist *Glasgow Herald* and the Liberal *Dundee Advertiser* were advocating a system of compulsory medical inspection for all school children and the provision of school meals at the public expense for necessitous children. On 17 July 1906 the *Herald* declared that 'notwithstanding the voluntary efforts of some [School] Boards, Scotland requires medical inspection of school children as urgently as England,'[12] while the *Advertiser* stated that under such a compulsory system 'many weaknesses unknown to parents and teachers' would be disclosed, 'precautions' taken, and 'the interests of the pupils more closely safeguarded than is possible under the present haphazard system'[13]. By late 1906, as lively debate continued on the Education (Provision of Meals) Bill, both of these newspapers had committed themselves to supporting the measure, with the *Herald* claiming that charitable agencies like the Poor Children's Dinner Table Society did 'not cover the ground', and asserting that publicly funded meals would constitute 'a step in advance'[14]. The *Herald* had come to accept the gravity of the situation and the need for radical remedies. In an editorial published on 7 December 1906 it announced that there could be no doubt that the general 'physical condition [of the nation] is unsatisfactory', and proposed that any publicly financed scheme of medical inspection should be extended to cover pre-school children and possibly even expectant mothers. 'When it is remembered', the *Herald* stated, 'that in 1904 the birth rate in Scotland was only 28.65 per thousand ... and that the marriage rate for the same year was below the mean of the rates for the previous ten years, the conviction grows that something needs to be done to stay the waste of life that is going on, especially among children of tender years born in poor districts'. It argued that:

> "our efforts after physical betterment should begin very early, and should be directed towards enveloping the period of infancy, and even the antenatal period, in a healthier atmosphere ... If we had in Glasgow a body of medical men specially charged with the supervision of children of school age, it would be a natural extension of their duties that they should devise means of enlightening the public as to the care of children before they are ready for school"[15].

Parliament showed little enthusiasm for the infant welfare scheme suggested by the *Herald*, but by 1906 there was all-party support in the House of Commons both for the principle of medical inspection of school children and for the provision of school meals for necessitous children. In the spring of 1906 George Barnes, Labour member for Glasgow Blackfriars, introduced a private member's Bill to oblige Scottish School Boards to provide meals for pupils. This Bill was referred to a Select Committee of the House of Commons, where it was incorporated or rather submerged in a similar private member's Bill for England and Wales, and its provisions rendered voluntary instead of mandatory. Thus transformed, the Bill won both government support and the tacit approval of most Unionists, while retaining the backing of the Labour Party. The Scottish opposition to the measure was led by Sir Henry Craik, Unionist member for Glasgow and Aberdeen Universities, the *Scotsman* newspaper, and the Edinburgh and Glasgow School Boards. Taking advantage of the complacency of the Bill's supporters, who made no efforts to ensure that favourable Scottish witnesses were called before the Select Committee, the House of Lords decided, on the motion of Lord Balfour of Burleigh, to throw out the Scottish clause on the grounds that the Education (Provision of Meals) Bill had no support in Scotland[16]. It was the last day of the parliamentary session when the Bill returned to the House of Commons, and faced with the probability of losing the whole Bill if they resolved to send it back to the House of Lords, the Commons decided, despite the protests of Keir Hardie and others, to accept the Lords' amendment. Scottish Liberal and Labour MPs were outraged by this outcome, and efforts were made to persuade the Government to bring in another Bill to deal with the problem in the next session. However, the parliamentary time table was congested, and the Liberal Government of Sir Henry Campbell-Bannerman would only consider such a measure as part of a general Scottish Education Bill[17].

The Education (Scotland) Bill, which came before the House of Commons in 1907, was a controversial measure which encountered much opposition from a variety of sources and for numerous reasons. By 19 March 1907 the Edinburgh School Board, which played a prominent part in organising opposition to the Bill, was claiming that of the 153 Boards which had replied to their circular letter asking for opinions on the proposed legislation, only six were 'in favour of placing the feeding of school children upon the rates'[18]. However, this claim misrepresented the views of the Scottish Boards, many of which were beginning to accept the necessity of providing children of blamelessly poor parents with free school meals paid for out of public funds. On 19 April 1907, at a conference in Edinburgh attended by 90 delegates from 34 of the larger Scottish School Boards, it was agreed by only 34 votes to 28 to oppose the clause in the Education Bill empowering Boards to provide accommodation, equipment, and services for the preparation and supply of meals to pupils[19]. By 1908, when the new Scottish Education Bill came before Parliament, even the Edinburgh School Board had decided to drop its opposition to the proposal. The change of mind undergone by one of the Board's members, a Mr Cunningham, was probably representative of that undergone by many others across the country. Cunningham:

"had been opposed to the proposal two years ago, but in the interval he had seen a great deal. He saw the necessity for the feeding of neglected children now, and he had seen that the voluntary fund proved inadequate. The supply of dinners was not sufficient"[20].

The Education (Scotland) Act of 1908, which required Scottish education authorities to organise schemes for the medical examination of all children attending public schools and empowered school boards to provide medical attendance, food and even clothes for those children whose parents through no fault of their own could not keep them fit for school attendance, met with less opposition than had once seemed likely. However, there was some opposition, particularly in rural areas, where some school boards argued that medical inspection of children was unnecessary. In April 1910 the *Caledonian Medical Journal* observed that: 'Some of the counties and burghs have had the question under consideration for a number of months, but do not appear to have arrived at any satisfactory working arrangements'. In some areas, the *Journal* commented sadly, parsimony and a 'proverbial Scottish caution' held the upper hand[21].

Part of this remaining opposition owed something to a fear that the 1908 Act would ultimately lead to even greater public involvement in health care. This apprehension was shared by some who welcomed the Act. The *Glasgow Herald*, for example, stated:

"if the children are to be helped, if society is to be benefited by such early attention to its youthful members as will make them healthy workers and protect them from premature inefficiency and thus save the community the cost of supporting them, remedial measures must follow the detection of defects calling for treatment. Who is to provide them? The London hospitals have refused to carry the burden that medical inspection of schools threatened to throw upon them; purely charitable institutions have declined on the special ground that they are not entitled to relieve a public authority of a natural duty. The consequence is that school clinics are being established for the treatment as well as the determination of physical defects. The problem is one of some nicety. It is probable that the ultimate effect of medical inspection will be the raising of the standard of health and a consequent quickening of parental responsibility. As a result the general practitioner will find himself more in demand among a certain class of parents, although it is certain that others will rely on the public services"[22].

It is difficult to overestimate the importance of the Education (Scotland) Act of 1908 and of the reports of the Royal Commission and the Interdepartmental Committee which preceded and, in part, inspired it. That the State should not only 'concern itself ... with the removal of specific conditions inimical to health', but also 'accept responsibility for measures to promote the health of the people'[23] was a major development in health policy. However, the full significance of the Education (Scotland) Act of 1908 probably only became apparent in retrospect. In 1931 Dr J. Parlane Kinloch, Chief Medical Officer of the Department of Health for Scotland, traced back a 'new concept' in health policy, which went 'far beyond the dreams of nineteenth century reformers', to the quiet revolution of 1908. The services which had been developed between 1908 and 1931, such as maternity and child welfare, school health and national health insurance, had been based, Kinloch pointed out, on the concept that any adequate health service must be concerned with the care of the individual. One of the fundamental aims of statecraft since 1908, he added, was the 'promotion of the health of the individual to the end that as a race we may grow in health and vigour'[24].

The Poor Law and Public Health

Poor Law medical relief represented in 1908 by far the biggest public commitment to medical care. Various administrative changes had been made since 1848 to improve the quality of the service, but the principles of the system as laid down in the Poor Law (Scotland) Amendment Act of 1845 had remained unchanged. By the turn of the century radicals were arguing that these principles were anachronistic and would have to be abandoned if a healthier and more efficient society was to be constructed. The Labour Party had already abandoned the idea of a special medical service for the poor, and was groping towards the concept of a comprehensive health service which provided the best available medical care for all. Of greater immediate political significance, however, was the fact that more conservative-minded Britons were becoming worried about the increasing number of paupers and the rapidly rising cost of maintaining and treating them. Indeed, it was a Tory, not a Liberal, government which appointed a Royal Commission in 1905 to investigate the Poor Law and recommend necessary reforms.

The Royal Commission on the Poor Laws presented its Scottish report in November 1909. While acknowledging that improvements had been made in the service since 1845[25], and commending the City of Glasgow for the provision of modern Poor Law hospitals, both the majority and minority reports criticised existing Poor Law medical services. Possibly the most trenchant criticism, however, came from Dr John C. McVail, Medical Officer of Health for Stirling and Dumbartonshire, who to the surprise and delight of Beatrice Webb[26], had been appointed to investigate the operation of Poor Law medical relief in England and Wales. McVail, whose findings could in broad terms be applied to Scotland as well as the rest of Great Britain, concluded that:

> "Poor Law medical relief, both urban and rural, is a cripple supported on two crutches – the general hospitals on one side and gratuitous medical work on the other. The general hospitals supplement the workhouse infirmaries, whilst the unpaid work of the district medical officers and other medical men supplements outdoor medical relief. The fact is that the whole system would break down if it were not thus assisted. But it is obvious that such charitable contributions in supplement of the Poor Law cannot be uniform throughout the country. Medical men are not all alike in their willingness to work for nothing, private charity does not equally abound everywhere, general hospitals are not equally well supported everywhere, and are not within convenient distance of every part of the country"[27].

Virtually everyone who looked at the existing system with a clear eye agreed that reform was necessary. The problem was that the Royal Commission could not agree on the reforms to be desired. The majority, led by Lord George Hamilton, shied clear of any radical changes. They advocated the abolition of the parish councils and the transference of Poor Law medical relief (or public assistance medical relief as they suggested it should be called) to county councils and large burghs, reasoning that larger scale administrative units would provide a more efficient service. However, while they recommended certain improvements in the quality of the service, such as the abolition of pauper nursing in poorhouse hospitals, the majority adhered to the idea of a separate Poor Law medical system which would deal only with the destitute[28].

A much more radical approach was adopted by the Fabian activist Beatrice Webb and her colleagues in the minority. They argued that the majority's remedies would be merely palliative, and proposed that the Poor Law should be abolished and its medical services transferred to the public health authorities. They were convinced of the importance of prevention as a principle in any service, and judged the Poor Law condemned because by definition it could not operate until the person concerned was already destitute and it was too late for prevention, and frequently even cure. The minority report stated that 'if we could prevent sickness, howsoever caused, or effectually treat it when it occurs; if we could ensure that no child, whatever its parentage, went without what we may call the national minimum of nurture and training; and if we could provide that no able-bodied person was left to suffer from long continued or chronic unemployment, we should prevent at least nine-tenths of the destitution that now costs the Poor Law Authorities of Scotland more than a million per annum'[29]. Webb and her colleagues eulogised the virtues of the public health approach, stating that:

> "it is a necessary condition of the public health medical service that there must be no delay ... in applying the necessary treatment; there must be no delay in the adoption of the appropriate hygienic habits. It is the consciousness of the importance of this 'early diagnosis', the immense superiority in attractiveness of the incipient over the advanced 'case', the overwhelming sense of the dire calamities that may come from a single 'missed case', that mark the characteristic machinery of the public health medical service – its notification; its birth, death and case visitation; its bacteriological examination; its domiciliary disinfection; its medical observation of 'contacts', and its prolonged domiciliary supervision of 'recoveries' and patients discharged from institutions in order to detect the 'return case' "[30].

The minority argued that the public health organisations were capable of being so developed as to do for the preventive treatment of diseases in general what they had already done for the preventive treatment of infectious disease. The public health service, they proposed, should become the centre of the preventive medical work of the whole community, directing and correlating the activities of all available agencies, both municipal and voluntary[31].

Not surprisingly the minority's recommendations had the backing of the notable public health officials of the day. Arthur Newsholme, Chief Medical Officer of the English Local Government Board, George Newman, Medical Officer of the English Board of Education, T.J. Stafford, Medical Commissioner of the Local Government Board of Ireland, Leslie

Mackenzie, medical member of the Local Government Board for Scotland, and John C. McVail, the Royal Commission's own medical investigator, all shared the minority's view that the public health approach to medical care offered the best way forward[32].

The *Scotsman* and *Glasgow Herald* greeted the publication of the Scottish Poor Law report with fierce editorial attacks upon the recklessness, financial extravagance, and demoralising tendency of the minority report's proposals. The minority report, the *Glasgow Herald* claimed,

> "embodies a wholly impracticable Socialism... The impracticability lies in devolving functions on different authorities which they do not exist to perform, and which they could not undertake without neglecting their legitimate duties and making a mess of those properly entrusted to them... What this transformation of agencies would cost in hard cash is incalculable. It would give the nation not one but half a dozen Poor Law authorities all dipping into the public purse, and dipping deeply... But the graver question is that which concerns the effects on the national character of this elaborate process of wholesale relief. To a large extent the present Poor Law has failed because it demoralises the people. The failure and tragedy of demoralisation would be colossal if we were so foolish as to adopt the recommendations of those who actually claim that their nostrums abolish the Poor Law"[33].

These opinions were echoed by the *Scotsman*, which stated that 'individual responsibility would be undermined by such a system of indiscriminate State largesse, which can commend itself only to Socialists and their hangers-on'[34]. However, not everyone shared the hostility of the Unionist newspaper press to the minority report, and, if a series of interviews published in the *Dundee Advertiser* of 3 November 1909 may be taken as representative of opinion in the Tayside region, it would appear that Mrs Webb's ideas had a significant level of support even in places such as Arbroath, which were not normally thought of as socialist hot-beds[35]. Moreover, Sidney and Beatrice Webb attracted large audiences to a series of meetings held in November 1909 to promote their views on Poor Law reform, and by 17 December 1909 the Scottish National Committee to Promote the Break-Up of the Poor Law was reported to have established branches in several of the principal towns and attracted a paid-up membership of nearly 900[36]. Nevertheless, the minority's proposals were apparently too radical for most, and were certainly too radical for the Liberal Government of the day and John Burns, President of the English Local Government Board, in particular.

In describing the response of more conservatively minded Scots to the controversial minority report it seems clear that a distinction should be drawn between the hostile and, arguably, doctrinaire reception accorded to the minority's general proposals; and the more pragmatic and

thoughtful stance adopted towards the specific plan to transfer the functions of Poor Law medical relief to the public health authorities. The
publication of Dr John C. McVail's erudite and lucidly argued report on
Poor Law medical relief in England and Wales forced the conservative
newspaper press, and probably many of its readers, to give the public
health approach to medical care serious consideration. The *Scotsman*,
while its attitude was less than welcoming (possibly because it feared that
the scheme represented the thin and acceptable end of a large and
unacceptable socialist wedge), conceded that the idea of transferring
Poor Law medical relief to the public health authorities 'is at least
logical'[37]. The *Glasgow Herald* gave the report a less guarded reception,
declaring that:

> "if the two services are to be brought together at all a com-
> plete unification is preferable to a complex scheme of co-
> ordination of doutbful practicability. We have previously
> expressed a preference for the proposals of the majority taken
> as a whole, and we in no way endorse the policy of 'breaking
> up'. But the case of medical relief is admittedly exceptional,
> and its reorganisation on the lines recommended by Dr
> McVail would only be the completion of a break begun long
> ago... It would seem that the experience of 60 years were
> forcing us back to the position of Thomas Chalmers, who
> tirelessly and without avail insisted that while the treatment
> of disease was properly a communal service, the relief of
> indigence must be placed on a different footing"[38].

This admittedly fragmentary evidence suggests that a chance was
missed in 1909 to form a consensus on the future direction of public
medical service policy. If such an opportunity was indeed missed, the
reason was almost certainly that no individual or grouping succeeded in
separating the health care issue from the wider and bitterly controversial
question of the overall reform of the Poor Law. Had such a separation
been accomplished, it is possible that legislation would have been passed
along the lines recommended by McVail. The case can be put no stronger, for it is important to emphasise that consensus on increased State
involvement in the promotion of health was hard to achieve in early
twentieth century Scotland or, for that matter, in England. Many Scots
of a conservative turn of mind (a category which included many Liberal
Party supporters as well as Unionists) clung tenaciously to what are
usually termed Victorian social values and could only be persuaded with
the greatest effort and difficulty to let go. The idea that individual
welfare was basically the responsibility of the individual, and that virtually any form of state or municipal involvement in social questions was
bound to demoralise the poor and create more problems than it solved,
was only slowly and reluctantly abandoned. When the *Glasgow Herald*
gave its less than totally enthusiastic support to McVail's plan to transfer

Poor Law medical relief to the public health authorities it sought to justify its stance by appealing to the ideas of the Rev Dr Thomas Chalmers[39] (which are usually associated with resolute opposition to state interference in matters social as well as ecclesiastical), while the *Scotsman* justified its violent opposition to the development of the early child welfare programme with arguments that Samuel Smiles, the Victorian author of *Self-Help*, might have employed. 'Impair the spirit of independence', the *Scotsman* stated,

> "accustom the individual to rely upon aid, either from private or public agencies, and you thereby improverish the common fund of integrity and efficiency... Medical service is being forced upon the pupils in every elementary and other public school; the Poor Law Commission tell how free medical relief has already affected the Scottish community. Its influence has been demoralising"[40].

If the public health approach to health care was rejected because it was treated as an integral part of a Webbian socialist package, the legislative improvements recommended by the majority report were blocked because the Liberal Government of the time refused to grasp the nettle of local government reform. Twenty years would pass before any Government came to grasp that particularly difficult nettle. However, while the influence of the Poor Law Commission was minimal in the short term, its longer term impact was marked.

The organisational structure of local authority health services laid down in the Local Government (Scotland) Act of 1929 was clearly based upon that advocated in 1909 by the Poor Law Commissioners. More importantly, the Poor Law reports put forward the idea that individual services concerned with health, although having different origins and separate stimuli, should be brought into closer association to form a health service. This concept was, as we shall see, to be at the very heart of much of the subsequent development of public medical care.

National Health Insurance

The lack of enterprise shown by the English Local Government Board and its President, John Burns, disgusted the Chancellor of the Exchequer, David Lloyd George, a committed and very capable social reformer. Long before the Poor Law Commissioners presented their reports, Lloyd George had become convinced that the State had to do something to improve the health of the poorer sections of society. He, along with the British Medical Association and others, saw that the existing health care provided by Friendly Societies and similar organisations was less than satisfactory. The general practitioners who were contracted to supply medical care to the Societies' members were poorly paid and were generally believed to provide an inadequate service. Moreover, chronic invalids and other high-risk patients were excluded from membership of the Societies, as were members' wives and children[41]. The key to improving health care, Lloyd George came to believe, lay in the type of state-supported health insurance scheme pioneered in Imperial Germany[42].

Lloyd George's National Insurance Act of 1911, which covered unemployment as well as health insurance, provided medical benefit to all employed persons and voluntary contributors earning less than £160 per annum. Those earning more than £160 per annum (or after the National Insurance Act of 1919 more than £250 per annum) were required to make their own arrangements. The medical care provided under the Act was restricted to that which could reasonably be provided by a general practitioner of average competence in his surgery or the patient's home, with drugs or appliances considered necessary by the doctor. Consultant, specialist and hospital services were not provided under the Act. Eligible employees contributed 4d (1.7p) per week into the insurance fund, while the employer and the general taxpayer paid in 3d (1.25p) and 2d (0.8p) respectively each week. The application of the scheme north of the Border was supervised by a body known as the Scottish Insurance Commission, whose members were specially appointed for the task. The scheme was administered by local insurance committees, on which the powerful vested interest of the Friendly Societies was dominantly represented[43]. This was a prudent concession on Lloyd George's part which did much to win over the Friendly Societies to the measure, but attempts to placate a medical profession jealous of its independence and equally fearful of both State control and Friendly Society tyranny met with little success in the short term.

The hostility of the medical profession, or at least of the British Medical Association, was vehement (although less so in Scotland than in England). However, it was not shared by the great bulk of the Scottish public, who gave Lloyd George's proposals a general welcome. In its editorial of 6 May 1911 the *Dundee Advertiser* accurately summed up the immediate Scottish response to the National Insurance Bill:

"The Chancellor of the Exchequer's great scheme of State insurance has had a very remarkable reception, which... divides itself into two moods following a very unusual line of cleavage. On the one hand we have the politicians of all parties, the newspapers of almost all categories, and the representatives of the working classes of all trades and grades, welcoming it effusively. There are, of course, the inevitable and altogether proper reserves. Details must be examined with critical care, actuarial wisdom must be consulted and deferred to, machinery must be most closely scanned. But as regards the thing aimed at... the classes referred to are

almost of one mind ... On the other hand stand the business
men. They cannot as a class be described as hostile, but their
attitude is distinctly that of disturbance"[44].

Some large employers gave their unreserved support to the scheme,
believing, on the basis of the German evidence, that it would help to
create a healthier and more efficient labour force, but others, notably the
Clydeside shipbuilders, the Dundee jute masters and the west of Scotland
coal-mine owners, expressed serious reservations and, in some cases, total
opposition. Perhaps the most outspoken critic of the scheme at this early
stage was Dr John Inglis of Messrs A. and J. Inglis, the shipbuilding firm,
who denounced it as an immoral measure designed to win politicians
votes by robbing employers. 'It was,' he told the *Glasgow Herald*, 'a case
of being liberal – with other people's money'[45]. Few, if any, businessmen publicly expressed their opposition in such terms, and most
contented themselves with arguing that the Bill would encourage malin-
gering, increase labour costs, adversely affect their competitiveness in
world markets, and possibly lead to economic disaster. Not surprisingly,
both the *Glasgow Herald* and the *Scotsman* drew attention to the anxieties
of these businessmen, and the *Scotsman* even hinted, in an editorial of 5
May 1911, that the proposed burden on industry and the general taxpayer should be reduced and that the proportion of the insurance fund
financed by workers' contributions should be raised[46].

A proposal to increase the share of national insurance borne by working people was unlikely to prove popular, but some industrial workers
probably shared their employers' fears that the increased financial burden on industry might damage British competitiveness in world markets
and lead to job losses. Moreover, it seems clear that a significant number
of working people, particularly farm workers, resented both the principle
of compulsion and what they considered the injustice of flat-rate contributions. The *Glasgow Herald* sympathized with such complaints, stating that 'if Mr Lloyd George had approached the question in a scientific
spirit, he would have seen that to impose an equal tax or contribution
on every man or woman was essentially unjust'[47]. In the largely agricultural constituency of North Ayrshire, the same newspaper pointed out,
'repudiation of compulsory blessings is most hearty and sincere'[48]. This
was no mere wishful reporting, for in the North Ayrshire by-election of
20 December 1911 the Unionist candidate, Captain Duncan Campbell,
defeated the sitting Liberal Solicitor-General A.M. Anderson, by 7,318
votes to 7,047, overturning a Liberal majority of 354. 'In North Ayrshire', the *Glasgow Herald* commented, 'it is clear that the agricultural
vote has gone against the Government because the farmer and the
labourer see that the Insurance Act deals inequitably with them and does
not take sufficient account of the special conditions of their industry'[49].
Opposition to the Insurance Act continued in Scottish agricultural communities, and on 25 October 1912 Mr James Kyd of Mains of Errol told

a meeting of farmers from Perthshire, Forfarshire, Kincardineshire, Aberdeenshire, Fife, Clackmannanshire, Kinross, and Stirlingshire that Lloyd George's Act was 'a gigantic swindle [applause] and a gross injustice to them as free citizens of the country, more especially as they knew that their ploughmen and domestics were far better provided for in sickness under the former conditions than they would be under that wonderful Act'. The meeting unanimously resolved to form a Scottish National Defence Association to resist the provisions of the Act which interfered with the relations of employers and employees, and to appoint a committee to organise a campaign which would aim at securing amendments to the Act[50]. However, it is significant that their object was not to remove agricultural workers from the national insurance scheme, but rather to secure fairer treatment for their industry under the scheme. By October 1912 the principle that employers and employees should be required by law to contribute to a national insurance fund seems to have been widely, if not universally, accepted.

While the principles underlying the National Insurance Bill won widespread support, the Bill's specific provisions regarding medical benefit generated considerable controversy and led to a debate on the future direction of public health service policy. As early as 11 May 1911 the *Scotsman* was arguing that:

> "it is not... easy to believe that the State can stop exactly where it has proposed to call a halt. The question of the hospitals, for example, cannot be ignored. Their position is very seriously prejudiced by the Insurance Bill, and it would not be surprising if the State were compelled before long to take them over. There are two considerations which lead to this conclusion. In the first place, it is natural to assume that voluntary contributions to hospitals will be diminished... As a consequence, hospitals now on the voluntary basis may languish and die for want of financial support, and the State may be forced to intervene with State grants to keep them in existence. But apart from the practical necessities of the situation, there are strong theoretical grounds for insisting upon State aid. The State has taken over the supervision of the health of the community – at least of the section of the community which is entitled to treatment in free hospitals – and has guaranteed free medical attendance. If, therefore, it is found necessary to remove to hospitals any of the State-insured during sickness, the State is logically bound to pay the bill, [for] it has pledged itself to supply to all its beneficiaries medicine and medical attendance"[51].

In an article dealing with the medical aspects of the National Insurance Bill in the *Glasgow Herald* on 22 May 1911 it was pointed out that, while clause 17 of the Bill authorised any Approved Society to subscribe to hospitals 'as it may think fit', it was extremely unlikely that such subscriptions would make good the expected shortfall in voluntary donations and subscriptions from employers and workpeople. Until wives and children were included in the scheme and contributions raised to meet the cost of a full medical service, the most likely solution to the financial problems of the voluntary hospitals, the author suggested, was a subsidy from public funds. Public funding, and the government control, or at least influence, over the voluntary hospitals which would necessarily accompany it, would, he continued, create numerous advantages. Hospitals would be built according to the needs of local communities, so that less populous areas as well as major cities would be adequately provided for, unpopular hospital projects (such as specialist provision for the treatment of venereal disease) would be more sympathetically dealt with, and the 'many desirable extensions of buildings and improvements in equipment [which] cannot be carried out' at present because of lack of funds would become financially feasible. Moreover, the full integration of hospital and general practitioner services would be of immense value in the efficient diagnosis and treatment of disease. 'The general practitioner', it was pointed out,

> "with his stethoscope and thermometer and other limited appliances, cannot provide the elaborate and costly apparatus and the special skill necessary for X-ray and Finsen light and electrical treatment generally which are obtainable at the hospital dispensaries. Such specialities, it may be assumed, will be more fully and systematically made use of when the sickness insurance scheme is linked up with the great hospitals"[52].

These and similar related issues were taken up by Dr Joseph MacGregor-Robertson, a noted Glasgow physiologist, in a powerfully argued series of articles published in the *Glasgow Herald* in December 1911. MacGregor-Robertson pointed out that the Bill made no provision to enable a general practitioner to take advantage of specialist equipment and skills in a difficult case. The omission of specialist and consultant services from the medical benefits obtainable under the Bill, he added, was regrettable and, indeed, unjustifiable. 'The Bill', he declared, 'so far as medical diagnosis and treatment are concerned, is drawn on lines that might have been satisfactory a quarter of a century ago, but are hopelessly inadequate now'[53].

The *Glasgow Herald* was convinced by the arguments of critics such as MacGregor-Robertson that the medical benefits provided under the Bill were inadequate. 'No part of the Insurance Bill', it declared in a leading article of 13 December 1911, 'has been more imperfectly planned than its central feature – namely, the provision of medical benefit'. It was, the leader continued, ludicrous to assume, as the framers of the Bill evidently did, that all sickness with the exception of pulmonary tuberculosis 'can be treated successfully by a friendly society doctor calling at the patient's home and prescribing a bottle of medicine or a truss', and illogical to exclude hospitals and their specialist facilities from the system of medical benefit. 'If the scheme is to be made workable', the *Herald* argued,

> "it is clear that hospitals will have to be brought into it . . .
> There is no reason why institutional treatment for one disease
> [i.e., tuberculosis] should be specially subsidised, while insti-
> tutional treatment for all other complaints is left to private
> charity . . . When the Bill is brought into operation it will at
> once be seen that the maintenance of the hospitals at a high
> degree of efficiency is essential to the administration of real
> 'medical benefit'. On the other hand, the hospitals cannot be
> maintained without some definite assistance from the State
> under a universal insurance scheme. These institutions, with
> a declining income, will not be able to keep all their wards
> open to insured persons from whom and on behalf of whom
> they receive nothing"[54].

Thus it is clear that, even before the National Insurance Bill reached the statute book, a broad band of informed Scottish opinion was convinced that the proposed scheme could not provide an adequate health service for the insured population. Even Unionist newspapers, which would normally have been decidedly apprehensive about any expansion of the State's involvement in health care, accepted that the scheme would have to be extended to include hospital benefit. Such organs remained, however, totally hostile towards any integrated State-run medical service. Their hostility was shared by the great bulk of the medical profession. Dr MacGregor-Robertson expected that the National Health Insurance scheme would eventually develop into 'a public medical service', and urged his medical colleagues to ensure that the service would be controlled by themselves and not by the State. 'If this revolution be not so directed', he warned, 'medical men will be but the servants, or slaves, of a system which, for a time at least, will be nothing but a State-crowned sham'[55]. His fears, if not his hopes, were shared by many. A public medical service, the *Glasgow Herald* stated, 'is an idea for which the country and the profession are by no means prepared'[56].

The advocates of a public medical service based upon the principles outlined in the minority report of the Poor Law Commission found little or no merit in the sickness insurance approach to health care. The Webbs had warned that:

> "what would tend to be provided under such a system would
> be, not preventive or curative treatment or hygienic advice,
> but, in the literal sense of the words, medical relief, and that
> wholly without conditions. On all these grounds, the pro-
> posal to supersede the poor law medical service by any system
> of universal medical insurance appears to us, not only polit-

ically impracticable, but also entirely retrograde in policy, and likely to be fraught with the greatest dangers to public health and to the moral character of the poor"[57].

In 1920 Arthur Newsholme declared that it was doubtful whether any system of sickness insurance had been an active auxiliary in the prevention of disease. It had been so, he stated, only to the extent to which the medical treatment of the mass of the population had been improved by it; and no such improvement could be claimed for British insurance. The wider possibilities of prevention of illness and elevation of the general standard of health by making each general practitioner a family adviser on health more than a practitioner in medicine had not been realised or even brought within sight[58]. However, while there was much good sense in Newsholme and the Webbs' argument, there can be little doubt that the National Insurance scheme effected some improvement in the quality of medical care in most, if not all, of the poorest areas of the country largely because it made practice in such areas more financially attractive than heretofore.

Health Services in the Highlands and Islands

The National Insurance Act was of little relevance to the sparsely populated Highlands and Islands of Scotland, where many of the inhabitants were self-employed crofters living barely above subsistence level, with little or no money to spare for health care. A separate solution had to be found for this quite distinct area, where medical services had long been recognised as totally inadequate. As early as 1852 the Royal College of Physicians of Edinburgh had published a report drawing attention to the paucity of medical services in the Highlands and Islands[59]. In subsequent years local authorities, public health officials, general practitioners and others frequently drew the central government's attention to the special difficulties of the crofting counties. In 1904, for example, Dr M. Mackenzie of North Uist told the Departmental Committee appointed by the Local Government Board for Scotland to inquire into the system of Poor Law medical relief that –

> "As I have frequently pointed out already, the want of sufficient medical attendance and nursing have a most prejudicial effect on the well being of the district. The loss of life, hardship and misery which this implies cannot be calculated. To a certain extent the physical evil is evident, while it tends to produce a callousness to suffering and death that becomes only too apparent in the number of uncertified deaths, especially among the aged"[60].

Little was done to remedy the situation, although there can be no doubt that by the early years of the century Scottish opinion was virtually unanimous in believing that only the intervention of central government could bring about any real improvement. In 1909 the *Scotsman* attacked the Poor Law Commission for its 'timid' refusal to offer any concrete proposals for the improvement of medical services in the Highlands and Islands, and suggested that a government grant of up to £35,000 per year should be made available 'for the purposes of public health . . . and for providing additional medical attendance or nurses'[61].

In August 1912 a committee was set up under the chairmanship of Sir John Dewar (later Lord Forteviot) to advise on how the special health care needs of the crofting counties might be met. After a flurry of well directed activity the committee produced its report in the December of the same year. The report provided a wealth of detail illustrating how the private enterprise of doctors was failing to meet the needs of the population. It was clearly shown that in the Highlands and Islands the scattered distribution of population, the poverty of those requiring medical attention, and the geographical difficulties of the area made it in many parts impossible for the population who could be reached from a given centre to remunerate adequately the services of their general practitioners. The main recommendation of the Dewar Committee was therefore that an Imperial grant should be made in order to induce a sufficient number of doctors to settle and practise in the crofting counties. Government grant monies, they advised, should be paid to doctors on the condition that they agreed to attend at reduced fees patients belonging to the crofter class, the dependents of insured persons, and persons of similar economic standing[62].

The Dewar Committee's findings startled many who had been blissfully ignorant of Highland problems, but, as the *Scotsman* pointed out, 'to those familiar with Highland conditions, the revelations of the Committee will be no surprise'[63]. Scottish opinion across the political spectrum welcomed the committee's recommendations, with the Unionist *Glasgow Herald* stating that it 'sets out the case for State aid in a manner both lucid and convincing'[64], and the Liberal *Dundee Advertiser* asserting that 'it is for the Imperial authorities to come to the rescue' of Highland communities[65]. The public response, in truth, could hardly have been otherwise, for once one accepted the size of the problem and the need to do something about it, there was simply no realistic alternative to central government funding of medical services in the Highlands and Islands. The Highland communities were too poor to support a rate-funded medical service, while, as the *Scotsman* put it, 'all that can be done by voluntary effort has already been done'[66].

The outcome was the Highlands and Islands (Medical Services) Act of 1913, under which an independent board, chaired by Sir John Dewar and including such distinguished men as W. Leslie Mackenzie, John C. McVail and Sir Donald MacAlister, was set up to administer the scheme. The board's first action was to ask local authorities to assess the needs of their respective areas. The Treasury granted the total sum requested,

£42,000, apparently without any quibble, but the outbreak of the first world war in 1914 placed severe restrictions on all non-defence expenditure and, consequently, much of the Highlands and Islands Medical Service scheme was put into cold storage for the duration. The advent of peace did not bring an end to the financial problems of the service. In the face of mounting economic difficulties, the economic orthodoxy of the period dictated that governments should prune their expenditure. Nevertheless, funds were eventually found to improve hospitals and provide specialist staff and services in the Highlands and Islands.

The Highlands and Islands Medical Service was the cherished concern of the Scottish Board of Health and of its successor, the Department of Health for Scotland. The scheme's administrators in Edinburgh enjoyed excellent relations with the doctors and others involved in providing the services. This cordial relationship did something to foster confidence among the medical profession in Scotland in the central department, which was to be important both during the setting up of the National Health Service in 1947–48 and subsequently[67].

The unique service provided in the Highlands and Islands area attracted much interest among those concerned with similar scattered populations elsewhere in the world. However, while a sub-committee of the Scottish Health Services Committee proposed in 1936 that the Highlands and Islands Medical Service, with its blend of central and local government control, should be treated as a model for wider application in Scotland (a suggestion which was quoted in the National Health Service White Paper of 1944)[68], this proposal does not appear to have found much favour. Given the undoubted success of the scheme, this lack of interest is perhaps surprising.

Child Health and Maternity Care

The last major piece of Scottish legislation relating to health care to be passed before Europe went to war in 1914 was the Education (Scotland) Act of 1913, which established the School Medical Service on a regular basis. Comprehensive medical inspection of school children had, since 1908, revealed a shocking amount of disease, much of which, it soon became apparent, was not being treated quickly enough. Alarmed by the problem, some School Boards had, on the basis of a liberal interpretation of section 6 of the 1908 Education Act, spent rate monies on the medical treatment of children in their areas, but in a test case brought against the Glasgow School Board the Court of Session had declared such expenditure illegal. In 1912 the Treasury made available to the Scottish School Boards a special grant of £7,500[69], but this was an emergency stop-gap measure. The situation was regularised by the Education (Scotland) Act of 1913 which made School Boards responsible for the pro-

vision of medical treatment for necessitous school-children. Half the cost
of this treatment, it was subsequently decided, was to be met by a central
government grant, the other half being raised from the ratepayers[70].

While certain ameliorative measures had been adopted prior to 1914,
it was the first world war that brought home to the nation the impelling
necessity for State action in the field of maternity and child welfare. The
Notification of Births (Extension) Act 1915 was passed against a background of high war casualties, falling birth rates and rising infantile
mortality. It rendered the adoptive provisions of the Notification of
Births Act of 1907 compulsory, and empowered local authorities to make
such arrangements as they thought fit, and were sanctioned by the
Scottish Local Government Board, for attending to the health of expectant mothers, nursing mothers, and children under five. By June 1918
some 50 schemes, covering areas with a total population of 1,250,000,
had been approved by the Scottish Local Government Board, and 24
others were under consideration[71]. Such was the urgency of the matter
and the priority accorded it by central government that some schemes
were being recognised for grant aid before they had been fully
approved[72]. The policy was not to replace the pre-existing voluntary
agencies in the field, but rather to utilise them fully, subsidise and extend
their activities and enlist the sympathetic co-operation of their management bodies. The degree of community involvement in the programme
excited contemporary comment. It was noted with pride that 'the number of enthusiastic women of all classes who have given themselves to the
work is really quite remarkable'[73].

The same anxieties which impelled the Notification of Births (Extension) Act lay behind the Midwives (Scotland) Act of 1915. This much
needed and long delayed measure provided for the registration of midwives and for the establishment of a Central Midwives Board for Scotland, with wide powers relative to the training and control of midwives.
Local authorities were charged under the terms of the Act with the
general supervision of all midwives practising within their districts, and
with reporting annually to the Central Midwives Board and the Local
Government Board for Scotland on the administration of the Act[74].

Despite these advances in the field of maternity and child welfare, the
later years of the first world war were marked by a continuing anxiety
about high infant mortality rates. On 30 July 1918 at a conference in
Edinburgh attended by local government representatives and others
interested in the establishment of a Scottish Child Welfare Institute, a
letter of apology was read from Robert Munro, Secretary for Scotland,
stating that

> "the importance of the proposal could not be gainsaid. The
> ravages of war had compelled them to recognise that the
> problems of maternity and child welfare were of national
> importance. A central institute would co-ordinate existing

activities and would be the power house to stimulate and energise them".

Munro's sentiments were echoed by Sir George McCrae, Vice President of the Local Government Board for Scotland, who declared that –

"there was no question which was of greater interest to the central authority than that of child welfare. It was one of increasing urgency and was vital to their national life"[75].

The Maternity and Child Welfare Act of 1918, which empowered local authorities to provide hospitals for the care of expectant mothers and children under the age of five years, represented only a part, and a fairly minor part at that, of the proposed solution to the persistent problem of high infant and child mortality. By the end of the first world war there was wide agreement that child health, and indeed adult health also, could only be significantly improved if, firstly, the physical environment of the poorer classes was dramatically improved, and, secondly, the public medical services were more efficiently organised and directed by a central government department devoted exclusively to the planning and administration of national health policy.

A Wartime Attempt to Control Venereal Disease

One of the groups of diseases to which servicemen, and through them the civilian population, are traditionally most prone in wartime is that of venereal disease. However, concern about venereal diseases, and congenital syphilis in particular, had been mounting even before the outbreak of war, and in 1913 the Government had appointed a Royal Commission to enquire into the prevalence of venereal diseases and the provision for their diagnosis and treatment. Reporting in 1916, the Royal Commission recommended the establishment of early diagnosis and treatment centres throughout the country, to be organised by the local authorities and supported by a 75 *per cent* Treasury grant. These recommendations were swiftly acted upon. In October 1916 the Local Government Board for Scotland introduced regulations under section 78 of the Public Health (Scotland) Act of 1897 which required local authorities to provide free, efficient, convenient and confidential treatment for persons suffering from venereal diseases. The Treasury provided a 75 *per cent* grant in support of approved expenditure on the scheme. Treatment centres were set up throughout the country, general practitioners were supplied with drugs and a considerable effort was put into a propaganda campaign to inform the public about venereal diseases[76]. Thus it took a major war to mute the taboos which had previously denied adequate provision for, and education about, the problem of sexually transmitted diseases. History was to repeat itself during the second world war, both in the promotion of more open discussion and in the provision of more effective surveillance for venereal diseases.

Housing and Health

The Royal Commission on Scottish Housing, which Dr W. Leslie Mackenzie later described as the 'most important that had sat in Scotland for
over a hundred years,'[77] presented its damning indictment of the
squalid state of much of Scotland's housing stock in October 1917. The
Royal Commission found –

> "unsatisfactory sites of houses and villages, insufficient sup-
> plies of water, unsatisfactory provision for drainage, grossly
> inadequate provision for the removal of refuse, widespread
> absence of decent sanitary conveniences, the persistence of
> the unspeakably filthy privy midden in many of the mining
> areas, badly constructed, incurably damp labourers' cottages
> on farms, whole townships unfit for human occupation in the
> crofting counties and islands, primitive and casual provision
> for many of the seasonal workers, gross overcrowding and
> huddling of the sexes together in the congested industrial
> villages and towns, occupation of one-room houses by large
> families, groups of lightless and unventilated houses in the
> older burghs, clotted masses of slums in the great cities"[78].

The correlation between bad housing and poor health struck every
objective observer. The one-roomed house had, for example, twice the
infant mortality and three times the death rate from tuberculosis of the
four-roomed dwelling. These were compelling statistics, for while less
than 8 *per cent* of the population of England and Wales lived in one- and
two-roomed houses in 1911, in Scotland the figure was 50 *per cent*[79]. The
Housing (Scotland) Act of 1919, which provided local authorities with
a State subsidy for the construction of approved council housing, was the
outcome of the post-war national determination to build 'homes fit for
heroes'. By 1923, however, only 25,000 houses had been built. The
Housing Act of 1923 altered the nature of the housing subsidy, providing
for a State payment of £16 for each house per annum for a period of
twenty years. This subsidy was increased to £9 per house, or £12.10s
(£12.50) in agricultural areas, per annum for forty years by the Housing
(Financial Provisions) Act of 1924. This Act, 'largely Scottish in conception and execution', was the work of John Wheatley, Labour MP for
Shettleston and Minister of Health in the first Labour Government. It
succeeded in stimulating the construction of council housing: the number
of houses built between 1925 and 1929 represented an increase of 140 *per
cent* over that for the preceding five year period[80]. However, the Act did
little for the slum dwellers who could not afford the higher rents of what
became known as 'Wheatley houses.' In 1930 the second Labour
Government's Housing (Scotland) Act shifted the emphasis towards
slum clearance. Slum clearance was also the priority of the Housing Act
of 1935, which partly restored the State subsidy, cut by the National
Government's Housing (Financial Provisions) (Scotland) Act of 1933.

Whereas the 1933 Act had reduced the subsidies of £9 and £12.10s (£12.50) available under the 1924 Act to £3 per house, the 1935 Act increased the subsidy to £6.15s (£6.75) per house per annum for 40 years in respect of houses erected to abate overcrowding[81].

Something like 337,000 houses, of which about two-thirds were council owned, were built between 1919 and 1939[82]. This was a substantial achievement, far in excess of the 250,000 houses recommended by the Royal Commission in 1917, but it was insufficient to meet the needs of the situation. In 1935, for example, it was discovered that 22.5 *per cent* of Scottish houses were overcrowded, while in some Clyde Valley towns the figure reached over 40 *per cent*. On the other hand, in England the national figure was 3.8 *per cent*, while the worst English locality was Sunderland, where 20.6 *per cent* of the houses were overcrowded[83]. The inadequacy of much of Scotland's housing stock could be illustrated in terms of health-related criteria other than overcrowding. In the burghs alone, as Tom Johnston, Labour MP for Stirling and Clackmannan, pointed out during a parliamentary debate on Scottish health policy on 14 July 1936, there were still 300,000 houses without modern sanitary conveniences[84]. It took concerted action during and after the second world war before Scottish water supplies and drainage were brought up to acceptable standards.

Establishment of a Central Health Department

Important as house building was deemed to be, it constituted but one part of a two-pronged attack upon the health problems of the nation. By the later stages of the first world war many had come to accept the validity of Lord Rhondda's claim 'that a Ministry of Health would save a thousand babies' lives a week,' and to urge that 'It is high time we commenced to save these future citizens'[85]. One propagandist, writing in the *Dundee Advertiser* on 2 August 1918, asked:

"How many of us know that at this moment there are four-teen Government departments responsible for the nation's health? They muddle the responsibility between them. It is anybody's job, and that, as we know too well, is nobody's job. None of these departments is primarily responsible for health; it merely happens to be one of their manifold duties, and hence cannot and does not receive the attention it merits. Thus we find that important health matters come under the control of two or three different departments".

The same author went on to complain about 'constant overlapping' of responsibilities and effort, and to argue that 'the work is not done so efficiently as if one Department had had entire responsibility'. He concluded that 'the more the question of national health is studied, the more one realises that the solution of the problem lies in a Ministry of Health, a new department whose *raison d'être* shall be health and health alone'[86].

Lloyd George's government had been committed in principle to the establishment of a Ministry of Health since 1917, but the demands of the war on Cabinet Ministers' time, and departmental frictions and jealousies in Whitehall, prevented any progress until the summer of 1918, when the Cabinet Home Affairs Committee was instructed to examine the whole business. All the time pressure was mounting on the government to introduce legislation to set up a Ministry of Health. In a leading article, dated 18 July 1918, the *Scotsman* declared that there was a 'universal acceptance' of the urgent need for a 'comprehensive reorganisation and expansion of the public health service'[87]. In Scotland, opinion was apparently unanimously in favour of the establishment of a separate Scottish Ministry of Health which would be independent of the proposed English body. During 1918 Scottish trade unions, the Convention of Royal Burghs, the County Councils' Association, the Association of District Councils and the Scottish Committee of the British Medical Association all lobbied Government in favour of a Scottish Ministry of Health[88].

By February 1919 Dr Christopher Addison, President of the English Local Government Board, had given in to pressure from Scotland and the Scottish MPs in London, and agreed to the introduction of a separate Bill setting up a Scottish Board of Health. The resultant Act followed the lines of the corresponding English and Welsh measure. Under its provisions the powers of the Local Government Board for Scotland, the Scottish National Insurance Commission, the Highlands and Islands Medical Service Board and the Scottish Education Department, in respect of the medical inspection and treatment of children and young persons, were transferred to the Board of Health. A Parliamentary Under Secretary, appointed for the purpose, was to be responsible, under the Secretary for Scotland, for the Board's direction. The Board was thus directly responsible to Parliament, but it was not packed with political appointees and could not be regarded as an explicitly political body.

Local Health Administration

The Scottish Board of Health Act of 1919 received a warm welcome, but there was strong criticism both in Westminster and Scotland of the fact that nothing had been done to reform local authority health care. During the debate on the second reading of the Bill on 1 April 1919, Joseph Johnstone, Coalition Liberal member for Renfrewshire East, expressed the hope that 'the setting up of this central authority in Scotland will lead to larger local areas being established'. He stated that 'we suffer just now in Scotland from having far too many small local health bodies', and urged that these bodies 'should be grouped or merged into larger areas, with a population of not less than 40,000 or 50,000'[89]. Johnstone's views had cross-party support. William Adamson, Labour member for West Fife and future Secretary of State for Scotland, objected that 'the Bill . . . is of far too limited a character', and regretted that 'no attempt has been made . . . to co-ordinate the local authorities'. He pointed out that there were no fewer than 310 local authorities administering public health in Scotland (some of which dealt with populations as low as 500), and argued that it would not 'be possible to carry out the ideas of the people of Scotland unless we have very much larger areas than we have at present'[90]. These criticisms were echoed by Lieutenant-Colonel Sir John Hope, Conservative member for North Midlothian. Hope regretted 'that the Secretary for Scotland has not found himself able to make some effort to provide for the co-ordination of local authorities, because we shall never get a satisfactory measure of health until not only the central authority, but the local authorities are co-ordinated'[91]. Sir Donald MacLean, Liberal member for South Midlothian and Peeblesshire and leader of the Liberal opposition in the House of Commons, focused his criticism on the issue of Poor Law medical service reform. He told the House of Commons that the reform of the Scottish Poor Law was a question 'not nearly so complicated as in England'. There may be 'points of contention', he added, 'but there is a real opportunity now, instead of deferring it, of dealing with the whole matter'[92].

Robert Munro, the Liberal Coalition Secretary for Scotland, did not dispute that local health administration, and the Poor Law medical service in particular, required reform. Indeed, he stated at the beginning of the second reading debate that 'the intention . . . is at the earliest possible moment to eradicate from health administration what has come to be known as the taint of the Poor Law', adding that he hoped 'the time is not far distant' when the question of local health administration is tackled. However, Munro believed that 'it would be a profound mistake to delay this measure by the insertion of provisions which might turn out to be highly contentious in their character'[93].

The Scottish Board of Health lost little time in taking up the issue of local health administration reform. However, recognising that 'the question of a unified local administration . . . is one of great difficulty and complexity', the Board called for expert advice from its Consultative Council on local administrative questions[94], one of four such consultative bodies established under section 5 of the 1919 Act. The Council's report, which appeared in 1923, stated that the need for reform was felt by all concerned with health administration in Scotland. Health administrators complained that many of the existing administrative units were too small, and that the distribution of responsibilities among different authorities in each area caused overlapping of services and waste. The Consultative Council cited the beneficial effects of amalgamating central government health responsibilities under the Scottish Board of Health, and argued that similar benefits would accrue from a similar reform of local government health administration. All local government health responsibilities, including Poor Law medical relief, the Council contended, should be administered by one authority, whose administrative area should be large enough to ensure efficiency. The recommended local authority units were burghs with populations over 50,000 and county councils. There should be no new *ad hoc* health authority, the Council advised, and powers should be transferred to existing authorities[95].

The Consultative Council's report was quietly shelved and apparently forgotten for nearly six years. Despite the Scottish Board of Health's evident commitment to local government reform, and despite the wide agreement among Scottish parliamentarians and local health administrators on the general direction which that reform should take, nothing was done until 1929. While small local authorities were generally reluctant to give up their jealously guarded powers and consequently represented a not insignificant obstacle to local government reorganisation, it is hard to excuse the inaction of successive Scottish Secretaries on this matter.

Proposals for Reform

In other areas too, apart from local health administration, the initial reformism of the period immediately after the first world war was to give way rapidly to inaction. One of the first actions of the Scottish Board of Health was to appoint a Consultative Council on Medical and Allied Subjects, under the chairmanship of Sir Donald MacAlister, MD, Principal of Glasgow University, which was instructed 'to make recommendations as to the systematised provision of such forms of medical and allied services as should ... be available for the community'. The Council's interim report, entitled *A Scheme of Medical Service for Scotland*, appeared in early December 1920. Like the more famous interim report of the English Ministry of Health's Consultative Council on the *Future Provision of Medical and Allied Services* (generally known, after the Council's chairman, the future Lord Dawson of Penn, as the Dawson report), the MacAlister report placed great stress on the family doctor as the key figure in the health services. At a time when the trend in Britain and elsewhere was towards specialism, the MacAlister report declared that

"we regard it as of primary importance that the organisation
of the Health Service of the Nation should be based upon the
family as the normal unit, and on the *family doctor* as the
normal medical attendant and guardian. It is not for disease
or diseases in the abstract that provision has to be made; but
for persons liable to or suffering from disease. The first essential for the proper and efficient treatment of individual

patients is therefore not institutional but personal service, such as can be rendered to the people in their own homes only by a family doctor who has the continuous care of their health'[96].

The general practitioner, in the Council's view, should not be 'isolated and self-dependent', but rather, as 'the recognised medical guardian of the family', should have 'the opportunity . . . of co-operating on behalf of its members with all the auxiliary health agencies established for the public benefit, and of acting as the professional intermediary between these and his patients'. Through the family doctor, the report argued, 'the resources of these public agencies will be mediated to the individual, and the present lack of continuity in operation and responsibility will be eliminated'[97]. The report urged the establishment of 'consultation clinics', which would be staffed by local general practitioners, who would see and treat patients, have access to laboratory facilities and specialist advice, and conduct research[98].

The MacAlister report envisaged the general practitioner taking his place at the very centre of what would have been not only a partly integrated but also a greatly expanded public medical service. It recommended that the scope of the National Health Insurance scheme should be expanded to include all dependent members of insured workers' families, and that the medical benefits available under the scheme should be extended to provide a complete medical service, including publicly provided specialist, consultant, and domiciliary nursing services, the services of health visitors and convalescent homes[99].

The immediate post-war determination to build a land fit for heroes had largely disappeared by 1920, and had been replaced by a desire for economic retrenchment in the face of mounting economic difficulties. The reception accorded to the proposals of the Consultative Council on Medical and Allied Subjects was consequently generally hostile. The prevailing attitude was perhaps best summed up by the *Scotsman*, which declared that 'it is a report born out of due season'. The same newspaper reproached the Council for writing 'their prescriptions as if in possession of a blank cheque on the Treasury,' and opined that the need of the times was for 'consistent, steady vigilance in the interest of economy'[100]. It is significant, however, that there was little or no attempt to defend the existing system of public medical services.

The Royal Commission on National Health Insurance, which reported in March 1926, made no attempt to defend the indefensible. Instead, its report followed the lines laid down in 1911 by some of the original critics of Lloyd George's Act and, later, in 1920 by the Mac-Alister and Dawson reports, in arguing ideally for a complete and unified health service. The majority report of the Royal Commission was, however, anxious to refute any charges of utopianism, and prudently accepted that, in the prevailing economic and political climate, the

Government would not contemplate any scheme which involved a significant addition to public expenditure. It proposed that extensions to the National Health Insurance scheme should only be attempted as and when funds became available, and argued that, by pooling some of the surpluses in the Approved Societies' funds, money could immediately be made available for consultant and specialist services[101]. The priority accorded to those services was in line with the expert evidence of Sir James Leishman, who told the Royal Commission that 'informed public opinion in Scotland in relation to health services ... is ... that the present insurance service, as far as it relates to health, is defective, and that the present medical service is merely a general practitioner service; and that in order to get the full benefit of the scheme ... it is imperative to extend that service to include ... all proper aids to diagnosis, all second opinions in the way of experts'[102].

The minority report totally rejected the cautious approach of the majority, arguing that the ideal of a complete and unified health service was attainable and that it was 'neither necessary nor proper to confine the developments of the National Health Insurance Scheme to such as can be paid for within the present financial resources of the Scheme'[103]. The minority proposed a socialist solution to the problems of health care, recommending that the full range of health services should be brought under local government control. Municipalisation, it was argued, would facilitate efficient planning and provision of health services, and eliminate wasteful overlapping[104]. The minority's recommendations found no favour with either the Conservative government of the day or the great majority of the medical profession to whom local government control was anathema, but the 'moderate' proposals of the majority report were well received by most sections of Scottish opinion. In the event, however, the Approved Societies set their face against the pooling of their surplus funds, and effectively blocked even the limited expansion of the National Health Insurance scheme proposed by the majority report.

Hospital Services

Shortly before the publication of the Royal Commission's report, the Scottish Board of Health's Hospital Services Committee had published its report. This Committee had been appointed on 21 June 1924 'To inquire into and report upon the extent and nature of the inadequacy of the present hospital and ancillary services in Scotland, and to make recommendations for the development and maintenance of those services to meet the needs of the community'. The causes of this worrying shortage of hospital accommodation were well known. While surgical and medical knowledge had increased remarkably since the late nineteenth century, and the advantages of treatment in a modern hospital were increasingly appreciated by the general public, hospital building programmes had been severely restricted during the first world war and subsequently hampered by high costs[105]. In short, both the demand for hospital treatment and the cost of providing it were increasing rapidly, and the voluntary hospital system was beginning to crack under the strain of trying to meet the needs of the situation. Waiting lists were growing in length, and it was discovered that 'overcrowding has come to be the normal condition of the large hospitals and of some of the smaller hospitals'[106]. The Hospital Services Committee found that

> "there are many persons in Scotland who, mainly because there are not enough hospital beds, are unable to get at the proper time the hospital treatment which they need. For all those persons, the shortage of beds means a prolongation of their suffering; for some it means that treatment is delayed beyond the stage when effective treatment is possible; and for a few, it may mean that they die before they can be admitted to hospital"[107].

All in all, the Committee estimated that 3,600 extra hospital beds were required in Scotland to meet the deficiency. Having reassured themselves as to the solvency of the voluntary system in Scotland, the Committee dismissed the arguments of those who favoured a State-financed and run hospital system, and proposed that the voluntary hospitals should provide 3,000 of the extra beds required[108]. However, while the Committee were confident that the voluntary hospitals could maintain those beds, they concluded that there was no likelihood of their finding all the money required to finance the proposed building programme. They recommended that the voluntary hospitals should be given a Treasury grant of £900,000 to meet 50 *per cent* of the estimated cost of the extension scheme[109]. Six months earlier the report of the corresponding English committee had recommended that 10,000 hospital beds should be provided in England and Wales (excluding London), and that a State grant of £2 million be paid to meet 50 *per cent* of the estimated cost. Successive Governments baulked at the prospect of finding almost £3 million to finance hospital expansion, and, in the event, no Treasury grant was ever made available. Without State assistance, the voluntary hospitals were unable to meet the target set by the Hospital Services Committee. By 1939 the total number of beds available in Scottish voluntary hospitals was 10,398, an increase of only 1,809 on the 1926 figure[110].

While the voluntary hospitals provided throughout the inter-war period 'much the bigger part of the institutional service for the treatment of acute medical and surgical conditions'[111], the services provided by the public authority hospitals were substantial and growing. 'The [largely voluntary] general hospitals', the Hospital Services Committee reported in 1926, 'have been relieved of groups of diseases, one after another, either by local authority hospitals or by special hospitals, and the poor law hospitals have grown in size and range of service until some of them occupy a place alongside the great voluntary hospitals'[112]. There were, by 1924, around 6,100 Poor Law hospital beds and, excluding municipal mental hospitals, 9,525 local authority beds in Scotland[113]. In all, therefore, the public sector provided nearly double the 8,589 beds in the voluntary hospitals. The annual running costs of the two sectors reflected, to some extent, their relative sizes. It was estimated that while the Scottish voluntary hospitals cost about £1 million a year to run in 1924, the local authority and Poor Law hospitals' annual running costs stood at £1.5 million[114].

Significant advances had taken place in the public authority hospital system since the beginning of the century. The Hospital Services Committee found that there had been 'a substantial improvement in many of the larger poorhouses and larger poorhouse hospitals' since the Poor Law report in 1909, although they added that 'only 3 or 4 [hospitals] would compare well, in staff, equipment and service generally, with modern general hospitals'[115]. Where parish councils, such as Glasgow, had endeavoured to bring their institutional treatment of the sick poor up to the standard of the voluntary general hospitals, working class reluctance to accept treatment in Poor Law hospitals had declined markedly. In the Committee's opinion, 'the development of the most progressive parish councils towards general hospital authorities' reinforced the already excellent arguments in favour of transferring the responsibility for Poor Law hospitals to local health authorities and, indeed, made such a transfer inevitable[116].

Important developments had also taken place within the local authority hospital system in recent times, although Scottish local authorities, being bound by the Public Health (Scotland) Act of 1897, were, unlike their English counterparts, legally prevented from operating general hospitals. The Hospital Services Committee stated that

> "The popular notion that the local authority hospitals are merely 'fever hospitals' has lingered long after the facts; the list of infectious diseases has been extended year after year until to-day several diseases [37 in all], including, for example, pneumonia, may be treated either in a voluntary or local authority hospital. Similarly in any given area there may be both local authority and voluntary provision for maternity and for diseases of children"[117].

The decline in the incidence of some infectious diseases, such as smallpox, typhus and enteric fever, had released accommodation which had 'gone some way towards meeting the need for increased accommodation for the new responsibilities of the local authorities', but a large amount of additional accommodation, particularly for the treatment of pulmonary tuberculosis, had had to be built, and much more was still needed. The Hospital Services Committee found that, while, 'on the whole, the accommodation for infectious diseases, including pulmonary tuberculosis, is adequate or is rapidly approaching adequacy,' the accommodation for non-pulmonary tuberculosis, pneumonia, maternity and diseases of children was insufficient[118]. No attempt was made to estimate the total deficiency of beds within the local authority hospital system, but the Committee did recommend that the local authorities should provide 600 additional beds for maternity and sick children.

The following decade saw a significant expansion in public authority hospital services, and by 1934 there were, excluding municipal mental hospitals, 18,227 beds in what were by then termed statutory hospitals[119]. Demand had, however, continued to outstrip supply, and the 1930s were as marked as the 1920s had been by a serious shortage of hospital beds. For example, while local authority hospitals had increased their provision of beds for maternity and sick children from 131 in 1924 to 658 in 1934, a commentator could note in 1937 that 'the supply of hospital beds [for such categories of patients] is notoriously inadequate for present needs'[120].

Development of Local Authority Services

The inter-war expansion of the public medical services was marked not only in the hospital service but also in the maternity and child welfare services and the school health service. The fact that the National Health Insurance scheme was not extended to cover dependants, the Cathcart Committee noted in 1936, prompted local authorities 'to develop their statutory services so as to fill the gap'[121]. In 1919 maternity and child welfare schemes were in operation in areas comprising 55 *per cent* of the population of Scotland, by 1929 the percentage had risen to 94, and by the end of 1935 'schemes were in operation in all areas' of the country[122]. While the amount of medical treatment provided at the various clinics was limited, the general practitioners regarded the development of local authority health services, which were staffed by salaried whole-timers, as an encroachment on their rightful territory. The general practitioners' concern was further heightened in the 1920s by the relaxation in the rules governing eligibility for Poor Law medical relief and the consequent expansion in the role of the Poor Law medical officer[123]. Being anxious to preserve their traditional professional status and independence, the general practitioners vigorously opposed local government control of medical services and the development of a salaried profession. The British Medical Association's proposals for a complete and unified public medical service, first put forward in outline form to the Royal Commission on National Health Insurance and subsequently elaborated in pamphlets published in 1929 and 1938, undoubtedly represented a public-spirited attempt to improve the nation's health, but may also be fairly seen as an attempt to defend the general practitioner against the threat posed by the expansion of local authority-run health services.

In its evidence to the Royal Commission on National Health Insurance the British Medical Association proposed that the National Health Insurance scheme should be extended 'so as to include complete consultant and specialist advice and treatment, full laboratory facilities for clinical purposes, residential treatment, ... dental advice and treatment' and all the personal health services provided by local health and education authorities. All the benefits, the British Medical Association argued, should be generally available[124]. In 1929 the Association published its *Proposals for a General Medical Service,* which were later revised and reissued in 1938. These pamphlets detailed and clarified the proposals made in 1926. The medical inspection of school children would continue, but all treatment would be carried out by the children's family doctors, and child welfare centres would become places of educational and social work, with their medical services being taken over by the general practitioners. Besides the child welfare educational centres and the medical inspection of school children, the local authorities' future health responsibilities would lie in the areas of environmental health, epidemiology, physical education, and some tuberculosis and venereal disease services. Not only did the British Medical Association make clear its determination to roll back the advances made in recent years by local authority health services, but it also restated the profession's opposition to salaried service, which in part was based upon memories of shabby treatment at the hands of the Poor Law authorities and the Friendly Societies, and voiced a recently discovered enthusiasm for the capitation method of remuneration as the best way to mediate State support of medical care[125].

While the medical staff employed by Scottish local authorities appear to have been quite satisfied with their conditions of service, it seems clear that many Scottish general practitioners fully shared the British Medical Association's views regarding local authority medical services. In February 1931 the Medical Practitioners Union, in a memorandum to Lanarkshire County Council, said:

> "The increasing encroachment upon the daily work of the general practitioner by the public health service, extending definitely to the therapeutic side of medicine, is noted, but it is pointed out that the development of the public health department in the county has now reached a point at which wider extension necessarily involves the appointment of general practitioners rather than specialists to its staff. This raises the question whether it is in the public interest that the public health service should continue to develop by the appointment of more whole-time officials until the ideal of a

State medical service is attained, or whether the general practitioner should be brought into closer association . . . The medical practitioners of the county . . . suggest that much clinical work, such as inspection and treatment of school children, maternity and child welfare, and domiciliary treatment of tuberculosis, could be efficiently performed by general practitioners on a part-time basis. After all, these represent the day's darg of every doctor in family practice. They also maintain that it is not in the interest of the public health service or of the people that this work should be undertaken by medical assistants whose experience and training is almost exclusively confined to the limited section of work in which they are engaged"[126].

The Local Government (Scotland) Act of 1929 accentuated the trend towards municipalisation of health services and thus heightened the anxieties of the medical profession and of general practitioners in particular. This long-overdue Act was a far-reaching measure which provided 'a completely new setting for local government'[127]. It sought to increase efficiency by unifying administration and spreading financial burdens, and to that end it enlarged local government areas and promoted co-ordination of services between different authorities. It abolished the District Committees, which had been responsible, in part, for the execution of the Public Health Acts, and the parish councils, which had been entrusted with the provision of both indoor and outdoor Poor Law medical relief, and transferred their powers to the 31 reconstructed county councils and the town councils of the 24 large burghs with populations of over 20,000. The major health services, including maternity and child welfare, and hospital provision for the treatment of infectious diseases, which had been provided by small burghs with populations of less than 20,000, were transferred to the county councils. The powers of the old education authorities, including those relating to the school health service, passed to the county councils and the town councils of Glasgow, Edinburgh, Dundee and Aberdeen[128].

The 1929 Act also effected a radical change in the method by which the Treasury provided financial support to local government. The old percentage grant in support of particular services was now replaced by a block grant. Whereas the structural reorganisation of local government was widely welcomed (although it did not go as far as the Association of County Councils in Scotland and various experts on Scottish local government would have wished in the direction of concentrating power in the hands of the county councils and town councils of the largest burghs), the change in the financial arrangements was highly controversial. Opposition to the block grant seems at bottom to have rested not on doubts as to the equity of the system itself, but rather on a belief that it had been introduced in order to curtail central government expenditure in support of expanding local government services. The fear was that the cost of any future expansion of local government services would have to be borne largely or entirely by the local authorities themselves, and that consequently only the wealthier authorities would be able to provide the expanded services that were generally agreed to be desirable. In the words of the Convention of Royal Burghs:

> "Almost without exception the financial officers of local authorities are satisfied that the substitution of the block grant system for the percentage grant system will... operate to the advantage of the Treasury and to the serious disadvantage of the local authorities. The fixing of the amount of the grant for fixed periods, based on a standard year, will tend to stop all progress, and, in the event of an industrial crisis or a period of severe unemployment, will place an overwhelming burden on the local ratepayers"[129].

The Government attempted to remove these anxieties by reducing the period of time between reassessments of the level of block grant, but the opposition remained unconvinced of the merits of the proposed new system. When the Bill reached its committee stage in the House of Commons, Ernest Brown, Liberal MP for Leith, moved an amendment excluding public health services from the operation of the block grant, stating that 'there is no single issue raised in the Bill which is causing more disquietude in the country... than the change-over as regards health services from the percentage to the block system'. Brown prophesied that the block grant would discourage the development of both new and existing health services. The block grant, he said, would lead to 'competition among idealists which will mean that one will want more money for tuberculosis treatment, another will want more for maternity and child welfare, another will want more for the treatment of venereal diseases, and it will leave local authorities with a very grave burden... and with the temptation that these moneys may be used for other local needs'. It would, he believed, 'hamstring the government's own scheme for the concentration and better working of the medical services'[130]. Brown's amendment was supported by the Labour opposition, and the Labour MPs for Edinburgh Central, Glasgow St Rollox and Edinburgh East all attacked the block grant as a retrograde measure which was introduced in the interests of economy and would prevent the development of much-needed but 'unpopular' services for the blind, the mentally defective and those suffering from venereal diseases[131].

In defence of the Government's proposals Walter Elliot, the Conservative Under Secretary of State for Scotland, maintained that, while the old percentage grants had supported only certain specified services, the block grant would cover all local authority services including the hugely expensive Poor Law services. The block grant, he explained, would be revised after three years, then at the end of four more years, and thereafter at intervals of five years, and would be raised on each occasion in proportion to the increase in local expenditure in the intervening period. Moreover, while the old percentage grant operated to the considerable disadvantage of poorer areas which could not afford to spend much on health services and therefore qualified for only a small grant, the block grant would be administered in such a way as to provide adequate funding of health services in necessitous areas. Finally, backward or irresponsible authorities which, in the Department of Health's view, did not provide a reasonable level of health services would be penalised by the withdrawal of grant support[132]. At the end of the debate the House of Commons divided on party lines and Ernest Brown's amendment was defeated[133].

Whether the introduction of the block grant system led to a reduction in the rate of increase of central government expenditure on local authority health services and consequently to a reduction in the growth rate of these services remains unclear, but what is clear is that the municipal health services continued to expand in the period between 1929 and the inception of the National Health Service. With hindsight it can be seen that the 1930s and early 1940s marked the zenith of local government responsibility for health service provision, but it appeared to many at that time that the future organisation of the health services would be based upon the Webbs' ideal of a municipal State Medical Service. In 1936, for example, the Cathcart Committee asserted that 'unless a policy is framed and developments guided by it, the local authority services are bound to extend further ... and ... influence if not determine the future medical organisation of the country'[134]. It was significant, the Committee believed, that 'the Corporation of Glasgow has now established a whole-time general medical service, with dispensaries and clinics, for the sick poor, and that it is intended to develop this service in association with the clinics and centres required for their other statutory services'[135]. Where Glasgow led, they thought, the rest of Scotland was likely to follow.

The Local Government (Scotland) Act effected important changes not only in the domiciliary and clinical services but also in the hospital sector. Section 27 of the Act made it 'competent for the County Council of a county or the Town Council of a large burgh to submit for the approval of the Department of Health a scheme for the reorganisation of the hospital facilities at the disposal of the Council, with a view to the provision of treatment for sick persons residing within their area'. In forming their judgment of such a scheme the Department of Health was required to 'have regard to any other facilities for treatment of any such sick persons, including those provided by any voluntary hospital or other institution'. The same section of the Act also made it 'competent for any such Council ... to make a representation to the Department of Health that the hospital facilities available are inadequate for the reasonable

requirements of sick persons residing in their area, and to submit a
scheme for the extension of such facilities'. As with the first provision, so
the second provision was hedged round with qualifications apparently
drafted after consultations with the Voluntary Hospitals Liaison Committee, and designed not only to ensure that the proposed hospitals were
properly located and of adequate size but also to protect the interests of
the voluntary hospitals. The clause provided that the Department, before approving any scheme of extension, 'shall satisfy themselves by
inquiry that hospital accommodation at the disposal of the Council,
together with the accommodation provided by voluntary hospitals . . . is
not reasonably adequate for the needs of the inhabitants of the area, and
that the Council have taken reasonable steps to seek and to continue to
secure full co-operation with every voluntary hospital, University, or
medical school within or serving the area of the Council'[136]. In effect
then, the voluntary hospitals were to be given something approximating
to a veto on the future expansion of the local authority hospital system.
The special status of the voluntary hospitals was acknowledged implicity
as well as explicitly: there was no requirement for voluntary hospitals to
consult with local authorities and secure the approval of the Department
of Health before embarking upon an extension programme.

Section 27 of the 1929 Act had a fourfold purpose. It sought, firstly,
by authorising local authorities to provide general hospitals apart from
the Poor Law, to facilitate the much-needed expansion of the hospital
system; secondly, to increase public willingness to use the hospitals provided by removing the stigma of the Poor Law; thirdly, to improve the
efficiency of the public hospital service by unifying its administration;
and, fourthly, to encourage co-operation between the local authorities
and the voluntary hospitals in planning and providing services within
their areas. The results, however, proved disappointing. Largely because
of financial difficulties arising from the depression, only four local authorities – Edinburgh, Dundee, Aberdeen, and the County of Bute – had
converted Poor Law infirmaries into general hospitals by 1936, although
Glasgow Corporation had three hospitals which functioned as general
hospitals while still being technically Poor Law institutions[137]. Even
this limited progress was not achieved without cost, for the conversion of
Poor Law infirmaries into general hospitals reduced geriatric provision
just at the time when, due to the ageing of the population, the need for
additional beds for the elderly sick and infirm was beginning to become
apparent. In the field of co-operation between local authorities and
voluntary hospitals, the hopes of the legislators of 1929 were largely
unfulfilled. Only in the North-East did there emerge the formal system
of regional planning and co-operation which the framers of the Local
Government (Scotland) Act had envisaged and which the *Glasgow Herald*
had declared, as early as August 1926, to be 'urgently necessary'[138].
The origins of the North-East scheme stretched back to 1925, when

Aberdeen County Council and Aberdeen County Education Authority brought all the public health services within the county under a Joint Committee and appointed a Chief Medical Officer to control the whole work, including the school medical service. The passage of the 1929 Act enabled this earlier scheme to be extended, and in 1930 Kincardineshire and the City and County of Aberdeen combined to form a North-East Regional hospital and public health service. Under this scheme key personnel and resources were shared, although no attempt was made to pool the costs, and each local authority, through its Public Health Committee, retained responsibility for the public health services within its area. A Liaison Committee was, however, set up and charged with reviewing the needs of the combined area and suggesting any necessary readjustments in the scheme[139]. The regional service was accounted a great success. A testimony to its value is found in the fact that it survived until 1950, by which time the National Health Service (Scotland) Act had reorganised hospital services in such a way as to make the scheme redundant[140]. The Cathcart Committee, reviewing the operation of the scheme in 1936, found that

> "The benefits of such a scheme are manifold. The city gains financially by the fuller use made of its facilities. The rural areas have made available to them those institutional and other facilities with their expert advice and treatment, which can normally only be provided at large centres. The scheme also ensures uniformity in the administration of the statutory services. The regional basis of the scheme, too, makes more readily attainable a full co-operation with voluntary agencies"[141].

The Department of Health for Scotland was optimistic that the Local Government (Scotland) Act of 1929 would lead to greater co-ordination of health service provision, and John Jeffrey, the Department's Secretary, believed that it might eventually facilitate the creation of a fully integrated health service. Addressing the Scottish Association of Insurance Committees on 28 September 1929, Jeffrey stated that the 1929 Act would allow 'an important advance ... in the co-ordination of the health services', and then went on to declare that

> "if they were to obtain the fullest and best use of all the resources at their disposal it seemed essential that the domiciliary medical services given under the auspices of the insurance committees should be brought into a close relationship with the public health and hospital services in Scotland ... It had always been a matter of regret to the Central Department that the general practitioner service under the Health Insurance Scheme had remained more or less detached from the service which had developed under the various Acts of Parliament administered by the local author-

ity, and no one could deny the advantages to be derived from breaking down any obstacles there might be in the way of full collaboration and consultation between the various experts who are treating the sick people.... The ultimate aim should be to create the most effective machine for the prevention and cure of sickness in all its forms. One would like, if possible, to secure for insurance practitioners an organic association with the voluntary and municipal hospitals, so that consultant services and specialised equipment might be made available to panel patients where necessary.... Was it not possible that within the new hospital organisation contemplated under the 1929 Act, the insurance service and the Local Authority and voluntary hospital services... would be able to bring to the aid of the insured patients all requirements in the way of equipment and specialist services available under the new hospital organisation?"[142].

Nothing came of the Department of Health's imaginative proposals for the implementation of its progressive, and apparently long-held, ideas on the future development of the health services, but action was taken in regard to a plan, also put forward by Jeffrey in his speech to the Scottish Association of Insurance Committees, for the compilation of morbidity statistics as an aid to the planning of health services. Each local authority produced its mortality statistics, Jeffrey noted, 'but apart from infectious diseases it had no knowledge of the prevalence of ordinary sickness among its inhabitants, or of the nature and causes of that sickness, and whether any action on the part of the Local Authority could prevent and reduce such sickness'. Now that Insurance Committees and public health authorities were to operate within co-extensive jurisdictions, he concluded, 'it seemed a matter for consideration whether steps could not be taken to remedy this obvious gap in the information at the disposal of the authorities responsible for looking after the health of the community'[143]. The Insurance Committees responded to the central Department's request, and the important data which was subsequently compiled revealed the now familiar pattern contrasting the frequency of the main causes of sickness with mortality data. It was found that the main causes of sickness were respiratory diseases, which accounted for about a third of the cases, diseases of the digestive system, accidents, rheumatism, and skin diseases. Later investigation was primarily concerned with unfitness for work and reviewed morbidity data for the years 1930 to 1938. The results of this investigation caused concern. They revealed an unsuspected amount of long-term or chronic sickness (the rate in 1936/37, for example, was 17.2 per 1,000 of the insured work force) and disclosed that between a fifth and a quarter of chronic cases were under 35 years of age. In 1936/37 the average number of days lost through incapacity for work was a startling 14.92[144].

The Cathcart Committee

The serious health problems of inter-war Scotland, and the relative slowness of progress in solving them, aroused widespread anxiety and stimulated some far-sighted thinking on health policy. 'The fact that our indices of disease and health show a slower rate of progress at several important points than England and some other countries have achieved,' the *Glasgow Herald* declared in an editorial of 6 April 1936, suggests 'that we have some way to go, in organisation, perhaps, and probably also in our personal habits and outlook, before it can be said that we have made full use of the victories already won by [medical] science'. Having noted that the forthcoming Report of the Scottish Health Services Committee was expected to be followed by the submission of 'a comprehensive health programme to the country', the *Glasgow Herald* went on to argue that this programme 'should receive the close and sympathetic consideration of the public, for... there is good reason to believe' that existing health services 'fall short of what is required to make full use of modern resources for the prevention of disease and the promotion of health[145].

The eagerly awaited Report of the Committee on Scottish Health Services, which was generally known after its chairman, Professor E.P. Cathcart, as the Cathcart Report, appeared on 1 July 1936. The Committee, which had been appointed in 1933 'to review the existing health services of Scotland in the light of modern conditions and knowledge, and to make recommendations on any changes in policy and organisation that may be considered necessary for the promotion of efficiency and economy',[146] produced an outstanding and comprehensive report. The Report was 'an unusually arresting document,' opined the *Glasgow Herald*, for 'it sets the problem of national health against its modern background, and for the first time enables one to view it as a whole'[147]. The theme of the Cathcart Report was the need for a national health policy. Existing health services, it was pointed out, had developed piecemeal at different periods and with widely different intentions. The need now was to produce a national health policy, which would promote the fitness of the people by means of the co-ordination of all the departments and agencies which influenced health. How best to achieve this end the Committee saw as the fundamental problem of their enquiry.

The Report was as comprehensive as its remit necessitated. It advocated major efforts in the area of health education and promotion, called for increased provision for physical recreation and training, criticised the diet of the Scottish people and stressed the need for improvement, urged the revision of public health legislation to combat environmental hazards, drew attention to the need for the codification of laws relating to sanitation (a task which is still outstanding), and pointed to the significance of an ageing population for health service planning.

So far as the provision of medical care was concerned, the Cathcart

Report accepted the submissions of the Scottish Royal Corporations and British Medical Association and followed the recommendation of the MacAlister Report of 1920 that 'the health service of the nation should be based upon the family as the normal unit, and upon the family doctor as the normal medical attendant and guardian'[148]. It argued that if health was a matter of reaction to environment, then it followed that the person best fitted to give expert advice to an individual on his health was the person who was most familiar with the individual and his environment. The Report adjudged the National Health Insurance scheme to have been a success, and urged that it should be extended to cover dependants[149]. It also argued that a separate domiciliary medical service for the poor was undesirable, and recommended that 'local authorities should be empowered to provide medical attendance for the necessitous'. The arrangements of local authorities should be such as to ensure that, 'as far as possible, poverty will not interrupt continuity of medical supervision by the family doctor'[150]. The co-ordination of general practitioner services with child welfare, school health, and other medical services would 'remedy one of the principal weaknesses of these services as they are organised at present'[151].

Co-ordination and extension of services were also the themes of the section of the Report dealing with hospitals. The Report's recommendations followed closely those of the Department of Health's Consultative Council on Medical and Allied Subjects which had been presented in January 1933[152]. The Cathcart Committee supported the Consultative Council's emphasis on the need to co-ordinate hospital provision. Co-ordination was required in order to avoid unnecessary duplication of buildings and equipment, to secure maximum use of specialised skills, to ensure the proper allocation of patients to the most appropriate hospital, to extend teaching facilities over as wide a range as possible and to facilitate consistent policies on recruitment of staff and payments by patients[153]. Regional hospital service committees, representing voluntary and statutory hospitals, the Report recommended, should be set up by statute for each of the proposed five Scottish regions to be centred on Glasgow, Edinburgh, Dundee, Aberdeen and Inverness. These committees were to be advisory bodies, whose primary function was to facilitate co-operation in the regions[154]. Proposals for the provision or extension of both statutory and voluntary hospitals were to be submitted to the regional committees for recommendation to the Department of Health[155]. The main financial responsibility for making up the long apparent and serious shortage of hospital facilities should be placed on the local authorities, 'for it would be unwise to endeavour to induce the voluntary hospitals to extend their financial commitments much further than at present'[156]. Being convinced that it was 'in the interest of the State to foster the voluntary hospital system', the Report recommended that a State 'teaching facilities grant' should be paid to the voluntary teaching hospitals, and that all voluntary hospitals should be exempted from the payment of legacy dues and be granted remission from rates[157].

The reaction to the publication of the Cathcart Report was somewhat less than enthusiastic. Of crucial significance, at a time when Stanley Baldwin's Conservative government was in power in Westminster, was the fact that Conservative opinion was unpersuaded of the merits of the Report's main recommendations. The Scottish conservative press, while agreeing that something had to be done to improve Scotland's deplorable health record, was deeply suspicious of the solutions offered by the Cathcart Committee. The *Glasgow Herald* said that 'practically every proposal of the Committee raises points of controversy', and expected that the report 'will provide material for much public discussion for a long time'[158]. The *Scotsman* expressed the view that the Cathcart Committee's 'whole system is really not far removed from a State medical service', and joined with Sir Andrew Grierson in expressing anxiety about the cost to the ratepayer and taxpayer of the Report's proposals[159]. These newspaper editorials appear to have been in tune with the prevailing views of Scottish conservative politicians. When the annual estimates of the Department of Health for Scotland were debated in the House of Commons on 14 July 1936 the debate was opened by Sir Godfrey Collins, Secretary of State for Scotland, who, while promising to give the Cathcart Report his fullest consideration, studiously avoided giving any indication of support for its main recommendations, and concentrated instead upon the housing issue, which he claimed was the most important in relation to public health. Collins boasted that more slums had been destroyed and more new houses erected during the three years since Baldwin's government had come to power that in the previous thirty years. A general improvement in public health, he claimed, was to be expected from the efforts now being made to remove slums and prevent overcrowding[160]. Collins' speech set the whole tone of the debate. Speaker after speaker, from both main political parties, rose to contribute his views on the housing problem and the government's endeavours to solve it, and, in the process, the wider issues raised by the Cathcart Report almost disappeared from sight. Ironically, it was a Conservative MP, James Guy of Edinburgh Central, who tried to persuade the House of Commons to broaden its horizons, and, by complaining that members had only had a week to study the Cathcart Report, reminded his colleagues in an oblique fashion that the debate should have been focused on Scottish health policy. Interestingly, Guy himself had found sufficient study time to pronounce that a definite line of advance for these services (ie, the health services) was now laid down and should be followed[161]. Guy's opinion was not widely shared, and Westminster quietly forgot about the main recommendations of the Cathcart Report.

Maternity Services

Only one of the Cathcart Committee's recommendations – the setting up of a comprehensive maternity service – was taken up before the outbreak of the second world war. Since at least as far back as 1929 official and public opinion had been worried by Scotland's high maternal mortality rate, and convinced by evidence from other countries where maternity services had been introduced that this rate could be dramatically reduced. 'Here is a case', declared the *Glasgow Herald* in a leading article of 6 April 1929 on the Annual Report of the Department of Health for Scotland, 'where public opinion is ready to say "if preventable, why not prevent?" '[162]. The challenge was taken up by the Department. In 1935, after a prolonged and systematic investigation by Drs Peter McKinlay and Charlotte Douglas, its Scientific Advisory Committee presented a Report on Maternal Morbidity and Mortality in Scotland, which found 'that in all areas of Scotland many women do not obtain obstetrical services of the amount and quality necessary to safeguard them to the maximum extent'[163]. The Committee were convinced that there was an 'urgent need for improvement in the standard of midwifery', and recommended the establishment of 'a comprehensive service designed to cover adequately the whole field of maternity provision in Scotland'. The aim, they stated, should be

"to ensure efficient maternity services for women at all stages of pregnancy, labour and puerperium. Such services should be available in patients' homes for those who may be properly cared for there; and in institutions for those who need institutional care. Where patients requiring specialist treatment cannot be removed to hospital, skilled obstetrical services should be provided in their homes. With these objects in view, the development of services suited to the circumstances and requirements of each area should be assisted and encouraged"[164].

These recommendations, which were endorsed and elaborated upon by the Cathcart Committee, formed the basis for the Maternity Services (Scotland) Bill which was introduced into the House of Commons by Sir Godfrey Collins on 27 July 1936[165]. The apparent intention behind this strange timing was to give all interested parties sufficient time over the summer to consider the measure before it was proceeded with in the autumn session, although in the event it was 28 January 1937 before the Bill received its second reading. The Scottish Bill was much more comprehensive than the recently enacted English Midwives Act, which, as its title suggests, related solely to midwifery. Under the Scottish Bill every expectant mother who desired to be advised in her own home would be entitled to retain the services of a midwife and a doctor, and, if the need arose, the doctor would be able to call in the services of a consultant obstetrician. The intention was that the midwife, general practitioner and consultant obstetrician would act in concert. Fees were to be charged to patients according to their economic circumstances, with the necessitous receiving the services provided free of any charge. The main financial burden of the scheme, however, was to be borne by local authorities and government, with the latter paying to the former a grant equivalent to approximately half the additional expenditure associated with the provision of maternity services[166].

The Maternity Services (Scotland) Act, which came into force on 16 May 1937, was widely and warmly welcomed. The medical profession, the newspaper press, the politicians and, in so far as it is possible to judge, the general public regarded it as a significant step forward which it was hoped would lead to a reduction not only in the maternal mortality rate but also in the number of infant lives lost and in the amount of 'invalidism' among mothers. The Act, it seems, was perceived as a bold and pragmatic solution to a problem which could no longer be ignored.

The Act undoubtedly contributed to the fall in the maternal mortality rate from 4.8 per 1,000 live and stillbirths in 1937 to a record low of 3.0 in 1944[167]. It seems clear, however, that factors other than the improved services offered by the Act were in part responsible for this impressive reduction. Largely due to a fall in deaths from puerperal sepsis associated with increasing recognition of the importance of droplet infection and the widespread employment of sulpha drugs, the maternal mortality rate had already fallen by 1.5 per 1,000 live and stillbirths in the two years preceding the passing of the Act[168].

The expected follow-up to the Maternity Services Act was the Registration of Stillbirths (Scotland) Act of 1938. This measure, which brought Scotland into line with England and Wales, and had been recommended by the Cathcart Committee, obliged the doctor or midwife in charge of a confinement resulting in a stillbirth to inform the authorities of the cause of death if known[169]. It enabled a start to be made to the epidemiological studies of stillbirth which have brought about steady progress in understanding and care.

Cancer Control

The last piece of health legislation relating to Scotland to be passed before the second world war was the Cancer Act of 1939, which was born of a growing concern (whose origins could be traced back to the beginning of the century) about the increasing incidence of cancer. The Act required local authorities to submit to the Department of Health schemes for the diagnosis and treatment of malignant disease. The outbreak of war put a brake on the implementation of the Act, although discussions were held, despite the prevailing difficulties, between the Department and representatives of local authorities in Glasgow, Edinburgh, Aberdeen and Inverness, as a first step towards the preparation or acceptance of interim schemes[170].

Looking back on the eve of the second world war, it was clear that there had been a significant improvement in the health of the Scottish people during the inter-war years despite the economic depression which had hung over the country for much of the period. However, there was, as we have seen, little or no room for complacency. Contemporaries were well aware of the serious nature of the health problems facing the country and of how badly Scotland's health record compared with that of similar industrialised nations. Much thought and effort had gone into understanding these problems and into recommending improvements, yet the advances which had undoubtedly been made during the inter-war period were of a piecemeal rather than a comprehensive nature. While the difficulties of the economy were frequently used as a justification for this failure to implement comprehensive reforms, it cannot be argued that Britain was a wealthier country in 1945 than in 1939. The chief impediment to progress, therefore, was not the economic depression, but rather the absence of the necessary political will within the country at large. That will was to be created by the experiences of the nation during Hitler's war.

Wartime Problems and Progress

After the passage of the Civil Defence Act of 1939 the Department of Health had to prepare itself to take an active role in the machinery of wartime administration. Hitherto it had been concerned with supervising the work of local authorities, but now it was faced with the possibility of having to administer and operate a large range of emergency services, and in certain fields, such as evacuation, to exercise much closer control over the work of local bodies.

One of the Department's major new concerns was the evacuation of children, their school teachers and, in the case of very young children, their mothers from vulnerable industrial areas. These evacuations, which took place at the beginning of the war and again in 1941 after the air-raids on Clydeside, shook up not only the routine operations of local administration, but also the social complacency of those involved in supervising them. Some alarming discoveries were made in what were termed the 'sending' and 'reception' areas, where arrangements had been made for the health screening and medical care of evacuees. The volume of infestation and infection – vermin, scabies, impetigo and the like – revealed by the screening procedure shocked the public health and voluntary workers involved, and 'aroused the conscience of the country'[171]. A privately instituted survey of the clothing of child evacuees revealed that 30 *per cent* was 'bad or deplorable', a figure which corresponded well enough with the 31 *per cent* of the children registered for evacuation in Glasgow who were found to be infested. Cleansing and treatment centres were established, and preventive measures of sanitary supervision and immunisation were adopted in response to the problem, but it was soon discovered that a discouraging number of children were re-infested by visiting relatives after being cleaned up. Perhaps even more shocking than the discoveries relating to the scale of infestation and associated infection was the revelation that between 5 *per cent* and 10 *per cent* of evacuated children were enuretic, and that dirty habits involving a failure to employ elementary methods of sanitation were not uncommon. Well could Dr A.K. Bowman of the Department of Health for Scotland conclude that 'as an index ... of unsatisfactory and in some cases of deplorable social conditions the experience [of war-time evacuation] was a valuable one'[172].

Although the fears of the central and local health authorities regarding the possibility of widespread epidemics were not realised, the war years did see significant increases in the incidence of certain diseases and increasing efforts to reduce them. As we have seen, scabies, with its associated conditions of impetigo and pediculosis, was revealed as a major problem by the evacuations of 1939 and 1941. In 1941 the Scabies Order (Scotland) was promulgated, giving Medical Officers of Health extended powers for the treatment and control of scabies and other verminous conditions, and by the middle of 1942 several authorities were able to report that the prevalence of the condition was decreasing. Thereafter the improvement was progressive[173]. In 1940 the prevalence of diphtheria rose sharply. Despite the fact that for some years before the outbreak of war immunisation had offered an effective method of reducing both the incidence and the mortality of this disease, immunisation programmes had been confined in the pre-war years to a few centres and had been carried out only fitfully. Wartime produced the resolution to do what should have been done earlier, and throughout 1941 and 1942 a massive propaganda campaign was waged in support of immunisation. By 30 June, 1942, 792,000 children (representing 73 *per cent* of the school and 58 *per cent* of the pre-school child population) had been immunised against diphtheria, and Tom Johnston, Secretary of State for Scotland, could inform the House of Commons that the rise of the disease had been checked. Thereafter, although the Department of Health remained worried about the relatively low level of immunisation among the pre-school population, the incidence of diphtheria continued to fall, reaching 5,679 cases in 1945 as against a peak of 15,069 in 1940[174].

The incidence of venereal diseases had remained fairly constant during the inter-war period and the early part of the war, but a marked rise occurred in 1941. The authorities responded with a campaign of public education, which was more forthright than peace-time susceptibilities would have tolerated, and with Defence Regulation 33B, which required any person named as a source by two or more people to undergo examination and, if found to be infected, treatment. Few twice-named contacts were revealed, but in a number of areas attempts were made, with frequently successful results, to persuade men and women who had been named once to attend voluntarily for examination and treatment. By 1944 the incidence of venereal diseases had been reduced to the pre-war level[175].

In contrast to the success in relation to venereal diseases, scabies and diphtheria, the failure to check the war-time rise in the incidence of pulmonary tuberculosis is striking. By 1940 the situation had become so worrying that the pre-war tuberculosis beds, which had been emptied at the start of hostilities to make way for the expected war casualties, were restored to their original function, and some wards of hospitals operating under the Emergency Medical Service were commissioned as supplementary tuberculosis units. By 1944 Scotland had 1,334 more tuberculosis beds than in 1939, and in the summer of 1944 the first mass radiography units were introduced in Glasgow and Lanarkshire in an attempt to obtain early diagnosis of the disease. A year earlier, in 1943, in order to encourage wage earners to accept treatment, the Department of Health for Scotland had made provision for the payment of special financial allowances to patients. Despite all these measures, the number of cases of pulmonary tuberculosis continued to rise, reaching a peak of 7,316 cases in 1945. Whatever the reasons for this increase, and it seems that there were many factors involved, 'nutrition, as such, would not appear to have been directly implicated'[176].

The importance of nutrition as a subject worthy of scientific investigation had only come to be generally appreciated in Scotland during the 1930s. In June 1935 the Minister of Health and Secretary of State for Scotland had requested the Advisory Committee on Nutrition 'to inquire into the facts, quantitative and qualitative, in relation to the diet of the people'. Around the same time Professor E.P. Cathcart of Glasgow and Sir John Boyd Orr of Aberdeen had conducted surveys of the Scottish diet. The latter, in his book, *Food, Health and Income*, had found that, although the Scottish diet had improved markedly since before the first world war, the diet of nearly half of the population, while sufficient to satisfy hunger, was deficient for the maintenance of health[177].

Much use was made of these investigations when it came to framing food and rationing policies during the second world war. These policies, which promoted a balanced diet and equal access to essential foods irrespective of income level, proved to be very successful. They were largely responsible, along with the full employment of war-time, for the improved levels of national health which were a feature of the period. The Secretary of State for Scotland's Scientific Advisory Committee, which from 1941 onwards investigated the feeding of the families of workers employed in heavy industries, found that 'compared with pre-war diet, the food of such workers – as well as of their families – had improved, and that no serious reduction in the intake of essential foods had occurred'[178]. The important place of milk as an article of food in the war-time dietary, particularly of children, expectant and nursing mothers and invalids, was well appreciated. Consumption of milk increased by 45 *per cent* during the war due to the development of the Milk in Schools scheme and the introduction, in 1941, of the National Milk scheme. By the end of the war 68 *per cent* of Scottish children attending education authority schools were participating in the Milk in Schools scheme, while over 75 *per cent* of pregnant women, nursing mothers and pre-school children were taking part in the National Milk scheme[179]. Although it is undoubted that other factors, such as the improved provision of school meals under the Education (Scotland) Act of 1942, had a sizeable effect, these schemes contributed significantly to the marked improvement in the health of infants and children during the war. The physical condition of children, as evidenced by their heights and weights on entering and leaving school, was maintained throughout the war, and in some areas an improvement on pre-war years was observed[180]. The improvement in the health and expectation of life of infants and pre-school children which took place between 1941 and 1946 was astonishing. The infant mortality rate declined by 35 *per cent* between 1941 and 1946, the greatest percentage reduction over a six-year period since records were first kept in 1855, while the stillbirth rate fell by a slightly less impressive 20 *per cent* between the same years[181].

The war years also witnessed significant advances in environmental health services. Progress towards the provision of a safe milk supply was marked by increases in the number of tuberculin-tested herds and by improvements in the efficiency of pasteurisation. The payment of a premium of 2¼d. per gallon to producers who possessed tuberculin tested herds (which was increased to 4d. per gallon in 1944), and the introduction of the attested herds scheme, did much to increase the number of tubercle-free animals. Between 1937, the year before the introduction of the premium payment scheme, and 1945 the number of tuberculin-tested herds increased from 769 to 3,762. Similarly, due to the joint efforts of the Department of Health and the dairy farmers, the number of milk producers holding a licence under the Milk (Special Designation) Order (Scotland) of 1936 increased between 1938 and 1945 from 2,000 to 4,700 out of an estimated total of 9,000 producers. Amendments to the Milk (Special Designation) Order (Scotland) in 1941 and 1944 led respectively to the introduction of the high-temperature short-time method of pasteurisation, and to the provision of new, more hygienic bottle-washing arrangements, bottle-filling machinery and other apparatus[182].

Progress was likewise made in extending the availability of safe water supplies during the war. An engineering survey of Scottish water supplies, which was begun in 1943, showed that many existing supplies were in need of improvement. The most pressing problem was to make piped water supplies available to the one-third of the rural population who were without such services, largely as a result of the inertia and lack of resources of the responsible sanitary authorities. A White Paper on *A National Water Policy*, published in April 1944, intimated that, as part of the general post-war reconstruction policy, a grant-in-aid of £6.375 million would be made available to assist local authorities to provide or improve water supplies, and to make adequate provision for sewage disposal in rural areas. These proposals were implemented by the Rural Water Supplies and Sewerage Act of July 1944[183].

Hospital Services in Wartime

It was the outbreak of war in 1939 and, in particular, the expectation of heavy air-raid casualties which led to the end of Scotland's chronic shortage of hospital beds. In 1938, as the threat of war became more imminent, existing hospital accommodation was surveyed. This survey formed the basis for the planning of the Emergency Medical Service (EMS) scheme, which greatly increased hospital accommodation, expanded the provision of specialist facilities and services, and brought together the various types of hospital authority on a regional basis. The scheme provided an additional 20,527 beds (representing approximately a 60 *per cent* increase in accommodation), of which 16,574 (located partly in annexes to existing hospitals and partly in new hospitals) were for general purposes and 3,953 (largely located in converted country houses) were for convalescence[184]. Seven new hospitals were built under the scheme, at Raigmore (near Inverness), Stracathro (near Brechin), Bridge of Earn (Perthshire), Killearn (Stirlingshire), Law (Lanarkshire), Ballochmyle (Ayrshire) and Peel (Selkirkshire)[185]. Pre-war investigations had revealed that along with a deficiency in general hospital accommodation there was a shortage of certain specialist facilities. The Cathcart Committee, for example, found 'that hospital facilities were seriously inadequate for patients who . . . required admission for specialist observation and diagnosis[186]. This deficiency was made good during the war by the Emergency Medical Service. Seven specialist orthopaedic centres, with a total of 1,980 beds, were established, while a further 28 centres, with 1,290 beds, were set up to cater for plastic surgery, psycho-neurosis, neurosurgery, eye injuries, and other specialisms[187]. These centres provided a great stimulus to specialist practice in Scotland. In the pre-war period the development of specialisation had been restricted by the heavy dependence of voluntary hospital doctors upon private practice. However, hospital doctors from the Emergency Medical Service were free from such restraints and could devote themselves entirely to their chosen specialism. Other special services were boosted by the demands of war-time planning. To supplement existing laboratory facilities an Emergency Pathological Laboratory Service was organised in Scotland, while in 1940 the Scottish National Blood Transfusion Association was formed to co-ordinate and develop existing blood transfusion services[188].

The expected numbers of military and civilian casualties never materialised, and in December 1940, in response to demands from the medical profession, the voluntary hospitals and the public, the Department of Health drew up a scheme to make Emergency Medical Service beds available to ordinary patients. 'It was obviously foolish', Tom Johnston, the Secretary of State for Scotland, wrote, 'to have the well-equipped hospitals often standing empty and their staffs awaiting Civil Defence casualties – which, thank God, never came – while war workers could not afford specialist diagnosis and treatment'[189]. The take-up of this scheme, which was restricted to short-stay surgical patients, was poor, and in January 1942 a 'perturbed' Tom Johnston extended it to include all categories of patients except chronic cases. By the middle of 1945 32,826 patients had been taken off the voluntary hospitals' waiting lists and treated in Emergency Medical Service hospitals[190].

Towards the end of 1941 the Department of Health began receiving reports suggesting that war strain, long hours of work, the blackout and other factors were beginning to affect the health of industrial workers in Scotland. It was clear to the Department that 'the manpower needs of the nation required the organisation of the civilian medical services on lines which would secure that early and correct diagnosis and treatment were available for any condition which threatened to impair the working capacity of war workers or leave a war aftermath of chronic invalidism'[191]. As there were staffed beds in EMS hospitals under the Department's direct control with full consultant and diagnostic facilities, the way was open to set up an interesting (and successful) experiment in preventive medicine which was to involve the close co-operation of the family doctors, consultants and hospital services. Thus, in January 1942, Tom Johnston launched the Clyde Basin Experiment. At first the experiment was limited to young industrial workers in West Central Scotland aged between 15 and 25 who were in a debilitated state or showing symptoms suggesting the need for expert diagnosis, but such was its immediate success that by the end of the year it was extended to cover war workers of all ages in the whole of Scotland except the Highland counties. Under the Supplementary Medical Service Scheme, as it was known after 1 December 1942, workers showing signs of a possible breakdown in health were referred by their general practitioners to a Regional Medical Officer, who arranged for an early and complete clinical investigation. Where necessary, the Regional Medical Officer arranged for the patient's admission to hospital for observation and diagnosis or, alternatively, to a convalescent home for a period of rest before resumption of work. In some cases, where it was believed that a change of occupation would be of benefit to health, consultations would be arranged between representatives of the Department of Health and the Ministry of Labour and National Service. In every case a full report was sent to the general practitioner for his future guidance and, in selected cases, follow-up work was undertaken. The scheme was appreciated by patients and practitioners alike, and by the end of 1945 22,174 patients had been referred to Regional Medical Officers under its provisions. 'The general conclusion was that the service as a whole had been both acceptable and beneficial'[192]. Tom Johnston, who seems to have been especially delighted at the conversion of 'the swagger hotel at Gleneagles' into a fitness centre, first for miners and latterly for all groups of workers, clearly regarded the utilisation of EMS hospitals for the treatment of ordinary civilian cases and the introduction of the Supplementary Medical Service Scheme as two of the greatest achievements of his time in office, and boasted, not unreasonably, that they 'blazed a trail for the National Health Service'[193]. Certainly, the EMS hospitals, with their net addition of 12,970 beds to Scotland's hospital accommodation and their much-needed specialist units, were as indispensable at the end of the war as Johnston had anticipated, and demonstrated to both the medical profession and the general public that a State-run hospital service could operate smoothly, with good relations between administration and staff.

Planning for the Future

On 9 October 1941 Ernest Brown, Minister of Health, announced to the House of Commons the outlines of the National Government's proposed post-war hospital policy. He proposed a comprehensive hospital service, organised on a regional basis, which would embrace both statutory and voluntary hospitals and provide treatment for all in need of it. The cost of the new service was to be largely borne by local authorities, although Treasury grants were to be paid in support of this expenditure. Voluntary hospitals, whose future was to be assured, were to be financially assisted by local authorities and also, in return for their educational services, by the Treasury. The principle that patients should make a reasonable contribution towards the cost of treatment, whether through contributory schemes or otherwise, was to be maintained[194].

By 1941 there was general agreement that hospital services should be organised on a regional basis and that the voluntary hospital system could only survive if it was supported by public money. A year earlier, on 23 October 1940, at a meeting of the representatives of voluntary hospitals in all parts of Scotland, discussions were held on how to accelerate the movement towards a co-ordinated regional system of hospital services. Progress towards this goal, leading speakers stressed, was essential. Robert Barclay, chairman of the Scottish branch of the British Hospitals Association, told the representatives 'that after the war it would not be possible for hospitals to return to the status quo ante, either financially or otherwise, and there was every reason why they should now consider what changes should and must be made rather than wait until a new organisation was forced upon them at the dictation of others who were not particularly interested in the continuation of the voluntary system'[195]. A matter of days after this conference took place the *Glasgow Herald*, in an editorial on 'The Post-War Hospital', stated that since the publication of the Cathcart Report four years previously 'the conviction had been growing that... the adequate hospital service necessary to public health can be provided only through the closest possible co-operation between the voluntary and statutory systems'[196]. Although the Scottish voluntary hospitals were generally in much better financial shape than their English counterparts, by the early 1940s it was generally acknowledged by even the most fervent supporters of the voluntary principle that the voluntary hospitals could only hope to maintain their traditional status as first-rate centres of medical practice with assistance from the public purse. While 'the complexities of modern medical treatment alone were imposing upon the voluntary hospitals burdens they could not possibly support indefinitely', the *Glasgow Herald* declared on 10 October 1941, 'the Government's plan seems to give a real chance of preserving the voluntary hospitals and maintaining a good deal of their independence'[197].

In the years following Brown's policy statement, planning for the post-war hospital system went ahead. In January 1942 Sir Hector Hetherington was appointed to chair a committee which was charged with making recommendations on the organisation of the proposed hospital system. The Hetherington Report, published on 13 October 1943, followed the Cathcart Report in recommending the establishment of five advisory Regional Councils, whose areas would be based on Edinburgh, Glasgow, Aberdeen, Dundee, and Inverness. The Regional Councils, which were to be composed of equal numbers of representatives from the local authorities and the voluntary hospitals, were to assess hospital needs in their areas and prepare outline schemes for the region as a whole. They were also to co-ordinate an efficient and adequate ambulance service, arrange for the maintenance of centralised clinical records and statistics, and 'participate' in the appointment of hospital medical staff. Unpaid medical service in the voluntary hospitals, the Report believed, would disappear, and in future, it recommended, hospital doctors should be paid according to a uniform salary scale. The EMS hospitals should be transferred on easy financial terms from the Department of Health to either voluntary bodies or local authorities. The Report's recommendations concerning the financing of the proposed hospital system were Byzantine in their complexity, but the essential point was that government grants would be provided to cover the greater percentage of the cost of hospital services[198].

In the same year as the Hetherington Committee presented its report, a survey of all Scottish hospitals (with the exception of mental hospitals, which were surveyed separately) was begun in each of the five proposed hospital regions. This survey, whose origins can be traced back to Ernest Brown's statement to the House of Commons on 9 October 1941 that a survey of hospital resources would be undertaken as a preliminary to the establishment of a comprehensive hospital service, took three years to complete, and its findings were published in early 1946. The detailed and highly expert surveys advised upon such extensions and modifications to hospitals as would be required to provide a comprehensive service, and recommended how the various hospitals could be fitted into a balanced regional scheme[199]. While, as we shall see, the under-financing of the National Health Service was to result in a failure to implement the more expensive of the surveys' recommendations, the surveys did prove useful to the Regional Hospital Boards which were set up by the National Health Service (Scotland) Act of 1947.

A National Health Service?

In the early years of the war some attention was devoted to the future overall shape of health service policy. Memoranda had been drafted within the Ministry of Health concerning the future expansion of general practitioner services to cover dependants of insured workers[200], while the British Medical Association's Medical Planning Commission, which included representatives of the English Royal Colleges and the Scottish Royal Corporations, had published a draft interim report in May 1942 proposing the establishment of a comprehensive health service providing everyone with all necessary services – general and specialist, domiciliary and institutional[201]. However, as one historian of the period has commented, these schemes 'seem to have about them a certain air of unreality, of the debating of abstract propositions which might – but more probably might not – one day take concrete shape'[202]. What transformed the climate of debate and 'introduced a note not only of realism but also of urgency' was the publication of the Beveridge Report on Social Insurance and Allied Services on 1 December 1942[203]. The Report proposed a single unified social security scheme which would insure against interruption of earning power whether because of sickness, disability, old age, unemployment, or injury. In return for flat-rate contributions benefits would be paid 'guaranteeing the minimum income needed for subsistence'. The whole structure rested on three assumptions, the second of which, the famous Assumption B, stated that a comprehensive health service would be made available to all. The Beveridge Report received a good press in Scotland and appears to have been generally welcomed. In a leading article on Scottish reactions to the Report, the *Glasgow Herald* said that 'if... as seems to be the case, the report has appealed to the imagination of the individual citizen, Parliament and the

Government must take note of the fact"[204]. The *Herald* was not surprised at the reception accorded to the Beveridge Report, explaining that

"Quite apart from the inspiriting tone of a document aiming at establishing 'freedom from want', it has made a deep impression because it is both comprehensive and imaginative. It appeals, for example, to the sense of community which is always fostered in war and which, in the kind of war we are fighting, is at once a necessity and a virtue... We are all in the war together, and we shall all be in the Beveridge plan together too"[205].

The Beveridge Report was the subject of a three-day debate in the House of Commons on 16, 17 and 18 February 1943. Expectation of early action along the lines recommended by Beveridge ran high, but the Government refused to be stampeded into what it regarded as premature legislation. Much, it was stressed, would depend upon the financial position at the end of the war and upon the other claims made on the country's resources. Nevertheless, the National Government was prepared to make a commitment in principle to Beveridge's Assumption B, and welcomed the concept of 'a reorganised and comprehensive health service', which it saw as 'the consummation of a general process which had been going on steadily, if piecemeal, under successive Governments for a great many years.' Sir John Anderson, Lord President of the Council, who sat as a member for the Scottish Universities, declared that 'the object is to secure, through a public, organised and regulated service, that every man, woman and child who wants it can obtain, easily and readily, the whole range of medical advice and attention'. The Government believed that the 'public health must not be many people's business and nobody's responsibility', and, Sir John Anderson continued, 'experience justifies putting this ultimate responsibility in any area on the well-tried local government machinery, working very often over larger areas perhaps and certainly working in consultation and collaboration with voluntary agencies'. He concluded by stating that

"with the war and the chances of post-war reconstruction there is an opportunity to pull together many of the loose strands of the last 20 or 30 years, and build up the whole service on rational lines until it justifies in every sense the word 'comprehensive'... It is an opportunity which must not be missed, and the Government do not intend to let it be missed"[206].

By early 1943, therefore, the National Government had committed itself to setting up a co-ordinated and comprehensive health service, but the details of the service remained to be settled by consultations between government departments, local authorities, voluntary hospitals and the medical profession. The Government preferred, as Anderson's statement to the House of Commons indicated, a service largely based on local authority control, but the British Medical Association made known at a relatively early stage of the consultations its opposition to this idea and its preference for a system of ad hoc authorities and central control. The Government's move towards acceptance of the idea of a primary care system based upon health centres staffed by whole-time salaried general practitioners also encountered strong resistance from a profession which expressed a clear preference for a system which would 'reinforce free choice by being related to work done or patients accepted by the doctor'. Moreover, while the Government was committed to the establishment of a service which was to be available to the whole population without limit of income and which was to be free at the point of delivery, the medical profession or rather its representatives were opposed to a '100 *per cent* service' and to the abolition of sale and purchase of practices[207]. Interestingly, Tom Johnston, Secretary of State for Scotland, was anxious to accommodate the general practitioners, believing that it was more important than anything else to win over the majority of doctors[208]. In urging concessions on the issues of local authority control and payment by salary, he ignored the official policies of his own Labour Party and anticipated the compromises made later by Aneurin Bevan as Minister of Health in the post-war Labour government.

On 17 February 1944 the National Government issued a White Paper entitled *A National Health Service*, which was more of a discussion document than a statement of policy and was intended to stimulate public debate and accelerate progress towards an agreement on the nature of the legislation to follow[209]. Nevertheless, the White Paper indicated how the National Government thought a national health service might be organised. The central organisation of the Scottish health service, it was proposed, should parallel that of its English counterpart. The Secretary of State would be directly responsible to Parliament for the administration of the new service, exercising his functions through the Department of Health for Scotland. He was to be advised by a Scottish Central Health Services Council which was to be composed largely of members of the medical profession, as was the Scottish Central Medical Board which was to be charged with 'the day-to-day administration of the general practitioner service'[210].

The local organisation of the proposed service would of necessity be radically different from that in England and Wales. 'In England and Wales', the White Paper explained

> "it is proposed to define areas of suitable size and resources for the direct administration of the hospital and consultant branches of the service and for the local planning of the service as a whole, and to secure suitable authorities to carry out these tasks by the combination of existing authorities [ie. counties and county boroughs] in the area. To do this in quite the same way in Scotland would usually be out of the ques-

tion since the areas which would have to be defined for the purpose would be so big as to be quite unwieldy and indeed destructive of local government administration"[211].

It was therefore proposed that, unlike England and Wales, there would be a separation between the co-ordination of the Scottish hospital service and the responsibility for its provision. The co-ordination of hospital services would be entrusted, as the Cathcart Report had recommended, to Regional Hospital Advisory Councils in five regions based upon Edinburgh, Glasgow, Aberdeen, Dundee and Inverness, while the responsibility for providing hospital services would be placed upon Joint Hospital Boards to be formed from such combinations of neighbouring counties and large burghs as would be required to supply an adequate service. These Boards, which would take over ownership of and responsibility for the public hospitals in their areas, would be required to consult with local voluntary hospitals in the planning of services. The continued existence of the voluntary hospitals, it was hoped, would be assured by the payment of large grants from central government and the Joint Hospitals Boards[212].

Unlike the new joint authorities to be set up in England and Wales, the Joint Hospitals Boards would not have planning functions outside the hospital service. Responsibility for the administration of the school health service would remain with the education authorities, while the maternity and child health service, including ante-natal clinics, the venereal disease service, the midwifery service and the health visitor service would remain the responsibility of the county councils and town councils of the large burghs. Only those clinic services which were 'nearly allied to the hospital service', most notably tuberculosis dispensaries and cancer clinics, were to be transferred to the new Joint Hospitals Boards[213].

In order that the general practitioner service would be linked up with the other parts of the new service, the White Paper proposed that Local Medical Services Committees covering the same areas as the Joint Hospitals Boards should be set up. These Committees were to be primarily advisory bodies (the general practitioner service, as we have seen, was to be centrally administered by the Scottish Central Medical Board) and were to be composed of representatives of both the local authorities and the medical profession. Moreover, unlike England and Wales, where it was proposed that health centres should be provided by the local authorities, the task of providing, equipping and maintaining health centres was to fall on the Department of Health[214]. However, while the government believed that a totally salaried service was not necessary, practitioners in health centres should be paid by salary, since competition for patients between health centre doctors would be intolerable[215].

The White Paper met with a largely hostile reception from the medical profession. The Council of the British Medical Association complained about an attempt 'to introduce by insidious means a State salaried service', since 'a clear majority' of the profession were 'opposed to the scheme of doctors working in health centres, remunerated by salary'[216]. The British Medical Association's fears were shared by the *Scotsman*, which saw in the White Paper's health centre proposals 'the thin end of the wedge of a State medical service'[217]. Not surprisingly, perhaps, the Secretary of the Glasgow branch of the Socialist Medical Council, Dr Donald G. Munro, took a somewhat different view. At a meeting in a Glasgow cinema on 25 June 1944 he advocated the advantages of health centres to the public. At present there was no real choice of doctor, he suggested, but at a health centre employing perhaps twelve doctors the patient would be able to express a preference. However, health centres which were mere accumulations of consulting rooms were not going to revolutionise our health. The emphasis should be on preventive medicine and the doctor's primary role should be that of a family adviser on health[218]. Similar criticisms of the lack of interest shown in preventive work were made by Lord Dawson of Penn and by Dr R.W. Craig, Scottish Secretary of the British Medical Association. The White Paper, Lord Dawson stated, was incorrectly described, for 'it is concerned with a sickness service and not a health service'. The 'gap between preventive and curative medicine', he added, 'remained wide open'[219].

Consultations between the Government and the representatives of the medical profession led to many important concessions by the Government. The price which the National Government was willing to pay for agreement with the profession included not only the abandonment of important elements of the scheme, such as controls on the distribution of doctors (which the White Paper had recommended should be exercised by the Central Medical Board and which the British Medical Association anathematised as an unacceptable attack upon professional freedom) and the rapid development of health centres, but also the creation of a planning and administrative system of almost unworkable complexity designed to allay medical fears of local authority control over the profession[220]. In the event, however, this revised scheme did not survive the election of a Labour government in July 1945.

The legislative measures introduced into Parliament by Aneurin Bevan, the new Minister of Health, in March 1946, and by Joseph Westwood, the new Secretary of State for Scotland, in December of the same year, were significantly different from those proposed earlier by the National Government. The English and Scottish Bills sought to nationalise all hospitals and to strip local authorities of those medical services, such as maternity and child welfare, which they had built up over the previous fifty or so years. The Bills also sought to re-emphasise the importance of the rapid development of health centres, reassert central control over the distribution of doctors, and introduce a salaried element in the remuneration of all general practitioners.

The National Health Service (Scotland) Bill had certain distinctive features. The Scottish teaching hospitals played such a large and important part in the services of their regions that the hospital service would have been quite incomplete without them. Consequently, unlike England, the Scottish teaching hospitals were included within the administrative structure of the hospital service, being administered by Boards of Management under the Regional Hospital Boards. While responsibility for the provision of health centres in England was to be in the hands of the local authorities, in Scotland that responsibility was to be vested in the Secretary of State. The Secretary of State was also to be responsible for the ambulance services which were to be organised nationally as a Scottish Ambulance Service.

The Scottish Bill received a generally warm welcome. The *Scotsman*, which, as a conservative newspaper, might have been expected to oppose the measure root and branch, welcomed the Scottish Bill as a distinct improvement on the corresponding English Bill. 'Though the main principles are similar', the *Scotsman* stated, 'the modifications suggest that the Scottish Bill has benefited from the criticisms made of the English measure, for the changes are, on the whole, in the right direction'. What particularly pleased the editorial writers was that 'some concessions' had been made in avoiding excessive centralisation and maintaining local independence in hospital administration, and that hospital endowments were not to be 'confiscated' but reallocated by an Endowments Commission in accordance with the spirit of the intention of the founder. The inclusion of the teaching hospitals within the general scheme was welcomed as a necessary step, and the *Scotsman* declared, perhaps grudgingly, that 'in its modified form the scheme will work better in Scotland than in England, at least as far as hospitals are concerned'[221]. A similar line was taken by the Scottish Branch of the British Hospitals Association. Addressing the annual meeting of the Association in London on 29 November 1946, Lt. Col. James Dundas, Secretary of the Scottish Branch of the British Hospitals Association, said that the Scottish Bill was 'better than we had expected'. Every effort would be made to secure an amendment giving the teaching hospitals more freedom in their internal administration, but, he added, once the Bill became law 'we shall ... give all the help we can to make it work'[222].

Much of the criticism of the Scottish Bill was focused on the administrative machinery proposed for the new service. The *Scotsman* and the *Glasgow Herald*, Conservative politicians, the British Medical Association in Scotland, local authorities, and even some independently minded Labour MPs criticised what they considered to be an excessively centralised system of management. The *Scotsman* considered that 'the danger of too much centralisation in St Andrews' House, with remote control by the Treasury which provides much of the cost, is latent in the scheme'[223]. while the *Glasgow Herald* declared that 'there can be little doubt... that the Scottish Bill, like the corresponding English Act, confers far too much power upon the Minister'[224]. The Glasgow Branch of the British Medical Association criticised 'the dictatorial powers' assumed by the Secretary of State for Scotland under the Bill, whereby he would nominate the members of all committees with the exception of a minority of local executive councils[225], while Mr Andrew Eunson, Honorary Secretary of the Board of Management of Edinburgh Royal Infirmary, suggested that the Scottish Bill showed 'a surprising distrust of the people and of popular representation'. No one, he added, was to be elected to the new Boards, all were to be appointed. It was, he concluded, hospital management by the officially approved[226]. The same theme was taken up by many Parliamentarians when the Bill received its second reading in the House of Commons on 10 December 1946. Conservative MPs argued that the Bill placed far too much power in the hands of the Secretary of State for Scotland. James Reid, Conservative MP for Hillhead, expressed the view that, while the Government must take a hand in the general planning of the services, they ought to keep out of the practical business of running the service and not pretend that they intended to have a universal grip on the services if, in fact, they did not intend to exercise it[227]. Walter Elliot, Conservative member for the Scottish Universities, said that the taking over of local authority hospitals constituted a 'serious inroad' into the responsibilities of local government, and went on to complain that the tendency was to remove all authority from the local authorities and vest it in boards and bodies wholly under the control of the Minister[228]. More interestingly, perhaps, the same complaint was voiced by James Carmichael, ILP member for Bridgeton, who stated that 'there was a danger of [the administration] encroaching unduly on democratic machinery', and argued that the diminution of the role of the local authorities, as envisaged by the Bill, was unwarranted by past experience[229].

Criticism by Scottish Medical Officers of Health and local authorities of the dismantling of local authority medical services was strangely muted. Dr W.G. Clark, Medical Officer of Health for Edinburgh, was one of the few who publicly expressed his misgivings about the Bill, saying that 'the Bill may be a progressive one in certain directions, but I think that it is going back in other directions, and it may be that experience will show the mistake and it will have to be remedied'. Clark's cryptic comments can only be understood within the context of what he went on to say. 'It is obvious', he added,

> "that the Bill is going to change the whole function of public health as we understand it. The system that has been built up by the Local Authorities and Medical Officers, with the help of the Government, will now cease to exist... The responsibility for infectious diseases, which has been the Local Authorities' function from the earliest days, has been taken from them. The tuberculosis service, with its clinics and hos-

pitals, has been taken away, the maternity and child welfare schemes have been taken also. Ante-natal clinics are going over to the new service, and the Local Authority is, roughly, left with the environmental care of the people"[230].

The local authorities were, if anything, more subdued in their public criticism of the Bill. The only evidence of such criticism to come to light is of a protest registered by the Fife County Finance Committee at its meeting on 10 December 1946 against the 'steam-rollering through Parliament of the second reading of the National Health Service (Scotland) Bill without giving Local Authorities the opportunity of expressing their opinion'[231]. It seems likely that the lack of opposition to the dismantling of the local authority medical services owed something to a realisation that opposition was useless. The English and Welsh Bill, with its similar provisions, had already become law, and, while there was undoubtedly room for amendments to the Scottish Bill, it was inconceivable that there could be any departure from one of the fundamental principles of Bevan's scheme.

The irony of course was that Bevan's scheme represented a volte-face on long established Labour Party policy on the future development of the health services. To some observers this about-face appeared both astonishing and reprehensible. Professor J.M. Mackintosh, for example, regarded Bevan's National Health Service as 'a frontal attack on... the basic principles of democracy', and quoted approvingly one writer on modern British government who referred to 'the spectacle of a Party which, in its missionary days, had preached an expanded municipalism as one of its major objectives, becoming an instrument for the greatest curtailment of local government functions which has taken place for 150 years'[232].

Why then did the Labour Government abandon its long-held commitment to a locally controlled national health service (a commitment which had been reaffirmed as late as April 1943 in a document entitled *National Service for Health: the Labour Party's Post-War Policy*)?[233] The answer, it seems clear, is to be found in the Government's perception of the political realities of the period. The fierce opposition of the medical profession to any form of administrative control by local government, and to any version of salaried general practice, persuaded Bevan and his colleagues that the old commitment to a municipally based and salaried service had to be jettisoned. Political expediency likewise dictated that the blow to local authorities occasioned by the loss of their medical services should be softened by permitting them to retain control over a number of community and environmental services, and that the general practitioners' strong preference for a separate administrative structure for their service should be respected. The consequence was that the tripartite structure of health services, 'so long and so heavily criticised', was retained. Had the Labour government felt able to 'take on' the doctors in 1946, 'the integration of services sought in 1974 would have existed from the outset, and there would have been participation in their administration by elected representatives of the community'[234].

The British Medical Association, which led the profession's campaign against the Act, concentrated its attack on the proposed terms and conditions of service for general practitioners, voicing opposition to the payment of a basic salary, to the ending of the sale and purchase of practices, and to any controls over the distribution of doctors. When, following a plebiscite of the profession in January 1947, it became clear that the Association's hostility was shared by a huge majority of doctors, the Government entered into serious negotiations with the profession's various representative bodies. Attempts to allay the fear that the Act would lead to the introduction of a full-time salaried State medical service proved fruitless, and in February 1948 another plebiscite of the profession confirmed that a large majority of doctors were still opposed to entering the new service. The Government now realised that, if the service was to commence on 5 July 1948 as planned, concessions would have to be made to the doctors. Acting on the suggestion of the Royal College of Physicians of London, Aneurin Bevan pledged, in the House of Commons on 7 April 1948, that amending legislation would be brought forward to prevent the introduction by regulation of a whole-time salaried service. As for the proposed basic salary of £300, Bevan now suggested that it should be available to new entrants for three years, after which each general practitioner would be permitted to go over to remuneration by capitation fee[235]. Bevan's concessions had a marked effect upon opinion within the medical profession. Whereas the plebiscite in February 1948 had shown only 9 *per cent* of the respondents in favour of the Act and 75 *per cent* against it, the results of May 1948 plebiscite revealed that 28 *per cent* were now in favour and 49 *per cent* were against. Moreover, a not insignificant minority of doctors failed to register any view on the Act and could therefore not be counted on to support any British Medical Association sponsored boycott of the service[236]. The British Medical Association accepted that, in Dr Guy Dain's words, 'The fight is over'[237], and advised the profession to co-operate in working the new Act. On 5 July 1948 the National Health Service came into existence.

References

(1)	*Report of the Royal Commission on Physical Training (Scotland)*. Cd.1507. (Edinburgh, 1903), p.7

(2)	Mackenzie, W.L. *First Report on the Medical Inspection of School Children in Scotland, by W. Leslie Mackenzie, M.A., M.D., LL.D., Medical Member of the Local Government Board for Scotland*. (London, H.M.S.O., 1913), p.3

(3)	*Report of the Royal Commission on Physical Training (Scotland)*. Cd.1507. (Edinburgh, 1903), pp.28–33.

(4)	*The Glasgow Herald*, Wednesday, 18 March 1903, p.8, col.E.

(5)   *The Scotsman*, Friday, 20 March 1903, p.4, cols.D&E.

(6)   *The Scotsman*, Saturday, 21 March 1903, p.10, col.H.

(7)   Mackenzie, W.L., and Matthew, E. *The Medical Inspection of School Children: A Text Book for Medical Officers of Schools, Medical Officers of Health, School Managers and Teachers.* (Edinburgh and Glasgow, 1904), p.1.

(8)   *The Scotsman*, Saturday, 21 March 1903, p.10, col.H.

(9)   *The Scotsman*, Monday, 1 August 1904, p.6, cols.D&E.

(10)   *The Dundee Advertiser*, Friday, 29 July 1904, p.4, col.C.

(11)   Knox W., Ed. *Scottish Labour Leaders 1918–1939. A Biographical Dictionary.* (Edinburgh, 1984), pp.22–26.

(12)   *The Glasgow Herald*, Tuesday, 17 July 1906, p.6, col.C.

(13)   *The Dundee Advertiser*, Tuesday, 17 July 1906, p.6, col.D.

(14)   *The Glasgow Herald*, Saturday, 24 November 1906, p.6, col.E.

(15)   *The Glasgow Herald*, Friday, 7 December 1906, p.8, cols.E&F.

(16)   The Parliamentary Debates. Fourth Series. Volume 167, cols.1662–1670.

(17)   *Ibid*, cols.1865–1881.

(18)   *The Glasgow Herald*, Tuesday, 19 March 1907, p.6, col.G.

(19)   *The Glasgow Herald*, Saturday, 20 April 1907, p.10, cols.G&H.

(20)   *The Glasgow Herald*, Tuesday, 21 April 1908, p.10, col.G.

(21)   *The Caledonian Medical Journal*, Volume 8, No.4, April 1910, p.141.

(22)   *The Glasgow Herald*, Monday, 20 September 1909, p.8, col.D.

(23)   Department of Health for Scotland. *Committee on Scottish Health Services Report.* Cmd.5204. (Edinburgh, 1936), p.19.

(24)   Quoted in Mackintosh, J.M. *Trends of Opinion about the Public Health 1901–1951.* (Oxford, 1953), pp.121–122.

(25)   *Royal Commission on the Poor Laws and Relief of Distress. Report on Scotland.* Cd.4922. (London, 1909), p.232.

(26)   On 28 January 1907 Beatrice Webb wrote in her diary that 'the ways of the Commission are past explanation. They appoint an investigator to look after and couteract me and my machinations to transfer medical relief to the Public Health authority, and they appoint an M.O.H.! I should not have dared to suggest it . . . and a Scotchman too, naturally biased in favour of domiciliary treatment'. Drake, B., & Cole, M.L., Editors. *Our Partnership by Beatrice Webb.* (London, 1948), p.370.

(27)   *Royal Commission on the Poor Laws and Relief of Distress.* Appendix Vol.XIV. *Report to the Royal Commission on the Poor Laws and Relief of Distress on Poor Law Medical Relief in certain Unions in England and Wales. By John C. McVail, M.D., LL.D., D.P.H.Camb.* Cd.4573. (London, 1909), p.148.

(28)   *Royal Commission on the Poor Laws and Relief of Distress. Report on Scotland.* Cd.4922. (London, 1909), pp.58–59, 71, 161–163.

(29)   *Ibid*, p.272.

(30)   Webb, S. and B. *The State and the Doctor.* (London, 1910), p.203.

(31)   *Royal Commission on the Poor Laws and Relief of Distress. Report on Scotland.* Cd.4922. (London, 1909), pp.262–263.

(32)   *Ibid*, p.262.

(33)   *The Glasgow Herald*, Tuesday, 2 November 1909, p.6, col.D.

(34)   *The Scotsman*, Tuesday, 2 November 1909, p.6, col.C.

(35)   *The Dundee Advertiser*, Wednesday, 3 November 1909, p.2, cols.A&B.

(36)   *The Glasgow Herald*, Saturday, 18 December 1909, p.13, col.B.

(37)   *The Scotsman*, Friday, 2 April 1909, p.6, col.D.

(38)   *The Glasgow Herald*, Thursday, 1 April 1909, p.6, col.F.

(39)   *Ibid*.

(40)   *The Scotsman*, Saturday, 13 November 1909, p.8, col.B.

(41)   Webb, S. and B. *The State and the Doctor.* (London, 1910), pp.136–38.

(42)   Braithwaite, W.J., *Lloyd George's Ambulance Wagon, Being the Memoirs of William J. Braithwaite 1911–1912. Edited, with an Introduction, by Sir Henry N. Brunbury, K.C.B. and*

with a commentary by Richard Titmuss. (London, 1957), p.22.

(43) National Insurance Act, 1911. 1&2 Geo.5.Ch.55. Part 1.

(44) *The Dundee Advertiser*, Saturday, 6 May 1911, p.6, col.B.

(45) *The Glasgow Herald*, Saturday, 6 May 1911, p.7, col.G.

(46) *The Scotsman*, Friday, 5 May 1911, p.6, cols.A&B.

(47) *The Glasgow Herald*, Wednesday, 6 December 1911, p.8, col.F.

(48) *The Glasgow Herald*, Saturday, 16 December 1911, p.6, col.E.

(49) *The Glasgow Herald*, Friday, 22 December 1911, p.6, col.E.

(50) *The Glasgow Herald*, Saturday, 26 October 1912, p.7, cols.C&D.

(51) *The Scotsman*, Thursday, 11 May 1911, p.6, col.C.

(52) *The Glasgow Herald*, Monday, 22 May 1911, p.9, col.I.

(53) *The Glasgow Herald*, Tuesday, 12 December 1911, p.11, col.H.

(54) *The Glasgow Herald*, Wednesday, 13 December 1911, p.8, col.F.

(55) *The Glasgow Herald*, Wednesday, 13 December 1911, p.13, col.B.

(56) *The Glasgow Herald*, Wednesday, 13 December 1911, p.8, col.F.

(57) Webb, S. and B. *The State and the Doctor*, (London, 1910), pp.149–50.

(58) Quoted in Mackintosh, J.M., *Trends of Opinion about the Public Health 1901–1951.* (Oxford, 1953), pp.90–91.

(59) Craig, W.S., *History of the Royal College of Physicians of Edinburgh.* (Oxford, London, Edinburgh, and Melbourne, 1976), pp.194–95.

(60) *Report of the Highlands and Islands Medical Service Committee to the Lords Commissioners of His Majesty's Treasury.* Cd.6559. (London, 1912), p.6.

(61) *The Scotsman*, Thursday, 11 November 1909, p.6, cols.B&C.

(62) *Report of the Highlands and Islands Medical Service Committee to the Lords Commissioners of His Majesty's Treasury.* Cd.6559. (London, 1912), pp.40–42.

(63) *The Scotsman*, Tuesday, 7 January 1913, p.6, col.B.

(64) *The Glasgow Herald*, Tuesday, 7 January 1913, p.6, col.E.

(65) *The Dundee Advertiser*, Tuesday, 7 January 1913, p.6, col.D.

(66) *The Scotsman*, Tuesday, 7 January 1913, p.6, col.B.

(67) Hamilton, D. *The Healers. A History of Medicine in Scotland.* (Edinburgh, 1981), pp.249–252.

(68) Ministry of Health. Department of Health for Scotland. *A National Health Service.* Cmd.6502. (London, 1944), p.72.

(69) *The Glasgow Herald*, Thursday, 27 February 1913, p.10, col.G. *The Glasgow Herald*, Saturday, 29 March 1913, p.8, col.F. *The Glasgow Herald*, Monday, 17 November 1913, p.9, col.B.

(70) Education (Scotland) Act, 1913. 3&4. Geo.5. Ch.12. See also *The Glasgow Herald*, Monday, 17 November 1913, p.9, col.B, for the reply from the Scottish Education Department to Dr William Chapple, the Liberal MP for Stirlingshire, who had written to the Department concerning the nature of the grant to be paid to local authorities in respect of medical treatment of school children in Scotland.

(71) *The Glasgow Herald*, Monday, 24 June 1918, p.4, col.G.

(72) *Ibid.*

(73) *Ibid.* See also Mackenzie, W.L. *Scottish Mothers and Children. Being a report on the physical welfare of mothers and children in Scotland.* The Carnegie United Kingdom Trust. (Dunfermline, 1917), p.537.

(74) Whyte, Sir W.E. *Local Government in Scotland. With complete statutory references.* 2nd Edition (Glasgow and Edinburgh, 1936), pp.395–97.

(75) *The Scotsman*, Wednesday, 31 July 1918, p.4, col.G.

(76) *Venereal Diseases. Circulars issued by the Local Government Board for Scotland on 31 October 1916 to (1) Local Authorities, (2) Parish Councils, and (3) Governing Bodies of Hospitals; The Public Health (Venereal Diseases) Regulations made by the Local Government Board for Scotland on 26 October 1916; and Memorandum on Schemes for the Diagnosis, Treatment and Prevention of Venereal Diseases.* (Edinburgh, 1916).

(77) *The Scotsman*, Monday, 25 February 1929, p.10, col.B.

(78) *Report of the Royal Commission on the Housing of the Industrial Population of Scotland Rural and Urban.* Cd.8731. (Edinburgh, 1917), p.346.

(79) Mitchison, R. *A History of Scotland.* (London, 1970), p.402. Harvie, C. *No Gods and Precious Few Heroes. Scotland 1914–1980.* (London, 1981), p.70.

(80) Harvie, C. *op. cit.,* p.71.

(81) Whyte, Sir W.E. *op. cit.,* p.435.

(82) Cramond, R.D. *Housing Policy in Scotland 1919–1964. A Study in State Assistance.* (Edinburgh, 1966), p.26.

(83) Harvie, C. *op. cit.,* p.70.

(84) *Parliamentary Debates: Official Report.* Fifth Series. Volume 314, col.1905.

(85) *The Dundee Advertiser,* Friday, 2 August 1918, p.6, col.C.

(86) *Ibid.*

(87) *The Scotsman,* Thursday, 18 July 1918, p.4, col.A.

(88) *The Scotsman,* Wednesday, 17 July 1918, p.4, col.F., and *The Scotsman,* Tuesday, 1 April 1919, p.7, col.C.

(89) *The Parliamentary Debates: Official Report.* Fifth Series. Volume 114, col.1147.

(90) *Ibid,* cols.1150–1151.

(91) *Ibid,* col.1158.

(92) *Ibid,* col.1142.

(93) *Ibid,* col.1140.

(94) *Second Annual Report of the Scottish Board of Health 1920.* Cmd.1319. (Edinburgh, 1921), p.17.

(95) Scottish Board of Health. *Reports by Consultative Councils on a Reformed Local Authority for Health and Public Assistance* (Edinburgh, 1923). Part I. Report by the Consultative Council on Local Health Administration and General Health Questions, pp.5–16.

(96) Scottish Board of Health. Consultative Council on Medical and Allied Services. *Interim Report. A Scheme of Medical Service for Scotland.* Cmd.1039. (Edinburgh, 1920), p.6.

(97) *Ibid,* pp.6–7.

(98) *Ibid,* pp.11–12.

(99) *Ibid,* pp.19–21.

(100) *The Scotsman,* Saturday, 4 December 1920, p.8, cols.B&C.

(101) *Report of the Royal Commission on National Health Insurance.* Cmd.2596. (London, 1926), pp.72–73, 119–24.

(102) *Ibid,* p.30.

(103) *Ibid,* p.327.

(104) *Ibid,* pp.327–28.

(105) Scottish Board of Health. Hospital Services (Scotland) Committee. *Report on the Hospital Services of Scotland.* (Edinburgh, 1926), p.17.

(106) *Ibid,* p.11.

(107) *Ibid,* p.7.

(108) *Ibid,* pp.33–43.

(109) *Ibid,* p.45.

(110) *Ibid,* p.10. *The Hospitals Year Book 1941. An Annual Record of the Hospitals of Great Britain and Ireland incorporating Burdett's Hospitals and Charities.* Central Bureau of Hospital Information. (London, 1941), pp.177–85. The figure of 10,398 beds represents the pre-war establishment, while the total number of beds (11,170) recorded on page 27 includes emergency beds.

(111) Ministry of Health. Department of Health for Scotland. *A National Health Service.* Cmd.6502. (London, 1944), p.68.

(112) Scottish Board of Health. Hospital Services (Scotland) Committee. *Report on the Hospital Services of Scotland.* (Edinburgh, 1926), p.8.

(113) *Ibid,* pp.20, 27, 30.

(114) *The Glasgow Herald,* Monday, 8 February 1926, p.10, col.B.

(115) Scottish Board of Health. Hospital Services (Scotland) Committee. *Report on the*

Hospital Services of Scotland. (Edinburgh, 1926), p.21.

(116) *Ibid*, pp.24–26.

(117) *Ibid*, pp.7–8.

(118) *Ibid*, p.33.

(119) Department of Health for Scotland. *Committee on Scottish Health Services Report.* Cmd.5204. (Edinburgh, 1936), Appendix IV, p.399.

(120) *The Glasgow Herald*, Thursday, 10 June 1937, p.10, col.C.

(121) Department of Health for Scotland. *Committee on Scottish Health Services Report.* Cmd.5204. (Edinburgh, 1936), p.325.

(122) *Ibid*, p.170. Ministry of Health. Department of Health for Scotland. *A National Health Service.* Cmd.6502. (London, 1944), p.71.

(123) Department of Health for Scotland. *Committee on Scottish Health Services Report.* Cmd.5204. (Edinburgh, 1936), pp.211–12.

(124) *Report of the Royal Commission on National Health Insurance.* Cmd.2596. (London, 1926), p.30.

(125) Pater, J.E. *The Making of the National Health Service.* (London, 1981). pp.18–19.

(126) Quoted in Mackintosh, J.M. *Trends of Opinion about the Public Health 1901–1951.* (Oxford, 1953), p.116.

(127) Whyte, Sir W.E. *Local Government in Scotland. With complete statutory references.* 2nd Edition. (Glasgow & Edinburgh, 1936), p.19.

(128) *Ibid*, pp.19–22.

(129) *Parliamentary Debates: Official Report*, Fifth Series. Volume 225, col.1401.

(130) *Ibid*, cols.1397–1403.

(131) *Ibid*, cols.1414–1429.

(132) *Ibid*, cols.1405–1407.

(133) *Ibid*, col.1436.

(134) Department of Health for Scotland. *Committee on Scottish Health Services Report.* Cmd.5204. (Edinburgh, 1936), p.162.

(135) *Ibid*, p.161.

(136) *Ibid*, p.238.

(137) *Ibid*, pp.234–35.

(138) *The Glasgow Herald*, Saturday, 7 August 1926, p.6, col.C.

(139) Department of Health for Scotland. *Committee on Scottish Health Services Report.* Cmd.5204. (Edinburgh, 1936), pp.403–04.

(140) Personal communication from the Archivist to Grampian Health Board.

(141) Department of Health for Scotland. *Committee on Scottish Health Services Report.* Cmd.5204. (Edinburgh, 1936), Appendix VI, p.404.

(142) *The Scotsman*, Monday, 30 September 1929, p.10, col.A.

(143) *Ibid.*

(144) *Second Annual Report of the Department of Health for Scotland 1930:* Cmd.3860. (Edinburgh, 1931), pp.127–31. Department of Health for Scotland. *Reports on Incapacitating Sickness in the Insured Population of Scotland, 1931–1937.* (Edinburgh, 1932–1939). The 1936–1937 figures are taken from the *Seventh Report on Incapacitating Sickness in the Insured Population of Scotland 1 July 1936 to 30 June 1937.* (Edinburgh, 1939), pp.5, 8, 59.

(145) *The Glasgow Herald*, Monday, 6 April 1936, p.10, col.B.

(146) Department of Health for Scotland. *Committee on Scottish Health Services Report.* Cmd.5204. (Edinburgh, 1936), p.9.

(147) *The Glasgow Herald*, Thursday, 2 July 1936, p.10, col.B.

(148) Department of Health for Scotland. *Committee on Scottish Health Services Report.* Cmd.5204. (Edinburgh, 1936), pp.150–56.

(149) *Ibid*, pp.156–63.

(150) *Ibid*, p.214.

(151) *Ibid*, pp.219–21.

(152) Department of Health for Scotland. Consultative Council on Medical and Allied Services. *Report on Hospital Services.* (Edinburgh, 1933).

(153) Department of Health for Scotland. *Committee on Scottish Health Services Report.* Cmd.5204. (Edinburgh, 1936), p.236.
(154) *Ibid*, pp.241–42.
(155) *Ibid*, p.241.
(156) *Ibid*, p.247.
(157) *Ibid*, pp.247, 287–88.
(158) *The Glasgow Herald*, Thursday, 2 July 1936, p.10, col.C.
(159) *The Scotsman*, Thursday, 2 July 1936, p.10, cols.B&C.
(160) *Parliamentary Debates: Official Report.* Fifth Series. Volume 314, cols.1897–1904.
(161) *Ibid*, cols.1981–1983.
(162) *The Glasgow Herald*, Saturday, 6 April 1929, p.8, col.C.
(163) Department of Health for Scotland. Scientific Advisory Committee: Clinical Sub-Committee. *Report on Maternal Morbidity and Mortality in Scotland by Charlotte A. Douglas, M.D., D.P.H., M.C.O.G., and Peter L. McKinley, M.D., D.P.H.* (Edinburgh, 1935), p.27.
(164) *Ibid*, p.25.
(165) *Parliamentary Debates: Official Report.* Fifth Series. Volume 315, col.1101.
(166) Maternity Services (Scotland) Act, 1937. 1 Edw.8. & 1 Geo.6. Ch.30.
(167) *Summary Report by the Department of Health for Scotland for the year ended 30 June 1945.* Cmd.6661. (Edinburgh, 1945), p.5.
(168) Macnalty, Sir A.S., Ed. *History of the Second World War. United Kingdom Medical Series. The Civilian Health and Medical Services.* Volume II. (London, 1955), p.236.
(169) *Ibid*, p.237.
(170) *Ibid*, pp.322–23.
(171) *Ibid*, p.252.
(172) *Ibid*, p.258.
(173) *Ibid*, pp.262–63.
(174) *Ibid*, pp.238, 264–65.
(175) *Summary Report by the Department of Health for Scotland for the year ended 30 June 1945.* Cmd.6661. (Edinburgh, 1945), pp.8–9.
(176) Macnalty, Sir A.S., Ed. *op. cit.*, pp.266–69.
(177) *Ibid*, p.234.
(178) *Ibid*, p.275.
(179) *Ibid*, p.278.
(180) *Ibid*, p.307.
(181) Titmuss, R.M. *Problems of Social Policy. History of the Second World War. United Kingdom Civil Series.* Hancock, W.K., Ed. (London, 1950), p.521.
(182) Macnalty, Sir A.S., Ed. *op. cit.*, pp.278–81.
(183) *Ibid*, p.274.
(184) Dunn, C.L., Ed. *History of the Second World War. United Kingdom Medical Series. The Emergency Medical Services.* Volume II (London, 1953), p.25.
(185) *Ibid*, p.25.
(186) Department of Health for Scotland. *Committee on Scottish Health Services Report.* Cmd.5204. (Edinburgh, 1936), p.234.
(187) Dunn, C.L., Ed. *op. cit.*, p.29.
(188) *Ibid*, pp.63–71.
(189) Johnston, T. *Memories.* (London, 1952), p.152.
(190) *Summary Report by the Department of Health for Scotland for the year ended 30 June 1945.* Cmd.6661. (Edinburgh, 1945), p.15.
(191) Ministry of Health. Department of Health for Scotland. *A National Health Service.* Cmd.6502. (London, 1944), p.69.
(192) Macnalty, Sir A.S., Ed. *History of the Second World War. United Kingdom Medical Series. The Civilian Health and Medical Services.* Volume II. (London, 1955), pp.288–91.
(193) Johnston, T. *op. cit.*, p.153.
(194) *Parliamentary Debates.* Fifth Series. Voume 374, cols.1116–1118.

(195) *The Scotsman*, Thursday, 24 October 1940, p.3, cols.F&G.
(196) *The Glasgow Herald*, Friday, 25 October 1940, p.4, col.B.
(197) *The Glasgow Herald*, Friday, 10 October 1941, p.4, col.B.
(198) Department of Health for Scotland. *Report of the Committee on Post-War Hospital Problems in Scotland.* Cmd.6472. (Edinburgh, 1943), pp.35–38.
(199) Macnalty, Sir A.S. Ed, *op. cit.*, p.323. Ross, J.S. *The National Health Service in Great Britain. An historical and descriptive study.* (Oxford, 1952), p.334.
(200) Pater, J.E. *The Making of the National Health Service.* (London, 1981), pp.36–38.
(201) *Ibid*, pp.38–39.
(202) *Ibid*, p.43.
(203) *Ibid*, p.43.
(204) *The Glasgow Herald*, Saturday, 5 December 1942, p.2, col.A.
(205) *Ibid*, p.2, cols.A&B.
(206) *Parliamentary Debates.* Fifth Series. Volume 386, cols.1661–1664.
(207) Pater, J.E. *op. cit.*, pp.62–67.
(208) Honigsbaum, F. *The Division in British Medicine. A history of the separation of general practice from hospital care 1911–1968.* (London, 1979), pp.197–98, 289.
(209) Pater, J.E. *op. cit.*, p.77.
(210) Ministry of Health. Department of Health for Scotland. *A National Health Service.* Cmd.6502. (London, 1944), p.42.
(211) *Ibid*, p.43.
(212) *Ibid*, pp.43–44, 46.
(213) *Ibid*, p.44.
(214) *Ibid*, p.45.
(215) *Ibid*, pp.31–32.
(216) *The Glasgow Herald*, Friday, 12 May 1944, p.6, col.C.
(217) *The Scotsman*, Friday, 18 February 1944, p.4, col.A.
(218) *The Glasgow Herald*, Monday 26 June 1944, p.2, col.D.
(219) *The Glasgow Herald*, Friday, 12 May 1944, p.6, col.D. For Craig's comments see *The Scotsman*, Friday, 18 February 1944, p.5, col.C.
(220) Pater, J.E. *The Making of the National Health Service.* (London, 1981), p.104.
(221) *The Scotsman*, Thursday, 7 November 1946, p.4, col.A.
(222) *The Scotsman*, Saturday, 30 November 1946, p.3, col.F.
(223) *The Scotsman*, Thursday, 7 November 1946, p.4, col.B.
(224) *The Glasgow Herald*, Wednesday, 11 December 1946, p.4, col.A.
(225) *The Scotsman*, Tuesday, 3 December 1946, p.4, col.E.
(226) *The Scotsman*, Monday, 18 November 1946, p.3, col.A.
(227) *Parliamentary Debates.* Fifth Series. Volume 431, col.1017.
(228) *Ibid*, col.1042.
(229) *Ibid*, cols.1055–1059.
(230) *The Scotsman*, Thursday, 7 November 1946, p.5, col.G.
(231) *The Scotsman*, Wednesday, 11 December 1946, p.4, col.G.
(232) Mackintosh, J.M. *Trends of Opinion about the Public Health 1901–1951.* (Oxford, 1953), pp.165–67.
(233) Pater, J.E. *The Making of the National Health Service.* (London, 1981), p.106.
(234) *Ibid*, p.184.
(235) *Parliamentary Debates.* Fifth Series. Volume 449, cols.164–166.
(236) *The Glasgow Herald*, Thursday, 6 May 1948, p.5, cols.A&B.
(237) *The Glasgow Herald*, Friday, 18 June 1948, p.5, cols.E&F.

3. *The National Health Service in Scotland: 1948–1984*

CONTENTS

THE SERVICE SINCE 1974

CONCLUSION

The National Health Service in Scotland: 1948–1984

THE NHS (SCOTLAND) ACT 1947

The organisation of the new service

At the centre of the new health service was the Secretary of State for Scotland who was charged with promoting 'the establishment in Scotland of a comprehensive health service designed to secure improvement in the physical and mental health of the people of Scotland and the prevention, diagnosis and treatment of illness'[1]. He was advised by the Scottish Health Services Council, the members of which were appointed by himself and comprised representatives of the medical, dental, and nursing professions, pharmacists, and persons with experience in hospital management and local government. The Council had a wide remit, for the Act laid down that 'it shall be the duty of that Council to advise the Secretary of State upon such general matters relating to the services ... as the Council think fit and upon any questions referred to them by him relating to those services'[2]. Advice on more specialised matters could be sought from standing advisory councils, which were composed partly of members of the Health Services Council and partly of persons appointed directly by the Secretary of State.

As we have seen, the National Health Service (Scotland) Act provided for the separate administration of hospital, general medical, and local health authority services. There were five hospital regions based on Edinburgh, Glasgow, Aberdeen, Dundee, and Inverness. Each region was administered by a Regional Hospital Board, whose members were appointed by the Secretary of State for Scotland after consultation with the relevant university, the local health authorities, and those organisations deemed representative of the former voluntary hospitals and the medical profession[3]. Medical Education Committees, 'not less than one third' of whose members were 'appointed by any university with which the provision of hospital and specialist services in the area is associated', advised the Boards on the administration of the service in so far as it related 'to the provision of facilities for undergraduate or post graduate clinical teaching or for research'[4]. Every Regional Hospital

Board was required to submit to the Secretary of State for Scotland a scheme for the appointment of Boards of Management which were to be established 'for the purpose of exercising functions with respect to the control and management of individual hospitals or groups of hospitals . . . and providing hospital and specialist services in the area'[5]. Before submitting such a scheme the Regional Hospital Board was required to 'consult any university with which the provision of hospital and specialist services in the area of the Board is or is to be associated'. Boards of Management were only to be appointed by the Regional Hospital Board after consultations with local health authorities, executive councils, and senior medical and dental staff employed at the hospital or group of hospitals[6]. In the case of teaching hospitals up to 40 *per cent* of the membership of the Board of Management was directly nominated by the teaching staff and the University. 84 Boards of Management were created to administer approximately 425 hospitals with accommodation for over 60,000 patients. The average board had a membership of between fifteen and twenty, which included doctors, representatives of local health authorities, persons with experience in the management of the former voluntary hospitals, and others with relevant knowledge.

The responsibility for providing maternity (excluding hospitals) and child welfare, midwifery, health visiting, and home nursing services was placed in the hands of the local health authorities, which for the purposes of the Act were the twenty four large burghs and the thirty one counties or groups of counties already recognised under the Local Government Act of 1929. Co-operation between local health authorities in the planning and provision of their services was encouraged by the Act which laid down that 'two or more local health authorities may, with the consent of the Secretary of State, combine for the purposes of all or any of their functions on such terms and conditions as may be agreed between them and approved by the Secretary of State'[7]. The Act also empowered the Secretary of State to order two or more local health authorities to combine if he believed the combination to be 'in the interests of the efficiency of any services provided' by them[8].

General practitioners retained their status as independent contractors under the National Health Service, but general medical services were administered by bodies known as Executive Councils. Twenty nine such councils were formed to administer the service in the four cities and twenty five counties or groups of counties. The Act charged the councils with making 'arrangements with medical practitioners for the provision . . . of personal medical services for all persons' in their respective areas. In exercising their functions, the Executive Councils were required to consult with committees deemed by the Secretary of State for Scotland to be representative of the local medical practitioners, dentists, and pharmacists. The Local Medical, Dental, and Pharmaceutical Committees, as these consultative bodies were known, appointed twelve of the twenty four members of the Executive Councils, with another eight being appointed by the local health authority and the other four being chosen by the Secretary of State. The Act provided no machinery to direct general practitioners to areas of greatest need, but it did set up a body known as the Scottish Medical Practices Committee which was empowered to refuse a general practitioner permission to set up practice in an area where 'the number of medical practitioners ... is already adequate'. The sale and purchase of practices was prohibited under the Act, and arrangements were made to compensate established practitioners for this loss[9].

Public Relations

The general public had to be instructed in the use of the new service, and a leaflet entitled *The New National Health Service*, which outlined the nature and scope of the service, was distributed to all householders during April 1948. Its first object was to make it clear that everyone could choose his own doctor, subject to the doctor's acceptance of him as a patient, and to ensure that the choice was made before the appointed day[10]. The National Health Service offered the people of Britain a comprehensive medical service, including general practitioner services, medicines and medical aids on doctors' prescriptions, dental services, spectacles, hearing aids, full treatment in general and specialist hospitals, a full maternity service, a health visitor service to advise mothers on the care of young children and to provide health education for the whole family, a home nursing service, and a home help service. Access to hospital and specialist services would be through the general practitioner. All this was provided free, in the sense that a patient did not have to pay for services, medicines, or other aids at the time he was given them. There were a few exceptions to this general rule. Hospital beds in single rooms or small wards, if available at the time, might be given to patients who were prepared to pay for more privacy either as 'private' or as amenity patients, and patients who wanted some special type of dental treatment or spectacles, beyond what was needed for health, had to pay the extra cost. These charges contributed little to the income of the National Health Service. The service was paid for mainly from national taxation (78 *per cent*), the rest of the cost being met by weekly contributions paid by employed people (18 *per cent*), by local taxation (3 *per cent*), for services provided by local health authorities, and by charges to patients (1 *per cent*)[11].

The new service was warmly welcomed in Scotland, with the British people, as the *Glasgow Herald* commented at the time, taking a pride 'in leading the world in progressive citizenship, and in demonstrating what unregimented democracy could achieve'[12]. The strength of public opinion on this matter was such as to convince conservatives of the need to be popularly perceived as the champions, and even progenitors, of the service. The *Scotsman* declared that:

> "Though the Socialists may be expected to take full credit for
> introducing an extensive social security system, they are
> building on foundations laid by the Coalition Government.
> On the principles of the new legislation there is widespread
> agreement among all parties, and criticism from the Op-
> position has been directed against the Government's method
> of operating the various schemes"[13].

However, while there was widespread agreement on the theoretical
merit of a complete public medical service offering 'free' treatment for
all, some people questioned whether the difficult period of post-war
reconstruction was the most propitious for embarking upon such an
ambitious project. The *Glasgow Herald* stated that:

> "a noble experiment is in danger of being bungled through
> inexperience and haste. In the interval between the vision
> and the realisation Britain has become a debtor nation whose
> highest aim for some years to come must be to maintain, far
> less improve upon, her present standards of life. The war has
> resulted in serious shortages of man-power in certain pro-
> fessions, including doctors and nurses. Thus the National
> Health Service starts off seriously, perhaps insurmountably,
> handicapped in this respect. The installation of health centres
> and the modernisation and reorganisation of hospitals, which
> were to have been the first fruits of the new scheme, have been
> indefinitely postponed"[14].

The *Herald* argued that the government should have proceeded more
cautiously and made 'a beginning by extending the provisions of the
former Health and Pensions Schemes to the families of the insured persons; then there would indeed have been every reason to regard its future
development with confidence'[15]. Similar doubts about the ability of
post-war Britain to supply all the services promised by the Act were
expressed by the *Scotsman*, which stated that:

> "As far as the health service is concerned it is certain that
> great difficulties will be encountered in the early stages ...
> Even with universal goodwill, the service could not work
> smoothly and give the public all the benefits it promises.
> There are not enough doctors to meet demands for treatment
> which may be expected to increase when treatment is free.
> Under present conditions hospital treatment cannot be pro-
> vided immediately for all who need it owing to the shortage
> of accommodation, of specialists, and of nurses. Waiting lists
> are likely to grow longer, when hospital treatment is, in
> theory, freely available to everyone ... A universal health
> service is a praiseworthy object, but its success may be preju-
> diced by introducing it without adequate preparations"[16].

Immediate reactions

That the National Health Service would not be able to provide immediately all the services promised was freely admitted by a Labour government anxious to lower popular expectations and by those charged with administering the service. Prime Minister Clement Attlee, broadcasting to the nation on the eve of the inauguration of the service, reminded his listeners that 'all our social services have to be paid for in one way or another from what is produced by the people of this country', and warned that in view of the economic difficulties facing the country the health service would 'take time to develop'. A 'full service', he added, would only become available 'when our present shortages have been overtaken', and, consequently, 'we shall have to be a bit lenient with the Service at first'[17]. The following day, Sir George Henderson, Secretary of the Department of Health for Scotland, issued a 'warning against expecting too much in the early days of the National Health Service'[18]. Even before the service was inaugurated, it was announced that there was no prospect of providing the health centres which had been envisaged as playing a central role in post-war Scottish health care. Instead of a full building programme, it was planned to establish only four 'experimental units' at Airdrie, Cowdenbeath, Dumbarton, and Sighthill in Edinburgh[19]. In the event, as we shall see, even this limited programme was cut, when it became clear that the public had no interest in the health centre idea and that the 'experiment' could be halted without creating a political storm. However, while restrictions on capital projects presented difficulties, the most serious problem facing the new service was probably the shortage of trained staff. There were barely enough doctors for general practitioner services and not nearly enough dentists. The services provided by local health authorities were seriously handicapped by a deficiency in the numbers of health visitors, assistant medical officers, and dental officers. In the hospitals the shortage of specialists was worrying, and that of nurses alarming. The latter problem had already prompted the experimental use of patients as nurses at Law Hospital, and, in July 1948, Sir Andrew Davidson, the Chief Medical Officer to the Department of Health for Scotland, asked the medical superintendents of every hospital in Scotland to consider introducing a similar system for patients to relieve the staffing problem[20]. The staffing problem was especially acute in those hospitals specialising in the treatment of pulmonary tuberculosis. The annual report of the Department of Health for Scotland for the year 1948 stated that there was a waiting list of some 2,500 respiratory tuberculosis cases, and that some 570 hospital beds which had been set aside for such cases were lying empty because of a shortage of nursing staff[21].

The problems associated with staff shortages were exacerbated by the unexpectedly heavy demand for the services provided, and the difficulties of the infant service soon began to generate concern and stimulate discussion of possible solutions. Addressing the annual conference of the Scottish Association of Executive Councils, in Aberdeen on 30 September 1949, Sir William Marshall, the chairman of the Lanarkshire Executive Council, drew attention to 'the heavy demands on the services of the doctors', which, he argued, were 'excessive and sometimes even unreasonable'. Overcrowded surgeries, he continued, inevitably led to 'delay and a danger of too hasty diagnosis and superficial treatment', and he urged that every effort should be made to reduce the burden of paper work on doctors in order that more of their time could be devoted to clinical work. Marshall reported that in the first year of the National Health Service the number of prescriptions issued had increased threefold to 15 million. Moreover, not only had the increase in the number of prescriptions greatly exceeded expectations, but the average cost of those prescriptions was 50 *per cent* higher than in the last year of the old National Health Insurance scheme. With regard to the dental service, Marshall stated, 'the present situation was disturbing'. The demand for dental services had been heavy and the cost of providing them had greatly exceeded expectations. Similarly, the demand for ophthalmic services had been 'overwhelming' (being five or six times what was estimated when the Bill was before Parliament), and had resulted in serious delays in the supply of spectacles. In Marshall's view, 'they had a duty at this time, when all were conscious of the heavy burdens which the country had to bear, to do their part in securing that these great benefits were not obtained at too heavy a cost, and it was their place to make certain that waste and extravagance were checked'. Marshall tentatively suggested that patients should be required to pay a proportion of the cost of dentures and spectacles. 'Whether it would be possible to make any charge in the case of drugs was more doubtful', he added, 'but with regard to appliances there might be some provision to entitle the Executive Council to insist on payment of at least part of the cost'[(22)].

Marshall's speech was welcomed by the *Scotsman*, which declared that while 'all parties are agreed that the health services are an investment that should yield a valuable return in the form of higher standards of national health', general support for the service:-

> "does not mean that expenditure can be allowed to rise without check. If reasonable economies are not introduced, the health services may well prove too heavy a burden for the straitened national economy. At present it is estimated that the cost is about 2s.6d [12½p] per person per week, whereas the original estimate was 1s.6d. [7½p] ... Probably considerable economies could be achieved by tightening up regulations in order to prevent abuse of the services by people who cannot resist the temptation of getting something for nothing. There might be a closer check on the repair of dentures and spectacles, although it is difficult to prove negligence ... It is

clear also that drugs are being supplied on too lavish a scale, and the prescribing of foods and toilet preparations should be restricted."[23]

A fortnight later Dr Guy Dain of the British Medical Association told the General Assembly of the World Medical Association in London that the British people had taken advantage 'to the uttermost extent' of a service which had been inadequately provided with doctors, nurses, hospital beds, and equipment. A method would have to be found, he suggested, of placing 'within reasonable control the demands of a free service'[24].

—And the Consequences

As Britain's post-war economic difficulties increased, producing a financial crisis which in turn led to a massive devaluation of sterling, the pressures mounted on government to check what were widely regarded as unacceptably expensive abuses of the National Health Service. Finally, Prime Minister Attlee announced his government's intention to reduce its planned expenditure by £250 million. While the housing budget was the most seriously affected by the Labour government's austerity programme, it was intended that the National Health Service would not escape unscathed. A prescription charge of 1s. (5p), it was announced, would be introduced in order to achieve savings of about £10 million in the cost of the service to the Treasury[25].

A new clause to enable the government to levy prescription charges was inserted into the National Health Service (Amendment) Bill, which had been brought forward in May 1949 in fulfilment of the Labour government's pledge to the medical profession that it would legislate to prohibit the introduction by regulation of a full-time salaried general practitioner service. The new clause was vaguely worded and raised more questions than it answered. Indeed, it bore the hallmark of crisis legislation. The Parliamentary Secretary to the Ministry of Health, Arthur Blenkinsop, defending the clause when it came before the House of Commons on 9 December 1949, explained that it had been 'drafted widely because the exact nature of the arrangements has not yet been settled'. He reiterated Attlee's promise that the charge would not exceed 1s. (5p), and assured the House that old age pensioners and those in receipt of war disability pensions would be exempted. 'Beyond that,' he added, 'I cannot say further than that we have under consideration the many representations which have been made by members of the House and others as to the detailed working of the scheme'[26]. The clause was not opposed by the Conservative opposition, but some opposition members could not resist the opportunity to make sport of Aneurin Bevan for introducing a measure which undermined the principle of a health service free at the time of use. Bevan, who apparently only agreed to the clause in the belief that he could manoeuvre later to prevent its powers being used, attempted to extricate himself from a ticklish situation by saying that the measure was not motivated by a desire for economy but by a determination to discourage abuse. The government's aim, he stated, was to 'reduce the queues at the surgeries and the unnecessary expenditure at the chemists' shops'[27]. While some back-bench Labour MPs predictably opposed the measure, arguing that it would deter some people from seeking early medical advice, there was no evidence of widespread indignation either within the parliamentary Labour party or among the party activists and trade union organisations. Moreover, it is noteworthy that not one Scottish Labour MP opposed the clause when it was debated in Parliament. At least part of the explanation for this behaviour may be found in the desire for party unity in the run-up to the general election of February 1950, and in the acceptance of the plain fact that as prescription charges would not be levied immediately there would be room for manoeuvre after the election to prevent their introduction.

In the event, Attlee's government did not introduce prescription charges. The Treasury, however, demanded and got approval for a ceiling to be placed upon National Health Service expenditure. In 1950 the Department of Health for Scotland began to preach retrenchment, warning hospital authorities that expenditure must be kept within pre-scribed and very narrow limits, and that savings made in one department of a hospital could not be used to provide better facilities in another[28]. It was relatively easy to impose limits on the hospital service, but ex-penditure on general medical services could only be controlled by means of persuasion. To that end the central department urged general prac-titioners to control the amount and cost of their prescribing and asked the public to exercise prudent restraint in their demand for medicines. This propaganda campaign proved less than totally successful. Hector McNeil, the Secretary of State for Scotland, told a press conference held to review the progress of the National Health Service in Scotland during 1950, that he was 'greatly concerned about the fact that the demand for doctors' prescriptions in Scotland is now approaching the rate of four annually per head of population, and he is being reluctantly forced to the conclusion that Scots are becoming too "medicine-bottle-minded".'[29]

The Introduction of charges

Treasury demands for retrenchment increased with the outbreak of the Korean War. The requirements of a substantial rearmament programme necessitated a series of austerity measures which Hugh Gaitskell, the Chancellor of the Exchequer, presented to the House of Commons on 10 April 1951. Gaitskell decided against introducing prescription charges, but he proposed that patients should be charged about half the cost of spectacles and dentures. It was calculated that these charges would result in savings of £2.7 million *per annum* from a national health service budget in Scotland of just over £43 million[30].

The controversial proposal received a mixed response. Opposition MPs and the conservative newspaper press welcomed what the *Glasgow Herald* considered to be 'a belated recognition of the fact that social services must be adjusted to economic realities', while criticising the charges for being 'too little and too late'[31]. Support for the proposal was also voiced by some prominent Scottish health administrators. Dr A.F. Wilkie Millar, the president of the Scottish Association of Executive Councils, had recommended the introduction of 'some small immediate charge' for spectacles and dentures during his address to the Association on 29 September 1950, while Sir William Marshall, the chairman of the joint committee of the Association of Executive Councils for England, Scotland, and Wales, who had argued along the same lines during his speech to the Scottish Association the preceding year, described Gaitskell's proposal as 'courageous and necessary'[32]. Other administrators disagreed. T.J. Addly, the recently retired former chairman of the Edinburgh Executive Council, described the decision to introduce charges as 'a very retrograde step'[33], while Walter Henderson, the chairman of the Glasgow Executive Council, expressed 'surprise at the drastic nature of the scale of charges proposed'[34]. The reaction of the Labour movement was on the whole less than welcoming, although the desire for party unity in the run-up to the general election, and the general feeling that the budget was not as stiff as had been feared, limited the opposition within the Parliamentary Labour Party to health service charges. Nevertheless, Gaitskell's rearmament budget proved too much for three members of the Government, provoking the resignations of Aneurin Bevan, the former Minister of Health who had been appointed Minister of Labour in the cabinet reshuffle of January 1951, Harold Wilson, the President of the Board of Trade, and John Freeman, the Under-Secretary at the Ministry of Supply[35]. Less than a week after these resignations, having heard John Johnson, the chairman of Glasgow Trades Council, describe the proposed charges as 'iniquitous', and James Carmichael, the Labour MP for Bridgeton, deplore 'the encroachment on the social services', the Scottish Trades Union Congress passed a resolution calling for a withdrawal of the proposed charges[36]. In an attempt to placate opposition within the party, Hilary Marquand, the Minister of Health, announced on 2 May 1951, during the committee stage of the National Health Service Bill (1951), that a new clause would be introduced at report stage to end charges for spectacles and dentures in April 1954 unless they were renewed before then by a resolution of the House of Commons. This announcement failed to silence back-bench criticism of the proposal, but it may have persuaded some Labour members to refrain from voting against their own government. The clause imposing the new charges was passed by 262 votes to 3, with an estimated

30 to 50 Labour MPs abstaining. Two of the three members to vote against health service charges sat for Scottish constituencies, namely, Archibald Manuel (Central Ayrshire) and James Carmichael (Bridgeton), while the two tellers against the Government were John McGovern (Shettleston) and Emrys Hughes (South Ayrshire)[37].

The latter months of 1951 witnessed a steadily worsening balance of payments problem and a serious fall in Britain's gold reserves. The new Conservative government, which had been elected in October 1951, decided that action was required to restore the health of the economy, and on 29 January 1952 R.A. Butler, the Chancellor of the Exchequer, announced a series of austerity measures including a 1s. (5p) charge for prescriptions, a charge of up to £1 for dental treatment (with children and expectant mothers excluded), and minor charges for medical appliances such as hearing aids and wigs. In Britain as a whole these charges were expected to bring in £20 million in a full year, while in Scotland the estimated yearly saving was £2.1 million, including £1.25 million on prescriptions and £750,000 on dental treatment[38].

The Scottish conservative newspaper press welcomed these measures. The *Glasgow Herald* declared that 'the decision to charge an initial fee for dental and medical services may restore some sense of proportion to those using the services and result in substantial saving with no harm to anyone'[39], while the *Scotsman* claimed that 'one of the factors standing in the way of our recovery is the burden of gross taxation which is absorbing about 40 *per cent* of the national income'[40], and asked those complaining about the charges to ponder Butler's observation that 'the real danger to the social services comes from the threat of bankruptcy'[41]. Opposition to Butler's proposals, however, was not slow in gathering force and making itself heard. Protests from the Labour Party (and in particular the 'Bevanites'), the Socialist Medical Association, the Scottish Trades Union Congress, and individual trade unions were only to be expected, but it soon became clear that a wide cross-section of the public were unhappy about the charges. Growing public anxiety generated some unease among Conservative back-bench MPs, and, faced with what the *Glasgow Herald* described as 'a rising tide of ... criticism', the Chancellor of the Exchequer and Harry F.C. Crookshank, the Minister of Health, addressed a private meeting of the parliamentary party's health committee on 19 February 1952 to defend and explain government policy. Butler and Crookshank did not have an easy evening. Back-bench Tories put forward their own alternatives for eliminating waste from the health service and suggested systems of charges designed to relieve the burden on the Exchequer without imposing hardship on the poor or discouraging people in need of treatment from going to the chemist[42]. Faced with this pressure, the Government decided to make some concessions. Free dental treatment was extended to everyone under twenty-one (instead of sixteen) and to old-age pensioners. Moreover, on

30 May 1952, the new Minister of Health, Iain Macleod, hinted that the remaining charges were only a temporary expedient. 'The Government', he declared, 'believe that there must certainly be charges now and for some time to come, but the Government in this Act do not declare, nor is it part of Tory policy or philosophy, that charges must remain a permanent part of the National Health Service'.

Prescription charges have in fact remained a permanent part of the National Health Service and have been steadily and substantially increased from time to time. With each increase there has been a good deal of public protest at the encroachment upon the principle of a 'free at the time of need' health service, but, while prescription charges are not and never have been popular, successive governments of different parties have agreed on their utility. A similar cross-party consensus has also existed on the need to exempt certain categories of patients, such as children and the poor, from prescription charges, and on the need to prevent charges from rising so high as to inhibit the less well off from seeking early medical advice. Whether this consensus can be maintained in a Britain in apparent economic decline is a question more easily asked than answered.

The Hospital Service

The economic difficulties of post-war Britain not only stimulated demands for health service charges, but also severely restricted the amount of money available for hospitals. The Regional Hospital Boards, upon which the responsibility for planning and developing the hospital service was devolved, had to carry out the twin task of combining many independent services into a unified hospital service and of providing hospital specialists in all areas of the country under less than easy financial conditions. Nevertheless, despite tight budgetary restrictions much was achieved in the decade following on the establishment of the service, and, when the purse strings were loosened in the more prosperous 1960s, the pace of progress noticeably quickened.

Throughout the whole of the post-war period significant changes have taken place in the character of acute hospital work. The period has been marked by a progressive increase in the rate of in-patient admissions, by a reduction in the average duration of in-patient treatment, and by a considerable development of out-patient services based in part upon the recommendations of the Standing Medical Advisory Committee's report of 1949 on out-patient facilities[44]. Specialist services, which prior to 1948 had been largely limited to the main centres, were increasingly provided in district hospitals, and the number of specialists was greatly increased. While in 1948 there had been some 900 specialist/consultants and senior medical officers working in Scotland, by 1973 that number had been almost doubled. However, the great expansion of the Scottish hospital service since 1948 is perhaps best illustrated by the increase in the total number of hospital medical staff. Between 1950 and 1973 the number of senior and junior hospital doctors increased by 76 *per cent* from 2,363 to 4,168[45].

A welcome relaxation—The White Paper

The most serious consequence of the financial difficulties affecting the National Health Service in its early years was the failure to provide new hospitals designed to meet modern requirements. Until the early 1960s the limited funds available for capital projects were almost entirely devoted to catching up with maintenance, which had been neglected during the war, to replacing the largely obsolete plant and equipment which had been inherited in 1948, and to adapting and improving existing hospitals to meet changing medical needs[46]. Such were the demands of these programmes and such were the limitations of the budget that only one new hospital, at Alexandria, was constructed during the first ten years of the service. In 1959, however, the central department asked Scotland's five Regional Hospital Boards to draw up plans for modernised hospital services in their areas, and, in 1962, the government issued a White Paper detailing its hospital policies for the next decade. The main objectives set by the White Paper were the provision of increased maternity hospital accommodation, more specialised surgical units, improved geriatric facilities for both long- and short-stay patients, modernised hospitals for the mentally ill, increased accommodation for the mentally deficient, and modernised laboratory and X-ray facilities in general hospitals[47]. All this was to be done within the context of a massive hospital building programme, costing £70 million, which was to involve the rebuilding of four key teaching hospitals, the extension and modernisation of four others, and the construction of ten new district hospitals. Priority was given to the rebuilding of teaching hospitals in Edinburgh, Glasgow, and Dundee (on which a third of the allocated money was to be spent), but the success of the plan depended upon the establishment, in the main centres of population outwith the four cities, of district hospitals. These hospitals, it was envisaged, would eliminate the service's over-dependence on the teaching centres, which had deprived the so-called peripheral hospitals of their due share of qualified staff. The new district hospitals would supply full consultant services, thus providing the populations they served with a higher standard of medical care, and dramatically reducing the need for patients and their visiting relatives to travel to the main regional centres[48].

The White Paper received a warm welcome, being regarded, as the *Glasgow Herald* put it, as a signal of 'the emergence of the hospital service from its long spell of improvisation into a period of genuine expansion'[49]. The unsuitability of Victorian and Edwardian hospitals, whether of voluntary or Poor Law origins, to modern medical needs was fully appreciated, as was the unsatisfactory dependence, particularly acute in west central Scotland, upon the great teaching hospitals. However, doubts existed as to whether the proposals would be carried out in their entirety within the planned timescale. The *Glasgow Herald*, having pointed out that the White Paper called for a doubling of the rate of capital expenditure on hospitals, remarked that 'until this is firmly guaranteed, which it is not, White Papers make unreliable timetables'[50]. The *Scotsman* shared these doubts, stating that:-

"It must be hoped ... that the hospital programme will be given a high place in the priority list of those making demands on the available resources. Otherwise the Government might find it only too easy to retreat from their programme on the grounds that the national economy is overstrained"[51].

These doubts were largely justified, despite the spending of increasingly large sums on hospital building year by year partly because the real costs of modern hospital building was grossly under-estimated after the long interval during which almost no new major hospital building had taken place. By 1974 only one new teaching hospital had been built, although the first phases of the rebuilding of three others had been completed, and work had begun on the redevelopment of another. A similar tale may be told regarding the district general hospitals. Only one had been completed by 1971, and work was underway at only three of the nine others promised in 1962. This near snail's pace progress, which was contrasted most unfavourably with that in comparable western countries, continued during the 1970s, and in 1979 the Royal Commission on the National Health Service, after reviewing the situation, recommended that 'the government should find extra funds to permit much more rapid replacement of hospital buildings than has so far been possible'[52]. The Royal Commission concentrated its attention on the hospital service in England and Wales, yet the situation in Scotland was, if anything, worse. In Scotland less than a third of the hospital accommodation has been built since 1948, and more than a third pre-dates 1900.

Nevertheless, while the rate of replacement and modernisation of Scottish hospitals has been unsatisfactory, and while serious structural problems have been discovered in some of the new hospitals, the picture of the Scottish hospital service since 1948 should not be made too gloomy. Between 1948 and 1974 the replacement and upgrading of outdated hospitals provided 11,000 beds in new buildings, over 100 new outpatient departments, and a variety of specialist units[53]. These improvements made it possible to keep pace, in some degree, with the rapid advance of medical knowledge, and went some way to making good the shortages of maternity and geriatric beds highlighted in the 1962 White

Paper. One of the most interesting and significant developments in recent years has been the establishment of some day hospitals and day centres, which have enabled geriatric and psychiatric patients to be treated within the community, although here also limited funds have restricted the scale of the developments. Ironically, the flow of funds into this and other urgent capital programmes has been restricted by the success of well-orchestrated public campaigns in delaying and in some cases preventing the closure of obsolete and uneconimic local hospitals.

General practice and the Charter

In its early years the National Health Service focused much of its effort on the provision of hospital and specialist services throughout the country. General practice seemed to occupy a lowly position in the new service, and there was considerable disappointment, especially amongst general practitioners, that the central role for the family doctor advocated by the MacAlister and Cathcart reports had been rejected. The keenest general practitioners in small towns and country areas suffered a severe setback with the ending of general practitioner surgery. A good case was advanced in support of this development, for the standards of general practitioner surgery varied enormously from place to place, and advances in investigative, anaesthetic and operative procedures required the provision of ever more expensive facilities and ever higher standards of surgical skill which, it was argued, could only be economically supplied by specialists in the major hospitals. These arguments were readily accepted by the public and by many practitioners, but the demise of general practitioner surgery was secured at a cost, for that surgery had formerly provided the 'spark,' not only to many rural practitioners, but also to the cottage hospitals where they performed, and following its ending many of those hospitals ceased to be active foci of local medical activity and degenerated into minor repositories of chronic and geriatric care. At the same time as general practitioners lost their stimulating and rewarding involvement in acute hospital work, they found themselves, with the removal of the old financial barriers, coping with a substantially increased demand for their services. The inevitable consequences were falling morale and rising resentment. Concern at the predicament of the family doctors under the National Health Service was felt outside the ranks of the medical profession. Commenting on a speech made by Dr A.F. Wilkie Millar, the president of the Scottish Association of Executive Councils, to the annual conference of the Association on 29 September 1950, which had laid emphasis on the necessity of enhancing the status of the family doctor, the *Glasgow Herald* stated:

> "A way must be sought of making general practice more attractive, not only as regards remuneration, but also in the opportunities it affords for personal effort to relieve suffering

and restore health – the true reward of everyone who devotes his life to medicine. Good doctors will not be bred by a system which, it is complained, is tending to offer an intelligent young man or woman, after years of arduous study, the prospect of becoming too often little more than a form-signing intermediary between the public and the specialist or the drug-store"[54].

Nevertheless, despite the seriousness of the problems facing general practice in those early years, there were some significant developments which seemed to point the way to a happier future. There was, for example, a steady growth in the number of partnerships, and an important change in the method by which a doctor usually entered general practice. The way of entering general practice began to change, with an increasing proportion of doctors applying for an assistantship, with a view to entering into a partnership, rather than applying for a single-handed practice vacancy. Also of importance were the adoption of policies encouraging the development of group practice and co-operation between general practitioners, health visitors and district nurses. Moreover, the central department also sought to improve the lot of general practitioners by encouraging Executive Councils to provide them with access to laboratory and other aids to diagnosis, and by promoting the establishment of links between groups of family doctors and particular hospitals for consultation references, clinical discussions, and ward visits[55]. Finally it may be noted that the Department of Health for Scotland made arrangements to promote an evenness of distribution of general practitioners and primary care services. In well-populated rural areas there were no problems in attracting general practitioners, but in remote areas of the Highlands and Islands, where small populations were scattered over large distances, special arrangements were necessary in order to provide an adequate service. The old Highlands and Islands Medical Services were continued and developed under the National Health Service, and, by a system of added inducement payments, the remuneration of general practitioners responsible for perhaps only a few hundred patients was brought up to a nationally agreed, and attractive, level[56].

However, despite these developments, the status and number of general practitioners continued to decline. The formation in 1953 of the College (subsequently the Royal College) of General Practitioners did something to arrest that decline, but it was only reversed in 1965 when agreement was reached on the so-called 'Doctors' Charter'. This critical intervention had its origins in general practitioner initiatives which led to negotiations between the central departments of England, Wales and Scotland, and the General Medical Service Committee of the British Medical Association. The outcome of those negotiations was an agreement on augmented terms of service for general practitioners, providing, among other things, financial support for the improvement of practice premises and the increased employment of supporting staff[57].

The charter provided a further spur to the development of group practice, and helped to stimulate the health centre programme. As we have seen, the financial difficulties of the country in the period following the end of the war prevented the development of health centres, where, the framers of the 1947 Act envisaged, general practitioners would practise side by side with the doctors, health visitors, district nurses, and other community staff of the local health authority. Thus, while it had been one of the stated aims of the National Health Service to promote the integration of community health services, precious little was achieved in the first seventeen years or so of the service. It was 1953 before an 'experimental' health centre in Sighthill, Edinburgh, was opened[58], and although this initiative was followed up two years later with a second centre in Stranraer, the 'experiment' was then seemingly abandoned. Nothing more was done until 1965 when, encouraged by an ambitious proposal for health centres drawn up by the Glasgow Local Medical Services Committee, the Scottish Home and Health Department (SHHD), with the support of the Scottish General Medical Service Committee of the British Medical Association, promoted a far reaching health centre programme. This programme gave priority to sites in central urban development areas where doctors' surgeries were endangered, to new towns, and to appropriate sites adjacent to hospitals where it was hoped to achieve closer integration of hospital and primary care services and obtain the benefits of shared resources. Such was the success of the programme that by 1983 one hundred and seventy health centres were in operation, accommodating approximately one in three general practitioners[60]. Recent years have seen health centre practice, and group practice, increasingly strengthened by nursing, health visitor, social work, secretarial, and receptionist support, and most general practitioners are now provided with direct access to X-ray and laboratory services. In an attempt to find ways of involving general practitioners in the hospital work which they had been almost totally denied since 1948, an interesting experiment was set-up in the later 1960s in Livingston New Town (West Lothian), where general practitioners were encouraged to combine their health centre responsibilities with half-time hospital appointments. This experiment was subsequently extended to other parts of the country, but its scale has been limited and general practitioners still complain bitterly about the lack of opportunity to become involved in acute hospital work.

The Local Authorities Health Services

The National Health Service Act of 1947 damaged the morale not only of general practitioners but also of the staff of local authority health departments. They lost their hospitals and the clinical responsibility which had been the basis of their daily contacts with local general practitioners and specialists. The Department of Health for Scotland in its annual report for 1949 stressed the continuing importance of the local health authorities' role and emphasised 'the extent of their responsibilities and opportunities in the promotion of better health',[62] but such exhortations gave small comfort to local authority medical staff who pointed out that it was difficult to practise prevention in a 'vacuum'. However, despite the difficulties arising from the loss of hospital responsibilities, much good work was done. Much effort was directed in the early years at improving the care of mothers and young children. New child welfare clinics were opened, and the number of health visitors was increased. The increased use of home nurses and home helps eased the strain on hospitals and allowed many children to stay at home during parental illness rather than be taken into the care of local authorities. Co-ordinated vaccination and immunisation programmes enabled diphtheria and poliomyelitis to be controlled and the incidence of whooping cough to be significantly reduced, and a contribution was made towards the decline of tuberculosis by local health authority measures which included the organisation of B.C.G. immunisation programmes and of a series of campaigns to persuade people to have a chest X-ray.

The high incidence of tuberculosis in Scotland throughout the later 1940s and early 1950s created serious problems for the health service. The Regional Hospital Boards found that they had insufficient beds and nurses to cope with the number of cases requiring treatment, and, while great efforts were made to remedy this unhappy situation, recourse had eventually to be made in 1951 to Swiss sanatoria which were contracted to provide treatment for Scots patients[63]. The flow of patients was increased by the success of radiography campaigns in detecting new cases. In 1957 a mass X-ray campaign of unprecedented scale was initiated, and 2565 previously undiagnosed active cases were identified and treated[64]. By this time, however, morbidity rates had declined and hospital provision had improved so as to eliminate the waiting list for tuberculosis treatment and allow the termination of the Swiss contract under which 1043 patients had been treated[65]. Many factors, including advances in diagnosis and treatment, contributed to the decline in tuberculosis which began in the mid 1950s and continued through the 1960s and 1970s, but much was undoubtedly owed to the success of the efforts of the local authority medical officers in promoting the B.C.G. vaccination and the mass radiography campaigns.

The post-war years have also seen significant developments in the field of environmental control. Atmospheric pollution had long been a serious problem in urban areas, contributing significantly to the high toll exacted by chest ailments. Effective action was, however, only taken after the public outcry against aerial pollution following on the infamous London 'smog' of 1952 which caused many deaths. The Clean Air Act of 1956, which tightened up controls on industrial smoke emission and authorised local authorities to issue orders declaring the whole or any part of their area to be smoke control districts in which the emission of smoke from any chimney would be an offence,[66] represented a landmark in environmental legislation. Its effectiveness may be well illustrated by comparison of aerial photographs taken in the early 1950s of urban areas shrouded in smoke with those taken in more recent years of the same areas which reveal the houses, streets, and business premises in total clarity.

The mid-1950s also saw the commencement of an experiment, supported by the Department of Health for Scotland, which aimed to assess the effects of fluoridation of water supplies upon children's teeth. A small research team was appointed to monitor the effect of fluoridated water upon the caries rates of Kilmarnock children, and compare them with the rates for children in the nearby burgh of Ayr where the water supply had not been fluoridated. Although it was demonstrated that the caries rates of Kilmarnock children fell progressively as a result of the addition of fluoride to the water supply, anti-fluoride propagandists persuaded the town council of Kilmarnock to abandon the experiment. As might have been predicted, the caries rates of Kilmarnock children then began to rise as steadily as they had fallen during the experiment[67]). Subsequent proposals to add fluoride to Scottish water supplies were generally blocked by the efforts of the emotive partisans of 'pure water', and, as yet, the numbers benefiting from fluoridated water have been small. An important test case was brought before the Court of Session in 1983 as a result of Strathclyde Region's announced intention to introduce fluoridated water supplies. This case resulted in a judgement declaring that the council's duty under the Water (Scotland) Act to provide wholesome water did not permit the addition of fluoride. However, the judge, Lord Jauncey, also declared that the expert evidence brought before him confirmed that the proposed concentration of fluoride of 1 part per million carried no risk to health, and would reduce considerably the incidence of dental caries. Following on this judgement, legislation is being prepared to clarify the powers of water authorities to add fluoride to water supplies on the recommendation of health boards[68].

While Scottish water supplies have been largely denied the prophylactic benefits of fluoride, they have unfortunately not been spared from lead pollution. The lead solvency of the softer waters of Scotland has been recognised as a health hazard for some time, but until recently little was done to deal with a problem which was especially serious in the Glasgow area. It was 1975 before Glasgow began hardening some of its water supplies to lessen their plumbosolvency, and encouraging the removal of lead pipes and tanks[69].

Perhaps progress towards improvement in the quality of the atmosphere and the water supply was hindered by the generally undramatic way in which lead and smoke pollution contributed to ill-health. There is nothing gradual and undramatic, however, about the effect of the typhoid bacillus, *salmonella typhi*, upon any population exposed to it. In 1964 a major epidemic of typhoid struck the city of Aberdeen, creating much anxiety. Although it was quickly brought under control, the concern created by the epidemic led to the establishment of a Communicable Diseases Unit in Glasgow with a staff of infectious disease epidemiologists available to help and advise throughout Scotland[70]. Had it not been for the 1964 epidemic, it may be doubted whether the Unit would have been set up at that time.

This is not the place to review the history of post-war Scottish housing, but reference must be made to a subject which closely involved medical officers of health, and which seemed to some of them to engross the attention of local authorities to the exclusion of virtually everything else. Medical officers of health might privately express dissatisfaction with what they conceived to be the exceedingly narrow views of their employers, but they did not question the need to tackle vigorously Scotland's acute housing crisis. Professor Thomas Ferguson of Glasgow University's Department of Public Health spoke for many, and probably most of Scotland's public health specialists, when, in his presidential address to the Royal Sanitary Association of Scotland on 5 October 1949, he drew attention to the great number of Scots still living in 'single ends', and declared that a 'healthy, decent life was no more possible under such conditions to-day than it was in the nineteenth century'. To pour social services into those wretched places, he continued, was certainly uneconomic and often quite useless. Bad housing, he believed, was still the greatest blot on Scotland's social welfare[71].

The response to the problem, once the immediate post-war shortages of labour and building materials were dealt with, was wholehearted, if less than inspired. Massive public funds were allocated to housing throughout the 1950s, the 1960s, and the early 1970s. Many of the old slums were cleared, significant reductions were made in the numbers of one and two roomed houses, and many Scots were able for the first time to live in houses with baths and indoor water closets. Yet, despite these undoubted improvements, the housing problem remained serious. The Cullingworth report pointed out in 1967 that a third of Scottish families were living in inadequate accommodation, and that much of this was deteriorating into slums[72]. The findings of the 1971 Census made even more depressing reading. Scotland was found to have 77.5 *per cent* of Britain's worst 5 *per cent* of socially deprived areas[73]. In Glasgow the Census revealed that, despite an 8 *per cent* drop in the population since 1961, the number of Glaswegians living in overcrowded houses had risen from 187,890 to 226,902. Perhaps most damning of all was the appearance of post-war housing estates, such as Easterhouse, in the Census statistics relating to overcrowding[74]. Since 1971 some initiatives have been taken to remedy the appalling mistakes of the past. The construction of high-rise housing, criticised by Richard Siefert, a leading architect of such housing, as 'socially evil', and productive of 'serious crime, loneliness, unhappiness, and mental disturbance',[75] has been halted. Urban aid programmes have been set up to ameliorate conditions in the most deprived areas, and the Scottish Office, apparently despairing of the ability of Glasgow District and Strathclyde Region to deal with Glasgow's housing problems, has established the Glasgow Eastern Area Renewal project (GEAR) in an attempt to transform an area which one delegate from the European Parliament described as 'like ... a bombarded city'[76]. Steps have also been taken to encourage the growth of home ownership, in the hope that higher levels of owner occupancy will not only change former tenants' political allegiances, but will also raise their expectations regarding the quality of housing.

As for personal social services, prior to the implementation in 1970 of the Social Work (Scotland) Act of 1967, medical social workers, successors of the almoners who had contributed so much over very many years to the hospital service, were in the employ of the National Health Service and had been specifically trained in medical work. The new Act replaced the medical social worker by the generic social worker employed by the Local Authority. In the long run the more general training of social workers may show advantages, but the initial impact of the Act has been to create a division in responsibility for medical care and social care with consequences not dissimilar to those created by the tripartite management structure of the National Health Service between 1947 and 1974. The Act also dealt a death blow to local health authority medical officers of health and their departments. This Act transferred responsibility not only for day care services, such as those for the disabled and mentally disturbed, but also for domiciliary services, such as home helps and 'meals-on-wheels' to local government Social Work departments[77]. With the loss of two of the most important responsibilities allocated to the local health authorities by the 1947 Act, and with the impending reorganisation of local government, public health doctors became willing to consider a new future as community medicine specialists in a reorganised National Health Service.

The Nursing Services

In the early years of the National Health Service a shortage of nurses obstructed the development of hospital services. It was quickly decided that, in the full employment conditions of the late 1940s and 1950s, the only way to increase recruitment of nurses was to improve salaries and conditions of service[78]. Such improvements, along with the introduction of subordinate grades and auxiliaries, have gone a long way to creating the nursing force required by modern hospital and community services.

The years following on the establishment of the National Health Service have also seen major changes in the organisation and training of nurses in Scotland. The General Nursing Council for Scotland was reconstituted under the Nurses (Scotland) Act of 1949, with the expectation that training regulations would be improved[79], while a similar intention lay behind the reconstitution of the Scottish Central Midwives Board effected by the Midwives (Amendment) Act of 1950[80]. In 1955 arrangements were completed for an experimental course of nurse-training in Glasgow, in which formal instruction was to be concentrated wholly in the first two years of the course, the third being spent as an intern year gaining hospital experience prior to registration[81]). The committee appointed to assess the experiment reported in 1960 'that the first of the principal objectives of the experiment – the preparation of the student nurse for the Final State Examination of the General Nursing Council for Scotland in two instead of three years – had been successfully achieved'[82]. In the same year, nursing education was boosted with the introduction by the University of Edinburgh, in agreement with the General Nursing Council for Scotland and the hospital authorities involved, of an integrated five-year course leading to an arts or science degree and registration as a Registered General Nurse[83].

The implementation of the Salmon and Mayston reports, of 1966 and 1969 respectively[84], and the unification of the organisation of the nursing profession following on the reorganisation of the National Health Service in 1974 gave nurses a place in the organisation of the service commensurate with their numbers and importance. The improved status of the nursing profession within the reorganised service is symbolised by the fact that the Chief Area Nursing Officer became an important member of the Area Executive Group. Far-reaching recommendations for the further reorganisation of nursing were made by the Briggs Committee in 1972[85], and these will take time to implement fully.

Postgraduate medical education and training

Important developments were also taking place in the training of the medical profession. Perhaps the most important development in postgraduate medical education in post-war Scotland was the establishment of the Scottish Council for Postgraduate Medical Education in 1970. This initiative was the culmination of a long-term movement towards a more planned and orderly process of preparation for specialist practice, which had been proposed by the Nuffield Provincial Hospitals Trust. The Royal Commission on Medical Education, which reported in 1968, strongly supported the movement's aims, and clearly and emphatically recommended the setting up of central bodies to co-ordinate the views of the profession, both service and academic, the health service, and the government on postgraduate medical education[86]. For a time, it seemed that a single such body covering the whole United Kingdom would be established. In the event, however, it was decided to set up, and support with central funds, a separate Scottish Council, to co-ordinate and stimulate the organisation and development of postgraduate medical education in Scotland, to provide a national forum for the discussion of matters relating to postgraduate education, and to supply government with authoritative advice on those matters. The Council met for the first time in May 1970 under the chairmanship of Dr Christopher Clayson[87].

Medical and Health Service research

Since 1948 the Scottish central department has initiated many important developments in support of medical research. In 1950 the Advisory Committee on Medical Research was established to advise on the initiation, direction, co-ordination and conduct of medical research. The Committee was appointed after consultation with the Medical Research Council, the Scottish Universities, and the Royal Scottish Medical Corporations, and worked in close co-operation with the Medical Research Council. It had no funds directly at its disposal, but it could suggest appropriate sources from which financial assistance might be available for particular projects, and could recommend projects to the Secretary of State as suitable for assistance from public funds under the National Health Service Act[88]. Over the years, with diligent support from its medical secretary, the Committee has not only promoted valuable research work in Scotland, but also created and fostered a good relationship between the central department and the academic and research community. In 1953 the Scottish Hospital Endowments Research Trust was set up to provide additional financial support for medical research. Working with monies transferred from the former voluntary hospitals' endowment funds, it provided, after consultation with the experts on the Advisory Committee on Medical Research in Scotland, financial assistance to research projects which were considered by the Committee to be worthwhile[89]. The next major development in research organisation took place following the publication of the Rothschild report on government-related research[90]. In 1973 Sir Andrew Kay, Regius Professor of Surgery in the University of Glasgow, was appointed part-time Chief Scientist at the Scottish Home and Health Department, and in the following year a Chief Scientist Organisation was established to co-ordinate the Department's contribution to all kinds of research likely to improve the health service. The Chief Scientist Organisation is responsible for advising the Secretary of State on the scientific implications of objectives proposed for the health service in Scotland, the promotion of research and development planned to improve the provision and operation of particular health services, the scientific merits of specific research programmes and projects, and the maintenance of balanced support for the different fields of research. To help achieve these ends, the Chief Scientist is supported by the Chief Scientist Committee, whose membership is drawn largely but not exclusively from the medical professoriate of the Scottish Universities, and by four sub-committees dealing with medical research, health services research, computer research, and equipment research[91]. One of the most successful committees was that concerned with health service research. Work in this field had been stimulated by the formation in 1965 of the Health Services Research and Intelligence Unit which was charged with collecting and analysing information about all aspects of the health services, studying long-term trends, and providing sound intelligence upon which policy makers could base their decisions[92]. Health service research has attracted an increasing amount of financial support in recent years as the importance of the work done by epidemiologists, statisticians, social psychologists, and others has come to be more fully appreciated.

Central Initiatives

The Scottish Home and Health Department has also been behind some major initiatives to improve Scotland's hospital services. The rapid increase in the hospital building programme in the 1960s rendered it essential that accurate information and sound guidance on the problems relating to the planning, design, organisation, and commissioning of hospitals should be made available to Scottish hospital authorities. Following on the establishment of the Hospital Design Team, the Scottish Hospital Centre was set up in December 1965 'to promote research into the functional design and operation of hospitals, to encourage research into the design of hospital equipment, . . . to compile a library of information primarily relating to hospital planning, and to prepare and publish reports and summaries bearing on research work' in relevant subjects[93]. In 1970, against a background of growing concern about the problems associated with 'long stay' care, the Scottish Hospital Advisory Service was set up to monitor and advise on the management and requirements of hospitals primarily concerned with the care and treatment of the mentally ill, the mentally deficient, geriatric patients, and the chronic sick[94]. The Service pursued its objective in a sensitive and co-operative fashion, and quickly established a good rapport with Regional Hospital Boards, Boards of Management, and hospital staff. It drew attention to the problems created by remote and defective management, low nurse/patient ratios, overcrowding, badly designed buildings and facilities (not all of them Victorian), inefficient supply and disposal services, and low staff morale, and supported management and staff in their endeavours to find solutions to these problems[95].

The Hospital Advisory Service was established in response to disquiet expressed about the care and treatment of the elderly and the mentally infirm. This disquiet emanated mainly but not exclusively from England, where the situation appears to have been worthy of particular concern. In Scotland, the interests of mentally disordered patients were, and still are, protected by the Mental Welfare Commission, a body set up under the Mental Health (Scotland) Act of 1960. The Commission is an independent body appointed by the Crown on the recommendation of the Secretary of State for Scotland, which exercises its protective functions by investigating and reporting to the appropriate authorities on such matters as deficiency in care or treatment, improper detention, ill treatment, and loss of or damage to patients' property. The Mental Health (Scotland) Act of 1983 strengthened the Commission and gave it the opportunity to take a broader and more active part in securing the welfare of patients[96]. Besides providing for the establishment of the Mental Welfare Commission, the 1960 Act swept aside the archaic provisions of the Lunacy (Scotland) Act of 1857 and the Mental Deficiency and Lunacy (Scotland) Act of 1913. Responding both to advances in medical knowledge and to changing public attitudes towards mental health and mental deficiency, the 1960 Act severely pruned the old powers providing for the compulsory detention and treatment of patients, placing the emphasis instead upon voluntary treatment, and sought to encourage the development of community care through the expansion of local authority mental health services[97].

Obstetric services

Significant improvements have been effected since the inception of the National Health Service in Scotland's maternity services in an attempt to reduce the nation's maternal and infant mortality statistics to levels similar to those of comparable European nations. One of the most notable of these was the Regional Obstetric Service pioneered in the north east by Professor Sir Dugald Baird of the University of Aberdeen. This service, guided by the findings of some detailed epidemiological and sociological research, effected a major reduction in the maternal and perinatal mortality of the region[98].

The maternal death inquiry, involving detailed reports on each maternal death, was a comparatively early and very successful venture into professional quality control which was adapted from earlier initiatives in England. The first report resulting from these inquiries was published in 1974[99]. A later development, along similar lines and with similarly effective results, was an inquiry into perinatal deaths, the findings of which were published in 1980[100]. Unfortunately, while organised and systematic self-scrutiny of clinical procedures as a means of achieving improvements in services is much discussed, it is still rarely practised. If it were more regularly and more widely practised, it is likely that great benefits would accrue to the health service.

One of the most socially controversial developments in recent years was the Abortion Act of 1967. This measure, which came into effect on 27 April 1968, permitted the termination of pregnancy on a number of grounds, the most important of which were where the pregnancy constituted a risk to the physical or mental health of either the woman or her existing children. An increasing number of Scottish women have availed themselves of the Act's provisions. The number of abortions performed in Scotland has increased from 3,544, or 3.9 *per cent* of live births, in 1969[101] to 8,419, or 12.9 *per cent* of live births, in 1983[102]. Somewhat less controversial than the Abortion Act was the Health Services and Public Health Act of 1968, Section 15 of which extended the existing powers of local health authorities in Scotland to enable them to provide family planning advice and services for people who required them on social grounds. While the authorities were authorised to charge for any contraceptive appliances or substances supplied or for any prescriptions issued in non-medical cases, in all other respects the service was provided free of charge[103].

Health Education

The 1960s also witnessed an important initiative in the field of health education. The Cohen Committee, which reported in 1964, recommended the establishment of a central, independent, and well funded health education agency[104]. In 1968 the Secretary of State for Scotland set up a separate Health Education Unit for Scotland. Its first objectives were to educate the public on the risks of smoking and of alcoholic excess, and on the importance of dental hygiene[105]. Following reorganisation of the health service in 1974, the new Health Boards were encouraged to appoint suitably qualified and properly supported Health Education Officers. In 1980 the Health Education Unit was combined with the Scottish Health Education Council to form the Scottish Health Education Group, and a Scottish Health Education Co-ordinating Committee was set up 'to consider the broad objectives for health education in Scotland, how they might best be achieved, and what co-ordination between the various agencies involved at central and local level might be required'. The health education priorities of the present day are much the same as those identified in the 1960s. There has, however, been a trend in recent years away from a negative emphasis upon the consequences of smoking, drinking to excess, and taking little or no exercise, towards a more positive stress on the benefits of a healthy lifestyle[106].

THE NHS (SCOTLAND) ACT 1972

The Reorganisation of the Service

For over twenty five years the tripartite administrative structure of the National Health Service remained unchanged. However, the failure to achieve greater co-operation between the different arms of service was a source of great disappointment, and the old administrative structure became the subject of increasing criticism. In 1962, after four years' work, a U.K. committee of the British Medical Association, the Royal Colleges, and the Society of Medical Officers, under the chairmanship of Sir Arthur Porritt, reported in favour of administrative integration under a complicated structure of Area Health Boards. The Committee found that 'the present tripartite administration has isolated doctors in the three main branches of the service', and recommended 'that the responsibility for the administration and co-ordination of all the medical and ancillary services in any area should be in the hands of one authority only – the Area Health Board'[107]. On 7 November 1967 the Secretary of State for Scotland, William Ross, announced that a 'thorough examination of the administrative structure of the health services in Scotland' would be undertaken 'in order to ensure that it is adequate to ensure the most effective development of these services in future'. The views of local authority, professional and other interests would be sought, he added, and a Green Paper would be published outlining the Government's tentative proposals[108]. The Green Paper, which was published on 12 December 1968, suggested that in place of the five Regional Hospital Boards, 76 Boards of Management, 25 Executive Councils, and 56 Local Health Authorities, some 10 to 15 Area Health Authorities should be responsible for the administration of all aspects of the health services. The question of whether such area authorities would form part of a new local government structure was left alone pending the report of the Royal Commission on Local Government in Scotland. However, the Green Paper did say that preliminary discussions showed that this solution would be unpopular with many health service interests[109].

The Green Paper received a mixed response. The British Medical Association and hospital administrators gave the Government's proposals a general, if somewhat cautious welcome, but local authorities and some medical officers of health were highly critical. Dr Ian MacQueen, the Medical Officer of Health for Aberdeen, favoured the administrative integration of public health and general practitioner services, but argued that the hospital service should be kept separate. 'If one combined the two', he said, 'one or the other would fall'[110]. A similiar line of argument was taken by Dr James Gilloran, the Medical Officer of Health for Edinburgh, who claimed that if the Government's proposals were adopted there would be a 'big danger' of creating 'a "national hospital service" instead of a National Health Service'. Gilloran feared that, under the proposed new structure, general practitioner and public health services would lose out financially to the ever more demanding hospital service[111].

The local authorities resented the charge of inefficiency which they believed had been levelled at the services they provided, and doubted the wisdom of entrusting the administration of the health services to un-democratic, bureaucratic health boards. Mr Frank Inglis, the secretary of the Association of County Councils of Scotland, suggested that the loss of local authority health services 'would create difficulties in many re-spects, including the tie-up with the social services under the new Social Work (Scotland) Act', and emphasised the general opposition of the county councils to the creation of *ad hoc* bodies such as those proposed in the Green Paper[112]. More forcefully expressed were the criticisms made by Mr Gordon Watson, the Town Clerk of Dundee, who stated:–

"It is claimed that the tripartite division of the National Health Service does not make the most efficient use of the resources available. However, much of the inefficiency and wasteful expenditure originates with the state-operated part of the service ... It is questionable whether the fusion of the services under one monolithic board will lead to greater efficiency. One certain result of such a merger would be to make the body responsible for the administration of the Na-tional Health Service even more remote from the electorate and therefore less answerable for its actions"[113].

Similar doubts about the lack of accountability of the proposed new health boards were expressed by the *Scotsman*. While welcoming the administrative integration of the health service on the grounds that 'with Area Boards it would be possible to make better use of medical resources and to plan developments on a bigger scale', the *Scotsman* argued that the health services should be handed over to the new regional authorities whose creation the Royal Commission on Local Government was ex-pected to recommend. Having asked why the health service should not be subject to the same democratic controls as other locally administered services, the same newspaper went on to suggest that the Government 'should discard the system of Ministerial appointment in favour of dem-ocratic participation'. The new Health Boards, the *Scotsman* proposed, should be composed of elected members of regional authorities and perhaps some co-opted specialists[114].

A convincing case for a local government-administered health service was presented to the Royal Commission on Local Government, but the Commission, while listing the arguments for as well as against this solu-tion, refused to make any recommendations on the matter and passed the problem back to government[115]. In truth, there was little enthusiasm within the ranks of what might be termed the establishment for the democratisation of health service administration. Well organised professional interest groups were as strongly opposed to local government control as they had been in 1911 or 1946–47, and neither the Conservative nor the Labour Party showed much interest in loosening the paternalistic grip of St Andrew's House. Thus, it came as no surprise when, in November 1970, Gordon Campbell, the new Secretary of State for Scotland, announced that the management of the National Health Service would be outside local government[116]. However, the opponents of administration by *ad hoc* bodies refused to give up the struggle. Both during the second reading debate and the committee stage of the National Health Service (Scotland) Bill of 1972, MPs such as William Baxter (Stirlingshire West), Robert Hughes (Aberdeen North), James Dempsey (Coatbridge and Airdrie), and, most notably and most ably of all, John Mackintosh (Berwickshire and East Lothian), argued the case for bringing the health service under the democratic control of the local authorities. Such efforts were doomed to failure, for the leadership of all the main parties were firmly opposed to entrusting local authorities with the responsibility for spending the vast budget of the National Health Service wisely[117].

While there were some serious misgivings about the lack of direct local democratic accountability, there were none, or next to none, about the utility of a unified administrative structure. Indeed, as early as 1969, 'it was clear ... that no important section of opinion felt that the existing division of the health services into three separate parts could now be supported'[118]. It was with some justice that David Steel (Roxburgh, Selkirk, and Peebles) declared the 1972 Bill to be 'an agreed Bill' and William Ross commented on 'the tremendous amount of agreement which exists about it'[119]. Not one voice was raised during the various parliamentary stages of the Bill in defence of the old tripartite administration.

Unlike the situation in England, where the equivalent 1973 Act was made the vehicle for schemes designed to improve management, the simplification of health service administration was not the main objective of the Scottish Act. In Scotland, the prime motivation behind the Act was the improvement of patient care by means of a fully integrated service. The National Health Service (Scotland) Act of 1972 instructed the Secretary of State for Scotland to 'secure the effective provision of an integrated health service in Scotland'[120]. To this end, Executive Councils, Regional Hospital Boards, and Boards of Management were to be abolished, and local authorities were to lose their responsibility for the provision of health services. The organisation and management of health services were to be united in each area of Scotland under a single Health Board appointed by and responsible to the Secretary of State for Scotland[121]. However, as one of the stated purposes of the Act was to provide for co-operation between the National Health Service and the services, such as social work, education, planning and development, and environmental sanitation, provided by local government, and as local government itself was in the throes of a massive reorganisation, it was found necessary to postpone the introduction of the new Health Boards until the boundaries of the regional and district authorities had been settled. Although local government reorganisation did not take place until May 1975, agreement was reached on the geographical areas of the new authorities in time to allow for the introduction of the reorganised health service on 1 April 1974.

Much preparatory work was necessary in relation to this reorganisation. Senior administrators in the three branches of the service underwent re-training programmes which sought to provide an insight into those parts of the service with which they were unfamiliar and to orientate them towards the new approach required in administering an integrated service. In addition to informal discussions between officers of hospital authorities, local health authorities, and Executive Councils on the problems to be confronted in the reorganised service, more formal training was provided in the shape of residential courses, seminars and 'attachments' through which administrators gained practical knowledge of those services and branches of services with which they were unfamiliar[122]. Doctors, dentists and nurses had also to adjust to the demands of the new service, and various working parties and groups were set up to investigate and report on the future organisation and role of these professions. The reports,[123] which appeared between 1971 and 1973, proved to be valuable discussion documents and assisted greatly in smoothing the way to reorganisation.

The Reorganised Service

The Scottish Home and Health Department (SHHD) remains the central Government Department responsible to the Secretary of State for Scotland for the running of the health service in Scotland. He is aided in his responsibilities for the administration of the service by a Minister of State and a Parliamentary Under-Secretary of State. A Health Service Policy Group of senior administrative and professional SHHD officers advises Ministers on policy and co-ordinates the work of the administrative divisions and professional groups of the SHHD, who are in constant liaison with the fifteen Scottish Health Boards[124].

The SHHD has a central role in the funding, administration, planning, and development of the health service in Scotland. While the Scottish Office receives an annually negotiated block grant from the Treasury, the allocation of that grant between the different areas of expenditure for which the Scottish Office has responsibility is primarily a matter for the Secretary of State. Under ministerial direction the SHHD is responsible for executing the Secretary of State's policies in the allocation of funds apportioned to NHS from the Scottish Office budget. This allocation is in part influenced by the objectives set, the policies formulated, and the priorities put forward for ministerial approval by the Department with the help of two creations of the 1972 Act, *viz* the Scottish Health Service Planning Council (SHSPC), which replaced the 1948 Scottish Health Services Council, and the National Consultative Committees (NCCs) of the health care professions[125]. Besides these tasks, the SHHD monitors the performance of the Health Boards and the Common Services Agency (for which, see below), involves itself in negotiations on pay and conditions of service for staff, advises on legislation, liaises with other government departments on matters relating to health, and sanctions consultant appointments and capital projects.

The SHSPC was intended to promote closer co-operation between the SHHD, the local Health Boards, and the health care professions in the planning and development of the health service[126]. Its chairman, and seven of its members, namely, five senior members of the SHHD, the chairman of the Common Services Agency, and a representative of the Scottish Association of Local Health Councils, are appointed by the Secretary of State, while one member is appointed by each of the fifteen Health Boards and by each of the four Scottish Universities with a medical school[127]. In addition to *ad hoc* planning groups and working groups, there are standing advisory groups which provide the Council with specialist advice on services such as scientific services, information and computer services, the epidemiological aspects of infections, and new developments in health care[128].

The responsibility for planning, organising, and providing health care services is delegated by the Secretary of State to fifteen Health Boards whose boundaries were drawn up to match those of regions or districts created by local government reform in 1975. There is a wide variation in the size of the population served by the Boards. At one extreme is the Greater Glasgow Health Board serving a current population of nearly one million, while at the other are Boards responsible for providing health services for the relatively tiny populations of the Western Isles, Orkney, and Shetland. The chairman and members of Health Boards are appointed by the Secretary of State, but in accordance with the proposals made in *The National Health Service and the Community in Scotland* the membership of each Board includes two doctors, a nurse or a midwife, two people employed by, or in contact with, Health Boards, at least one person nominated by the appropriate university, two trade unionists, and persons nominated by local authorities[129]. Each Board was to be served by a team of chief officers consisting of a Secretary, the Chief Administrative Medical Officer, the Chief Nursing Officer, and the Board Treasurer. The chief officers were responsible to the board for the activities associated with each of their disciplines. Meeting together as an Area Executive Group, they took corporate responsibility for the running of the health services in their board's area and for preparing policy and planning options for the board's consideration. The four officers were from time to time joined on the Area Executive Group by the Chief Administrative Dental Officer and the Chief Administrative Pharmaceutical Officer. Until a relatively recent further reorganisation, some of the larger boards had a subordinate administrative tier of districts managed by a group of officers standing in what management science describes as line relationship to the Area Chief Officers. Below district level the service was organised in units and sectors[130].

The importance of maintaining and fostering the close links between the Scottish Universities and National Health Service was recognised in the National Health Service (Scotland) Act of 1972. Section 15 of the Act provided for the establishment of University Liaison Committees for any health board area or combination of areas. The purpose of these committees was, and is, to advise the relevant Boards on matters relating to clinical teaching or research in so far as they affect the administration of the service, and both the boards and the universities on any other matters of common interest to them. At least one third of the members of each committee are appointed by the relevant university, with an equal proportion being chosen by the appropriate board or boards[131]. At national level, the interests of the universities are looked after by statutory representation on the SHSPC and the National Consultative Committees formed by the health care professions.

National Consultative Committees (NCCs) have been established by the medical, nursing, dental, paramedical, pharmaceutical, optical, and scientific professions, and recognised by the Secretary of State for Scotland. These committees, having been formed by the professions themselves independent of all external interference, are regarded as the principal sources of advice on matters relating to professional interests. They have two main functions. They provide professional advice to the SHSPC on matters under consideration by the Council and its substructure of groups and committees, and, secondly, they advise the SHHD directly either at the request of the Department or on their own initiative[132].

Similar professional advisory committees exist at health board level. While the membership of these local committees may sometimes overlap with that of their national counterparts, the committees are not directly linked and have a different function. The area professional committees are involved in the evolution of plans for the development of services within their health board area, and boards must consult them on matters affecting their interests[133].

The interests of the public as users of the health service are, at least in theory, represented by local health councils. Since 1974 forty-eight of these councils have been set up in Scotland. Their membership is in part directly appointed by local authorities, and in part by the Health Boards from nominations received from a large number of voluntary organisations. The councils have certain prescribed rights relating to what information they may obtain from Health Boards, when they are to be consulted, and what forms of representation they may make to the boards. They were intended to be not merely a channel of criticism on existing facilities but a persuasive force for the improvement of those facilities[134]. However, from the beginning, serious doubts were expressed about the effectiveness of local health councils. For example, the *Scotsman*, in its review of the proposals outlined in the 1971 White Paper, pointed out that comparable 'consumer' bodies had 'a poor record of effectiveness'[135], while David Steel doubted in 1972 whether, in view of the limited role of the councils, 'many people will be willing to devote time, ability, and energy to them,' and argued that rather than setting up such bodies it would be better 'to concentrate on giving the Health Boards a larger democratic element.'[136] Efforts have been made to increase the effectiveness of the health councils, most notably in 1977 when the Association of Scottish Local Health Councils was set up to provide a national forum for the exchange of views and information between councils both about local health service consumer trends and about broader developments in the service which might affect them generally[137]. However, despite these measures, the effectiveness of health councils is still a subject of considerable criticism.

The National Health Service (Scotland) Act of 1972 created a new office, that of Health Service Commissioner, for the further protection of the public. The Act empowered the Commissioner to investigate complaints made against National Health Service bodies by any person who alleges that he has suffered injustice or hardship because of a failure in a service, or failure to provide a service, or in consequence of maladministration. Although there is direct access to the Commissioner, he will not normally investigate a complaint unless he is satisfied that the health service body concerned has had it brought to its notice and has had reasonable opportunity to investigate and reply to the allegations. The aim of this provision is to ensure that matters which can and should be put right promptly at local level are not unnecessarily referred to the Commissioner. Matters for which pre-existing procedures or courts of law provide appropriate means of redress, such as complaints against general medical practitioners, general dental practitioners, pharmacists, or opticians, are excluded from investigation by the Commissioner[138]. Over the years the number of complaints made under any procedure has been relatively small, but whether this is owing to public satisfaction with the service or to less happy reasons is unclear.

Another creation of the 1972 Act was the Common Services Agency (CSA), which has no equivalent in England. This agency is designed to serve both the Secretary of State for Scotland and the Health Boards, and is responsible not only for the provision of certain services for which various health service bodies were formerly responsible but also for certain functions previously carried out, either directly or through *ad hoc* bodies, by the central department. The services taken over by the CSA are those which can be provided on an all-Scotland basis. Dental estimates, pricing of prescriptions, the ambulance and blood transfusion services, and the planning, design, construction, and commissioning of health service building are all handled by the CSA. The agency has also taken over responsibility for a variety of functions, including those of the Scottish Hospital Centre, the Central Legal Office for the Hospital Service, the Scottish Hospital Staffs Committee and Nursing Staffs Committee, the Catering School, the Health Education Unit, and the Research and Intelligence Unit which had been the responsibility either of *ad hoc* bodies or, in the case of the last two named, the SHHD. Certain aspects of other important services relating to information, supplies, management services, specialised scientific support, and manpower questions were also transferred to the Agency[139].

The growing cost of health provision

The modern National Health Service makes substantial and apparently ever growing demands upon the Treasury. The total net cost of the service in Scotland for the financial year 1983–84 was £1,727 million, which, after allowing for changes in the value of money, represents a threefold increase in the cost of the service since its introduction in 1948. It is instructive to analyse current health service expenditure, such analysis being most conveniently displayed in the form of a statistical table[140].

Expenditure for the financial year 1983–84 in £millions

Hospital and Community Services		1245.9	(including 96.7 on capital projects)
General Medical Services		106.7	
General Dental Services		40.3	
Ophthalmic Services		12.2	
Pharmacological Services		159.0	
Common Services Agency		54.8	(including 8.3 on capital projects)
General Administration		61.6	
Other Services		46.5	
	Total	1727.0	

Two important points emerge from this table, firstly, the low cost of administration relative to comparable health care systems in other countries, and, secondly, the massive proportion of funds devoted to hospital and community services. It is unfortunately impossible, from the information available, to separate totally the sums of money expended on the hospital service from those spent on community services. However, it is possible to state that current expenditure on hospital services amounted to £1,046.1 million in the financial year 1983–84[141], and that those services cornered a very large percentage of the £96.7 million spent on capital projects over the same period. Thus, something like 70 *per cent* of the total National Health Service budget is allocated to hospital services. Both the central department and the health boards, who are largely responsible for allocating current expenditure in their areas, can and do exercise tight controls over hospital costs. The case is somewhat different with family practitioner services which are largely demand-determined. The independent contractor status of the general practitioner was preserved by the 1972 Act and, consequently, the level of service he provides is by and large not susceptible to administrative control. However, an important innovation designed to improve control over the cost of general medical services was introduced in 1985. Until then the drugs bill was largely determined by professional habit and public demand, although prescription charges helped to offset the gross cost and some effort was made by the central department to influence the pattern of prescribing. The introduction in 1985, after prolonged consultation, of a limited list of prescription drugs was intended to limit costs by substituting, where possible and medically acceptable, cheaper generic drugs in place of more expensive proprietary equivalents.

Manpower as the greatest element of cost

Manpower costs constitute the most important item in the National Health Service budget. The service is the largest single employer in the country, employing approximately 1 in 8 in the working population of Scotland, and it has tended, for reasons which will be explained later, to increase its manpower steadily despite the financial constraints imposed by recent national economic difficulties. The manpower characteristics of the post-reorganisation National Health Service in Scotland are shown in the table on page 139.[142]

Before analysing the service according to the categories of staff given above, two general points may be made about staffing requirements and policies. Health service staffing policies have countervailing and paradoxical tendencies, for, while narrowing specialisation promotes rigidity, technological change demands flexibility of job specification, which is not easily promoted in the face of the detailed specifications of Whitley Council and other negotiated terms and conditions of employment. The second general point is that the health service is heavily dependent on female staff. If the female labour market is slack, the service reaps enormous financial benefits not only because wage and salary levels may be kept down but also on account of the greater availability of women willing to work part-time who are employed when the work-load is heaviest and for that period only.

	1975	1980	1983
Total Staff & Practitioners	*113,143*	*123,432*	*129,344*
Medical & Dental Staff & Practitioners	*9,886*	*10,690*	*11,204*
Hospital Doctors	4,766	5,173	5,366
Consultants	1,623	1,774	1,834
General Practitioners	4,190	4,536	4,853
Nurses & Midwives	*52,540*	*58,603*	*62,396*
Qualified	24,246	28,028	32,232
In Training	11,096	12,414	12,402
Unqualified	17,198	18,160	17,762
Scientific & PSM	*2,977*	*3,858*	*4,356*
Technical	*3,775*	*4,217*	*4,390*
Works	*673*	*820*	*869*
Administrative & Clerical	*12,365*	*13,256*	*14,088*
Ancillary	*26,601*	*27,100*	*26,970*
Tradesmen	*2,486*	*2,795*	*2,889*
Pharmacists & Opticians	*371*	*447*	*487*
Ambulancemen	*1,291*	*1,646*	*1,696*
Others	*178*	–	–

N.B. Totals are given in whole time equivalents. PSM are Professions Supplementary to Medicine, e.g., radiographers and physiotherapists.

The constitutional elements of manpower
General Practitioners

The status of the general practitioner was not altered by the 1972 Act[143]. He is not an employee of the health service, but an independent contractor who has undertaken to provide an agreed range of services within it in return for various fees and allowances. The training of the general practitioner has been improved in recent years, and it is now compulsory for a doctor to have a specified period of prescribed experience in hospitals and general practice before he can become a principal in general practice. The basic role of the general medical practitioner, however, has not changed. He is based within the community and is responsible for providing primary care and advice informed by his knowledge of individual patients and the environment in which they live. The hospital consultant service provides the general practitioner with the specialist opinion and help he may require, and within the National Health Service the patient normally only has access to specialist services through his family doctor.

Hospital Doctors

Those doctors who wish to specialise in one branch of medicine and make a career in the hospital service undergo a long and rigorous training which takes them through the various junior grades of senior house officer, registrar, and senior registrar before they reach the most senior position of consultant. Not all doctors working in hospitals are employees of the National Health Service. Some general practitioners work a number of sessions each week in a hospital, or in a special unit within a hospital where patients are attended by their own family doctors, while still continuing with their practices, while in teaching hospitals associated with university medical schools, some of the medical staff are university employees who hold honorary appointments in the health service so that they may have access to patients. Hospital specialists are paid by salary according to the number of sessions they work in the service, but salaries are supplemented by a system of 'merit awards', administered by the profession, which rewards those deemed to be the most distinguished and deserving. Hospital medical staffing is controlled by the Advisory Committee on Hospital Medical Establishments, the membership of which is drawn from the Health Boards, the profession, and the central department. Numbers in the different training grades are reviewed annually in an attempt made to avoid promotion bottle-necks. The procedure has been more successful in Scotland than in England and Wales, partly because of the more manageable size of the operation in Scotland, but also partly because the honorary NHS contracts of University staff in Scotland have been included in the totals and the establishment in each grade adjusted accordingly. For some years now the senior registrar and honorary senior registrar establishment has been strictly controlled so that any doctor becoming a senior registrar can be confident of getting a consultant appointment somewhere without excessive delay. Attempts are being made to adjust the registrar establishment in the same way, but there are many conflicting factors to be taken into account and it cannot be said that attainment of registrar grade can be regarded as the *entree* to a specialty.

The Community Medicine Specialist

While the general practitioner and the hospital specialist are concerned with the treatment of individual patients, the community medicine specialist is concerned with the broad questions of health and disease in populations. Each Health Board employs community medicine specialists who, while they have particular responsibility for measures to control communicable diseases, are primarily concerned with identifying the health needs of the local population so that priorities may be established for the promotion of health, prevention of disease, and the provision of medical care. In addition to their health board duties, community medicine specialists advise local authority departments on environmental health and on health matters related to the responsibilities of education and social work departments.

The title 'community medicine' was a compromise accepted by the

Royal Commission on Medical Education[144]. In Scotland, the Joint Working Party in preparing its Report 'Doctors in an Integrated Health Service'[145] were well aware that it would take some time for the specialty, consisting as it did of former Medical Officers of Health, former hospital medical administrators, and academic and research workers in epidemiology, medical sociology and other relevant fields, to be understood, to find itself, and to make its full contribution to health care. The University Departments of Community Medicine are playing an important part in organising training courses for the specialty, and there is little doubt that, as a new generation of specialist emerges with more appropriate training, the specialty will be able to play its full part in health service planning and management as well as in health service research and epidemiology.

Dentists

Except for those few employed in health centres, general dental practitioners are independent contractors who, unlike their medical counterparts, are paid not by capitation fees but according to the number of different types of treatment they have provided for their patients. The scale of fees, which is kept under review, is intended to enable the general dental practitioner to earn a specified net income after deduction of practice expenses. Dentists who enter the hospital service after qualifying may specialise in restorative dentistry, orthodontics, or oral surgery, and have a career structure and training programme similar to that of hospital doctors. They are paid by salary as are those dental officers who provide treatment for pre-school children, children at school, pregnant women, and nursing mothers.

Pharmacists and Opticians

Although a small number of opticians and pharmacists are directly employed by health boards to provide appropriate services for hospital patients, most members of the two professions enjoy, like general medical and dental practitioners, the status of independent contractors to the National Health Service. These independent pharmacists and opticians are paid fees for the medicines, appliances, and spectacles they dispense, the scales of fees being nationally negotiated by their representative bodies.

The Nursing Staff

The nursing staff form the largest single group employed in the health service. They work not only in hospitals, but also in the community where they provide health care in the home for certain categories of non-acute patients including, principally, young children and the elderly. Aside from their traditional responsibilities, nurses, midwives, and health visitors also play a prominent role in the early detection of illness and in health education. Both within the hospital and the community, nursing has become more specialised and highly skilled in recent years, and this has increased the demands made upon the profession. For example, while the health visitor still has basic responsibility for the welfare of pre-school children, the role has now been enlarged to include, among other things, special responsibilities for the elderly.

Other Health Professionals

Of all the groups employed in the National Health Service, that of the scientists and the professions supplementary to medicine has experienced the largest percentage growth in numbers employed in recent years. Between 1975 and 1983 the number of scientists and PSMs working in the Scottish service increased by 68 *per cent*. The growth in the number of biochemists, physicists, and other scientists, medical laboratory scientific officers, medical physics technicians, and others reflects the increasing contribution made by science and technology to clinical research, diagnosis, and treatment. There have been and will continue to be arguments as to whether in certain cases the scientist should be as eligible as his medical colleagues for the role of having responsibility for the laboratory. Recent years have also seen a greater awareness of the importance of the role played by the paramedical professions and of the need to expand the services they provide. Thus, the number of occupational therapists, physiotherapists, remedial gymnasts, chiropodists, dieticians, orthoptists, speech therapists, orthodontists, prosthetists, dental hygienists, and the like, has increased quite significantly.

Administrative etc. Staff

Administrative and clerical staff, who comprise about 11 *per cent* of the total work force of the health service, undertake a large number of duties, the full range of which is not immediately apparent from their generic description. This heterogeneous group are responsible, among other things, for providing high-level management skills, supplying professional legal advice to management, acquiring and distributing equipment and supplies, administering hospitals, health centres, and clinics, paying staff salaries and bills, processing claims for payment submitted by dentists and pharmacists, providing clerical support in out-patient clinics, acting as ward clerks and relieving nurses of non-nursing duties, and supplying the specialist skills required of such functions as work study, computing, and commissioning new hospitals. In addition, a variety of specialist functions are performed by hospital wardens, press and publicity officers, and managers of catering, laundry, and domestic services, hospital sterile supply departments, and farms. However, the vast majority, over 75 *per cent*, of administrative and clerical staff are typists, personal secretaries, and clerks.

The Common Services Agency employs a number of architects, quantity surveyors, engineers, and others who play an essential part in the provision of new hospitals and other buildings and in the maintenance of existing health service properties. The Building Division of the Common Services Agency acts on behalf of the Health Boards to provide the professional and technical expertise involved in the design and management of new building projects.

Domestic and manual workers, and maintenance tradesmen are employed mainly in and around hospitals. They are the second largest group of hospital staff, and their widely varying duties include housekeeping, laundry, catering, and the maintenance of hospital equipment, buildings and grounds, as well as the operation of essential services such as heating and lighting. This grouping also includes mortuary and theatre attendants, plaster orderlies, central sterile supply department assistants, orthopaedic appliance makers, and others undertaking similar duties. Recently, the Government has encouraged Health Boards to invite external contractors to tender for these services. Competitive tendering is expected to lead to greater efficiency, but moves to 'privatise' ancillary services have met with strong opposition, particularly from the unions who claim that ancillary workers' wages will be reduced and that services will deteriorate; little has so far been achieved in Scotland.

Remuneration

With a few exceptions, most notably doctors, dentists, and tradesmen, the salaries and conditions of service of staff working in the health service are determined for the whole U.K. by a number of negotiating bodies known as Whitley Councils, all but one of which were set up in 1948. Staff are dealt with, as far as possible, in broad groups, such as nurses and midwives; professional and technical staff; administrative and clerical staff; ancillary staff and ambulance men. The wide range of work undertaken by National Health Service staff necessitated the creation of nine 'functional' Whitley Councils to settle the rates of pay and conditions of service of each of the groups. A General Whitley Council supervises the working of the 'functional' Councils and deals with certain matters of common interest to all groups, such as the application of industrial relations legislation to the National Health Service. The membership of Whitley Councils comprises representatives of the employers, central department, trade unions, and professional organisations. If both sides fail to reach agreement, recourse may be had to independent arbitration, or, exceptionally, the Secretary of State may unilaterally promulgate terms and conditions of service.

The remuneration of doctors and dentists in the National Health Service is kept under review by an independent body, appointed by the Prime Minister, whose recommendations are based upon evidence submitted by the professions and the health departments, and also upon its own enquiries into the earnings of comparable professional groups. A similar independent body, also appointed by the Prime Minister, is responsible for reviewing nurses' remuneration. Other terms and conditions of service are usually negotiated directly between the health departments and the representatives of the doctors, dentists, and nurses.

THE SERVICE SINCE 1974

No shortage of problems

The reorganised health service made possible an improved and integrated system of health care, but it had a difficult passage in its early years. A centralised service is difficult to change except by ordinances which apply throughout, and there is little opportunity for a gradual, piecemeal, or experimental approach to change. The opportunity afforded by the 1974 reorganisation was therefore seized upon to introduce a number of innovations which were not strictly related to the more clinical aspects of the service. It soon became clear, however, that the complexity and multiplicity of innovations were beyond the capacity of the service to accommodate swiftly. The result was confusion. For example, the increased emphasis on functional management in such ancillary services as engineering works, catering, supply, and personnel led to apparent conflict with the authority of unit and district administrators, and made it difficult for health workers to locate the correct decision-makers within the management structure.

A further difficulty stemmed from the determination of various interest groups within the health care professions to secure direct representation on the health service's consultative committees. The resultant consultative structure was over elaborate and unwieldy, and led to unacceptable delays in decision making. Yet more difficulties arose from the introduction of consensus management in area and district administration, for it took some time before Area and District Executive Group members learned to distinguish between those matters which were properly the responsibility of individual officers and those issues where group decisions were required. Slow as it was to prove itself, consensus management has considerable value in overriding inter-professional sensitivity and rivalry, and it should remain the essential foundation for future management systems such as those which are now being proposed in the wake of the Griffiths' report[160].

Dissatisfaction with the reorganised service also arose because of the concentration of managerial power in the hands of the Health Board officers. While reorganisation saw English hospital clinicians and general practitioners serving as full members of district management teams, Scottish clinicians on the whole shunned management responsibility, although the chairmen of area medical committees sometimes sat in on meetings of their Area Executive Groups and Health Boards. In Scotland, a nostalgic hankering after the old medical superintendent system (which was seldom praised in its day) led to community medicine specialists serving as intermediaries in general hospitals between the clinicians and the unit management.

While clinicians shied clear of full involvement in health service management, the lay members of the Health Boards were prevented from maintaining the level of their former involvement. More significant than the reduction in the number of lay members of health authorities from over 1,500 to only 276, was the instruction to board members to concern themselves not with day to day problems, but with major policy issues, strategic planning decisions, broad questions of allocation of resources, and matters of substantial interest to the community. As the power of Health Board officers increased, that of lay members contracted. In practice, lay members were restricted to the difficult task of approving policy and monitoring performance in the absence of specific objectives and measures of output, and not surprisingly many became very critical of their allotted role.

In addition to the problems arising from administrative reorganisation, there were other factors creating confusion and discontent within the service. After a period of substantial economic growth, during which the National Health Service had become accustomed to annual growth rates of between 3 *per cent* and 4 *per cent* in real terms, the British economy was plunged into recession following the Middle East oil crisis. As a result of these economic difficulties, the health service had to make do with an annual growth rate, in real terms, of just over 1.5 *per cent*, which was barely sufficient to meet the 'insidious' costs due to an ageing population and the committed expenditure on existing services. While economic expansion first slowed and then, in the mid-1970s, came to a virtual halt, the financial and professional expectations engendered by the prosperous 1960s remained high. The National Health Service found itself unable to satisfy the demands of some health workers for greater professional status and higher pay, and, as frustration increased among its staff, the rather rudimentary industrial relations skills of the service proved incapable of preventing conflict. The growing unrest was made evident by the expansion of trade union membership amongst professional and white collar workers, and by the increasing militancy of formerly quiescent employees, such as the junior hospital doctors who went on strike in 1975[146].

The Royal Commission

As a result of this turbulence, anxiety about the well-being of the National Health Service grew, and in 1976 a Royal Commission was appointed under the chairmanship of Sir Alec Merrison 'to consider in the interests both of the patients and of those who work in the National Health Service the best use and management of the financial and manpower resources of the National Health Service.'[147] Throughout the period of the Royal Commission's investigations and deliberations, criticism of the service mounted. Much of this criticism was well founded. The Royal College of Physicians of Edinburgh, in its memorandum of evidence to the Commission, argued that the service's management structure was top-heavy, that the district tier of administration should be abolished so as to promote direct contact between area boards and the units providing clinical care, and that the service's committee structure was 'extravagant of time, energy and money'[148]. Similar submissions were made by other witnesses, such as, for example, the South-Eastern District (Greater Glasgow) Local Health Council which contended that there were 'too many time consuming committees and overlapping functions which delay decision-making even on minor issues'[149]. Some of the criticism, however, which was levelled at the service was quite unjustified. As W.P. Blyth, the former chairman of the Argyll and Clyde Health Board, put it,

> "The public are rarely given the true or fair picture of the National Health Service in Scotland. The picture usually painted by the 'popular' media, aided and abetted by some members of the medical profession, applies mainly to England where the position is not the same... The vast and overwhelming majority of the criticism of the reorganisation of the Health Service has emanated from the English three-tier system – Regional, Area and District".

Blyth concluded that 'despite all the problems which face the Health Service, it is *not* falling apart at the seams'[150].

This was a verdict with which the Royal Commission agreed. In their report, which was published on 18 July 1979, Sir Alec Merrison and his colleagues passed an emphatic vote of confidence in the National Health Service, rejecting alarmist claims that it was suffering from 'a mortal disease susceptible only to heroic surgery'[151]. Nevertheless, the Royal Commission found that certain improvements were desirable. While some of its recommendations, such as those calling for the abolition of health service charges and the introduction of the option of a salaried general practitioner service, were not taken up, others were acted upon.

The following years saw the introduction of a 'limited list' of prescription drugs, the trimming of functional management, the reconstruction of the advisory committee structure so as to make it less unwieldy and more responsive, and the development of improved information systems for health service planning and management.

Major developments

Reorganisation, despite the difficulties which followed in its wake, allowed a more purposeful and better informed approach to policy-making than had previously been possible, and undoubtedly facilitated some major developments in the Scottish health service, most notably in regard to planning and the location of resources among Health Boards of greatly varying size. In 1977 a Scottish Home and Health Department working party issued a report recommending that the allocation of revenue resources to Health Boards should be decided according to a formula involving the use of weighted area populations modified by reference to cross-boundary flow of patients and the services provided by the four Health Boards with teaching hospitals[152]. This working party had been set up in 1976, the same year as the Scottish Home and Health Department issued a discussion document entitled *The Way Ahead* which outlined the priorities of the Scottish health service for the first time[153]. This was a timely production, for it had become clear, as financial stringency had driven home the lesson that demand for health care was always liable to outstrip supply, that health service planning had formerly owed too much to individual advocacy and influence and would in future require to be formulated according to objective criteria. The priorities advocated in *The Way Ahead* anticipated those called for by the Scottish Health Service Planning Council's Health Priorities Working Party in its report which was published in 1980. *Priorities for the Eighties*, as the report was called, recommended three levels of priorities for the Scottish Health Service. The first priorities were preventive services, health services for the multiply deprived, community nursing, care of the elderly, care of the elderly suffering from mental disability, the mentally ill, the mentally handicapped, and the physically handicapped. The second level priorities were primary dental services, the maternity services, the general medical service, and the general ophthalmic service, while child health, the acute hospital services, and the general pharmaceutical service were nominated as third level priorities[154].

The major thrust of *The Way Ahead* and *Priorities for the Eighties* was away from the acute hospital services and towards increased provision for community care and long-term services for the elderly and the mentally disordered. It has, however, proved easier to state objectives than to achieve them. Some progress has been made in building up geriatric services, but little has been achieved in the way of improving services for the mentally disordered. This lack of success is in part owing to the severe financial constraints imposed upon the service in recent years, but it owes something also to the vigorous defence mounted on behalf of the prestigious acute hospital service. Health Boards have encountered great difficulties in closing hospital facilities in the face of determined and well-organised public opposition. Unless more funds are made available to the Health Boards or the public come to accept that resources should be transferred from acute hospital services to finance the expansion of community and long-stay services, it seems clear that progress towards the goals set by *Priorities for the Eighties* will continue to be unacceptably slow.

Economic concerns and managerial responsibilities

While the mounting costs of medical care have created concern in many developed countries, that concern has become particularly acute in a Britain which has experienced increasing economic difficulties and has been in relative economic decline for some decades. The National Health Service in the United Kingdom now accounts for about a tenth of national expenditure. Its real costs have risen by over 300 *per cent* since its inception in 1948, and its share of Gross National Product has increased from 3.92 *per cent* in 1949 to 6.20 *per cent* in 1984[155]. The Scottish health service, which is relatively better financed than the service in the rest of the United Kingdom, consumed 15.4 *per cent* of identifiable public expenditure in Scotland and 8.1 *per cent* of the country's Gross National Product in the financial year 1982–83[156]. Experience has therefore disproved the theory, popular in 1948, that the National Health Service would so improve the nation's health as to lower demand for medical care and thus reduce the cost of providing that care. The growing health care needs of an ageing population, the increase in remuneration of health service personnel due in large measure to a movement towards equal pay for women and increased unionisation, the introduction of new technologies involving higher capital and running costs, the expansion in the number of doctors and dentists per 1,000 of population, and greater public expectations of health have all contributed to the apparently remorseless increase in the cost of the National Health Service[157]. This ever increasing cost has, in a Britain beset with economic difficulties, led to attention being focused on a search for savings to be obtained from better and more efficient planning and management of the health service.

As far back as 1956, the Guillebaud Committee's report revealed the potentially unlimited demand for health care and the necessity of containing that demand within a finite budget[158]. Following this report, various management skills, such as 'work study' and 'organisation and method,' were developed in an effort to promote efficiency. In more recent years the increasing financial constraints upon the National Health Service have intensified the search for savings deriving from improved management which would fund desirable, but otherwise unaffordable, new developments. The 1974 reorganisation in England was aimed principally at improving the management of the health service[159], and a similar objective lay behind the 1983 Griffiths' Report to the English Minister of Health[160]. The principles of this report were adopted by the Government in Scotland, and in 1984 the Secretary of State issued a consultative paper proposing the appointment of General Managers at both Health Board and Unit level[161].

There has been a tendency for doctors in the National Health Service to lose contact with and interest in the financial implications of their actions. Before 1948, most specialists were made well aware of these implications by their experience both in private practice and in voluntary hospitals where limited funding required that every penny be counted. Doctors who came into the National Health Service from that background continued to be cost-conscious (sometimes to a fault), but the succeeding generation never experienced the discipline of working in the old voluntary hospitals, and were inclined to be motivated by the therapeutic imperative, i.e. that whatever seemed to offer some improvement in diagnosis or treatment should necessarily be provided[162]. The current intention is to restore, in a somewhat more positive way, the former connection in medicine between care and cost by bringing clinicians into a financial relationship with their work through a system of budgeting at clinical unit level. Much of the success of the new management arrangements will depend upon whether this can be achieved. Various attempts have been made in the past with little success, but the application of computer technology makes it more likely that financial and clinical data can now be combined satisfactorily at clinical unit level.

The introduction of health service General Managers reflects a governmental preoccupation with the analogies of industrial line management, where decisions at the centre are carried down the line to a subordinate and unquestioning point of performance on the production line. The analogy with the health service is, however, far from satisfactory. Higher management can determine the allocation of resources and influence priorities, but the product, *viz.* patient care, is decided and delivered by high prestige workers in the treatment and caring professions who cherish their traditional freedoms. The challenge facing the post-Griffiths' health service is to find measures of productivity combined, by means of clinical audit, with measures of quality and effectiveness which will be acceptable to management and the health care professions[163]. In facing this challenge, however, there is a serious risk of becoming pre-occupied with the minutiae of management and financial control. So far the health service in Scotland, unlike its counterpart in England, has been largely concerned with maximising the effectiveness of the acute treatment and caring services rather than with strengthening managerial control in order to minimise the costs of these services. It would be sad indeed if the National Health Services in Scotland lost sight of its old goal.

A Crisis in the National Health Service?

Over the last decade and more, there has been much written, especially in the popular press, about crises or even *the crisis* in the National Health Service. More often than not, however, these reports are based on particular events which are alleged to have taken place in England, the relevance of which to the Scottish health service has not always been accurately construed by the press. Perhaps surprisingly, the public's confidence in the health service does not seem to have been shaken by this plague of sensationalist and alarmist reports. Various opinion polls, including those commissioned by the Royal Commission on the National Health Service[164], have consistently reported high levels of public satisfaction with the services provided by both hospitals and general practitioners. It may be objected that, as similar opinion polls in other countries have resulted in similar findings, there is a tendency for the public to support the health care system with which they are familiar, but it is surely of some significance that relatively few complaints about the National Health Service have been received by the Health Boards and the health service Commissioner.

Clearly, however, all is not well with the National Health Service in Scotland. The problem of community participation, as we have seen, still awaits resolution, as does that of co-operation between local authorities and the health service. This latter problem is still one of great importance despite the removal of certain health functions from local authorities following reorganisation in 1974. Local authorities are responsible for a wide range of services which bear directly on the health of the population, including the control of communicable diseases and atmospheric pollution, food hygiene, housing, water supplies, and sewage disposal, and there are also close links between the local authorities' social work services provided by the Health Boards. That the general relationship between local authorities and Health Boards following reorganisation was somewhat less than satisfactory was strongly suggested by the report in 1977 of a working party which recommended the establishment of a national body and local liaison committees to advise on the planning and operation of services of joint concern[165]. While the national body recommended in 1977 has not as yet been set up, many efforts have been made to improve co-operation. Joint Liaison Committees have been set up with representatives of the Health Board meeting members of the Regional and District Authorities to discuss matters affecting health and social work. Nevertheless, much more still requires to be done. For example, some patients are being kept in hospital simply because there is no support available to look after them in the community, others who should really be in hospital are being cared for in the community because hospital beds are not available, and others still are being discharged from hospital before proper arrangements are made for home support. Greater co-operation between local authorities and the health service, however, cannot of itself solve all these problems. Community care is not an inexpensive option, and substantial resources will have to be made available to improve Scotland's social services if it is to be implemented properly.

CONCLUSION

Ageing

The problems facing the health service in Scotland have been, and still are, immense. As is the case throughout the developed world, one of the most important of these problems has been that of an ageing population. The number of people aged sixty-five and over has risen every decade since 1901 and had tripled by 1981. However, until the Second World War the age distribution of the population aged sixty-five and over remained stable. From 1951 it became increasingly more elderly, with the number of Scots over eighty years of age doubling between 1951 and 1981[166]. Thus, the National Health Service was introduced just at the time when the proportion of the very old in the population was beginning to grow. Making provision for the increasing number of the elderly is a major problem not only because of the greater liability of older people to suffer chronic illnesses and to lose domestic support, but also because some of today's costly technological developments such as hip joint replacements create new demands on the service. It has been calculated that the average elderly person over seventy-five is eight times more demanding on the National Health Service than the average adult in middle life[167].

Vital Statistics

Many of the problems confronting the National Health Service in Scotland cannot, however, be attributed simply to the ageing of the population. The health service in Scotland has to provide for a population with a greater volume of ill-health, as evidenced by mortality rates, than most other parts of the United Kingdom or Western Europe. Death rates from coronary heart disease, cancer and strokes, the three main causes of death, are among the highest in Western Europe, while expectation of life at birth for both male and female Scots is among the lowest[168]. This unhappy state of affairs is in large measure owing to the unhealthy lifestyle of the Scottish people. The nation has a most unenviable record in relation to poor diet, cigarette smoking, and alcohol abuse. Moreover, the health problems attributable to this record have undoubtedly been exacerbated by a standard of housing which is among the worst in the United Kingdom and probably also Europe. A report published by the Department of the Environment in 1976 showed that the situation in Scotland generally, and Clydeside particularly, was very much worse than in other parts of the United Kingdom in relation to overcrowding and lack of exclusive use of household amenities, such as water closet and bath[169].

Positive improvements

Faced with these problems, the National Health Service's most notable contributions to the health of the population have been the steady expansion of a specialist hospital service, and, after initial faltering, the strengthening of general practice as the essential foundation of the health care system. There have been some improvements in the field of tertiary and secondary prevention, most notably in the antenatal and child health surveillance services, while the way to possible further improvements through close collaboration between the hospital and community services has been pointed out by interesting pilot studies carried out under the auspices of the Royal College of Physicians of Edinburgh and by far-sighted reports from the Royal College of General Practitioners.

Prevention

Despite the fact that health promotion offers the most likely means of the National Health Service effecting a beneficial and radical change in the lifestyle of the population, and despite the fact also that health promotion and prevention of disease are the first of the stated objectives of the service, they have received relatively little attention. Prevention is, however, becoming a higher priority, as shown by the Department of Health and Social Security and the Scottish Home and Health Department's publication in 1976 of a booklet entitled *Prevention and Health: Everybody's Business*[170]. The increased interest in, and support for, health education is perhaps the most obvious sign of the growing recognition of the importance of prevention. The identification of cigarette smoking as the biggest avoidable health hazard and the discovery that Scotland spends more on tobacco per household than any other part of Britain led to a health education campaign to persuade people to stop smoking. This campaign provided a stimulus to further endeavours, for example, in regard to alcohol-related problems, and most recently to a more positive approach to health education stressing the benefits of an active, healthy lifestyle. The results of these campaigns, while hardly giving grounds for unrestrained joy, are on the whole encouraging. While the situation in regard to alcohol abuse has deteriorated throughout the United Kingdom in recent years, the situation in regard to cigarette smoking has been improving slowly in Scotland, although it is still worse than in other parts of the United Kingdom[171]. There is, perhaps most encouragingly, clear evidence of growing public interest in and knowledge of the health benefits of good diet and exercise. It is perhaps doubtful, however, if much more can be achieved in preventive measures without the general public becoming more involved in the priorities and politics of health.

A case for local involvement?

The Royal Commission on Local Government made an excellent case for transferring responsibility for the health service to the reorganised local authorities, and, having made it, dropped it, just as Aneurin Bevan had dropped it over thirty years earlier. There are major obstacles to the democratisation of the health service, most notably the medical profession which is probably as hostile now as it was in 1946. Yet especially if the way forward for health care in Scotland lies in the direction of a fundamental change of emphasis from institutional care to community care with all that that implies for individuals and families, some way must surely be found in future to generate effective local involvement in the health service.

References

(1)   National Health Service (Scotland) Act, 1947. 10 & 11 Geo.6. Ch.27. Part 1 Section 1, Sub-Section 1.
(2)   *Ibid*, Part I, Section 2, Sub-Section 1.
(3)   *Ibid*, Part II, Section 11, Sub-Sections 1 and 2, and Fourth Schedule, Part 1.
(4)   *Ibid*, Part II, Section 11, Sub-Section 3, and Fourth Schedule, Part 2.
(5)   *Ibid*, Part II, Section 11, Sub-Section 4.
(6)   *Ibid*, Part II, Section 11, Sub-Section 5, and Fourth Schedule, Part 3.
(7)   *Ibid*, Part III, Section 20, Sub-Section 2.
(8)   *Ibid*, Part III, Section 20, Sub-Section 8.
(9)   *Ibid*, Part IV, Sections 32–37, and Sixth Schedule.
(10) Ross, J.S. *The National Health Service in Great Britain. An Historical and Descriptive Study.* (Oxford, 1952), p.120.
(11) Department of Health for Scotland. *Scottish Health Statistics 1958.* (Edinburgh 1959), Section XI, Table 2, p.189. The figures are for the financial year 1948/9.
(12) *The Glasgow Herald*, Monday 5 July 1948, p.2, col.A.
(13) *The Scotsman*, Saturday, 3 July 1948, p.4, col.A.
(14) *The Glasgow Herald*, Monday, 5 July 1948, p.2, col.A.
(15) *Ibid*.

(16)   *The Scotsman*, Saturday, 3 July 1948, p.4, col.A.

(17)   *The Scotsman*, Monday, 5 July 1948, p.5, col.C.

(18)   *The Glasgow Herald*, Tuesday, 6 July 1948, p.3, col.D

(19)   *The Glasgow Herald*, Monday, 5 July 1948, p.2, cols.C&D.

(20)   *The Glasgow Herald*, Wednesday, 21 July 1948, p.4, cols.C&D.

(21)   *Report of the Department of Health for Scotland for the year 1948*. Cmd.7659. (Edinburgh, 1949), p.32.

(22)   *The Scotsman*, Saturday, 1 October 1949, p.6, col.G.

(23)   *Ibid*, p.6, cols.A&B.

(24)   *The Scotsman*, Saturday, 15 October 1949, p.8, col.G.

(25)   *Parliamentary Debates*, Fifth Series. Volume 468, col.1019.

(26)   *Parliamentary Debates*. Fifth Series. Volume 470, col.A.

(27)   *Ibid*, col.2263.

(28)   *The Glasgow Herald*, Tuesday, 28 November 1950, p.4, col.A.

(29)   *The Glasgow Herald*, Monday, 25 December 1950, p.5, cols.F&G.

(30)   *Parliamentary Debates*. Fifth Series. Volume 486, cols.851–852. *The Scotsman*, Wednesday, 11 April 1951, p.6, col.B.

(31)   *The Glasgow Herald*, Wednesday, 11 April 1951, p.4, col.A.

(32)   *The Glasgow Herald*, Saturday, 30 September 1950, p.5, col.G. *The Glasgow Herald*, Wednesday, 11 April 1951, p.5, col.D.

(33)   *The Scotsman*, Wednesday 11 April 1951, p.9, col.F.

(34)   *Ibid*.

(35)   Foot, M. *Aneurin Bevan. A Biography. Volume Two: 1945–1960*. (London, 1973), pp.317–339. Harris, K. *Attlee* (London, 1982), pp.473–480.

(36)   *The Glasgow Herald*, Saturday, 28 April 1951, p.5, col.F.

(37)   *Parliamentary Debates*. Fifth Series. Volume 487, cols.1314–1315, 1372–1376

(38)   *Parliamentary Debates*. Fifth Series. Volume 495, cols.54–55. *The Glasgow Herald*, Saturday, 2 February 1952, p.5, col.G.

(39)   *The Glasgow Herald*, Wednesday, 30 January 1952, p.4, col.A.

(40)   *The Scotsman*, Saturday, 2 February 1952, p.6, col.A.

(41)   *The Scotsman*, Wednesday, 30 January 1952, p.6, col.A.

(42)   *The Glasgow Herald*, Wednesday, 20 February 1952, p.5, col.E.

(43)   *The Glasgow Herald*, Saturday, 31 May 1952, p.5, col.C.

(44)   Scottish Home and Health Department. *Health Services in Scotland. Report for 1974*. Cmnd.6052. (Edinburgh, 1975), p.17. *Report of the Department of Health for Scotland and of the Scottish Health Service Council 1949*. Cmd.7921. (Edinburgh, 1950), p.109.

(45)   Scottish Home and Health Department. *Health Services in Scotland. Report for 1974*. Cmnd.6052. (Edinburgh, 1975), p.15.

(46)   Scottish Health for Scotland. *Hospital Plan for Scotland*. Cmnd.1602. (Edinburgh, 1962), p.12.

(47)   *Ibid*, pp.20–22.

(48)   *Ibid*, pp.19–20.

(49)   *The Glasgow Herald*, Wednesday, 24 January 1962, p.8, col.B.

(50)   *Ibid*.

(51)   *The Scotsman*, Wednesday, 24 January 1962, p.8, col.B.

(52)   *Royal Commission on the National Health Service. Report*. Cmnd.7615. (London, 1979), pp.140–142.

(53)   *Scottish Home and Health Department. Health Services in Scotland. Report for 1974*. Cmnd.6052. (Edinburgh, 1975), p.17–18.

(54)   *The Glasgow Herald*, Saturday, 30 September 1950, p.4, col.B.

(55)   *The Report of the Department of Health for Scotland and of the Scottish Health Services Council 1949*. Cmd.7921. (Edinburgh, 1950), pp.16–18. *Reports of the Department of Health for Scotland and the Scottish Health Services Council 1952*. Cmd.8799. (Edinburgh, 1953), pp.18–20.

(56)   *Report of the Department of Health for Scotland and of the year 1948*. Cmd.7659, pp.14–15.

Report of the Department of Health for Scotland and of the Scottish Health Services Council 1949. Cmd.7921. (Edinburgh, 1950), pp.18.

(57)   Scottish Home and Health Department. *Health and Welfare Services in Scotland Report for 1965.* Cmnd.2984. (Edinburgh, 1966), p.45.

(58)   *Reports of the Department of Health for Scotland and the Scottish Health Services Council 1953.* Cmd.9107. (Edinburgh, 1954), p.32.

(59)   Scottish Home and Health Department. *Health and Welfare Services in Scotland Report for 1965.* Cmnd.2984. (Edinburgh, 1966), p.59. Scottish Home and Health Department. *Health Services in Scotland Report for 1974.* Cmnd. 6052. (Edinburgh, 1975), p.52.

(60)   Scottish Home and Health Department. *Health in Scotland 1983.* (Edinburgh, 1984), p.18.

(61)   Duncan, A.H. ed. The Livingston Project—The First Five Years. *Scottish Health Service Studies, no.29.* (Edinburgh, Scottish Home and Health Department, 1973). Munro, H.D.R. ed. The Livingston Scheme: A Ten Year Review. *Scottish Health Service Studies, no.43.* (Edinburgh, Scottish Home and Health Department, 1982).

(62)   *Report of the Department of Health for Scotland and of the Scottish Health Services Council 1949.* Cmd.7921. (Edinburgh, 1950), p.10.

(63)   *Report of the Department of Health for Scotland and the Scottish Health Services Council 1951.* Cmd.8496. (Edinburgh, 1952), p.17.

(64)   *Report of the Department of Health for Scotland 1957.* Cmd.385. (Edinburgh, 1958), p.35.

(65)   *Report of the Department of Health for Scotland 1956.* Cmd.140. (Edinburgh, 1957), p.30.

(66)   *Ibid,* p.113.

(67)   *Reports of the Department of Health for Scotland and the Scottish Health Services Council 1955.* Cmd.9742. (Edinburgh, 1956), p.50.

(68)   Scottish Home and Health Department. *Health in Scotland 1983.* (Edinburgh, 1984), p.36.

(69)   Scottish Home and Health Department. *Health Services in Scotland Report for 1975.* Cmnd.6506. (Edinburgh, 1976), p.15–18.

(70)   Scottish Home and Health Department. *Health and Welfare Services in Scotland Report for 1964.* Cmnd.2700. (Edinburgh, 1965), p.9. Scottish Home and Health Department. Scottish Health Services Council. *Health Services in Scotland Reports for 1969.* Cmnd.4392. (Edinburgh, 1970), p.13–14.

(71)   *The Scotsman,* Thursday, 6 October 1949, p.7, col.E.

(72)   Scottish Development Department. *Scottish Housing in 1965 by J.B. Cullingworth.* (Edinburgh, 1967), pp.7,9.

(73)   Harvie, C. *No Gods and Precious Few Heroes. Scotland 1914–1980.* (London, 1981), p.155.

(74)   Adams, I.H. *The Making of Urban Scotland.* (London, 1978), p.231.

(75)   *Ibid,* p.181.

(76)   *Ibid,* p.233.

(77)   Scottish Education Department. Scottish Home and Health Department. *Social Work and the Community. Proposals for reorganising local authority services in Scotland.* Cmnd.3065. (Edinburgh, 1966), pp.10–11. Social Work (Scotland) Act, 1968. 16 & 17 Eliz.2. Ch.49. Section 1, Sub-Section 4.

(78)   *Report of the Department of Health for Scotland and of the Scottish Health Services Council 1949.* Cmd.7921. (Edinburgh, 1950), p.40. *Report of the Department of Health for Scotland and the Scottish Health Services Council 1950.* Cmd.8184. (Edinburgh, 1951), p.45.

(79)   *Report of the Department of Health for Scotland and of the Scottish Health Services Council 1949.* Cmd.7921. (Edinburgh, 1950), p.40–41.

(80)   *Report of the Department of Health for Scotland and the Scottish Health Services Council 1950.* Cmd.8184. (Edinburgh, 1951), pp.46–47.

(81)   *Report of the Department of Health for Scotland and the Scottish Health Services Council 1955.* Cmd.9742. (Edinburgh, 1956), p.11.

(82)   *Report of the Department of Health for Scotland 1960. Part 1. Health and Welfare Services.*

Cmd.1320. (Edinburgh, 1961), p.73.

(83) *Ibid*, p.74.

(84) Ministry of Health. Scottish Home and Health Department. *Report of the Committee on Senior Nursing Staff Structure.* (London, 1966). Department of Health and Social Security. Scottish Home and Health Department. Welsh Office. *Report of the Working Party on Management Structure in the Local Authority Nursing Services.* (London, 1969).

(85) Department of Health and Social Security. Scottish Home and Health Department. Welsh Office. *Report of the Committee on Nursing.* Cmnd.5115. (London, 1972).

(86) *Report of the Royal Commission on Medical Education 1965–1968.* Cmnd.3569. (London, 1968), pp.80–81.

(87) Scottish Home and Health Department. Scottish Health Service Council. *Health Services in Scotland Reports for 1970.* Cmnd. 4667. (Edinburgh, 1971), p.36.

(88) *Reports of the Department of Health for Scotland and the Scottish Health Services Council 1950.* Cmd.8184. (Edinburgh, 1951), pp.16–17.

(89) *Reports of the Department of Health for Scotland and the Scottish Health Services Council 1953.* Cmd.9107. (Edinburgh, 1954), p.21.

(90) *A Framework for Government Research and Development.* Cmnd.4814. (London, 1971).

(91) Scottish Home and Health Department. *Health Services in Scotland Report for 1974.* Cmnd.6052. (Edinburgh, 1975), pp.9–10.

(92) Scottish Home and Health Department. *Health and Welfare Services in Scotland for 1965.* Cmnd.2984. (Edinburgh, 1966), p.24.

(93) *Ibid*, p.64.

(94) Scottish Home and Health Department. Scottish Health Services Council. *Health Services in Scotland Reports for 1970.* Cmnd.4667. (Edinburgh, 1971), pp.67–69.

(95) Scottish Home and Health Department. Scottish Health Services Council. *Health Services in Scotland Reports for 1972.* Cmnd.5323. (Edinburgh, 1973), p.97.

(96) Scottish Home and Health Department. *Health in Scotland 1983.* (Edinburgh, 1984), p.21.

(97) *Report of the Department of Health for Scotland 1960. Part 1. Health and Welfare Services.* Cmd.1320. (Edinburgh, 1961), pp.31–38.

(98) Too many communications to list..

(99) Scottish Home and Health Department. *A Report on an Inquiry into Maternal Deaths in Scotland, 1965–1971.* (Edinburgh, 1974).

(100) McIlwaine, G.M., Howat, R.C.L., Dunn, F., and Macnaughton, M.C. Scottish Perinatal Mortality Review 1979. *Health bulletin*, Volume 39, No 1 (January, 1981), pp.39–44.

(101) Scottish Home and Health Department. Scottish Health Services Council. *Health Services in Scotland 1969.* Cmnd.4392. (Edinburgh, 1970), p.79.

(102) *Scottish Health Statistics 1983.* (Edinburgh, 1984), pp.51,53.

(103) Scottish Home and Health Department. Scottish Health Services Council. *Health Services in Scotland Reports for 1970.* Cmnd.4667. (Edinburgh, 1971), p.28.

(104) Ministry of Health. The Central Health Services Council and the Scottish Health Services Council. *Health Education. Report of a Joint Committee of the Central and Scottish Health Services Councils. (London, 1964).*

(105) Scottish Home and Health Department. *Health and Welfare Services in Scotland Report for 1968.* Cmnd.4012, (Edinburgh, 1969), p.55.

(106) Scottish Home and Health Department. *Health in Scotland 1980. (Edinburgh, 1981), pp.6–7,* 27–28.

(107) *A Review of the Medical Services in Great Britain. The Report of the Medical Services Review Committee.* (London, 1962), p.162.

(108) Scottish Home and Health Department. *Health and Welfare Services in Scotland Report for 1967.* Cmnd.3608. (Edinburgh, 1968), pl.

(109) Scottish Home and Health Department. *Health and Welfare Services in Scotland Report for 1968.* Cmnd.4012. (Edinburgh, 1969), p.2.

(110) *The Glasgow Herald*, Friday, 13 December 1968, p.24, col.C.

(111) *The Glasgow Herald,* Wednesday, 18 December 1968, p.9, col.E.

(112) *The Glasgow Herald,* Friday, 13 December 1968, p.1, col.D., and p.24, col.C

(113) *The Scotsman,* Friday, 13 December 1968, p.7, col.G&H.

(114) *The Scotsman,* Friday, 13 December 1968, p.12, col.A&B.

(115) *Royal Commission on Local Government in Scotland 1966–1969. Chairman: The Rt. Hon. Lord Wheatley. Report.* Cmnd.4150. (Edinburgh, 1969), pp.127–130.

(116) Scottish Home and Health Department. Scottish Health Services Council. *Health Services in Scotland Reports for 1970.* Cmnd.4667. (Edinburgh, 1971), p.1.

(117) *Parliamentary Debates. House of Commons Official Report. Standing Committees. Session 1971–72.* Volume XIII. Scottish Grand Committee. National Health Service (Scotland) Bill (Lords), 2 and 4 May 1972, Cols.20–77. For the views of the Scottish Leadership of the Labour Party on this issue, see the comments of William Ross and Bruce Millan, IBID, cols.20–21, 89–90.

(118) Scottish Home and Health Department. Scottish Health Services Council. *Health Services in Scotland Reports for 1969.* Cmnd.4392. (Edinburgh, 1970), p.98.

(119) *Parliamentary Debates. House of Commons Official Report. Standing Committees. Session 1971–72.* Volume XIII. Scottish Grand Committee. National Health Service (Scotland) Bill (Lords), 2 May 1972, Cols.33 and 15.

(120) National Health Service (Scotland) Act 1972. 20 & 21. Eliz.2.Ch. 58, Part I, Section 1, Sub-Section 1.

(121) National Health Service (Scotland) Act 1972. 20 & 21. Eliz.2.Ch. 58, Part II, Section 13, and Schedule 1, Part 1.

(122) Scottish Home and Health Department. Scottish Health Services Council. *Health Services in Scotland Reports for 1972.* Cmnd.5323. (Edinburgh, 1973), pp.5–6.

(123) *Doctors in an Integrated Health Service. Report of a Joint Working Party appointed by the Secretary of State for Scotland.* (Edinburgh, 1971). *Nurses in an Integrated Health Service. Report of a Working Group.* (Edinburgh, 1972). *Community Medicine in Scotland. Joint Working Party on the Integration of Medical Work. Report of a Sub-Group on Community Medicine.* (Edinburgh, 1973). *General Practitioners in the Hospital Service. Joint Working Party on the Integration of Medical Work. Report of a Sub-Group on General Practitioners in Hospital Service.* (Edinburgh, 1973). Towards an Integrated Child Health Service. Joint Working Party on the Integration of Medical Work. Report of a Sub-Group on the Child Health Service. (Edinburgh, 1973). *Organisation of a Medical Advisory Structure. Joint Working Party on the Integration of Medical Work. Report of a Sub-Group on Medical Organisation.* (Edinburgh, 1973). *Maternity Services: Integration of Maternity Work. A Joint Sub-Committee of the Standing Nursing and Midwifery Advisory Committee and the Standing Medical Advisory Committee of the Scottish Health Services Council.* (Edinburgh, 1973).

(124) Pendreigh, D. *The National Health Service in Scotland.* (Typescript, Usher Institute, University of Edinburgh, 1982), p.6. Scottish Home and Health Department. *Health Services in Scotland Report for 1974.* Cmnd.6052. (Edinburgh, 1975), p.9.

(125) National Health Service (Scotland) Act 1972. 20 × 21. Eliz.2.Ch.58, Sections 17 and 18.

(126) Scottish Home and Health Department. Scottish Health Service Council. *Health Services in Scotland Reports for 1972.* Cmnd.5323. (Edinburgh, 1973), pp.2–3.

(127) National Health Service (Scotland) Act 1972. 20 × 21. Eliz.2.Ch.58, Schedule 2.

(128) Scottish Home and Health Department. *Health Services in Scotland Report for 1974.* Cmnd.6052. (Edinburgh, 1975), p.8.

(129) Pendreigh, D. *The National Health Service in Scotland.* (Typescript, Usher Institute, University of Edinburgh, 1982), p.6. Scottish Home and Health Department. *The National Health Services and the Community in Scotland.* (Edinburgh, 1974), pp.4–5.

(130) Scottish Home and Health Department. *Health Services in Scotland Report for 1974.* Cmnd.6052. (Edinburgh, 1975), pp.4–5.

(131) National Health Service (Scotland) Act 1972. 20 × 21. Eliz.2.Ch.58, Section 15 and Schedule 1, Part II.

(132) *Ibid*, Section 18. Scottish Home and Health Department. *Health Services in Scotland Report for 1974.* Cmnd.6052. (Edinburgh, 1975), pp.8–9.

(133) National Health Service (Scotland) Act 1972. 20 × 21. Eliz.2.Ch.58, Section 16.

(134) *Ibid*, Section 14. Scottish Home and Health Department. *Health Services in Scotland Report for 1974.* Cmnd.6052. (Edinburgh, 1975), p.7.

(135) *The Scotsman*, Friday, 30 July 1971, p.10, cols.A&B.

(136) *Parliamentary Debates. House of Commons Official Report. Standing Committees. Session 1971–72.* Volume XIII. Scottish Grand Committee. National Health Service (Scotland) Bill (Lords), 2 May, 1972, Cols.33–34.

(137) Scottish Home and Health Department. *Health Services in Scotland Report for 1977.* Cmnd.7237. (Edinburgh, 1978), p.32.

(138) National Health Service (Scotland) Act 1972. 20 × 21. Eliz.2.Ch.58, Sections 42–48.

(139) *Ibid*, Section 19. Scottish Home and Health Department. *Health Services in Scotland Report for 1972.* Cmnd.5323. (Edinburgh, 1973), pp3–5. Scottish Home and Health Department. *Health Services in Scotland Report for 1974.* Cmnd.6052. (Edinburgh, 1975), Appendix B.

(140) *Scottish Health Statistics 1983.* (Edinburgh, 1984), pp.123–126.

(141) *Ibid*, p.124.

(142) *Ibid*, pp.100,112.

(143) The whole section on manpower is based upon *The National Health Service in Scotland 1948–1978*, pp.12–17. This booklet was produced by the Scottish Home and Health Department to mark the thirtieth anniversary of the National Health Service.

(144) *Royal Commission on Medical Education 1965–1968. Report.* Cmnd.3569. (London, 1968), pp.66–69.

(145) Scottish Home and Health Department. *Doctors in an Integrated Health Service. Report of a Joint Working Party appointed by the Secretary of State for Scotland.* (Edinburgh, 1971), pp.31–40.

(146) *Royal Commission on the National Health Service. Report.* Cmnd.7615. (London, 1979), pp.160–164.

(147) *Ibid*, p.1.

(148) *The Scotsman*, Thursday, 10 March 1977, p.9, cols.F&G.

(149) *The Scotsman*, Friday, 4 February 1977, p.9, col.G.

(150) *The Scotsman*, Friday, 16 March 1979, p.7, cols.F&G.

(151) *Royal Commission on the National Health Service. Report.* Cmnd.7615. (London, 1979). p.355.

(152) *The Scottish Health Authorities Revenue Equalisation (S.H.A.R.E.). Report of the Working Party on Revenue Resource Allocation.* (Edinburgh, 1977).

(153) Scottish Home and Health Department. *The Health Service in Scotland: The Way Ahead.* (Edinburgh, 1976).

(154) Scottish Home and Health Department. *Scottish Health Authorities Priorities for the Eighties. A Report by the Scottish Health Service Planning Council.* (Edinburgh, 1980), pp.72–73.

(155) Office of Health Economics. *Compendium of Health Statistics.* 5th Edition, 1984, Table 2.

(156) *Scottish Health Statistics 1983.* (Edinburgh, 1984), p.123.

(157) Abel Smith, B. Cost Containment in 12 European Countries, in *World Health Statistics Quarterly*, Volume 37, No. 4, (1984), p.352.

(158) *Report of the Committee of Enquiry into the Cost of the National Health Service.* Cmnd.9663. (London, 1956).

(159) See *Management Arrangements for the Reorganised National Health Service.* Department of Health and Social Security. (London, 1972).

(160) Department of Health and Social Security. *National Health Service Inquiry.* Leader of Inquiry: E.R. Griffiths. (Typescript, 6 October, 1983).

(161) *British Medical Journal*, Volume 288, 23 June 1984, p.1934.

(162) McIntosh, D. The Doctor and Resource Allocation, in *Scottish-American Conference on the 250th Anniversary of the founding of the University of Edinburgh Medical School.* (Nuffield Provincial Hospital Trust, 1976).

(163) Klein, R. Auditing the NHS, in *British Medical Journal*, Volume 285, 11 September 1982, pp.672–673. Steele, R. Clinical budgeting and costing—friend or foe?, in *British Medical Journal*, Volume 288, 19 May 1984, pp.1549–1551.

(164) *Royal Commission on the National Health Service. Report.* Cmnd.7615. (London, 1979). pp.13–14.

(165) Scottish Home and Health Department. *Report of the Working Party on Relationships between Health Boards and Local Authorities.* (Edinburgh, 1977). Scottish Home and Health Department. *Health Services in Scotland Report for 1977.* Cmnd.7237, (Edinburgh, 1978), pp.31–32.

(166) See Mr S. Sklaroff's chapter.

(167) Pendreigh, D. *The National Health Service in Scotland.* (Typescript, Usher Institute, University of Edinburgh, 1982), p.5.

(168) Pisa, Z., and Luemara, K. Trends of mortality from ischaemic heart disease and other cardiovascular disease in 27 countries, 1968–1977, in *World Health Statistics Quarterly*, Volume 35, No.1, (1982), pp.11–47. *World Health Statistics Annual* (W.H.O., Geneva, 1984), pp.40–41, and 350–351.

(169) EcUR Division. Department of the Environment. *Census Indicators of Urban Deprivation.* Working Note No.6. Great Britain, p.16 and Appendix F, Table 8.

(170) Department of Health and Social Security. *Prevention and Health: everybody's business. A reassessment of public and personal health.* (London, 1976).

(171) *Health education in the prevention of smoking-related diseases. A Report by the Scottish Health Education Co-ordinating Committee.* (Edinburgh, 1983), pp.2–12. *Health education in the prevention of alcohol-related problems. A Report by the Scottish Health Education Co-ordinating Committee.* (Edinburgh, 1985), pp.7–23.

PART II:
The Three Branches of the NHS

CONTENTS

1. *General Practice*

James Hogarth

CONTENTS

About the Author

JAMES HOGARTH CB., MA.

James Hogarth, joined the Department of Health for Scotland in 1938, and was concerned with the National Health Service from 1952 until 1974, when he retired as an Under Secretary in the Scottish Home and Health Department.

He is the author of *'Payment of General Practitioners'*, (1963).

Author's Note

This essay traces the development of private practice from the early 20th century pattern – a mingling of private practice, "contract practice" and various forms of charitable provision – through the state-sponsored National Health Insurance system introduced in 1913, which provided insured persons with improved medical care and improved the financial status of general practitioners, to the wider concept of general medical services as the central element in primary health care which has evolved under the National Health Service. Although the limitations of National Health Insurance were widely recognised, the pattern remained practically unchanged for 35 years. In contrast to this has been the steadily developing pattern of general medical services under the National Health Service, which in spite of financial constraints has seen a constant striving by the medical profession and the public authorities concerned towards the fuller integration of general practitioners to use their particular skills and increasing therapuetic resources more effectively for the benefit of their patients.

In the transformation of general practice from an under-equipped "cottage industry" into an effective primary care service, John Brotherston played a major part. He promoted with enthusiasm such pioneering developments as the Livingstone experiment, and it is not too much to say that he saw the integration of the National Health Service administrative structure in the early 1970s primarily as a means of providing a setting in which general practitioners could play their full part.

General Practice

Nineteenth Century Origins

The concept of general practice emerged in Britain in the early nineteenth century to describe the work of a doctor who did everything for his patients of which he and the medical knowledge of the day were capable. 'The GP was to be a one-man medical service'[1]. In England and Wales the development of general practice was long hampered by the traditional distinction between the roles of the physician (who could claim to belong to a learned profession), the surgeon (who practised a craft) and the apothecary (who followed a trade). Scotland was more fortunate. There the surgeons and apothecaries had joined forces as early as the seventeenth century, producing a breed of surgeon-apothecaries who were trained in both surgery and medicine and can be regarded as the first general practitioners in anything approaching the modern conception of the term; they were more widely distributed throughout the country than the physicians, who catered for the wealthier patients in towns[2]. To this basic stock of practitioners trained by apprenticeship were added the graduates of the Scottish university medical schools, with a general training which included medicine, surgery and midwifery. During the nineteenth century these schools greatly increased their output, so that by around 1880 some two-thirds of the doctors practising in Scotland were graduates.

The second half of the nineteenth century saw great advances in medical science which affected the position of the general practitioner. When medical resources and techniques were relatively limited in their power to provide specific treatment for disease the general practitioner could plausibly be thought of as a one-man service, since there was little that a hospital could do that he could not, whether in terms of physical medicine or surgery: indeed the danger of infection might make hospital treatment less safe than domiciliary treatment or surgical intervention ('kitchen-table surgery') by a general practitioner. Many general practitioners thus developed special interests of their own, notably in surgery. The situation changed with the rapid development of anaesthetic procedures after the discovery of the use of ether and chloroform in mid century, followed by the adoption of Lister's antiseptic techniques in the 1860s. Rapid advances in surgery now became possible, using apparatus and skills which could be economically provided only in hospital. Later in the century came the emergence of bacteriology, the use of X-rays and other developments, all pointing in the same direction. The result was a steady trend towards specialism and a reduction in the scope of the general practitioner: to such an extent that when Dr Joseph Bell, a general practitioner who made a great name for himself as a surgeon (and incidentally gave Conan Doyle the inspiration for Sherlock Holmes) died in 1911 he was described in his obituary as 'a supreme example of a type that, for good or ill, is fast passing away, the type of the general practitioner who develops a speciality'[3].

(In fact the demise of the general practitioner/surgeon took another forty years, the final *coup de grâce* being administered by the establishment of the National Health Service in 1948.)

The second half of the nineteenth century also saw a great increase in the number of doctors in Scotland. In 1861, soon after the Medical Act of 1858, there were 1,870; in 1901 this figure had almost doubled to 3,696, giving Scotland (whose population had increased by some 45 *per cent* over the period) one doctor for every 1,220 of population, compared with one for every 1,350 in England and Wales. This is an advantage which Scotland has maintained ever since[4].

The Growth of Contract Practice

But the growth in population during the nineteenth century, combined with the redistribution brought about by increasing industrialisation, had a profound effect on the pattern of medical practice. All general practitioners depended for their income on private practice; and traditionally, in pre-industrial communities with a reasonable mix of the more prosperous and the poor, doctors had commonly tended their poorer patients free of charge, recouping themselves by the fees they charged those better able to pay. The industrial revolution changed this pattern, creating large agglomerations of population living in insanitary conditions and in greater or lesser poverty, in which the principle of robbing Peter to pay Paul could no longer apply. This led to the growth of 'medical aid associations'; this was the collective term for a large and miscellaneous collection of bodies which set out to offer what was in effect a form of insurance for medical care. The better paid workers were catered for by the friendly societies, which had a long tradition[5] of providing sickness and funeral benefits for their members and during the nineteenth century moved into the provision of medical care for working men (and later women) on a large scale, contracting with practitioners to give medical attendance and medicines to their members in return for a fixed annual fee of a few shillings per head. By 1892 there were 1,320 friendly societies in Scotland, with a total membership of 128,000. In addition there were a variety of 'clubs', less formally organised than the friendly societies, which collected a modest weekly subscription – commonly a penny (.4p) per head, and a halfpenny for children – from their members and arranged with a doctor for their treatment in case of need. Sometimes the club might be organised by the doctor himself; it might be a 'works club', confined to workers in a particular factory; not infrequently it consisted of the *habitués* of a public-house (with the landlord, it was said, sometimes levying his toll on the subscriptions). The very poor who could not afford to belong to a club had to rely for medical care on the poor law or on a 'dispensary' or other charitable organisation. The medical aid associations, and the friendly societies in particular, had two attractions for doctors: this 'contract practice' provided a regular, if modest, income, and it offered the doctor the prospect of private fees for the treatment of members' families and the opportunity of making himself known in the district. From the professional point of view it had the disadvantage of exposing doctors to control by the societies, concerned to minimise the issue of sickness certificates which involved the payment of benefit, and at least the theoretical objection that it deprived patients of their free choice of doctor. A more serious grievance, however, was that the friendly societies increasingly tended to take in members who could well afford to pay doctors' fees, and thus deprived them of income. The increased numbers of doctors in the latter part of the nineteenth century created a competitive situation which enabled the societies and clubs to keep their fees low, and this was demoralising to the profession. Practitioners also felt themselves threatened by competition from the out-patient departments of hospitals, which provided free treatment, and by the various provident dispensaries and other charitable organisations in working-class districts: in 1890 more than two-fifths of the population of Edinburgh, including many people well able to help themselves, were said to be receiving free medical advice from the city's medical charities[6].

The low fees paid by friendly societies and clubs tempted doctors to take on too many patients or to neglect their society and club patients in favour of private work. The physical conditions of practice were all too often unsatisfactory and the standard of care low, particularly in the larger towns. Looking back half a century later, a prominent Glasgow practitioner recalled that 'general practice was at a very low level in the industrial areas . . . There was little pretence at real prescribing. The club contract included attendance and medicine, which was usually supplied from one of six mixtures suitably diluted'[7]. Standards of midwifery were low, with early use of forceps and frequent damage to the mother. Another observer reported spending an evening with a Glasgow panel doctor who saw over seventy patients in the course of three hours, the patients being shown in three at a time towards the end of the evening[8].

The difficulties were not of course confined to contract practice, which was estimated in the early years of the twentieth century to cover more than half the working population of the country. Apart from the medical care provided for the poorest members of the community by the poor law and other public services and by various charitable institutions there was still a very substantial volume of private practice, catering for the more prosperous classes. For the poorer members of the population who did not belong to an approved society or club there were the 'sixpenny doctors' who provided a low standard of medical care, including medicines, for 6d (2.5p) a time, which was a rate of remuneration well below even that paid by the friendly societies and clubs. Conditions naturally varied from area to area, but clearly many general practitioners were working in unsatisfactory conditions even by the standards of the time. This was particularly true of working class districts in towns, but rural areas had their special problems. Many Scottish country practitioners complained of the long distances they had to cover in caring for their patients, over poor roads and often no roads at all.

The problems of contract practice became particularly acute towards the end of the nineteenth century, when the *Lancet* carried out a series of investigations of club practice, under the general heading of 'The Battle of the Clubs'.[9] These were concerned mainly with conditions in English industrial towns, and made only passing reference to difficulties in Scotland (Glasgow); but the controversy left its mark on the attitudes of the profession, and led the British Medical Association in 1903 to undertake a major enquiry into contract practice.

The report of the BMA's investigation, presented in 1905[10], confirmed some of the complaints about club practice but also found practitioners who were reasonably content with the system, and on the whole was remarkably moderate in tone. This was perhaps because the poor response to the questionnaire issued to practitioners (only 1,548 out of the 12,000 practitioners to whom it was sent replied to the questionnaire, and only 856 of these were actually in contract practice) suggested that professional discontent with contract practice was not as deeply or as widely felt as the publicity given to the 'battle of the clubs' might have implied. The report found that the commonest rate of remuneration for doctors in contract practice was between 4/- and 5/- (20p and 25p) per member per year; but the real grievance among practitioners appeared to be not so much the rate of remuneration as the fact that people who could afford to pay privately for medical care were able to obtain treatment at these cheap rates. There was therefore strong feeling in favour of an upper income limit for membership of friendly societies and clubs, the limit most commonly suggested ranging between £1 and £2 a week. There was also objection to the increasing practice of admitting women and children to membership of clubs, which meant more work as well as the loss of private fees. The report expressed the anxiety of practitioners about the control of medical men by a non-medical organisation and about the lack of security enjoyed by club practitioners. It concluded by making a number of fairly general recommendations, which assumed the continuance of some form of contract practice, preferably in a 'public medical service' run by the profession themselves. Whatever the form of service, however, it called for proper medical control, the agreement of the general body of practitioners to the terms of contract practice in any area and a right of participation for all practitioners in the area.

Such evidence as is quoted in the BMA report suggests that practitioners in Scotland were in general rather less well paid by approved societies and clubs than their English colleagues, but were less disposed to complain of their lot. (This disparity between Scotland and England was noted by a later commentator[11], who observed that the difference in medical remuneration was perhaps not so great as it seemed, 'the Scotch being understood to be less fond of drugging than the English'.)

The report on contract practice had surprisingly little impact. Its recommendations were generally approved by the BMA's annual representative meeting in July 1906 and commended to the Association's Divisions. A central emergency fund was set up to help practitioners in disputes over contract practice, but the voluntary contributions which were called for do not appear to have materialised on any large scale. Some success was achieved in improving the terms of the practitioners' contract in certain areas, but on the whole there was little change in the conditions of practice until matters were brought to a head by the Liberal government's proposals for a national health insurance scheme.

The Coming of National Health Insurance

Lloyd George's proposals on national health insurance did not originally include the provision of medical care, but were centred on financial benefits (sickness, invalidity and widows' and orphans' pensions). By the end of 1908, however, they had been extended to include medical benefit, which, like the financial benefits, was to be administered by the friendly societies. The estimated cost of medical attendance and medicines was set at 4/- (20p) per insured person per year, a figure evidently related to the level of cost under existing contract practice arrangements.

The medical profession were not at first brought into Lloyd George's consultations, which were mainly with the friendly societies and industrial insurance interests; but as the government's proposals developed they grew increasingly concerned. They were strongly against the administration of medical benefit by friendly societies, which would continue to expose practitioners to control by a non-medical body and would deprive patients of the right to choose their own doctor, and they were anxious to ensure that the income limit for insurance purposes was fixed low enough to exclude all those who were able to pay private fees. They were not opposed to the health insurance scheme as such; a remarkably even-handed 'Report on the Organisation of Medical Attendance on the Provident or Insurance Principle'[12] circulated by the BMA for consideration by their Divisions in March 1911 accepted the case for an insurance scheme, in a form satisfactory to the profession, as a means of remedying the defects of the existing system.

Professional opinion hardened, however, when the National Insurance Bill was published at the beginning of May 1911. It provided for a contributory insurance scheme covering all manual workers and all other employed persons with incomes under £160 a year, with medical benefit administered, like the cash benefits, by friendly societies, now to be known as 'approved societies'. The government offered a capitation fee of 6/- (30p) for medical attendance and medicines. By the end of the month the BMA had set out its minimum conditions for entry into the National Health Insurance scheme in the form of 'six cardinal points';

(1) an income limit of £2 a week;

(2) free choice of doctor by the patient;

(3) medical benefits to be administered not by the friendly societies but by the local health committees provided for in the Bill, and all questions of medical discipline to be settled by purely professional committees;

(4) the method of remuneration in each area to be decided by the profession;

(5) the amount of remuneration to be adequate – an annual capitation fee of 8/6d (42.5p) was claimed; and

(6) the profession to have adequate representation on all National Health Insurance administrative bodies.

To strengthen the profession in the fight for these principles the BMA organised mass meetings of doctors, collected undertakings from individual doctors (eventually reaching a total of over 27,000) not to accept service under the new scheme save on terms 'satisfactory to the medical profession and in accordance with the declared policy of the BMA', and (with rather less success) called for contributions to a fighting fund.

The doctors' campaign against the Bill continued throughout 1911 and 1912, with much violent and emotional language. The main points of difficulty were financial: the income limit for insured persons and the level of doctors' remuneration. The government did not give way on the income limit, which remained at £160 a year, and the question of remuneration remained in dispute until the very eve of the 'appointed day' for the commencement of the new scheme. As regards the administrative framework of the scheme, however, the profession's objections were met. Medical benefit was to be administered by the 'local health committees', renamed insurance committees, with which individual doctors would be in contract, and not by approved societies; insured persons were to be free to join the list of patients of any doctor in contract with the insurance committee for their area; the method of payment in each area, although technically a matter for decision by the insurance committee, was in practice to be settled according to the preference of the local practitioners; and provision was made for medical representation in the running of the scheme, in particular by the establishment (under an amending Act of 1913) of 'panel committees' representing doctors engaged in insurance practice ('on the panel' – the list of practitioners from which insured persons could choose their doctor) in each insurance committee area. As Dr Alfred Cox, secretary of the BMA during this period, later said when recollecting the emotion of 1911 in tranquillity, the profession had 'really done very well' in the argument; and he went on to quote a comment in the *Westminster Gazette* to the effect that, while people admire a man who does not know when he is beaten, the trouble with the BMA was that it did not know when it had won[13].

The National Insurance Act passed into law in December 1911, but the battle over remuneration raged right up to the end of 1912, with the appointed day for the operation of the new scheme already set for 15 January 1913. Against the government's original proposal of a 6/- (30p) capitation fee, to cover medical attendance and medicine, the British Medical Association had claimed 8/6d (42.5p), excluding drugs. In October 1912 the government raised its offer to 9/- (45p), including drugs. Of this sum 7/- (35p) was to go to the doctors for the treatment of insured persons, 1/6d (7.5p) was to be set aside to meet the cost of drugs and a further 6d (2.5p) which became known as the 'floating sixpence', was to be available in each area to meet the cost of drugs if it was over 1/6d per head but would go to increase the doctors' remuneration in so far as it was not required for that purpose. Although this offer fell short of the profession's claim it was a great improvement on current rates of payment of contract practice – which an enquiry carried out on behalf of the government and the profession by a prominent accountant, Sir William Plender, had shown to average only 4/5d (22p), including both treatment and drugs – and opinion within the profession moved towards acceptance of the government's proposals. Hostile demonstrations continued to the end, and as late as 21 December 1912, only three weeks before the appointed day, a special representative meeting of the BMA voted by an overwhelming majority not to accept the government's terms. But the leaders of the profession were clearly out of touch with the general body of practitioners, who were now joining the scheme in large numbers, and on 17 January 1913 the BMA conceded defeat and released doctors from their undertaking not to accept service, most of them having already anticipated their release.

Scottish doctors seem to have been less hostile to the new scheme than their colleagues in the south. Since rates of payment for contract practice had tended to be lower in Scotland than in England the capitation fee offered by the government no doubt appeared relatively more attractive; and the mileage payments offered to doctors in the Highlands and Islands and in other sparsely populated Scottish areas – £10,000 for the highland areas and £16,000 for the lowlands, out of a total of £50,000 a year for the whole country – could be described as generous. There was much vociferous opposition by the local divisions and committees of the BMA, and in April 1912 a Scottish Medical Insurance Council, with a membership representing general practitioners, the medical corporations, the universities and the BMA, was established to defend professional interests threatened by the National Insurance Act; but the Scottish front was far from solid. When towards the end of 1912 the BMA sought the views of its members on whether the profession should refuse to give service under the Act on the final terms offered by the government, 7 out of 22 Scottish divisions and branches voted against refusal, compared with only 12 out of 165 in England and Wales; and the Scottish Medical Insurance Council made so little impact that it was dissolved in June 1913. Attitudes varied in different parts of the country: Dundee, some areas in the central belt and Glasgow Central (but not other parts of Glasgow) favoured acceptance of the government's terms, while Aberdeen was against acceptance and Edinburgh, a stronghold of private practice, was strongly opposed. But at the end of the day doctors all over the country agreed to operate the new scheme, although in Edinburgh the proportion of practitioners 'on the panel' long remained much lower than in other parts of the country.

National Health Insurance in Operation

The First World War

Under the medical benefit provisions of the National Health Insurance

scheme which came into operation on 15 January 1913, general practitioners entered into a contract with the insurance committee for their
area to provide medical care for all insured persons who applied to join
their 'list' (the register of those for whom they accepted responsibility).
The patient had a free choice of doctor – a freedom necessarily qualified
by the availability of doctors in the area – and the doctor was equally
free to accept, or not to accept, a particular person on to his list. Provision
was made for a patient to change his doctor, or for a doctor to have a
patient removed from his list. The care which a doctor was required to
give his patients was defined as treatment 'of a kind which can consistently with the best interests of the patient be properly undertaken by a
general practitioner of ordinary professional competence and skill'. It did
not include maternity services (attendance at a confinement or post-
natal care). Where a patient needed treatment beyond the competence
of a general practitioner the doctor was required to advise the patient on
getting such treatment. Procedures were laid down for determining
whether particular forms of treatment fell within a doctor's obligations;
and boundary problems of this kind subsequently occupied much administrative and professional time.

The question of general practitioners' remuneration, which had
bulked so largely in the discussion of the NHI scheme, was dealt with in
a complex set of regulations; but basically the pattern was simple. The
agreed capitation fee, multiplied by the number of insured persons to be
cared for, was to be paid into a central pool, which was then to be divided
up into local pools for each insurance committee area and distributed to
the doctors in each area on a basis accepted by them. The regulations
provided a wide range of options: after the deduction of certain sums to
meet particular circumstances like the treatment of emergencies the local
pool could be distributed to doctors in the form either of a capitation
payment for each patient on a doctor's list, or of an attendance fee for
consultations, visits and certain special services, or of various combinations of capitation and attendance fees. In practice doctors showed little
interest in this variety of choice, and capitation rapidly became the
accepted method of payment throughout Scotland, even in conservative
Edinburgh, where general practitioners had voted in June 1912 against
the capitation principle and in favour of attendance fees.

Whatever reservations the profession had had about the NHI medical
benefit scheme, it was immediately popular with the public. In the first
quarter of 1913 the number of insured persons registered in Scotland was
over 1,450,000, with some 1,800 general practitioners in contract with
insurance committees to care for them. This average of 800 insured
persons per doctor (plus varying but on average greater numbers of
private patients) was more favourable than the ratio south of the Border,
even allowing for the special difficulties of Scottish geography; but it did
of course conceal wide variations from area to area. In the cities some

general practitioners, inheriting the competitive traditions of contract practice, had very large lists of patients, and in the early years of NHI there was no limit on the number of insured persons a doctor could accept. But the difficulties were local and mainly transitional, and by the end of 1913 the National Health Insurance Commission for Scotland was able to report that in general the numbers of practitioners on the local panels were adequate. In the following year they claimed that the panel service 'had in general reached a fairly high standard when compared with the best tradition of private practice'.

There were, inevitably, teething problems. Doctors found themselves involved in a good deal of paperwork in registering the flood of patients seeking to join the list, and they were unhappy about the need to write prescriptions in triplicate (one respect in which Scottish administrative procedures were more demanding than English). The very enthusiasm of patients for the new scheme brought problems: a doctor in Edinburgh complained that many patients coming to register with him took advantage of the opportunity to have an unnecessary consultation, while others sought to get their money's worth by asking for a retrospective prescription to deal with a condition which had been cured before the introduction of the scheme.

There were no restrictions on the drugs a doctor could prescribe, and from the beginning of National Health Insurance there was concern about the mounting cost of the drugs bill and the apparent over-prescribing by some doctors; this in spite of the prospect held out by the 'floating sixpence' of getting more money for doctors' remuneration if less was spent on drugs.

From the outset the profession were given the full share they had asked for in the administration of National Health Insurance. In each area they had two committees to look after their interests in their dealings with the insurance committee: a local medical committee representing all qualified practitioners in the area, which the insurance committee was required to consult on all general questions affecting the administration of medical benefit, and a panel committee representing insurance practitioners in the area, which also the insurance committee was required to consult. In addition there was a medical service committee, half professional and half lay, to deal with complaints against practitioners. It was soon found unnecessary to have both a local medical committee and a panel committee, and it became normal for the panel committee to be recognised also as the local medical committee. These arrangements for involving the profession in the administration of the service may be said to have stood the test of time, for more than seventy years later, under the NHS, the pattern is still recognisably the same.

After the excitement of the years leading up to the introduction of National Health Insurance the new scheme settled down to a brief period of normal functioning before the outbreak of the first world war brought fresh problems. The profession's apprehension about the evils of a State-run system were not realised, and doctors were now assured of a steady income which, together with fees from a still substantial volume of private practice, brought the average general practitioner a considerably higher standard of living: one estimate put the average doctor's NHI income at £320, with probably at least as much again from other sources[14]. This represented a distinct improvement on the incomes of pre-NHI, contract practice days. Significantly, it was reported that the going price for medical practices – which doctors were still able to buy and sell – had increased by about 50 *per cent*[15]. The considered view of Dr Alfred Cox, looking back after seven years of National Health Insurance, was that the National Insurance Act had been a blessing to the medical profession, having practically doubled the income they had been getting for their contract patients and raised the standard for all medical remuneration, including private fees[16].

In terms of medical coverage the population of Scotland was now well served. In August 1914, just before the outbreak of war, there were 2,172 general practitioners in Scotland, including 1,796 insurance practitioners. This represented a population of 2,192 persons per general practitioner; but this average figure concealed wide variations between different parts of the country. Leaving aside the Highlands and Islands with their sparse and scattered populations, the range extended from Edinburgh, relatively favoured with only 1,728 potential patients for every practitioner, through Glasgow (2,188 per practitioner) to Dundee (2,786 per practitioner) and Lanarkshire, with no fewer than 2,948 per practitioner[17].

In spite of the increased financial security which National Health Insurance had brought, doctors complained about being harassed by regulations and circulars, about excessive clerical work, about interference with treatment or the overruling of medical certificates by approved societies, concerned to protect their funds, and about not being paid fully and promptly. As time went on some of these difficulties were ironed out; the arrangements for calculating the remuneration pool and for paying it out were simplified and expedited; and the war which was soon to come led to further streamlining of NHI machinery.

The immediate effects of the outbreak of war in August 1914 were to reduce drastically the numbers of general practitioners available to care for the civilian population – by the end of 1914, 162 of Scotland's 1,796 insurance practitioners had left to serve with the forces – and to diminish the supply and increase the cost of drugs. The burden on those doctors who remained in civilian practice was increased by the need to look after the patients of absent doctors; and in addition the profession as a whole had undertaken to treat, free of charge, the necessitous dependants of men serving with the forces. At the same time it became necessary to safeguard the interests of doctors whom the war had called away from their practices.

The medical profession in Scotland was quick to recognise the need for action to deal with these problems, and at a meeting of representatives of the different branches of the profession in Edinburgh on 12 August 1914 – only a week after the outbreak of war – a Scottish War Emergency Committee was formed 'for the purpose of assisting to meet the immediate difficulties in regard to medical practice among the civil population ... owing to the departure of practitioners summoned to take up military duty'. The Committee took a wide and constructive view of its functions, for in addition to watching over the adequacy of the country's civilian medical resources and evolving arrangements for protecting the practices of absent doctors it developed into an effective instrument for operating, in collaboration with the military authorities, the arrangements for ensuring that the medical manpower requirements of the forces were met without leaving the civilian population inadequately cared for. (It was only in January 1915 that the profession south of the Border, taking note of this action in Scotland, resolved to follow the Scottish example).

Under the general pattern that emerged for the protection of serving doctors' practices the patients of such practitioners were looked after by those who remained, the remuneration in respect of these patients was shared between the absentee doctor and the doctor doing the work, and there was a ban on the permanent transfer of patients from one doctor's list to another's for the duration of the war.

As the war went on the need for doctors to serve in the forces became ever more acute. The British Medical Association prepared a register of all doctors, indicating their availability for war service; a Central Medical War Committee, with local committees, was established to co-ordinate recruitment for the forces with the medical needs of the population; and there were repeated appeals to the local committees to seek more and more doctors for the forces. By 1917 the number of panel doctors left in Scotland had fallen to only 1,229, which was a third less than before the war. To make the best use of the manpower available 'medical bureaux' were established in some Scottish cities. These were embryo health centres with doctors attending on a rota system, and a member of staff on duty day and night to call out a doctor if required. The idea was first put into practice in August 1914 in Dundee, and proved extremely successful as a means of economising medical manpower; this example was followed by Aberdeen and by Edinburgh, where three such bureaux were brought into operation in 1917, and also by three English towns. An experiment in Glasgow, however, was less successful.

The extent to which the medical strength of the general practitioner service had been reduced, and the burden on practitioners increased, can be seen by comparing the average population per practitioner in November 1918 with the corresponding figures for August 1914. Over Scotland as a whole the figure had increased by 80 *per cent*, from 2,192 to 3,966;

different parts of the country had fared differently, with Edinburgh showing an increase of 120 *per cent* (from 1,728 to 3,792 persons per practitioner), Glasgow increasing by 105 *per cent*, Dundee improving its relative position with an increase of only 68 *per cent* and Fife becoming the most under-doctored area with 5,731 persons per general practitioner, an increase of 112 *per cent* over the August 1914 figure[18].

Reflecting the reduction in the number of doctors, and perhaps also in patient demand, the average number of consultations and visits per insured person showed a declining trend. The expenditure on medicines, however, rose steadily until the beginning of 1915, when a checking bureau was set up to allow over-prescribing to be monitored. The effect was shown at once, with a sharp fall in the Scottish drug bill in the three following years, from £100,000 to £90,000, £80,000 and £73,000, after which it started to rise again. During the war years the argument about general practitioners' remuneration was put on one side, and the capitation and other fees for medical benefit remained unchanged, though war bonuses were paid in 1918 and again in 1919. A 'necessitous districts' fund was introduced in 1914 to supplement the incomes of doctors in sparsely populated lowland areas. In addition the mileage fund for doctors in rural areas was increased in 1917 and 1918, and increased provision was made for practice expenses in 1918.

By the beginning of 1917, however, thoughts were being turned to the future. In January of that year the BMA invited their divisions and branches to consider the whole system of National Health Insurance and make suggestions for its improvement, taking account of the views of insured persons as well as of doctors. The results of this opinion poll showed a remarkable degree of unanimity. The general pattern of NHI was approved, with criticism directed mainly to points of detail; insured persons were found to be generally satisfied with the service they received; but there was a large body of medical opinion in favour of extending the scheme to cover the dependants of insured persons and to provide all medical, surgical and special facilities and treatment, not merely general practitioner care.

With the end of the war in November 1918 the demobilisation of doctors began at once and general practitioners were able to return to their practices, to cope with the influenza epidemic that was sweeping the country and to confront the problems of the postwar world.

Between the Wars

The immediate post-war years were a period of readjustment to peacetime conditions and changing costs of living, and also of new beginnings, although some of the new ideas canvassed during this period were not to reach fruition for many years. The establishment of the Scottish Board of Health in 1919 held out the prospect of action to develop wider and more co-ordinated health services for the people of Scotland; and there was a movement of opinion in favour of extending medical benefit to cover a wider range of population and/or a wider range of services. But at the same time there was apprehension among practitioners that this development might take the form of bringing the provision of medical benefit under the control of local authorities, or might lead to the establishment of a State medical service, with doctors paid by salary and subject to bureaucratic control. In fact none of these fears were realised, and the established pattern of medical benefit under the National Insurance Acts continued in being, with little essential change, until the Second World War.

Although there was a continuing undercurrent of dissatisfaction with some aspects of the medical benefit system, and recurrent arguments about the remuneration of insurance practitioners, the profession as a whole accepted that it had brought benefits to both patients and doctors. Scottish practitioners were apparently less concerned about the defects of the system than their counterparts south of the Border: the correspondence columns of the *British Medical Journal* between the wars regularly contain critical or complaining letters from doctors in insurance practice, but very few from Scottish addresses.

Increases in income levels and in the cost of living were reflected in the raising of the income limit for insured persons from £160 to £250 under the National Health Insurance Act 1919 and by additional bonus payments to insurance practitioners. Mileage payments and the allowance for practice expenses were also increased. These interim remuneration arrangements were followed by discussion of a consolidated capitation fee and revised terms of service for insurance practitioners. The new capitation fee was finally agreed in 1920 at 11/- (55p). The revised terms of service provided that the number of insured persons on a doctor's list should not exceed a maximum, to be fixed locally, of not more than 3,000; the maxima actually fixed ranged from 1,500 upwards. (It should be remembered, on the one hand, that these maxima applied to the numbers registered on doctors' lists, which were estimated to be inflated by duplicate registrations and 'dead souls' to the extent of 20 *per cent*; and on the other that, allowing for the treatment of dependants of insured persons and other private practice, the care of insured persons probably accounted for rather less than half of the average insurance doctor's practice). The 'floating sixpence' was now abolished, and the whole of the 2/- (10p) per insured person contributed to the central drug fund became available for meeting the cost of drugs and appliances.

An important development at this period was the appointment by the Scottish Board of Health of five medical referees to provide a check on cases of incapacity. The role of these officers – originally known as District Medical Officers, later as Regional Medical Officers – was seen also as offering practitioners the opportunity of obtaining a second opinion on difficult cases at their own request, and was eventually to expand into a general advisory function and a means of contact between the central department and the individual practitioner.

The year 1920 also saw much discussion of forward-looking plans. In England and Wales the Dawson report had recommended what in effect was the outline of a national health service with domiciliary services based on primary health centres from which general practitioners could practise if they wished, and in Scotland there was the even more progressive MacAlister report, perhaps the most important feature of which was its resounding statement of the central role of the family doctor in the health services, already quoted in the Introduction.

The MacAlister report made a number of specific proposals on the role of general practitioners and the facilities that should be available to them. They should supervise maternity cases, with midwives as their auxiliaries; co-operation between general practitioners should be promoted; they should have access to the services of 'district consultants' in acute medical cases and to laboratory services; and 'consultation clinics' should be established at which they could see and treat patients and obtain specialist advice. As an example of what they had in mind the Consultative Council referred to the Institute of Clinical Research established at St Andrews in 1919 by Sir James Mackenzie after a distinguished career as a general practitioner and later a heart specialist. The institute was staffed by the local general practitioners, who held surgeries there and had access to laboratory facilities and specialist advice, while their records were used as the basis of research into the relationship between the environment, slight ailments and subsequent disease. This pioneering institution continued in operation until the Second World War. It does not appear, however, to have attracted emulation elsewhere in Scotland.

Professional reaction to the MacAlister report was mixed. There was some support for its proposals; but doctors generally, and general practitioners in particular, were still apprehensive about a possible State medical service and the more immediate threat of control by local authorities. These feelings, combined with the financial stringency of the time, ruled out any immediate prospect of making progress with the MacAlister recommendations or with the proposals of the Dawson report in England. With the fall in the cost of living in the immediate post-war years the capitation fee for 1922 and 1923 was reduced from 11/- (55p) to 9/6d (47.5p) and there was a fear that the government might seek to reduce it still further. In 1923 the government did indeed propose a reduction in the capitation fee from 1924 onwards, offering doctors the alternative of 8/6d (42.5p) for three years or 8/- (40p) for five years. Both alternatives were rejected by the profession, who thereupon threatened to withdraw from panel practice. The crisis was finally resolved by referring the matter to a special court of enquiry, which in 1924 recommended a capitation fee of 9/- (45p). This was accepted by both sides, and remained in force until reduced by 10 *per cent* under the National Economy Act 1931. The cut was restored in 1935, and thereafter the capitation fee remained at 9/- until increased during the Second World War.

Through all these wider discussions the medical benefit scheme continued to operate with reasonable smoothness. There was a good deal of administrative argument, under the provisions of the NHI Act, about the scope of the services to be expected of a general practitioner under the scheme; an important decision promulgated by the Scottish Board of Health in 1921, after reference to a special committee of enquiry, was that prophylactic treatment fell within the scope of an insurance practitioner. Various changes were made to the terms of service of practitioners. In 1923 patients were given the right to change their doctor at any time (instead of only at the end of each half-year), and the maximum list was reduced from 3,000 to 2,500. The range of service to be given by an insurance practitioner was redefined as 'all proper and necessary medical services other than those involving the application of special skill and experience of a degree or kind which general practitioners as a class cannot reasonably be expected to possess, and as including the administration of anaesthetics, or rendering of other assistance at operations of certain defined kinds and subject to defined conditions.'

During this period Scottish general practitioners made less complaint about their lot than their colleagues south of the Border. They were more numerous in relation to the population to be served; a considerable section of the country was agreed to be well served by the Highlands and Islands medical service; doctors in rural areas outside the Highlands had the advantage of the 'necessitous districts' scheme which gave them modest additional remuneration over and above their normal mileage payments, an advantage envied and sought after by their English counterparts; and the paperwork involved in the medical benefit scheme appeared to be less for Scottish than for English doctors.

In evidence to the Royal Commission on National Health Insurance of 1924–1926 the BMA referred to the 'immense gains' which had resulted from the medical benefit scheme. Large numbers of people were receiving medical attention which they did not get before and the doctor/patient ratio in densely populated areas had increased: in England the number of doctors had increased by more than a fifth since 1911, in Scotland by more than two-fifths. Illness was coming under observation and treatment at an earlier stage; doctors' work had an increased bias towards prevention; clinical records were being kept which could be useful in the fields of medical research and public health; co-operation among practitioners was being encouraged, and there was a more marked recognition of the collective responsibility of the profession to the community in all health matters. The approved societies, representing the interests of the patients, recorded their view that the medical profession as a whole had rendered 'competent and conscientious service' to insured persons. The chairman of the Scottish Board of Health, Sir James Leishman, stated in evidence that there was 'absolutely no justification' for suggestions that panel patients got inferior treatment to private patients, and reported that complaints against doctors by patients were, relatively, only about a third as numerous in Scotland as in England. Some adverse criticisms were received, but on the whole the Royal Commission were able to conclude that there was nothing seriously amiss in the scheme other than the limitation on the scope of medical benefit to cover only general practitioner services.

In practice the report of the Royal Commission made little impact on the pattern of general medical services: the time was evidently not ripe even for the cautious recommendations it put forward. Concern was periodically expressed by the Board of Health about laxity in the issue of certificates of incapacity by some doctors and the high levels of prescribing in some areas, and the doctors for their part were still worried about the 'disciplinary' procedure for dealing with complaints by patients against doctors The Board issued guidance to doctors on certification and prescribing; the numbers of references to District Medical Officers (DMOs) on certification were increased; and in order to protect doctors who refused to issue unjustified certificates the terms of service were amended in 1927 to restrict the insured person's right to change his doctor. The insurance committees tried to improve the efficiency of their registers of insured persons by purging them of the 'dead souls' which had accumulated over the years, although this was not always appreciated by doctors who saw their rate of payment apparently reduced in consequence.

In 1929 the Department of Health for Scotland, which had now succeeded the Scottish Board of Health, set out to promote a closer relationship between its Regional Medical Officers (RMOs) and insurance practitioners. More time was to be devoted by the RMOs to visiting practitioners, who it was hoped would come to regard them as colleagues able to offer advice and a second opinion on difficult cases and not merely as referees concerned to control certification. For some time, however, doctors were slow to seek consultation with the RMOs, and it was only with the establishment of the National Health Service that they were to come fully into their role as advisers and consultants.

The following year saw the publication of the BMA's proposals for a 'general medical service for the nation'. These proposals still raised in some practitioners' minds the spectre of a State-run – and no doubt salaried – health service, so much so that the BMA were compelled to deny that in the preparation of their proposals there had been any collusion with the Ministry of Health. In their discussion of the general practitioner services the BMA reaffirmed the central role of the general practitioner or family doctor, but stressed that he should be able to treat patients in 'home hospitals', which would give him contact with the specialist staff of larger hospitals, should have access to non-institutional services like home nursing, home helps and domiciliary visits by specialists, and should be responsible for maternity care.

A factor in the BMA's desire to stimulate progress in the wider discussion of health services may well have been the feeling that more progress was being made in Scotland than in England. In 1932 the Department of Health for Scotland had agreed with the BMA and the Scottish local authorities to establish a committee to discuss the co-operation of private practitioners in the statutory health services; but this proposal was overtaken by the appointment in June 1933 of the Committee on Scottish Health Services (the Cathcart Committee).

The report of the Cathcart Committee in 1936 quoted the view of the MacAlister report on the central role of the family doctor in the health services, which they found generally accepted by all branches of the medical profession in Scotland; and they recorded the opinion of the Royal College of Physicians of Edinburgh that there was 'probably no country in the world in which the standard of general practice is higher than it is with us'. More forthright than the Royal Commission on National Health Insurance, they saw an 'irresistible case' for making medical benefit available to dependants of insured persons and others in similar circumstances, and they thought that this could be achieved by extending the existing insurance scheme. They recommended that general practitioners should have access to specialist, diagnostic and other facilities, that they should act as a liaison between their patients and the other health services, that they should provide maternity services and that their training should be designed to develop a preventive outlook. As regards the administration of the general practitioner services, however, the Committee recommended, like the Royal Commission on NHI, that the functions of insurance committees should be transferred to local authorities.

The Cathcart Committee's recommendations, like other far-reaching proposals before them, were destined to run into the sand. Some limited progress was made along the lines sketched out by the Committee. In 1936 general practitioners in Ayrshire set up what was in effect a pilot scheme of extended medical benefit on Cathcart lines by undertaking to provide services for the dependants of insured persons in return for weekly contributions ranging between 4d (1.7p) and 1/- (5p) according to the number of dependants. In 1937 the Maternity Services (Scotland) Act provided a framework within which, under arrangements made by local authorities, general practitioners could provide antenatal and postnatal services and attend confinements if called in by the midwife; and under these arrangements they were also able to bring in obstetric specialists if required.

The Cathcart recommendations were also taken up in the BMA's revised proposals on a 'general medical service for the nation', published in April 1938. These cited MacAlister and Cathcart in support of the principle that every individual should have a general practitioner, and noted that the NHI scheme had been, in spite of its defects, an 'undoubted success'. The BMA proposals also gave credit to Scotland for possessing a more comprehensive maternity scheme than England, thanks to the 1937 Act.

Once again hopes for the development of the general practitioner services were to be frustrated by the pressure of events. The Second World War was approaching, and both the Department and the medical profession became involved in defence plans. Nevertheless discussion of the possibility of health service development continued right up to the very eve of the war. At the BMA's Annual Representative Meeting in July 1938 the proposals for a general medical service for the nation had been approved, after a discussion which showed some support (from Glasgow among other places) for a State medical service.

In the early months of 1939 a fresh stimulus was given to the discussion by a proposal put forward by Dr E.R.C. Walker of Aberdeen (later Scottish Secretary of the BMA) for a part-time salaried general practitioner service run by regional councils, with provision for access to consultant advice and all necessary diagnostic facilities. The idea received support from some leading Scottish general practitioners, but also elicited some critical comment. The BMA's Annual Representative Meeting in July 1939, held at Aberdeen, saw some further Scottish initiatives. The Edinburgh division put forward a motion inviting the BMA Council to consider the possibility of a health service financed by the State rather than by insurance contributions and administered by regional health committees, not by local authorities; it was proposed that general practitioners would continue to be paid by capitation, but with modifications to recognise experience and ability. A similar motion was put forward by the Aberdeen division, which also invited the Council to consider the remuneration of doctors by 'graded and adjusted salary with pension'. Surprisingly, perhaps, in view of earlier professional attitudes, both motions were carried, in spite of a speech opposing the Aberdeen motion by one of the great elder statesmen of the BMA, Sir Henry Brackenbury.

These fresh initiatives, however, were overtaken by the outbreak of war a few weeks later, which brought general practitioners more immediate problems to deal with.

1939 to 1948
With the outbreak of war in September 1939 the attention of those concerned with and engaged in general medical services turned to the arrangements for the care of the population in a situation in which many practitioners had been called away to war service.

At the request of the government the BMA had prepared a register of doctors indicating their availability for war service, and by July 1939 the BMA's Scottish Central Emergency Committee had notified individual doctors of their provisional allocation to the services or to civilian work. When war came many general practitioners left their practices, inevitably involving more work for those who remained. Regulations were made allowing insured persons whose doctors were absent on war service to select another doctor without being permanently transferred to his list; and under the 'protection of practices' schemes adopted in most areas the absent doctor drew half his 1939 share of the medical fund for the area.

The NHI capitation fee remained at its 1935 level of 9/- (45p) for the first years of the war. In 1942 it was increased to 9/9d (48.75p) to take account of the wartime increase in practice expenses and the loss of private practice income following the increase in the NHI income limit from £250 to £420 in that year. In 1943 it was increased again to 10/6d (52.5p), a figure which was accepted by the profession on the understanding that it would be reviewed after the war.

In spite of the pressures of war conditions and the additional work they threw on the reduced numbers of general practitioners who remained in civilian practice, the Department of Health for Scotland was able to report that medical benefit had been maintained at a satisfactory standard, and the health of the people remained good. New opportunities opened up for general practitioners, bringing them into closer contact with the other health services. Some became visiting medical officers to the auxiliary hospitals run by the Department in country houses, receiving an honorarium for this work; and the Clyde Basin Experiment, a scheme initiated in 1942 for the rehabilitation of young industrial workers, involved close co-operation between general practitioners and the hospital and specialist services; by the end of the year it had been extended to the rest of Scotland apart from the Highland counties.

Once the medical services had adjusted to a war footing, thoughts began to turn again to the future. In 1942 the BMA set up a Medical Planning Commission to study wartime developments and the country's medical services both present and future. In parallel with this there was much discussion in the medical press of possible patterns of health services, including the pros and cons of a State medical service. Although this found little favour, the mere continuation and extension of the NHI scheme was felt to have defects from the point of view of the general practitioner. Its basis was still the single-handed doctor, whereas it was now recognised that 'medical treatment was too big for one man'; the machinery of NHI would be a cumbrous means of covering the whole population; and the evils involved in the buying and selling of medical practices, tolerable in a limited scheme, would be unacceptable in a wider service.

The Medical Planning Commission's draft interim report, published as a basis for discussion in June 1942, stressed, like so many earlier reports, the general practitioner's sense of isolation, the pressure of work which prevented him from pursuing postgraduate study or special interests and the need to integrate his work with that of the other health services. It cited once again the view of the MacAlister report in 1920 – now generally accepted by the profession – that any system of national health services should be based on the family as the normal unit and on the family doctor as their normal medical attendant and guardian. It returned to the idea of health centres accommodating both general practitioner and local authority services. But it still saw the service it contemplated as being for the benefit only of those under the NHI limit of £420 a year.

Early in 1943 the government announced their acceptance in principle of the famous 'Assumption B' of the Beveridge report – that a comprehensive national health service covering 100 *per cent* of the population would be established – and invited the various professions and other interests involved to enter into discussion. This the medical profession agreed to do; but they took strong objection to the government's original ideas, which contemplated a salaried general practitioner service based (at any rate in urban areas) on health centres and controlled by local authorities. The government thereupon undertook to reconsider their proposals.

The White Paper setting out the government's revised proposals, issued in February 1944, postulated two principles on which the general practitioner service should be based: patients should be free to choose and to change their doctor, and doctors should be free to use their knowledge and skill in the way they felt best. It stressed the value of 'grouped practice', though recognising that this was not suitable everywhere, and suggested that grouped practice could best – though not exclusively – be realised in health centres, which would be provided in England and Wales by local authorities but in Scotland, at any rate initially, by the Secretary of State. It saw a strong case for paying general practitioners in health centres by salary, and suggested, more tentatively, that payment by salary might also be appropriate in grouped practices; but otherwise practitioners would continue to be paid by capitation. As regards administrative structure, it did not seem practicable to extend the scope of the existing NHI machinery to cover the whole population. Instead, doctors would be in contract with a Central Medical Board, which would have local committees to take over the functions of insurance committees. Co-ordination between the general practitioner service and other health services would be achieved by having local authority representatives on the Board's local committees and by the establishment of Local Medical Services Committees in the new and larger areas to be formed in Scotland for running the hospital and specialist services. The administrative structure proposed for England and Wales was more closely aligned to the local government pattern.

In order to secure a better distribution of doctors the White Paper proposed that the Central Medical Board would have power to control entry into general practice. It was not proposed to ban the sale of practices, except in over-doctored areas, when compensation would be paid; and compensation would also be paid when a doctor gave up his practice to enter a health centre.

Although the White Paper proposals were more moderate, and more tentatively expressed, than the government's original proposals they were still not acceptable to the profession.

Discussion continued actively throughout 1944 within the profession and between the profession and the Health Departments. The BMA's Scottish Committee, while taking the same general line as their colleagues in the south, recognised that the administrative machinery proposed for Scotland was better than that contemplated in England and Wales. The Committee noted that the successful Highlands and Islands scheme was the nearest approach in the United Kingdom to a complete medical service, and that the Maternity Services (Scotland) Act 1937 had produced a good example of a service founded on the family doctor, supported by nursing, consultant and hospital services in contrast to the corresponding English service, which was essentially a midwife service.

A conference of Scottish BMA divisions and panel committees in October 1944 set out the views of the profession in Scotland in more detail. They favoured an extension of the NHI scheme to cover dependants of insured persons and to include consultant and specialist services and hospital and laboratory facilities; but the administration of the scheme must not be handed over to local authorities, and it must provide for adequate participation by general practitioners. They were against the extension of the scheme to the whole population, at any rate until they knew more about the proposals for safeguarding private practice, which must be preserved. They insisted that the terms of service and method of payment of general practitioners must be the same whether they worked in separate or in grouped practices; and compensation must be paid for the loss of capital value of practices.

Faced with this professional opposition, the government gave way, and in the early months of 1945 put forward revised proposals which gave the profession most of what they wanted. The plan for a Central Board would be pursued only if the profession wanted it, and the alternative of retaining a machinery of NHI type was left open. Health centres would be provided only on an experimental basis, and practitioners working in health centres would be paid in the same way as those working in their own group surgeries. The question of having a part salary element in remuneration (perhaps as a means of attracting practitioners to under-doctored areas) was left open for consideration; the wider issues of remuneration would be considered by a committee; and the question of retaining or banning the sale of practices would be left until the new service was in operation.

These proposals were accepted by the BMA, though they still had reservations on certain points; but once again external events intervened. A general election was imminent; the Labour Party's manifesto referred to the general practitioner services in terms which seemed to imply payment by salary and a ban on private practice; and in July 1945, after the end of the war in Europe, a Labour government came into power.

The end of the war made possible the release of doctors from the forces to return to civilian work. At first slow, the process was greatly speeded up by the end of 1945 and continued at a steady pace throughout 1946. Newly qualified doctors were recruited into the services after a short period of hospital experience to permit the return of older doctors to their practices. Refresher courses for doctors returning to civilian practice were organised by the Universities and financed by the Department; and when the demand from ex-service doctors slackened off towards the end of 1946 these courses were made available to other practitioners. The 'protection of practices' scheme which had operated in most Scottish areas since the outbreak of war was now unwound; and as a transitional arrangement it was decided that for up to 18 months after a service doctor's return to panel practice his share of the medical fund was not to be less than his 1939 share. In order to facilitate a better distribution of doctors the medical benefit regulations were amended to give people who had been put onto a practitioner's list during the war complete freedom to change their doctor during a period of three months, or six months for people transferring to a doctor who had been on war service.

One matter requiring immediate attention was the question of general practitioners' remuneration for their NHI work, pending the establishment of the National Health Service which was now so much in the air. The capitation fee had remained at 10/6d (52.5p) since 1943 on the understanding that it would be reviewed after the war. In the meantime a committee under the chairmanship of Sir Will Spens had been appointed (in February 1945) to recommend the appropriate level of remuneration for general practitioners in a publicly organised service, and in August 1945 the profession accepted a government offer of a capitation fee of 12/6d (62.5p) from January 1946 as a payment on account, on the understanding that the amount recommended by the Spens Committee would be backdated to that date. The committee reported in April 1946, in effect recommending a capitation fee of 15/6d (77.5p), and by the end of the year this recommendation had been accepted by the government and the profession.

Establishment of the National Health Service

The profession had awaited with some apprehension the new Labour government's proposals on a National Health Service. When these were made public in the (English) National Health Service Bill in March 1946 they turned out, in relation to general practitioner services, to be less radical, and less objectionable to doctors, than perhaps they had feared in the light of earlier Labour Party views. General practitioners were not to be forced into a salaried service but were to continue to be paid by the familiar capitation fee, though there was a provision for a 'basic salary' (plus capitation fees) to help young doctors setting up in practice or to attract doctors to otherwise unattractive areas; they were to be free to practise privately; and they were not to be made subject to local authority control, but were to be in contract with Executive Councils – rather unimaginatively named bodies, half professional in membership – which bore a remarkable likeness to the insurance committees of the National Health Insurance scheme. It was contemplated that health centres would feature prominently in the organisation of general practitioner services. The sale of practices was to be abolished, subject to the payment of compensation. A Medical Practices Committee was to keep the distribution of general practitioners under review, with power to restrict entry to over-doctored areas.

The National Health Service (Scotland) Bill was based on the same principles and provided a similar administrative structure. The main difference so far as general practitioner services were concerned was that health centres were to be provided by the Secretary of State rather than by local authorities as in England and Wales: a variation welcomed by the profession.

Nevertheless professional opinion, as represented by the BMA, was hostile to the government's proposals, claiming that the legislation gave Ministers unduly wide powers, that the Medical Practices Committee's powers amounted to direction, and that it would stilll be open to Ministers under the Acts to introduce a full-time salaried service at some time in the future. This feeling was reinforced by a remark of Aneurin Bevan's during the second reading of the NHS Bill which was interpreted as meaning that although the time was not yet ripe for a salaried service it might be ripe one day: 'there is all the difference in the world between plucking fruit when it is ripe and plucking it when it is green'.

Even after both NHS Bills had become law (the English Bill in December 1946, the Scottish Bill in May 1947) and the 'appointed day' for the establishment of the National Health Service had been fixed as 5 July 1948 the BMA's objections were maintained and reinforced, and there was much discussion and negotiation in an attempt to meet them. A plebiscite of the profession in February 1948 showed a large majority against coming into the NHS, though the proportion approving the Act in Scotland was slightly higher than in England and Wales, the proportion disapproving was considerably lower and the proportion not voting at all considerably higher. Thereafter the government sought to remove apprehensions about a salaried general practitioner service by undertaking to introduce amending legislation which would make it impossible to introduce such a service by regulations and would limit the scope of the proposed basic salary. A further plebiscite of the profession in May 1948 still showed a majority against entering the NHS, though this time the majority was much smaller and again the profession in Scotland was less hostile. The BMA had previously resolved that the decision whether or not to co-operate in the establishment of the NHS would depend mainly on the views of the general practitioners: if 13,000 of them voted against joining, the profession as a whole would refuse to co-operate. In the May plebiscite the number of general practitioners against accepting service was just under 8,500; and the BMA was obliged to withdraw its opposition. In any event substantial numbers of general practitioners had by this time individually agreed to join the service: 37 *per cent* of all practitioners in Scotland, 26 *per cent* in England. The NHS duly came into operation on 5 July 1948, and general practitioners found themselves in contract with the new Executive Councils.

The new pattern of general medical services represented a great advance for those members of the population who had been excluded from the NHI scheme, and was immediately so popular that it led to increased demands on doctors who were not adequately equipped for the new comprehensive service: some 60 *per cent* of Scottish principals still practised single-handed, with little or no ancillary help and with surgery accommodation which often left much to be desired. By the end of 1949 over 95 *per cent* of the population of Scotland were on doctors' lists and only about 2 *per cent* of general practitioners were not in the NHS. Private practice thus no longer made a significant contribution to the average general practitioner's income, and only a few doctors in certain areas (relatively fewer than in England) continued to have any substantial number of private patients. Scotland retained its advantage over the southern part of the kingdom in having a relatively greater number of doctors; with average lists of some 2,000 patients compared with 2,400 in England and Wales, Scottish general practitioners were subject to less pressure than their colleagues in the south, and there were relatively few complaints from patients.

One other difference between the Scottish and the English situations is worth noting. The Scottish tradition had been that doctors' prescriptions were normally dispensed by pharmacists, and it was only in areas remote from a chemist's shop that general practitioners dispensed as well as prescribed for their patients. In England, however, there were relatively more 'dispensing doctors', often in areas which could hardly be regarded as remote, who might earn a substantial income from this source. Scottish practitioners in general were much less affected by what might be regarded as a distraction from their main responsibilities and one which made additional demands on their time.

The number of NHS patients a doctor might have was limited to 4,000. In the early days of the NHS some doctors – relatively fewer in

Scotland than in England – found themselves with more than this number of patients and had to be given temporary dispensations. This proved, however, to be merely a transitional problem.

The National Health Service in Operation

The administrative structure of the new service, so far as it concerned general practitioners, was not very different from that of the old NHI scheme, with the executive council replacing the insurance committee and a local medical committee still representing the practitioners' interests. Much of the detail of the doctor's terms of service was carried over from the old service to the new, and many regulations first drafted in the early days of NHI could still be recognised in their 1948 counterparts, and for many years thereafter. The change of management, therefore, created no particular difficulties for practitioners, except for the volume of paperwork involved in the registration of a flood of new patients on their lists.

Although there was little complaint from patients about the quality of the care they received from the NHS and surprisingly little reaction by general practitioners apart from complaints of overwork and excessive demands by patients in some areas, there were some discordant notes. A minor thunderbolt was launched by Dr J.S. Collings, an Australian doctor who visited numbers of practitioners throughout Britain and published his findings on 'General Practice in England Today' (with an appendix on Scotland) in the *Lancet* in 1950[19]. He concluded that the standard of general practice in Britain was low and was still deteriorating. It had for many years adapted itself to the development of the hospital and other medical services but had not itself developed concurrently; there was little co-ordination between general practitioners and other health care services, and little thought was given to the lines on which general practice should develop. He found that the establishment of the NHS had made little difference to general practice apart from increasing doctors' work-load.

Collings did, however, take a more favourable – though still in some respects critical – view of general practice in Scotland. He found that Scottish general practitioners had a more co-operative attitude to the central and local authorities concerned with health services than their colleagues in the south[20], whereas his discussions with English practitioners had centred mainly on problems of remuneration, work-load, etc. He found Scottish doctors more interested in professional issues, like the quality of medical care, relationships with the hospital and specialist services and the development of health centres; and they appeared to keep better records, to organise their work better, to conduct better examinations of patients and to show less readiness to refer cases to hospital outpatient departments. He commented also on the fact that

Scottish practitioners had retained some responsibility for midwifery, making the Scottish general practitioner much more the family doctor.

Collings' report was criticised by the *British Medical Journal* as inaccurate and unfair; but at any rate it provided a form of shock treatment which helped to dispel any feeling of complacency over the very real achievement of developing a limited insurance service into a general medical service for the whole population. The BMA was stimulated into setting up a major enquiry into general practice. One of their officers, Dr S.J. Hadfield (later Scottish Secretary of the Association), was commissioned in 1951 to carry out a field survey of general practice based on a random sample of practices; his report[21] classified 44 *per cent* of the practices he visited as 'good', another 44 *per cent* as 'adequate' and 7 *per cent* as 'inadequate'. Still another survey of general practice was carried out by Dr Stephen Taylor, whose book *Good General Practice* was published in 1954; this was not a random survey like those of Collings and Hadfield but designedly a study of good practices with the idea of pointing the way forward for others. To some extent, too, both Hadfield's report and Taylor's book served as morale-boosters for the profession: a leading article in the *BMJ*[22] claimed that they would 'do much to restore confidence in general practice'.

A more important development was the foundation in November 1952 of the College of General Practitioners, with the object of restoring the status of the general practitioner and promoting the development of general practice. The College – granted the status of Royal College in 1967 – has continued to play its part in enhancing the quality of general medical care through its *Journal* and other publications, the promotion of discussion and the exchange of information, the encouragement of research, etc.

Discussions of the general medical services, however, continued to be dogged by the problem of remuneration. The Spens Committee had been asked to recommend what ought to be the range of total professional income of a doctor in a publicly organised service of general medical practice, and, reporting in 1946, had recommended £1,300 (in 1939 values) as the mid point of a range designed to concentrate incomes in the middle part of the range, with fewer in the lower ranges than there had been in 1939 and a substantial number in the highest range. Overall, the Spens recommendations represented an average net income in 1939 values of £1,111, an increase of almost 20 *per cent* on the average income of a pre-war general practitioner. This was accepted by the government and the profession as a basis for negotiation; but disagreement arose over the 'betterment' factor required to bring the £1,111 up to 1948 values. The government took a factor of 20 *per cent* (against the 100 *per cent* claimed by the profession), and used it in building up the new NHS remuneration pool. This was done by taking the Spens figure of £1,111, multiplying it by the number of general practitioners practising in 1939, increasing the total by 20 *per cent*, adding the accepted estimate of 1939 practice expenses increased by a betterment factor of 55 *per cent* and finally adding another 3 *per cent* to take account of the increase in population since before the war. The total thus arrived at (for Great Britain) was £42.7 million, or about 18/- (90p) per head of the estimated 1948 population. The quarterly remuneration pool was then calculated by taking a quarter of this amount and multiplying it by 95 *per cent* of the estimated population (on the assumption that 5 *per cent* would remain as private patients). This sum, less an amount set aside for mileage payments, was divided between England and Wales on the one hand and Scotland on the other and distributed to Executive Councils, mainly on the basis of population but allowing also for the number of temporary residents. These local pools were then distributed to doctors, after deduction of 'fixed annual payments' of £300 for new entrants to practice, fees for temporary residents, the treatment of emergencies, etc., in the form of capitation fees (which might thus vary slightly from area to area according to the amount of deductions). In addition there was a mileage fund (£2 million for Great Britain), distributed under a separate and very complicated scheme.

On top of the pool thus arrived at the Exchequer provided additional money for certain specific services, for example an inducement fund to increase the incomes of doctors in remote or otherwise unattractive areas, a contribution to the mileage fund, payments for maternity services, drugs dispensed by general practitioners, etc. Altogether this added another £6.5 million to the Exchequer commitment, and in effect amounted to a 'betterment' factor of something over 50 *per cent*.

Although general practitioners as a whole were thus apparently better off than before the war, some doctors in middle-class areas found their income reduced as private patients switched over to the NHS. Temporary arrangements were therefore made to help them by additional payments out of the unspent balance of money set aside for inducement payments and 'fixed annual payments'.

The profession as a whole, however, remained dissatisfied with the government's application of the Spens report. In particular they claimed that the 'betterment' factor was still not high enough to take account of the changed value of money, and that in order to realise the Spens conception of a guaranteed averge income the pool should be adjusted according to changes in the number of doctors, not changes in the population. After protracted discussions between the profession and the health departments it was agreed to refer the matter to adjudication, with Mr Justice Danckwerts as Adjudicator. A joint working party was also established to recommend adjustments in the method of distributing the remuneration pool so as to discourage unduly large lists, improve the position of doctors with small practices, make it easier to enter general practice and stimulate group practice.

The result of the adjudication, published in March 1952, was very favourable to the profession. It fixed the betterment factor at 100 *per cent* for 1950–51 and 85 *per cent* for the two preceding years; it decided that the pool should vary according to the number of doctors rather than the number of potential patients; and it laid down that the amount of money to be paid into the pool was to be determined by calculating the size of the 'all-in' pool of total professional income and deducting from this the amount of income (ascertained or estimated) from sources outside the NHS pool (private practice, local authority and hospital appointments, etc.). Inducement payments were to remain outside the pool as a separate Exchequer responsibility.

The working party on distribution, reporting in June 1952, fixed the basic capitation fee at 17/- (85p); recommended a supplementary capitation fee ('loading') for all patients from the 501st to the 1,500th on a doctor's list, with the object of encouraging medium-sized practices; in order to promote the formation of partnerships, it introduced the idea of 'notional loadings', allowing partners to obtain loadings on the most advantageous basis, as if the maximum possible number of patients were included in the 501–1,500 range; replaced the fixed annual payment of £300 by larger 'initial practice allowances' designed to help doctors setting up in single-handed practice in under-doctored areas; and it set aside a sum of £100,000 (£12,000 for Scotland) from the pool for the purpose of encouraging group practice. The working party also tried to promote a more even distribution of patients by recommending a reduction of the maximum list from 4,000 to 3,500 for a single-handed practitioner.

Meanwhile only limited progress had been made in achieving some of the wider aims of the new service. Earlier hopes for a major development of group practice in health centres were dashed by financial stringency and lack of interest among general practitioners. At the outset it was possible to contemplate only one health centre in Scotland, at Sighthill in Edinburgh, and this was not to come into service until 1953. Failing the establishment of health centres, Executive Councils were invited to consider, in consultation with Local Medical Committees, how to develop arrangements for mutual aid between practitioners, co-operation with local authority nurses and health visitors, the provision of laboratory and diagnostic facilities and contacts between general practitioners and hospital doctors. There were also local initiatives aimed at promoting co-operation between general practitioners and the hospital and specialist services: the Northern Regional Hospital Board launched a postgraduate training scheme providing a combination of hospital and general practice experience for young doctors proposing to enter either of these fields; and, under an apprenticeship scheme operated in Aberdeen, 5th or 6th year medical students were attached to general practices for periods of a month at a time.

Later, in 1956, and with the agreement of the profession, the Department put forward a scheme to encourage doctors to combine general practice and hospital work, based on a two-year training period, half in general practice and half in hospital, after the pre-registration year; it was also proposed that entry into general practice on a part-time basis should be made easier, so that general practitioners would be able to combine two fields of activity. These proposals, however, made little immediate impact, though they can be seen as foreshadowing the Livingstone experiment of ten years later.

Although first reactions to the Department's attempts to promote group practice were disappointing, a trend towards increased partnership practice did begin to establish itself; the proportion of principals practising in partnership rose from around 40 *per cent* at the start of the National Health Service to 59 *per cent* in 1954, and thereafter continued to rise slowly but steadily. Further encouragement was given to the establishment of group practices by a scheme of interest-free loans for the provision of group practice premises which came into operation in 1954. The Sighthill health centre was able to report a successful first year's operation which had promoted co-operation between general practitioners and other health services, and the construction of another health centre was now under way at Stranraer. But for the next few years the health centre programme was to make little progress. Finance, as always, was a difficulty; but the impulse for the development of health centres had essentially to come from the general practitioners themselves, and this was still lacking. By 1965, after seventeen years of the NHS, there were still only four health centres operating in Scotland.

As an alternative, and less costly, means of promoting co-operation between general practitioners and the hospital services the Department, with financial support from the Nuffield Provincial Hospitals Trust, established a 'family doctor centre' in the Grassmarket, Edinburgh, in which general practitioners had access to laboratory and radiographic facilities for their patients, while continuing to practise in their own surgeries. The centre, catering for some eighty Edinburgh general practitioners, came into operation in 1959.

Ten years after the establishment of the NHS the number of general practitioners in Scotland had risen by 10 *per cent*, from 2,400 principals in 1948 to 2,640 in 1958, and the proportion practising in partnership had increased very substantially, from 40 *per cent* to 66 *per cent*. The average number of patients on doctors' lists was around 1,985 (compared with 2,267 in England and Wales,) and there was a better distribution of patients among doctors, with more patients on the lists of medium-sized practices. (The average number of patients in fact overstates the true figure, since there was still some inflation in the Executive Councils' registers, though much less than in the days of NHI. Periodic efforts were made, with some success, to purge the registers; but in considering figures of average list size under the NHS allowance must always be made for some degree of inflation).

The cost of doctors' prescribing had been a matter of constant concern under NHI, and the problem became increasingly urgent in the NHS, as a result of the steadily rising costs of drugs, the increasing numbers of new and powerful drugs which now became available, the availability and popularity of proprietary preparations and the greater expectations – and indeed sometimes demands – of a wider and better informed public. In the first year of the NHS some 15 million prescriptions were dispensed in Scotland, at an average cost of 44d (18.3p) and a total cost of £2.75 million; and from the outset these figures showed a steady upward trend.

The main thrust of the activity directed to the control of excessive prescribing took the form of providing information about drugs and about doctors' prescribing costs: doctors were not banned from prescribing any particular drugs, though if their costs were high they might be called on to justify them, and in the last resort might have a sum withheld from their remuneration if they were found by the Local Medical Committee to have incurred unjustified excessive prescribing costs. Doctors were periodically given statistics of their prescribing costs as compared with the average – figures which showed surprisingly wide variations between different areas and within a particular area – and 'Prescribers' Notes' giving information about the cost and effectiveness of drugs were issued, together with information on the comparative costs of proprietary and standard preparations. In 1952 the problem was approached from the other end, by the imposition of a charge, payable by the patient, of 1/- (5p) for each prescription form (which might cover a number of items). This brought about a temporary fall in the number of prescriptions issued and a reduction in the cost to the Exchequer; but these effects were soon overtaken by the rising trend. By 1955 the number of prescriptions dispensed had risen to 21.2 million and the net cost to the Exchequer (allowing for prescription charges) to £5.1 million. At the end of 1956 the prescription charge was increased from 1/- per form to 1/- per item. Again, this temporarily checked the trend, reducing the number of prescriptions in 1957 to 20.9 million, with a net cost of £6.2 million; but by 1958 these figures had risen again to 22 million and £7.7 million.

Meanwhile remuneration continued to be a problem. Spens and Danckwerts had not provided a means of keeping doctors' pay in line with increasing costs, and as time went on general practitioners became increasingly dissatisfied. In 1956 the profession put foward a claim for a 24 *per cent* increase in remuneration, which in the economic circumstances of the time the government felt unable to consider. Discussions between the two sides proving unfruitful, a Royal Commission was appointed in 1957, under the chairmanship of Sir Harry Pilkington, to consider the whole question of doctors' (and dentists') remuneration. Pending their report the Danckwerts target of £2,222 was increased to £2,333 in 1957 and again to £2,426 in 1959, with corresponding increases in capitation fees and 'loadings'.

During the argument on remuneration the BMA had – not for the first time – prepared a scheme for a withdrawal by general practitioners from the NHS if their claim for increased remuneration was not settled, and had appointed a committee to consider an alternative means of providing medical services on the doctors' own terms. In 1958, in an unexpected and perhaps ill-judged move, they invited a retired senior civil servant, Sir Frank Newsam, to consider the deficiencies of the arrangements for providing general medical services and to suggest modifications in, or alternatives to, those arrangements; and were somewhat dashed by his finding that it was 'unrealistic' for general practitioners to think of withdrawal from the NHS.

The Royal Commission, reporting in 1960, recommended a substantial increase in general practitioners' remuneration. They set the target net income at £2,425 from January 1960, but added that in the calculation of the NHS pool no deduction should be made for practitioners' estimated income from private practice or for Exchequer superannuation contributions. They also recommended that the £100,000 set aside annually for interest-free loans to encourage group practice should come from the Exchequer and not from the pool, and that the Exchequer should also provide an additional £500,000 a year for 'distinction awards' to general practitioners, similar to those available to consultants in the hospital service. Allowing for the changes in the method of calculating the pool, the Commission estimated that their recommendations would mean a real increase of about 23 *per cent* over the Danckwerts level. Finally they recommended that a standing Review Body should be established to advise the government on doctors' and dentists' remuneration.

The remuneration levels proposed by the Royal Commission were designed to achieve a reasonable relativity between general practitioners and their consultant colleagues. This was a matter on which practitioners were understandably sensitive, more particularly in view of a rather tactless suggestion by Lord Moran, a prominent consultant, in evidence to the Royal Commission, that general practitioners were doctors who had fallen off the ladder leading to the (consultant) heights of their profession: an ill-judged remark[23] which Lord Moran was subsequently at some pains to explain away[24].

The Royal Commission's recommendations were accepted by the government; general practitioners received arrears of payment amounting to £11 million; and arrangements for the distribution of the new and larger pool were agreed by a working party of the Health Departments and the profession. The standard capitation fee was increased from 18/- (90p) to

19/6d (97.5p) and there were corresponding increases in other payments. It was also agreed that the fund for encouraging group practice should be doubled by adding another £100,000 from the pool to the £100,000 contributed by the Exchequer.

In the event general practitioners felt unable to accept the principle of distinction awards. They did, however, agree in 1962 to set aside £1 million from the pool to encourage good general practice. Three-quarters of this sum was distributed in the form of increased 'loadings' for the 1,001st to the 1,500th patients on doctors' lists; the rest was used to provide grants (in addition to the expenses already covered by the Exchequer) to doctors taking postgraduate courses.

Although the problems of remuneration inevitably feature prominently in any account of these years, the day-to-day work of general practitioners in providing primary medical care continued, showing steady if unspectacular progress. The number of practitioners continued to increase slowly until the mid 1960s, and the proportion of doctors practising in partnership continued to rise, reaching 75 *per cent* by 1966. The average doctor's list in Scotland, after allowing for inflation of the registers, remained below 2,000, compared with 2,400 in England and Wales. There were some indications, however, that with their smaller numbers of patients Scottish general practitioners did relatively more work (more surgery consultations, more home visits, more night calls) than their colleagues in the south[25].

A further stimulus was provided in 1963 by a report on 'The Field of Work of the Family Doctor' produced by a sub-committee of the (English) Central Health Services Council under the chairmanship of Dr Annis Gillie. This stressed once again the importance of the general practitioner as a family doctor and the need to provide him with the tools to do his job: the time had come to get away from the 'cottage industry' approach to general practice and develop the idea of the general practitioner as the leader of the primary health care team. Early in 1964 the Health Ministers, concerned by the dissatisfaction in the profession, set up a joint working party of the Health Departments and the profession to consider the Gillie report and carry out a wide-ranging review of general practice in the National Health Service with the object of securing the best standards of practice; only the quantum of remuneration was excluded from the working party's scope. The working party set about their task at once, operating on a Great Britain basis but with parallel discussions in Scotland to consider specifically Scottish interests and attitudes, and by the early months of 1965 had produced the first of a series of 'commentaries' dealing with particular aspects of the general medical services.

The Family Doctors' Charter

In spite of the co-operative atmosphere in which these discussions were carried on, particularly in Scotland, a major crisis blew up in 1965. The new Review Body had recommended a substantial increase in 1963, bringing the average net professional income of a general practitioner to £2,765; but their response to a further claim put forward in the following year was less satisfactory to the profession. Reporting in 1965, they found no evidence that remuneration had been seriously inadequate since 1948, as the profession claimed; but they did recommend that some increase was justified because the population was growing faster than the number of doctors and that doctors' income from local authority, hospital and government appointments should be excluded from the calculation of the pool. They accordingly concluded that the pool should be increased by £5.5 million, which should be largely earmarked for partial direct reimbursement of doctors' expenditure on ancillary help and practice premises; and they supported the Pilkington recommendation that a scheme of distinction awards for general practitioners should be devised.

Dissatisfied with the Review Body's recommendations, the BMA delivered what was in effect an ultimatum, publishing in March 1965 a 'Charter for the Family Doctor Service' and securing notices of withdrawal from the National Health Service (undated, to be held in reserve as the profession's ultimate weapon) from a substantial proportion of practitioners.

The Charter began by setting out four principles for the future of general practice – all expressed in the form of the practitioner's 'rights', and three of them referring to his remuneration. The four rights were the right to practise good medicine in company with doctors in other branches of the profession, from suitable and properly equipped premises staffed by trained medical and non-medical personnel, with adequate remuneration and a minimum of interference with the doctor's independence; the right to practise to the best of his ability with the least possible intrusion by the State, protection from misuse by patients and safeguards against unjustified disciplinary procedures; the right to enjoy proper payment, based on responsibility and work load; and the right to financial security after retirement and for his dependants.

The Charter went on to work out the detailed implications of these principles. Among other things it called for a capitation fee of 36/- (£1.80), plus additional payments for night calls and weekend work. Although accepting that the bulk of doctors' practice expenses must be included within this gross capitation fee – since to meet them directly would involve an unacceptable degree of administrative control – it asked that there should be direct reimbursement of doctors' expenditure on ancillary help and the provision of practice premises.

The proposals in the Charter were accepted by the government as a basis for negotiation, and in the meantime it was agreed that the £5.5 million recommended by the Review Body should be added to the remuneration pool, not earmarked for any particular purpose but in the form of additions to the capitation fee, which now became 22/6d (£1.125), and other standard fees. The negotiations which followed resulted in agreement between the Health Departments and the profession on a new form of contract which broadly gave effect to the Charter proposals, relating general practitioners' remuneration more closely to their work-load and responsibility and to their experience, conditions of service and practice expenses. In addition it was agreed to set up a General Practice Finance Corporation to make loans for the provision or improvement of practice premises; and the government agreed to reduce the volume of certification required of general practitioners. The Health Departments proposed that provision should be made for 'merit awards' to a proportion of general practitioners; but once again this was turned down by the profession.

The Review Body was invited to 'price' the new form of contract, and in 1966 recommended an increase of £24 million (more than a third) in the net annual remuneration of general practitioners. The government accepted this recommendation but proposed that the additional £24 million should be paid in two stages, in April 1966 and April 1967. Following a general standstill on prices announced by the government in July the payment of the first instalment was deferred to October 1966, with a firm undertaking that the second instalment would be paid on the due date.

The new remuneration arrangements which came into effect in October 1966 meant the abolition of the 'pool' system which had governed general practitioners' remuneration under National Health Insurance and the National Health Service since 1913: the cost of providing general medical services was now to be met by the Exchequer without any ceiling on the total amount. Although the bulk of general practitioners' income was still to come from capitation fees (the standard fee for 1966 being fixed at £1, with a higher rate for older patients) and 'loadings', plus a 'basic practice allowance' of £925 (payable to doctors with at least a thousand patients), other payments were more directly related to a doctor's particular circumstances and experience. There were additional payments for practice in certain areas designated as in need of more doctors; for group practice; for seniority; for doctors who had taken vocational training and for attendance at postgraduate training courses; for the employment of an assistant; for acceptance of 'out-of-hours' responsibility at nights and weekends; and, as before, for the provision of maternity medical services and the treatment of temporary residents and emergencies. In addition there were direct payments towards the cost of employing ancillary staff and the provision of practice premises. Taken as a whole, the new remuneration pattern represented a major improvement in general practitioners' terms of service[26] and offered the prospect of developing the family doctor service without the recurring arguments about pay which had dogged it in the past.

The number of general practitioners in the National Health Service had reached a peak in 1963, and thereafter for a year or two had shown a tendency to decline. As a result of the steps taken to increase the output of doctors from the medical schools, combined with the boost given to recruitment by the new remuneration pattern, the number of general practitioners now maintained a steady upward trend, with the average list size showing a corresponding decline: the number of patients per doctor in Scotland remained under 2,000 – still very comfortably below the English average. Within ten years, between 1966 and 1976, the number of general practitioners (principals) had risen from just under 2,600 to rather over 2,800, and the move towards partnership rather than single-handed practice continued: whereas in the earlier year a quarter of Scottish general practitioners were still single-handed, ten years later the proportion had fallen to a seventh, and the trend was still downwards. Evidence collected by the Royal College of General Practitioners, however, showed that general practitioners spent relatively more time with their patients (more consultations, more visits) in Scotland than in the South[27].

The second half of the 1960s also saw an upsurge of interest in health centres among general practitioners. In 1967 two new ones were opened, and – more significantly – no fewer than 48 others were at various stages of consideration. By the end of 1975 the number of health centres in operation had risen to 75, serving a population of nearly a million, 16 were under construction and another 89 were at various stages of planning. In many, if not most, cases the initative had come from the general practitioners themselves. A major initiative was taken in Glasgow in 1965, when a joint committee representing the general medical, local authority and hospital services was set up to plan the future provision of health centres, taking account of the large development plans then under way in the city.

1965 also saw the launching of what came to be known as the 'Livingstone experiment', initiated by the Department in consultation with the various professional interests and administrative bodies concerned. This new town in West Lothian was seen to offer the opportunity for developing the general practitioner services in the closest possible association with hospital and local authority services. A joint committee representing the central department and the various local interests was established to plan a fully integrated service by the creation of joint hospital and general practitioner posts and the provision of general practitioner, local health authority and, where appropriate, hospital facilities in a number of purpose-built health centres associated with the new district hospital to be built in the area. The first doctor combining general practitioner and hospital duties took up his post early in 1966. Encouraging aspects of the early years of the project were the high quality of the doctors recruited, the goodwill shown by the various health service authorities and the satisfaction of the population served; but the building up of the full community health team proved to be a slow process, mainly because of the tripartite NHS structure[28].

The Move Towards Integration

Scottish general practitioners were now impatient to push on the process of integrating services. In March 1966 the General Medical Services Committee (Scotland) adopted a resolution recording their view that the future of general practice depended on the closest functional integration of all parts of the health service, and that, where the geographical situation made this appropriate, the best method of achieving integration was by the provision of health centres; and invited the Department to arrange a meeting of all those concerned to discuss the forward planning of integrated services. The Department welcomed this initiative, and a joint working party of the Committee and the Department was set up to carry the matter forward; their discussions, completed in 1968, played a significant part in shaping the government's proposals for the reorganisation of the National Health Service in Scotland. The 'green paper' (a discussion document) of December 1968 which set out these proposals hardly needed to argue the case for integrating the general practitioner services with the other health services; and the proposed establishment of a new type of area authority responsible for all health services raised no difficulties for general practitioners, who would have the same contractual relationship with the new bodies as with the existing councils, while no change was required in the functions of the Medical Practices Committee. The transfer of the Secretary of State's direct responsibility for the provision of health centres to the area health authorities was a logical consequence of the new pattern. Rather enviously the *British Medical Journal* commented in a leading article in May 1969, after noting that the Scottish green paper was not the 'twin' of the corresponding English document published in July 1968 but was the result of prolonged informal discussions between the Scottish health department and the professions: 'Good relations have existed between doctors and the (Scottish) Department for some years, and this contrasts with the more sceptical attitude that English doctors often adopt to proposals from the Elephant and Castle ... Scottish doctors have for years differed from their colleagues in the south in several respects – for example, by their ready acceptance of the value of health centres. So Scotland is likely to lead the way to a unified service'[29].

One notable respect in which the Scottish proposals differed from the English ones was that Scottish general practitioners were to be in a direct relationship with the new area health authority – a more evidently 'integrated' arrangement than the English proposals – to establish an independent Family Practitioner Committee to administer the general practitioner services. The chairman of the General Medical Services Committee (Scotland) was compelled to defend the Scottish pattern against criticism by the English GMS Committee, insisting that this was what Scottish general practitioners wanted and was not an idea forced on the profession by the central department. (It may be added that Scottish general practitioners were felt by some of their colleagues in England to be getting rather too far ahead of the rest of the profession in discussing integration with the Department.[30])

Meanwhile some of the problems of the existing service persisted. The cost of general practitioners' prescribing continued to grow at an alarming rate, in spite of the flow of information on costs issued by the Department and the measures for controlling excessive prescribing. By 1961 the net cost to the Exchequer (after allowing for the charges payable by patients) was £7.6 million, and an increase in the prescription charge from 1/- (5p) to 2/- (10p) in that year failed to reverse the rising trend. By 1964 the net cost had risen to £9.5 million, and the abolition of prescription charges by the Labour government early in 1965 was followed by a further massive increase of 16.7 *per cent* in the number of prescriptions (from 21.95 million to 25.62 million) and an increase in the cost to the Exchequer from £9.5 million in 1964 to £14 million in 1965. In 1966 the number rose to 27.53 million and in 1967 to 28.21 million, with a cost to the Exchequer of £16.91 million. In June 1968 the Conservative government reintroduced a prescription charge of 2/6d (12.5p) per item, with exemption for children, old people, expectant and nursing mothers, and certain other categories; but the rising trend was now so well established, with the sharply increasing costs of drugs, that this produced little effect. In 1970 the number of prescriptions was just under 29 million and their net cost just under £20 million, and even a further increase in the prescription charge to 20p in 1971 was insufficient to halt the continuing rise in cost, to £24.45 million in 1972 and £28.4 million in 1973.

In 1968 the Department's annual report was able to record some progress in the improvement of general medical services. The decline in the number of principals had been arrested, group practice was still increasing, the use of appointments systems was increasingly common and there had been an increase in the number of ancillary staff employed by general practitioners.

Remuneration, however, remained a regular preoccupation. In 1968 the Review Body recommended that no increase in general practitioners' remuneration was called for, but proposed various adjustments designed to offset increased practice expenses, encourage older doctors to remain in practice and promote the employment of ancillary help. In 1969 they recommended an increase which fell within the (Labour) government's 3½ *per cent* 'ceiling' on pay increases, and this was given effect to, but when in the following year they recommended a further increase of 30 *per cent* the government decided to refer this to the National Board for Prices and Incomes which they had established: whereupon the British Medical Asssociation imposed sanctions, involving a refusal by general practitioners to sign certificates and co-operate on NHS administrative bodies, and the Review Body resigned. Then, after a general election, the new (Conservative) government offered to withdraw the reference to the Prices and Incomes Board and appoint a new Review Body, and agreed to a restricted increase of 20 *per cent*, which was accepted by the profession. The new Review Body recommended an increase of 8 *per cent* in 1971 and a further 7½ *per cent* increase in 1972, bringing the target average net income of a general practitioner to £5,575. In the two following years the Review Body recommended further increases, taking into account the government's incomes policy, which brought the target net income to £5,750 and £6,127.

In July 1971 the Conservative government put forward its proposals for reorganisation, following the broad lines set out in the previous government's green paper. It said little – in the light of the earlier discussions there was little that needed to be said – about the general practitioner services, beyond noting that the new health service structure would not involve any change in the 'independent contractor' status of general practitioners and that the local medical committees which had long represented general practitioners in their relationships with executive councils provided a pattern for the professional committees representing the profession as a whole which were to be established under the new structure.

In preparation for the new integrated health service a working party of representatives of the medical profession in Scotland had been appointed in December 1969, under the chairmanship of the Chief Medical Officer, Sir John Brotherston, to 'consider how medical work in the National Health Service might best be organised to promote the full development of all aspects of health care'. Its report, 'Doctors in an Integrated Health Service', published in July 1971, stressed the importance of general practice as the mainstay of the health care system, but insisted that it must be strengthened so that general practitioners were equipped in terms of both training and resources to undertake greater clinical responsibility. They must have better supported places of work with adequate diagnostic facilities – most readily provided by the continued development of the health centre programme – and should increasingly have access to beds in which they might care for some of their own patients in hospital. In the longer term the report foresaw the emergence of a new style of general practitioner trained and equipped to do much of the work of the general physician. If general practitioners were to have the time to make these developments possible a closer partnership would be required with the other health care professions (nurses, health visitors, social workers, professions supplementary to medicine).

As the working party recognised, the wider role now contemplated for general practitioners made it necessary to ensure that they were properly trained for the task, both before and after qualification. The Royal Commission on Medical Education which reported in 1968 had already stressed the need to include experience of general practice in the basic education of medical students; and the working party drew particular attention to the importance of providing adequate postgraduate vocational training and continuing education for general practitioners. This point had also been made by the Royal Commission, and their recommendation was followed up by the establishment, early in 1971, of the Scottish Council for Postgraduate Medical Education, charged with a general responsibility for supervising and promoting the provision of a comprehensive programme of refresher courses: a form of training which had been steadily gaining in popularity among general practitioners, with financial assistance provided by the Scottish Home and Health Department. By the end of the year the Council had produced a report recommending a scheme of post-registration vocational training in general practice (one year in general practice and two years in hospital, with a common path during the initial postgraduate training for all doctors, whatever branch of medicine they were aiming at).

The Act which provided the statutory basis for the integration of the NHS administrative structure became law in August 1972. So far as general practitioners were concerned there was little change in the day-to-day arrangements for running the service, but the potentiality for change in the pattern of general practitioner services was considerable, with the removal of the administrative barriers which had hitherto made co-operation between general practitioners and their colleagues in other parts of the NHS more difficult to achieve. Significantly, the report of the Scottish Home and Health Department contained, for the first time, a section devoted not to the general practitioner services but to primary health care, defined as 'the advice and care given to members of the public on health matters by multi-disciplinary professional teams responsible for providing a service at the point of first contact and continuing through the treatment, rehabilitation or terminal phases of illness when these take place in the community'.

The Department's report went on to note that the essential primary care services were those provided by the general practitioner and the nurse, health visitor and midwife, but that this basic team was increasingly being supported by professional and other colleagues, forming a multi-disciplinary group with shared responsibility for providing personal and community health care. The formation of primary care teams had been facilitated by the development of group practice – by 1974 some 62 *per cent* of general practitioners were practising in partnerships of three or more, compared with only 48 *per cent* in 1968 – and teams of this kind were expected in future to be increasingly based in health centres, the planning of which should be facilitated and speeded up by the new integrated structure of the National Health Service.

There were other encouraging features. The number of general practitioners practising in the National Health Service was now rising, and was to continue rising steadily if unspectacularly. The number of principals in the Scottish NHS in 1974 was 2,745, with an average list of 1,973. Increased interest in general practice was also signalled by the establishment of a chair of general practice in Glasgow University (Edinburgh had had one – the first in the United Kingdom – since 1963). The Livingstone experiment in combining general and hospital practice seemed to be going well, in spite of financial stringency; a report on the first ten years of the scheme was to refer to a 'continuing flush of success'[31].

But once again the problem of doctors' remuneration came to the fore. The Review Body had continued to recommend annual increases, though they were now expected to have regard to the government's incomes policy. In June 1974 they recommended an increase designed to bring the average net remuneration for a principal to £6,147, and this was implemented for the year from April 1974; but when, later in the year, the profession put in a further pay claim the Review Body recommended no change in general practitioners' net income, though they recognised that it would have to be brought up to date as from the following April. Thereupon the General Medical Services Committee fell back on the tactics they had used before, invited general practitioners to submit undated resignations from the NHS and set about drafting a new form of contract. The crisis passed, however, when the Review Body in a further report (April 1975) recommended a substantial increase in pay, bringing the average net remuneration of a general practitioner to £6,377: whereupon the British Medical Association was able to claim triumphantly that over the previous ten years average net remuneration had increased by 178 *per cent*, against an increase in the index of retail prices of only 113 *per cent*. The standard capitation fee now became £2.15, and the additional demands made by older patients were recognised by the introduction of two higher-level fees – £2.80 for patients aged between 65 and 74, £3.45 for those over 75.

In 1976 legislation was passed by Parliament providing for the introduction of a requirement that any doctor seeking to enter general practice as an 'unrestricted' principal (i.e. one not limiting the scope of his practice) should have had three years full-time vocational training after registration, with at least a year as a trainee in general practice and the rest of the time in approved posts in hospital and community medicine; thus giving effect to the recommendations put forward by the Scottish Council for Postgraduate Medical Education in 1971. Before this requirement could come into operation time had to be allowed for the necessary preparations to be made, and it was 1982 before the full requirements for vocational training became mandatory. Meanwhile the number of doctors taking vocational training voluntarily continued to increase; though attendance at the short-term postgraduate refresher courses for general practitioners was now declining.

Towards the 1980s

During the 1970s the team approach to the provision of primary health care showed steady development, the basic elements in the team being the family doctor and the nurse. The 1975 report of the Scottish Home and Health Department referred to this as 'one of the most successful developments in modern clinical organisation', and the Royal Commission on the National Health Service which reported in 1979 also saw the growth of teamwork in primary care as a development of great significance. The Royal Commission noted that the grouping of practices and the spread of health centres had brought general practitioners into closer working contact with each other and with their nursing and administrative colleagues, and also with dentists, pharmacists and social workers.

This development was promoted by the steady growth in the number of health centres, which were more popular with general practitioners – and, in general, with patients – in Scotland than in England and Wales. By 1982 there were 157 health centres in operation in Scotland, and another 56 were at various stages of construction or planning. Almost a third of Scottish practitioners were now practising from health centres, which varied in size and facilities according to local circumstances, catering for anything between one and 36 practitioners.

The number of general practitioners working in the NHS in Scotland also continued to increase – slowly, perhaps, but steadily. From its low point of 2,592 in 1968 it rose each year to reach 3,040 in 1982, with a corresponding fall in average list size (i.e. the number of people for whom each practitioner was responsible) from 2,106 to 1,778. The number of general practitioners in relation to population remained considerably higher in Scotland than in England, and the average list size correspondingly lower.

Throughout the 1970s and early 1980s the problem of general practitioners' (and other doctors') remuneration continued to loom large. The Review Body was still producing regular annual reports recommending appropriate levels of remuneration; but for much of the period the difficulties of settling remuneration were increased by government policies of pay restraint. In spite of these restrictions the average net remuneration of a general practitioner, as recommended by the Review Body, had risen by 1979 to £12,327, though the Review Body made it clear that but for the government's pay 'guidelines' the figure would have been £13,695. Once again the representatives of the profession put themselves into a defensive posture, and the General Medical Services Committee devised a scheme for financing general practice in the event of general practitioners' withdrawal from the National Health Service.

In 1980, however, the pay guidelines were relaxed and relations between the profession and the government became rather easier. The Review Body's recommendation of £16,290 as the average net remuneration of a general practitioner was accepted, and the basic practice allowance now became £4,725, with standard capitation fees ranging between £4.15 and £6.65.

The reorganisation of NHS management structures which took place in 1981 made no difference to the administration of the general practitioner services in Scotland, which continued on the established pattern within the organisation of the health boards. (This contrasted with the situation south of the Border, where it was now proposed to establish the family practitioner committees as independent health authorities). Meanwhile the number and cost of prescriptions issued by general practitioners had continued to rise. By 1978 the number of prescriptions was 35.85 million and the net cost to the Exchequer £81.7 million. In July 1979 the prescription charge payable by the patient was increased from 20p to 45p; and although the number of prescriptions issued in 1980 fell slightly to 35.61 million the net cost rose steeply to £108.58 million. The corresponding figures for 1982 were 36.33 million and £139.61 million, for 1983 37.08 million and £156.21 million – and this in spite of further increases in the prescription charge which brought it to £1.40 in 1983. The rising trend in cost appeared to be irreversible, for although the number of prescriptions was now being held or increasing only slowly the cost of drugs continued to increase and the proportion of expensive proprietary drugs prescribed, already high (84 *per cent* in 1974), was still rising. Early in 1985, therefore, the government made a further effort to halt the trend, increasing the prescription charge to £2 and introducing restrictions on the prescribing of some categories of proprietary drugs.

By 1985 the level of average net remuneration recommended by the Review Body had risen to £23,440 – ten and a half times the figure recommended in the Danckwerts award for 1948. As an indication of the complexity of the pattern of remuneration which had evolved over the years it is of interest to consider the range of fees and allowances recommended by the Review Body to achieve this level of income.

First there was a basic practice allowance, payable to every general practitioner, of £7,065. This was supplemented by designated area allowances of £2,185 or £3,335 for practice in areas to which it was necessary to attract doctors; initial practice allowances ranging up to £19,650 for doctors setting up their first practice; an allowance of £1,225 for doctors practising in a group; seniority allowances ranging from £1,690 to £4,560; an allowance of £1,450 for doctors who had taken vocational training and a postgraduate training allowance.

The second main element in remuneration was the capitation fee – £6.85 for patients under 65, £8.85 for those between 65 and 75 and £10.90 for those over 75.

These payments covered only services given during normal working hours. For practitioners accepting 'out of hours' responsibility there was a supplementary practice allowance of £1,405 plus a supplementary capitation fee (for all patients beyond 1,000) of £1.91 and a night visit fee of £15.55. (In practice all doctors accept this responsibility, though they may meet it with the help of a deputising service or other arrangement for providing a deputy.)

The various allowances accounted for rather more than a quarter of the average practitioner's income, capitation fees for something like a third. In addition there were a variety of 'item of service' fees, making up perhaps an eighth of average remuneration: for the provision of maternity services (£105, plus night visit fees if required), vaccination or immunisation, contraceptive services, cervical cytology tests, emergency treatment and the treatment of temporary residents, the provision of an anaesthetist to give a general anaesthetic and the arrest of dental haemorrhage.

Direct reimbursement of particular practice expenses – on ancillary staff, practice premises, dispensing, etc. – contributed another quarter of the average practitioner's remuneration. And finally for doctors practising in rural areas there were mileage payments from the rural practices fund.

Complicated though it may be, the system of general practitioners' remuneration under the National Health Service now reflects much more closely than in the past the different circumstances and skills of individual practitioners. It has made it easier for doctors – particularly those not practising from health centres – to finance improvements in their practice premises and equipment and has encouraged the employment of ancillary staff; and it has fostered the continuing trend towards partnership and group practice. In recent years the arrangements for keeping the level of NHS remuneration under review have operated without any major crisis, though there has been complaint about government 'phasing' (i.e. postponement) of increases recommended by the Review Body. At any rate the remuneration appears to have been sufficient to attract doctors into general practice at a rate which has been steady if not spectacular. In 1983 the number of 'unrestricted' principals (i.e. those not limiting their list to patients in particular categories) in the National Health Service in Scotland was 3,106, with an average list size of 1,739. Of these practitioners only 331 (10.5) were in single-handed practice, and 1,634 (52.5) were in partnerships of four or more. (The move towards partnership practice since the establishment of the National Health Service has been rather more marked in Scotland than in England and Wales: in 1983 some 24 *per cent* of practitioners south of the Border were single-handed and 48.6 *per cent* were in partnerships of four or more).

The general practitioner's ability to provide effective care for his patients has been enhanced by improvements in practice premises and equipment, increased support from ancillary staff and the availability of more powerful therapeutic resources. The steady increase in the drug bill has been a cause of concern throughout the history of the National Health Service; but this increase has only partly been due to careless or excessive prescribing. In the main it reflects the continuing development of new and more effective drugs which have transformed the general practitioner's armamentarium and enabled him to do much more for his patients. At the same time better access to diagnostic facilities has made it possible for him to retain control of treatment in cases where previously referral to hospital would have been necessary. Many practitioners, too, run clinics for particular groups of patients, taking over a function performed in the past by other health service agencies. (But conversely, largely as a result of the closure of small cottage hospitals, general practitioners have lost opportunities they formerly enjoyed for caring for patients in hospital.)

These developments have increased the content of the practitioner's work and offered greater personal satisfaction; but they have also tended to increase his work load, and sometimes encouraged patients to make greater demands (e.g. for particular drugs or forms of treatment). The trend towards transferring the care of chronic and geriatric patients so far as possible from institutions to the community has also increased the general practitioner's responsibilities.

Another recent development which works both ways – reducing work in one direction but also opening up new fields of action – is the application of computer technology. Some 10 *per cent* of Scottish general practitioners now have the use of a micro-computer, even though they may not exploit its full potentialities. Its commonest use is probably for controlling and processing repeat prescriptions, but it can also be used for patient registration, the supervision of chronic disease, recall procedures for immunisation and screening, drug intelligence and research of various kinds. Some of these operations save time and trouble; others, while increasing the content and value of the general practitioner's professional role, will involve him in more work if he takes full advantage of them. But clearly the impact of the computer on general practice is only just beginning to make itself felt.

In recent years general practitioners have increasingly become involved in family planning and in giving contraceptive advice: a field which enhances their role as family doctors but brings problems of its own. Against this, their work in the field of maternity services has been reduced over the years by the trend towards hospital confinement, now the almost invariable rule.

The extent to which increases in the practitioner's work load have been counterbalanced by better ancillary support, technical facilities and practice organisation is difficult to assess. A general impression would be that there has not been much change in absolute work load in recent years, though there is sometimes a feeling that patients have become more demanding. Much evidently depends on the relationship which each individual doctor establishes with the patients on his list.

One respect in which the call on the general practitioner's time has been reduced is the decline in the number of home visits in favour of surgery consultations. Night calls are less of a problem than they used to be; the growth of partnership and group practice has made it possible to spread the load of 'out of hours' calls in general; and in some areas (Glasgow, Edinburgh and neighbouring counties) there are now organised deputising services, though these are less used in Scotland than in some parts of England and Wales (under a quarter of Scottish practitioners having obtained authority to use a deputising service, compared with something over two-fifths in England and Wales).

Demanding or not, patients in general seem to be well satisfied with the service they get from their general practitioner. Complaints are few, and the obvious remedy for dissatisfaction – a change of doctor – is little used. A recent survey reported in 1981[32] found a high degree of stability in people's attachment to their family doctor, the great majority changing practices only when they moved away from the district or the practice ceased to operate. An opinion poll in 1985[33] found 89 *per cent* of those questioned satisfied with the service given by their family doctor.

How general practitioners themselves feel about it is more difficult to assess. Are they functionaries of the welfare state, hamstrung by government regulation? Are they, as has recently been suggested[34], a 'relatively well rewarded, non-competitive monopoly', 'the most stultifying impediment to change' in the provision of primary care? In this most individual branch of an individualistic profession it is not easy to make generalisations; but it is probably true to say that most general practitioners have a satisfying and challenging job, with its compensations as well as its frustrations. The enhanced standing of general practice and its increased self-confidence have been demonstrated and symbolised by the activities and the increasing influence of the Royal College of General Practitioners; and general practice, paradoxically, has come to be regarded as a specialty in its own right – a development which may perhaps have tended, to some extent, to emphasise the divide between general practitioners and their colleagues in hospital.

This can only be an interim report, since the general practitioner services, like the rest of the National Health Service, are in process of constant development; and the coming years will present them with fresh challenges – the problems of an ageing population, changing patterns of disease, advances in pharmacology and medical technology. This account has traced the difficulties and problems which have accompanied their development; but through it all there has been a steady push for improvement – for enhancing the status and resources of the family practitioner and the quality of the services provided for the people of Scotland. This is a task which involves both the government, represented by the central health departments, and the profession. Although the two sides have sometimes been at odds over questions of finance and remuneration they have always been conscious of their common responsibility and their common achievement in building up the general practitioner services; and they can both find some satisfaction in the conclusion reached in a booklet published by the British Medical Association in December 1983 under the title 'General Practice: a British Success':

> "There are grounds now for claiming that the ideal of a well-organised service manned by doctors maintaining high skills and yet retaining a personal approach to patients as well as a flexible approach to new medical needs has largely been achieved"[35].

References

(1) Brotherston, J.H.F., 'Evolution of medical practice', in *Medical History and Medical Care*, pub. for the Nuffield Provincial Hospitals Trust by the Oxford University Press, 1971, p.88.

(2) Hamilton, David, *The Healers*, Edinburgh, 1981, pp.62, 98.

(3) *Edin. Med. J.*, 1911, p.462.

(4) The figures are taken from an article in the *Lancet*, 1905, 1, p.593.

(5) A longer tradition in Scotland than in England. The earliest recorded friendly society in Britain was the Incorporation of Carters of Leith, founded in 1555.

(6) *Lancet*, 1890, 2, p.372: correspondence referring to an article in the *Scotsman* of 9 August 1890.

(7) Grant, I.D., 'Status of the General Practitioner Past, Present and Future', *Brit. Med. J.*, 1961, 2, pp.1279–82.

(8) Brend, W.A., *Health and the State*, 1917, p.180.

(9) The first skirmish in the 'battle' took place in Cork in 1894, when the club doctors used the recently devised Irish technique of the boycott, withdrawing their services from the club and setting up an organisation of their own: the first medical use of a tactic followed by the profession in later conflicts with the National Health Insurance and Health Service authorities.

(10) 'An Investigation into the Economic Conditions of Contract Medical Practice in the United Kingdom', Supplement to *Brit. Med. J.*, 1905, 2, pp.1–96.

(11) Article in *Glasgow Herald*, 25 May 1911.

(12) *Brit. Med. J.*, Supplement, 1911, 1, pp.81–122.

(13) Cox, Alfred, "Seven Years of National Health Insurance in England", *J. of Amer. Med. Ass.*, 1921, 2, p.1311.

(14) Gilbert, B.B., *The Evolution of National Insurance in Great Britain*, London, 1966, p440.

(15) *National Insurance Gazette*, 13 December 1913.

(16) Cox, Alfred, *op. cit.* (note 11), p.1398.

(17) The figures are conveniently summarised in Currie, J.R., *The Mustering of Medical Service in Scotland 1914–1919*, Edinburgh, 1922, p.10.

(18) Currie, J.R., *op. cit.*, p.193.

(19) *Lancet*, 1950, 1, pp.555–585.

(20) It is fair to say that relations between the profession and the central department in Scotland were not bedevilled by arguments on remuneration, which was for the most part dealt with on a Great Britain basis in London.

(21) *Brit. Med. J.*, 1953, 2, pp.683–706.

(22) *Brit. Med. J.*, 1954, 1, pp.746–748.

(23) Comment by a general practitioner: 'Hitherto I have considered myself devoid of superstition, but, after reading some of the evidence to the Royal Commission last week, I shall think twice before walking under a ladder – you see, there might be a consultant at the top of the ladder, and he may drop a brick'. Letter in *Brit. Med. J.*, Supplement, 1959, 1, p.48.

(24) *Brit. Med. J.*, Supplement, 1959, 1, pp.29 and 36–37.

(25) Article by Stevenson, J.S.F., *Brit. Med. J.*, 1964, 1, pp.1370–73.

(26) Under the new pattern, with the further increases recommended by the Review Body in subsequent years, the average net income of general practitioners rose by 103 *per cent* between April 1960 and April 1970, against an increase of 46.7 *per cent* in retail prices over the same period. Forsyth, Gordon, *Doctors and State Medicine: A Study of the British Health Service*, 2nd ed., 1973, p.60.

(27) Royal College of General Practitioners, *Present State and Future Needs of General Practice*, 1st, 2nd and 3rd editions, 1965, 1970 and 1973.

(28) Duncan, A.H., *The Livingstone Project: the First Five Years*, Scottish Health Service Studies No. 29, 1973.

(29) *Brit. Med. J.*, 1969, 2, p.331.

(30) Report of Annual Representative Meeting of BMA, *Brit. Med. J.*, Supplement, 1969, 3, p.13.

(31) Munro, H.D.R. (ed), *The Livingstone Scheme: a Ten Year Review*, Scottish Health Service Studies No. 43, 1982.

(32) Ritchie, Jane, Jacoby, Ann and Bone, Margaret, *Access to Primary Health Care*, HMSO, 1981, p.58.

(33) Poll conducted by MORI, November 1985. Sample: 1,058 adults aged 18 and over in 53 sampling points throughout Scotland. *Scotsman*, 28 November 1985.

(34) Marinker, Marshall, *Developments in Primary Health Care in a New NHS Act for 1996?*, Office of Health Economics, London, 1984, p.19.

(35) *General Practice: a British Success*, British Medical Association, 1983, p.27.

2. *The Hospitals*

John Kinnaird

CONTENTS

About the Author

JOHN KINNAIRD

John Kinnaird held a number of senior hospital posts in hospitals before and after the Second World War, in which he served as a non-medical officer in the R.A.M.C. He was a WHO Fellow of the University of Minnesota in 1961, after which he was Senior Lecturer in Medical Services Administration at the University of Edinburgh.

Author's Note

The following pages trace the stages by which a miscellany of separate Scottish institutions, designed in the nineteenth century for the care of the sick poor and the ailing pauper, developed during the twentieth century into a national system for the application of a sophisticated medical technology to the treatment of diseases of the whole population. The emergencies of two world wars promoted both the astonishing medical advances of the period and, in breaking old moulds of thought and habit, the rationalisation of the contributions of local institutions and central government. By the second half of the twentieth century, the hospitals, with their concentrations of medical and nursing skills and technical resources, had taken their place among the principal institutions of modern society. In the light of their remarkable achievements in curing or alleviating many previously intractable or fatal conditions, they were deserving of substantial support from the nation's resources, far beyond the modest demands which they had made on the public in earlier times. Thereby they came into strong competition with other claimants upon these extensive, yet limited, resources.

During the century, the administrative structure seen to be appropriate to the funding and supervision of hospital services developed as the hospitals themselves were developing; the concept of informal association was eventually replaced by that of a formal hierarchical structure encompassing the country. Within the national dimension, the variety and complexity of medical care, the need for the effective association of hospital and community services, the disparities in social and demographic conditions in the different parts of Scotland, set problems as to the appropriate spans of administration at lower levels. These were to be the subject of repeated efforts to match the circumstances.

Erudite in medical history, concerned for the Scottish identity, and conscious of the necessary interdependence of medical practitioners of the various professions involved in health care, and of the three branches of the tripartite service, John Brotherston played his unique part in the most ambitious of these efforts.

The Hospitals

Part One: Towards a Co-ordinated Hospital Service

The Separate Strands

By the beginning of the twentieth century that small seed,which the physicians of Edinburgh, in partnership with its Town Council and benevolent citizens, had sown 170 years earlier with the opening of a 6-bed infirmary[1], had grown and multiplied until the great cities and many of the towns throughout Scotland had their infirmaries (Glasgow having three). Burdett lists 21 Scottish infirmaries founded between 1729 and 1881, with a total in the year 1900 of nearly 4,000 beds. In the cities these general hospitals had been supplemented by special hospitals, some catering for a particular clientele, for example women, children (or both together), and others for specified forms of care-maternity or the treatment of diseases of particular organs or types: for example diseases of the eye, ear, nose and throat, cancers and venereal diseases. Burdett lists a score of these, opened between 1793 and 1893, with, by the turn of the century, some 700 beds. Throughout the rural areas cottage hospitals, funded by local appeal or generous bequest, had been springing up. Of such, Burdett lists more than 40, founded between 1836 and 1897, with a total of some 600 beds[2].

These voluntary hospitals, with honorary medical staffs, which in the main institutions included physicians and surgeons of great distinction, gave their patients the benefit of the medical knowledge of the time. The smaller institutions might cope only with minor complaints and chronic ailments, but in the major institutions the application of the principles of antisepsis and asepsis had permitted a revolution in surgery. In Glasgow, for example, whereas only 310 operations were undertaken in its Royal Infirmary in 1865, in 1900 that figure had been multiplied over 14 times to 4,531 operations between its then three infirmaries, Royal, Western and Victoria[3]. With such an expansion of activity the directors of the largest hospitals sought to appoint Superintendents of high calibre to act as intermediaries between the management boards and the medical staffs. These medical administrators recognised that the new treatments demanded nursing care for which systematic training was necessary. On taking up his duties as Superintendent of the Edinburgh

Royal Infirmary in 1871, Deputy Surgeon-General Fasson, the first of a line of Superintendents with military titles[4], secured the engagement of a nurse trained at St Thomas's to supervise the organisation and training of the nurses[5]; as did Dr Robert Sinclair at the Dundee Royal Infirmary in 1874[6] in the person of Mrs Rebecca Strong who four years later accepted the appointment of Matron at the Glasgow Royal Infirmary where she introduced patterns of nurse training which had an international influence[7].

With expenditure rising continuously as they endeavoured to cope with the needs of a growing population and the additional costs of more effective treatments, the voluntary hospitals had developed, in varying degrees, the systematic collection of subscriptions which generally, for a specified minimum sum, qualified subscribers to recommend patients for admission to the institution. Increasingly, organised contributions from working people, in mills, factories, engineering works or shipbuilding yards were forthcoming for the hospitals' support, Scotland being notable in this respect[8], while income from invested funds, accumulated from special donations and bequests, was making an important contribution to the revenues of the more prominent institutions.

The infectious diseases, whose periodic epidemics during the nineteenth century had frequently disrupted the work of the general infirmaries, were now being provided for by local authorities, urged thereto by the Board of Supervision for the Poor Law[9] and its successor, the Local Government Board for Scotland, which by the Public Health (Scotland) Act of 1897 had been granted mandatory powers in this respect[10]. The endemic scourge of the period, tuberculosis, was the object of a strategic attack initiated by Dr Robert W. Philip (later Sir Robert) which became known as the Edinburgh Co-ordinated Anti-Tuberculosis Scheme[11], exemplifying, relative to a single disease, the comprehensive organisation of treatment which was eventually to be the goal for every form of illness.

As to the care of the sick poor, the Scottish tradition of the poorhouse as an almshouse which offered a refuge for the more respectable of the aged and infirm poor had, with the operation of the Poor Law in the circumstances of the economic and social turmoil of the nineteenth century, become confused with concepts applicable to the English workhouse for the destitute of all sorts[12]. Accommodation for the genuinely sick was inadequately differentiated, nursing was undertaken by healthier paupers, and the attraction for medical men of the task of treating mainly chronic and degenerative diseases was limited. Facilities for the efficient care of acute illnesses were less developed than in the voluntary hospitals – the major infirmaries had the added stimulus of providing medical education – and any serious surgery was generally performed under primitive conditions. Yet young men might accept the work for short periods to obtain experience. Dr William Macewen was appointed as the first Medical Superintendent of the Glasgow Fever Hospital at Belvidere in 1870, an office which included clinical responsibilities. He followed this within a year with a period of independent practice which included an appointment as a district medical officer with the Parochial Board, evidence that Poor Law employment was acceptable to men of the highest calibre. Indeed Dr Alexander Robertson, the capable physician-superintendent in the Glasgow poorhouse at Parliamentary Road, was able to offer Macewen facilities for surgical work there, the beginning of a great career in that discipline[13]. (The medical administrators in both Municipal Fever and Poor Law hospitals differed from their colleagues in the voluntary infirmaries in that additionally they carried clinical responsibilities. Dr Robertson himself was later to be appointed a Physician in Glasgow Royal Infirmary.)[14]

When, from the 1870's onwards, the voluntary hospitals were awakening to new possibilities in hospital care, some of the Poor Law authorities began to take similar measures. In 1878 the Board of Supervision reported the observation of one of its Visiting Officers, who deplored the low standard of nursing in the Scottish poorhouses compared with that in the Scottish infirmaries and suggested that the pauper as the recipient of a legal provision for his relief – dealt out to him under Government supervision and to some extent under Government control – had claims not inferior to the infirmary patient, who was in many instances the recipient of charity[15]. In 1880 the Board were able to report the introduction of satisfactory arrangements for skilled nursing in the Barnhill Poorhouse of Glasgow's Barony Parish[16] where a two-year training for nurses was soon introduced[17]. In 1885 the application to the cost of employing trained nurses of a portion of the medical grant was authorised. Governing bodies of poorhouses were slow to take advantage of the concession but by 1902 twenty-nine poorhouses participated to the extent of employing 152 trained nurses[16]. By that date four poorhouses had hospitals which were training schools for nurses: Dundee, Govan and two in the Glasgow Parish–City and Barnhill[18]. The Local Government Act of 1894 had transferred the Poor Law function of Parochial Boards to popularly elected Parish Councils. The new Glasgow Parish Council boldly assumed its responsibilities, adopting in 1899 an imaginative and far-sighted plan for a large general hospital of around 1,200 beds, including a sanatorium for consumptives of 200 beds, and two smaller district hospitals. Stobhill General Hospital, which was to make a notable contribution to hospital care in Glasgow then and in later years, resulted in 1902. It was capable of accommodating about 1,800 patients in an emergency. In 1904 the Western District Hospital (Oakbank) with 320 beds and the Eastern District Hospital (Duke Street) with 312 beds followed. Between 1902 and 1905 the neighbouring Govan Parish Council provided over 700 beds in good modern hospital accommodation including a children's block, siting this in the grounds of Merryflats

Poorhouse[19]. The twentieth century was already beginning to add its contribution to the Victorian legacy. Yet that legacy was to be of no small importance to the Scottish National Health Service. When the Service was entering the last quarter of the present century 143 of its 349 hospitals (including mental institutions) were found to date from before 1900[20].

Occasions for Co-operation

Thus the hospitals of the late nineteenth century fell into distinct categories according to the strictly defined functions for which they were founded and maintained by independent agencies. Within these categories the individual institutions were separate entities with their own purposes. Yet the critical emergency might excite ready co-operation. Thus, in 1878 when Glasgow's Royal and Western Infirmaries were overwhelmed by pressures for admission, the Town Council made an old Fever Hospital available for the reception of medical cases, and for a period of four months it was managed by Royal Infirmary staff, the Council giving financial aid with a grant of £500[21]. In the following year the same premises were placed at the disposal of the Maternity Hospital for lying-in cases until the completion of the reconstruction of that hospital early in 1881[22,23].

The mutual concerns of local authorities and voluntary institutions could be given recognition by the representation of the Town Council on the management committee of a voluntary hospital[24], and co-operation was facilitated through the authorisation of Parochial Boards to subscribe to any public infirmary, dispensary or lying-in hospital, or to any lunatic asylum or infirmary for the blind or deaf and dumb[25]. This enabled them to cater for needs which they could not meet themselves. Later this authorisation was extended to subscription to convalescent homes[26].

New Vistas

In 1904 the Report of the Departmental Committee was produced. The Committee had been appointed by the Local Government Board for Scotland to inquire into the system of Poor Law Medical Relief and into the Rules and Regulations for the Management of Poorhouses; it noted with approval the new practice of some of the larger parish councils of subscribing to convalescent homes for the accommodation of their child patients, but warned against the over-generous extension of this benefit to adults, as possibly fostering pauperism and risking objection from ratepayers who could not afford such a facility for members of their own families[27]. The Report expressed satisfaction with the larger poorhouse hospitals which had gradually been coming into line with the more advanced general hospitals or infirmaries in the country. As a consequence the reluctance of the poor to enter a poorhouse hospital for treatment of their illnesses had lessened, and even non-paupers who failed to gain admission to an infirmary were finding the poorhouse hospital an acceptable alternative. The Committee recommended that the sick should always be housed in a building detached from the rest of the poorhouse. For new poorhouses this should be the rule, and in existing poorhouses 'if the cost be not too great' a similar provision should be made. An amalgamation of poorhouse combinations should be organised in order to secure the efficiency of sizeable hospital units. Such units could justify the employment of trained nurses. In the larger hospitals only, operating rooms were called for, having regard to the frequency of surgical operations, an aspect of treatment which was also important in nurse training[28]. Nursing by paupers should be completely abolished[29]. (The English Local Government Board had issued an Order in 1897 which prohibited nursing by pauper inmates in workhouses, but the Scottish Board had felt unable to do this because of the many small poorhouses with only limited or occasional need for skilled nursing, and in 1902 twenty-seven poorhouses were to be found which still had only pauper nurses, with the number of sick in these ranging from one to forty-two[30].) It was in response to a recommendation of the Departmental Committee that three years later the Local Government Board instituted a syllabus of nurse training with the award of certificates of proficiency[31].

Other recommendations of the Departmental Committee were being implemented when the members of the Royal Commission on the Poor Laws and Relief of Distress reported in 1909. The Royal Commission noted that the development of hospital facilities in Scottish poorhouses between 1860 and 1908 had resulted in an increase from 13.3 per cent to 30.4 per cent in the proportion, in some districts, of poorhouse inmates who were sick[32]. Accordingly, the number of cases sent by the Poor Law authorities to voluntary hospitals had declined. But it was evident to the Commission that the amount of hospital accommodation was generally insufficient for the needs of the local communities, and that in the interests of economy and of the patients themselves any expansion of the hospital system must be accompanied by closer co-operation between the voluntary hospitals and the Poor Law[33]. The Commissioners took the view that disability to earn a livelihood should no longer be essential for eligibility for Poor Relief and that any person should be eligible for Public Assistance who was, for the time being, without directly available material resources which were appropriate for the satisfying of his physical needs[34]. They proposed changes in the administrative structure appropriate to this new policy for the dispensing of what would be titled 'Public Assistance'[35].

A Minority Report emanating from four members of the Commission took no satisfaction from the improved state of present conditions. The absence of provision for the sick poor, 'in thousands of cases', was 'a disgrace to twentieth century administration'[36]. As for the conditions of the poorhouse hospitals the Minority Report remarked: 'it is difficult to believe that we are speaking of a civilised country in the twentieth century'[37]. The dissidents regarded the proposals of the majority as a superficial and ineffective way of tackling a scandalous state of affairs and felt the need for a more radical approach, involving the transfer of Poor Law medical responsibilities to the Public Health authorities (and likewise the transfer of other Poor Law functions to appropriate existing government agencies).

The two Reports from the Royal Commission were thought-provoking. They sowed a seed, but many years were to pass before the seed flowered. Schemes calling for large changes in customary practice, however excellently conceived, must struggle against misunderstanding, apathy and vested interest. That was the experience of the Liberal Government in the promotion of the National Insurance Scheme which crystalised in the Act of 1911. This reform was attained through political compromise with strongly entrenched pressure groups. So far as institutional care was concerned, insured persons were to receive sanatorium benefit and concurrently Government Grants were forthcoming for the construction of sanatoria[39]; but Sir Henry Burdett's campaign to secure an extension to cover hospital care met with no response from the Government; it was more concerned about the support which the Daily Mail was giving to the London ladies who were campaigning against a statutory requirement that their maidservants lick insurance stamps on their premises[40]. The Act conceded only that payments to hospitals in respect of maintenance and treatment of members might be one of a number of additional benefits which the approved societies holding the insurance funds might decide to provide out of the surplus which might be thrown up at the periodic valuation of their respective funds[41]. In the event the voluntary hospitals gained little from this concession, which the Mackenzie Committee found to depend upon the willingness of the managers of voluntary hospitals, to enter into a contractual arrangement with a society for the professional treatment of its members[42]. Yet the new scheme did affect the hospitals, for in promoting primary care for a designated section of the population, referrals to the hospitals by the panel doctors for consultant opinion and specialist treatment inevitably increased, justifying Burdett's quip that the panel doctors were acting as recruiting sergeants for the hospitals[43].

The National Insurance Act of 1911 had an early effect on the medical services in the Highlands and Islands when the Scottish Insurance Commissioners made representations to the Treasury regarding the difficulty of ensuring satisfactory services for insured persons in that area of Scotland[44]. The Highlands and Islands Medical Service Committee, appointed in July 1912, recognised that hospitals were indeed complementary to general practice. It found that, apart from the Northern Infirmary in Inverness which had 68 beds functioning, there were 19 cottage hospitals in the area, their bed complements ranging from 2 to 22 beds (with an average of 11). Having regard to the distances involved and the costs and dangers of travel, the Committee called for more small cottage hospitals located suitably for the access of patients and for medical attendance. It argued for the subsidising, as necessary, of existing cottage hospitals and stressed the clamant need for additional accommodation for tuberculosis cases[45]. The Highlands and Islands Medical Board was consequently appointed, but only from 1916 onwards was a small part of its annual grant available to supplement the uncertain revenues of the hospitals; the Belford Hospital in Fort William was given the bulk of this support to prevent its closure through lack of funds[46].

The First World War

The Great War of 1914–18 was an emergency which disrupted the routines of most Scottish hospitals as much as it affected the rest of the nation. At the outbreak of hostilities there was an immediate outflow of members of medical and nursing staffs to join the armed forces and ancillary services. The many recently qualified house officers who left their positions in the teaching hospitals were replaced for the remainder of the war by senior medical students[47].

Not only was there a mass exodus of professional and non-professional volunteers; the Territorial Army scheme transferred to military service from big infirmaries their principal administrative officers when, on 10th August 1914, a general instruction was issued for the opening of all military hospitals in the United Kingdom[48]. Of the 27 Territorial Force general hospitals, four were in Scotland. The 1st Scottish General Hospital, located in Aberdeen, occupied four of the City of Aberdeen School Board's schools, to provide 34 beds for officers and 1,385 beds for other ranks. The 2nd Scottish General Hospital, located in Edinburgh, occupied the buildings of Craigleith Poorhouse, to provide 30 beds for officers and 1,002 for other ranks. The 3rd and 4th Scottish General Hospitals occupied the new Glasgow Parish Hospital at Stobhill with 1,163 and 1,180 beds respectively, all for other ranks[49].

At the Royal Hospital for Sick Children in Glasgow, for which new premises had been opened at Yorkhill on 7th July 1914, its 200 beds making it the largest children's hospital in the United Kingdom after London's Great Ormond Street, 4 of the 12 wards were requisitioned. Here the substitution of military men for child patients required more extensive re-equipping than elsewhere! The unit was designated Yorkhill War Hospital and was administered for officer patients as part of the military hospital at Stobhill[50]. (The Aberdeen Children's Hospital, on the other hand, was evacuated from January 1915 to November 1917, because its proximity to the docks seemed to expose its patients to the risks of enemy action[51].) Other War Hospitals were those of Dundee, Perth, Merryflats (Govan, Glasgow), Oakbank (Glasgow), all in poorhouse premises; at Leith and Crookston in Poor Law infirmaries, and at Bangour (Bathgate) in the new asylum buildings[52]. In Aberdeen, the Parish Council's Oldmill Hospital (later named Woodend Hospital) was evacuated to be used entirely as a military hospital[53]. Robroyston (in Glasgow), whose construction as accommodation for infectious diseases had commenced in 1914 but was suspended for part of the War, was completed in 1918 and was occupied as a military hospital until June 1919[54]. At Cromarty, on the north side of the Moray Firth, a hutted hospital of over 200 beds, designated Cromarty Military Hospital, was added to the hutted camp there[55]. Two large hospitals were established in Glasgow by the Scottish Branch of the Red Cross Society[56]. Sir William Macewen, then Surgeon-General in Scotland, gave his support to a successful campaign in Glasgow for the provision of a hospital for limbless service men. As a result the Princess Louise Scottish Hospital for Limbless Soldiers and Sailors was opened at Erskine in October 1916, with 200 beds. Within two years it had a complement of 400 beds[57]. Throughout Scotland there were as many as 180 Red Cross Auxiliary Hospitals in premises ranging from parish halls to mansion houses. In all, over 300 private houses and other adapted buildings were in use within Scottish Command for the sick and wounded[58]. From the outbreak of hostilities, the managers of voluntary hospitals had readily offered to the military authorities accommodation for sick and wounded servicemen. In August 1914 the Inverness Infirmary undertook to set aside 100 beds for wounded sailors, but in May 1915 this allocation was reduced to allow the provision of 50 beds for soldiers[59]. The extent to which the facilities of the teaching hospitals were in demand is made evident by the income of over £30,000 which their care generated in 1918 for infirmaries in Edinburgh, Glasgow (Royal and Western), Dundee and Aberdeen[60], where the treatment of service patients was paid for by the Government at daily rates per occupied bed[61]. Elsewhere not all offers of accommodation were taken up. The offer of beds by the Directors of the small Chalmers Hospital in Edinburgh was not accepted and the hospital continued to provide its customary service for civilian cases, although to replace its absent practitioners it was obliged to employ final year male medical students or 'in the last extremity' women doctors[62]. Women doctors, nurses and other staff were to win renown in the battle zones, under the leadership of Dr Elsie Inglis and her associates, in the service of the Scottish Women's Hospitals on the Eastern Front, with the Serbian and Russian forces, whose military defeats aggravated the often grim conditions which the women courageously encountered[63]; also in France, where twenty-three members were awarded the Croix de Guerre by the French authorities[64].

High Technology and its Promoters

The War interrupted further improvements in the peacetime services. Its sad results, in the thousands of casualties brought to the hospitals for treatment, stimulated efforts to make the fullest use of the new technologies which had recently appeared on the hospital scene. After the discovery of Roentgen Rays in 1895, the city infirmaries and a number of smaller institutions were quick to exploit their use in new electrical departments. Glasgow Royal Infirmary had the distinction of being the first hospital in Britain to instal an X-ray apparatus for diagnostic purposes through the advocacy of laryngologist Dr John MacIntyre in 1896. Its rebuilt main block, opened in 1914, included the King George V Electrical Institute[65]. At Aberdeen Royal Infirmary an ophthalmic surgeon, Dr J. Mackenzie Davidson (later Sir James) was to become the most celebrated of the early radiological specialists[66]. The medical superintendent might become personally involved in this invention, as in the case of Dr D.J. Mackintosh at the Glasgow Western infirmary[67]. (Dr Mackintosh's comprehensive grasp of the requirements of effective hospital care was to bring him into great prominence in the ensuing years, as an expert adviser to other hospital managements in Scotland, and to the central authorities[68,69].) Dr D.O. MacGregor, superintendent at the Glasgow Victoria Infirmary, developed a similar interest, to the extent that in 1919 he was formally appointed the Victoria's radiologist[70].

It was not to be long before even Shetland and the Outer Hebrides would have the benefit of this first example of high technology. When, in 1919, the Scottish Board of Health assumed the functions of the Scottish Local Government Board, the Scottish Insurance Commissioners and the Highland and Islands Medical Service Board, it honoured an obligation of the last named body in contributing to the cost of extensions, which included X-ray facilities, at the Gilbert Bain Memorial Hospital, Lerwick[71]. In 1926 it gave a substantial grant for the construction of new surgical and X-ray facilities at the Lewis Hospital, Stornoway[72]. Both projects were important to the provision of effective surgical services in the respective islands.

For the staffing of such technical departments the professions of radiography and physiotherapy were emerging. During the war years and the post-war years the demand was increasing for their skills in diagnostic and therapeutic radiography, in electrical treatment, and in massage and gymnastics. The Western Infirmary opened its School of Massage, Medical Electricity and Remedial Exercise in 1918, with examinations under the auspices of the Incorporated Society of Trained Masseuses, which, on receipt of a Royal Charter, was renamed in 1920 the Chartered Society of Massage and Medical Gymnastics[73]. In the same year the Society of Radiographers was founded[74]. Other professionals, supplementary to medicine, were beginning to make their important contributions to hospital care: occupational therapists, dieticians, and, to assist with social problems, almoners. In 1919 the status of nursing was confirmed by the establishment of the General Nursing Council for Scotland[75], with its register and examination requirements. Training programmes for nurses, which at the leading hospitals came to include Preliminary Training Schools, for the growing sophistication of hospital treatment, and the introduction of shorter hours (generally no more than 56 hours weekly) and longer holidays, all contributed to an expansion of nursing staff[76]. Residential accommodation for nurses (with single bedrooms for both trained nurses and probationers) had a high priority in capital expenditure plans[77,78].

The Shortfall in Accommodation

The arrival of peace brought new beginnings in the governmental agencies also, with the establishment of the Ministry of Health in London and, as already mentioned, the Ministry's partner in Edinburgh, the Scottish Board of Health. Reports commissioned by the Health Departments are important for an understanding of the relationship between the ideal and the actual provision of hospital services at this period. In October 1919 the Ministry appointed a Consultative Council of Medical and Allied Services under the Chairmanship of Lord Dawson of Penn. The Interim (and only) Report of the Council, the 'Dawson Report', presented with haste in May 1920, offered a radical blueprint for the organisation of the medical and allied services which, in the Council's opinion, should be available to the inhabitants of a given area[79]. It recommended a system comprising three classes of institution, each with appropriate outpatient and inpatient facilities, widely distributed 'primary health centres' staffed by the general practitioners of each district, with visiting consultants and specialists and an efficient nursing service, 'secondary health centres' of a more specialist nature sited in urban concentrations, and, thirdly, a teaching hospital associated with a medical school[80]. This system, under a single Health Authority of some sort, on which the medical profession would be represented, should encompass all services, preventive and curative, educative and investigative, all being supported by financial grants as necessary[81].

Such was the thinking of forward-looking medical men of the time. The principle of unified control, involving the assimilation of Poor Law health services to those of the local authorites, was accepted by the Ministry, but the Council's radical blueprint was not accepted. Indeed, most of the post-war schemes for the reorganisation of the economic and social life of the country were laid aside in face of the financial stringency of 1921. Long term planning was lost sight of in the preoccupation of the politicians with current problems[82].

In Scotland the Board of Health received advice from several Consultative Councils and *ad hoc* committees. Growing concern regarding the inadequacy of hospital bed provision led to the appointment in 1924 of a Hospital Services (Scotland) Committee chaired by Lord Mackenzie, with Sir Norman Walker and Dr D.J. Mackintosh as leading members. After an extensive review of the available facilities of all types throughout Scotland, the Committee produced its recommendations in January 1926. It remarked on the response to the extraordinary revolution in hospital care, instancing the change in Glasgow. In that city in 1841 admissions to its then single infirmary had been 17 per 1000 of its population, whereas in 1924 admissions to its then three infirmaries, its Poor Law hospitals and its local authority hospitals amounted to 44·9 of its population[83]. In particular it noted the phenomenal growth in surgery, Glasgow's three infirmaries treating 6,000 medical and 21,000 surgical cases in 1924 compared with 4,000 medical and 9,000 surgical cases in 1901[84]. Throughout Scotland, whose population was estimated by the Registrar General to be 4,891,300 in mid 1925, 131 voluntary hospitals were providing 8,589 beds[85], which were classified as follows:

In 6 hospitals associated with medical schools	3,256 beds
In 18 other hospitals of 100 or more beds,	2,463 beds
In 18 hospitals having 50 but under 100 beds,	1,228 beds
In 89 hospitals having less than 50 beds,	1,642 beds

Urgent cases would always be admitted, even if this sometimes meant serious overcrowding, but many patients with subacute conditions might suffer a long, often indefinite, delay in receiving attention. Some 30 convalescent homes with over 1,800 beds contributed little to easing these pressures, since they catered for patients who had already progressed to the stage of discharge from hospital. Auxiliary hospitals, which could receive patients who still needed a measure of care, would be of some help[86].

Much of the evidence received by the Committee indicated a need for the provision of pay beds in voluntary hospitals for persons of moderate means who could pay for maintenance and treatment in a general hospital. Nursing home facilities, as offered by the McAlpine Nursing Home in Glasgow, Queen Mary Nursing Home in Edinburgh, and some small or cottage hospitals, fell far short of meeting the demand for such accommodation[87].

Of the 6,000 beds in Poor Law institutions, only 4,285 were in buildings detached from the main poorhouse, whether in the poorhouse grounds or located elsewhere. These were in the following units:

Hospitals	Beds
Glasgow, Stobhill Hospital, (of which 400 were in use for children)	1,784
Glasgow Eastern District Hospital	315
Glasgow Western District Hospital	228
Govan, Southern General Hospital	586
Edinburgh, Craiglockhart Poorhouse Hospital	400
Paisley, Poorhouse Hospital	193
Dundee, Eastern Hospital	374
Aberdeen, Oldmill Hospital	405

Although there had been a substantial improvement in the standard of nursing in many of the larger poorhouses since the Royal Commission reported in 1909, only 3 or 4 of these would stand comparison, in general staffing and facilities, with modern general hospitals. In this the efforts of the Glasgow Parish Council were specially commended. Only in Stobhill and Oldmill Hospitals, however, were there significant numbers of vacant beds which could be placed at the disposal of a wider hospital service[88].

The Committee observed that Scottish Local Authorities, unlike their English counterparts, had not been empowered to provide general hospital services, but their contribution to hospital accommodation was already substantial. The incidence of some infectious diseases had declined, but a large amount of additional accommodation, particularly for the treatment of pulmonary tuberculosis, had been erected, although much more was still needed. In treating pneumonia and some other conditions, the Local Authorities were beginning to go beyond their established roles. With some 5,500 local authority beds (mainly for infectious diseases, excluding tuberculosis and smallpox, with a few for maternity and child care)[89], it was estimated that in 1924 the running costs of the Local Authority and Poor Law hospitals together amounted annually to £1.5 million compared with £1 million for the voluntary hospitals. The Committee regarded it as inevitable that responsibility for the care of the sick poor should be transferred to the Local Authority. This would facilitate full co-operation between voluntary and statutory authorities, which was essential if the common objective of a complete and efficient hospital service within the reach of all was to be attained[90]. To examine the matter of adequacy of beds the Committee found it convenient to divide Scotland into five regions, centred in Inverness, Aberdeen, Dundee, Edinburgh and Glasgow respectively[91], a geographical division to be adopted later for administrative purposes. The national shortage of beds was estimated to be 3,600, of which 1,040 were lacking in the south-eastern and 1,720 in the western regions. For maternity cases and for sick children 600 beds might be provided by the local authorities, leaving the balance of 3,000 beds to be provided in voluntary hospitals[92]. The capital expense of adding 3,000 beds to the voluntary sector was estimated at £1.8 million, of which it was suggested the Treasury should contribute half, the balance to be raised by the hospitals[93]. (The corresponding English committee had recommended that the Treasury meet half of the cost of 10,000 additional beds in England and Wales estimated at £4 million.) Likewise the additional maintenance cost might be met partly from the National Insurance Fund and also from some minor sources, the balance being met through the generosity of the public[94].

In its Annual Report for 1926 the Scottish Board of Health welcomed the Mackenzie Report. It accepted the importance of co-operation be-

tween voluntary bodies and local authorities, and praised the proposals
for the financing by the Local Authorities of maternity wings in new
infirmaries in Stirling and Falkirk. It noted the Committee's concern
that the Poor Law hospitals remained outside the general hospital services, having regard to what, if improved, they could contribute to
patient care and to medical teaching and research, and expressed satisfaction that Stobhill Hospital had opened its surplus accommodation to
the managers of the Glasgow Royal Maternity Hospital[95].

. The Board of Health considered the Mackenzie Committee's estimate
of a shortage of 3,600 hospital beds nationally to be a cautious and
conservative figure but, in view of the substantial costs envisaged, saw the
current condition of central and local finance as the obstacle to rapid
progress[96]. Without such State assistance the voluntary hospitals were
unable to expand sufficiently. Their bed numbers in 1939 were 10,398,
being only 1,809 over the 1924 figure[97], and although the public
authority services had attained 18,227 beds (excluding the municipal
mental hospitals) by 1934, demand continued to outstrip supply. The
local authority provision for maternity and sick children had increased
from 131 beds in 1924 to 658 beds in 1934, yet a commentator could
observe in 1937 that 'the supply of hospital beds [for such categories] is
notoriously inadequate for present needs'[98].

Enabling Powers

The hopes of the Board of Health relative to Poor Law reform were to
be encouraged by the passing of the Local Government (Scotland) Act
1929, under whose enabling powers hospital treatment could eventually
be dissociated from the Poor Law. (In 1929 also, the Scottish Board of
Health was replaced by the Department of Health for Scotland.) Parish
councils, education authorities, district committees and district boards of
control were abolished on 15 May 1930, their functions, together with
the major health services and certain other functions of small burghs,
being transferred to county councils and town councils of cities and large
burghs (with population of 20,000 or more)[99].

The terms of the Act enabled the local (health) authorities to reorganise their hospital facilities so as to provide for the sick within their
areas, including the possibility of expansion of those facilities to remedy
deficiencies in their own and voluntary hospital provision[100]. (But the
established interests of the voluntary hospitals were given preferential
protection, for in approving such schemes the Department of Health had
to be satisfied that reasonable steps had been taken to seek and to
continue to secure full co-operation with every voluntary hospital, university or medical school serving the council's area[101], whereas there
was no corresponding requirement that voluntary hospitals consult with
local authorities and secure the approval of the Department before

embarking on extension programmes.) Two or more councils might join together and submit a scheme. Thus the stage was set for what the Mackenzie Committee envisaged: the provision of an adequate service for the community through the association of voluntary and statutory agencies.

Already, in 1928, the Town Council of Aberdeen, anticipating the powers to be granted by the 1929 Act, had arranged with the Parish Council to take full control of the Oldmill Poor Law Hospital, converting it into a municipal hospital of 324 beds and renaming it Woodend[102]. By the end of 1932 the Edinburgh Corporation was operating three municipal general hospitals with a total of some 900 beds. Pilton, Craigleith and Seafield Hospitals had been renamed the Northern General, Western General and Eastern General Hospitals, and had been suitably equipped and staffed. The University Professors of Medicine, Surgery, Obstetrics and Gynaecology, and Child Life and Health were in charge of four units for patient care and teaching. The Corporation imposed charges as required by the Act and fixed these, according to means, at up to 25s. per week for Edinburgh citizens, £2.12s.6d. for patients from other local authority areas, and £3.3s.0d. for private patients[103].

An important point in the public provision of hospital facilities had been reached. Yet full advantage of these facilities was not taken. Professor (later Sir) Stanley Davidson observed in his inaugural lecture that, on taking up his duties in October 1938, he found a waiting list of 81 patients for admission to his medical wards in the Edinburgh Royal Infirmary, many of whom were seriously ill, while there were hundreds awaiting admission to the surgical side. At the same date the three municipal general hospitals, served by highly qualified physicians and surgeons, had 218 vacant beds. This anomaly was the consequence of the survival of old attitudes to buildings which had been associated with the Poor Law, and of the retention of established medical connections with the voluntary hospital. The absence of charges at the voluntary institution was no doubt a factor in the balance of choice[104].

The Department of Health's Consultative Council on Medical and Allied Services, its Chairman Sir Norman Walker and its Vice Chairman Dr A.K. Chalmers (formerly Medical Officer of Health in Glasgow), examined the possibilities of the new situation and set itself up to offer guidelines for progress. Reporting in January 1933 the Council postulated a single hospital system in a given area, attained not by absorption or common control but by co-ordination of the various institutions. A pre-requisite of effective co-ordination was the assimilation of key features of these institutions, paying no regard to the fact that they might be administered by different agencies. Unhampered by the Poor Law stigma of pauperism, local authority hospitals should be able to collaborate simply on medical grounds according to the nature of the care required. This called for assimilation to common standards of quality of staff and of equipment and, in the financial sphere, uniformity in the payment of staff, and adoption of similar policies in respect of charges to patients who had the means to contribute to the cost of their care[105]. The Council noted that the Consultative Council on Local Health Administration had recommended in 1923 that the units to be administered for the purpose of area health services should be as consistent as possible with the Scottish system of local government[106]. The Act of 1929 had provided accordingly but the Council observed that in general hospital services there was, in practice, a tendency to ignore such narrow boundaries in favour of the regional organisation, around a teaching centre, of district hospitals, and beyond the district hospitals the smaller cottage hospitals. (Thus the theoretical system recommended in the Dawson Report was appearing naturally in the patterns of hospital provision and medical referral.) The Council urged the further development of this web of relationships. It also noted that the Department of Health had established a central liaison committee in order to sound voluntary hospital opinion. Each region of Scotland, in the view of the Council, should have a committee which could represent statutory authorities, voluntary hospitals, medical schools and the medical profession. With the benefit of the advice of such committees the development of an efficient and co-ordinated hospital service for Scotland could be secured[107].

Slow Progress

The Department of Health was finding that the attainment of an efficient co-ordinated service through voluntary co-operation in a period of economic depression was not to be easy. The system of local government prior to the 1929 Act had involved 33 county councils, 98 district committees, 201 town councils and 869 parish councils[108]. With the operation of the Act in 1930 this structure was greatly simplified but the possibility of local friction remained. The Department's Annual Reports present an uncertain picture. In Ayrshire, when the County Council proposed the construction of a large new hospital at Kilwinning for infectious diseases, maternity, and ultimately for other purposes, the Town Councils of Ayr and Kilmarnock protested that this would leave vacant beds in their hospitals. An attempt to reach agreement on a scheme based on the Ayr and Kilmarnock hospitals failing, the Department sanctioned the County Council's proposal which gave the promise of a comprehensive hospital service of a high standard for three-quarters of the population of Ayrshire[109]. In Lanarkshire a scheme to provide general, maternity and infectious disease hospitals for its half million population was accepted by the County Council but by only three of the five town councils. It was, however, approved by the Department and was eligible to receive a government grant through the Commissioner for the Special Areas of Scotland[110], (although the construction of the general hospital was eventually delayed when the grant proved insufficient). For the Greenock area the County Council, the Greenock Town Council and the Directors of the Greenock Royal Infirmary discussed co-operation in the provision of a new hospital but the Port Glasgow Town Council took exception to the proposals for representation on the management of the hospital and would not participate[111]. Negotiations for co-operation between Perth Town Council and Perthshire County Council broke down after reaching a 'hopeful stage'[112]. On the other hand Dumbarton County Council and the Town Councils of Dumbarton and Clydebank reached agreement on the joint provision of a general hospital of 150 beds and an infectious disease hospital of 150 beds on the same site, and the Commissioner for the Special Areas agreed to give their construction financial support[113]. In Inverness the County Council and the Inverness Town Council agreed on the joint management of three hospitals[114]. Together with the County Councils of the other northern counties and the managements of the Royal Northern Infirmary and the Inverness District Asylum, they also agreed to the appointment of a Consultant Physician to the Infirmary who would provide a consulting service in their areas, half his salary being met by the Highlands and Islands Fund[115].

In the south-west, after a survey by their Medical Officers of Health, a measure of agreement was reached between the local authorities, Dumfries Town Council and Dumfries, Kirkcudbright, and Wigtown County Councils, regarding the need for new hospital provision for maternity cases, and for other specialties, and on the desirability of joint action. An approach was thereupon made to the Directors of the Dumfries and Galloway Royal Infirmary regarding the possibility of locating these beds at the Infirmary[116].

That element of co-ordination which depended on the transformation of Poor Law hospital beds into general health service beds proceeded at a painfully slow rate. The Department's Report for the year 1934 stated that there were still 59 Poor Law hospitals with 5,570 beds, figures which give only a bare indication of the heavy burden which the local authorities were carrying in the care of the chronically sick and the incapacitated elderly. Of these 59 hospitals, 55 with 3,270 beds were located in mixed poorhouses, only 4, with 2,300 beds, being separate hospitals[117]. Schemes formulated in terms of Section 27 of the 1929 Act had produced 5 general hospitals open to any sick person, with a total of 1,577 beds. These were, in Edinburgh, the Northern, Western and Eastern General Hospitals; in Dundee, Maryfield Hospital; and in Aberdeen, Woodend Hospital[118]. (The re-organisation by the County of Bute of a small hospital at Millport had also been approved[119].) The Department restated principles of health service re-organisation which it had enunciated three years earlier in its Report for 1931, when it had asserted that 'the modern view is that, given the standard of medical administration that is of the essence of any well-conducted hospital, there is no medical necessity for providing separate hospitals for special types of patients. Comprehensive units, by avoiding duplication of equipment and staff, should provide the most economical service and, because of the resources at their command, should give the patients the best chance of recovery'[120].

The Department's Report for 1935 again remarked on the slow progress in the abolition of mixed poorhouses. Apparently despairing in that regard, the Department turned its attention to the need for an adequate staff of trained nurses in such units, commenting that the 'matron' responsible for the nursing was often not a qualified hospital nurse[121].

The Cathcart Committee

In 1936 the Report of the Committee of Scottish Health Services, appointed in 1933, and chaired by Professor Cathcart of Glasgow, stated that advances in medicine called for a new order of facility, where the more active skilled treatment and nursing now known to be effective could be dispensed. The small infectious diseases hospitals, catering for three diseases – diphtheria, scarlet fever and enteric fever – were obsolete in most areas in view of the development of modern transport[122]. The Committee noted that about 5,500 beds were by then allocated to tuberculosis patients in sanatoria and infectious diseases hospitals, but recently developed techniques demanded a greater concentration of resources. The Committee looked for the establishment of regional centres from which all treatment of pulmonary and non-pulmonary tuberculosis in an area would be supervised[123].

As to the hospital services of Scotland as a whole, long waiting lists, even if they could not be accepted at their face value, offered one piece of evidence as to the insufficiency of hospital facilities. The physical enlargement of voluntary hospitals would put a further strain on their maintenance income, which was already overburdened. This being so, the Committee saw the public authorities as the appropriate vehicle for the necessary extensions to the services. The Local Government Act should be amended to give powers to the central department to oblige local authorities to augment existing hospital facilities, the Exchequer giving grants of 50 *per cent* or more in aid of capital costs[124].

The Cathcart Committee paid a warm tribute to the public service rendered by the voluntary hospitals and recognised that it was not in the interests of the State to weaken their contribution. Eighteen of the principal voluntary hospitals in Glasgow and the West of Scotland had submitted a memorandum of evidence in which they called for official recognition by the State. At the same time they baulked at any suggestion of control. However, one of their representatives, Mr R.F.

Barclay, Chairman of the Royal Hospital for Sick Children, Glasgow, eventually agreed that exception would not be taken to something in the nature of regulation and control, including the regulation of proposed extensions, which had as its object the securing of the co-ordination and co-operation which all agreed were necessary[125]. (Perhaps Mr Barclay had in his mind the lesson of 1861 when the original campaign for the building of a Hospital for Sick Children in Glasgow collapsed in face of the declared opposition of the Royal Infirmary's Directors who were apprehensive about competition from a children's hospital in the raising of funds![126]) The Committee recommended that all proposals for the extension of hospital facilities, whether statutory or voluntary, should require the approval of the Department, asserting that central supervision of this nature need not, and indeed ought not to, interfere with the autonomy of each hospital in its internal management. It recommended also that each of the five regions in Scotland should have a Hospital Services Committee which would include representatives of both the voluntary and the statutory hospitals. These committees would meet at regular intervals to discuss matters of common interest, such as waiting lists, staffing, equipment and contributions from patients[127].

Developments in Patient Care

Financial stringency was hampering developments in the voluntary sector no less than in the public authority sector during the interwar years, the years of economic depression. Nevertheless the system did respond to medical advances in the shape of new patterns of organisation and further specialisation.

The recognition of the value of convalescent facilities, both to ensure full recovery after treatment and to relieve pressure on the acute hospitals, led in 1923 to the foundation of the Astley-Ainslie Institute, in association with the Edinburgh Royal Infirmary. There, with an average length of stay of 11 weeks, compared with 17 days in the Infirmary, patients were receiving the benefits of open-air living, remedial exercises, massage, electrical treatment and occupational therapy[128].

Physical medicine and orthopaedics were developing their scope from the treatment of war casualties to that of accidents and also in the surgery of non-pulmonary tuberculosis. A voluntary institution, the Princess Margaret Rose Hospital for Crippled Children, opened in 1932 on the southern outskirts of Edinburgh; it offered a specialist centre of treatment and advice from which orthopaedic surgeons could supervise cases attending a constellation of clinics in the Lothians, Borders, Fife and Clackmannan. It also received patients sent by local authorities from even greater distances[129]. Leonard Findlay in Glasgow[130] and John Thomson in Edinburgh[131] had pioneered the child health specialty of paediatrics in the pre-war years. Professorial chairs in the specialty were established in Glasgow in 1924[132] and in Edinburgh in 1931[133]. Advances in obstetric practice and the growing tendency of women to prefer to be delivered in a hospital or maternity home rather than in their often unsuitable domestic environment called for more accommodation for maternity cases. Local authorities throughout the country produced additional maternity beds[134]. Privately run maternity homes offered their services, their uncertain standards necessitating the passing of the Midwives and Maternity Homes (Scotland) Act in 1927, which introduced registration with, and inspection by, the local authority of the area[135]. The Nursing Homes (Registration) Scotland Act of 1938[136] empowered local authorities to set standards of qualification for those superintending nursing in maternity homes and for persons giving professional attendance. By that time there were 148 registered maternity homes in Scotland, accommodating about 1,200 patients, while local authority institutions provided for 800. In voluntary institutions there were 630 beds for maternity cases[137]. Notably, in 1939, the Simpson Memorial Maternity Pavilion was opened in the grounds, and under the management of the Edinburgh Royal Infirmary, replacing the obsolete mid-Victorian premises of the Edinburgh Royal Maternity and Simpson Memorial Hospital nearby[138]. Extensions, reconstructions and new equipment were frequently necessary in the infirmaries to cope with rapid advances in the technologies of X-ray diagnosis and deep and superficial X-ray therapy, and in the diagnostic and research techniques of bacteriological and biochemical laboratories. National radium centres were established at the Royal Infirmaries in Edinburgh, Glasgow, Aberdeen and Dundee and at the Glasgow Western Infirmary[139]. Blood transfusion services, which at first relied on the commitment of individuals, became organised on a wider basis. The Edinburgh Blood Transfusion Service was launched in 1936 at a public meeting called by the Lord Provost[140]. By mid 1939 a regional blood transfusion service had been established in the West of Scotland to serve the five principal hospitals: the Glasgow Royal; the Western and Victoria Infirmaries; and the Southern General and Stobhill Hospitals[141].

The most remarkable scheme in the inter-war years was a project brought to fruition in Aberdeen, for the concentration of hospitals and the Medical School on one site.

Dr Matthew Hay, Professor of Medical Jurisprudence and Medical Officer of Health for the City of Aberdeen, proposed this scheme in 1920 to the Medico-Chirosurgical Society. A conference, at which the Society, the City Corporation, the University Court and the governing bodies of the Aberdeen Royal Infirmary and Royal Hospital for Sick Children were represented, approved the scheme. On an extensive site which was then available at Foresterhill, a new Royal Hospital for Sick Children, of 134 beds, was opened in 1928, a new Royal Infirmary of 500 beds was opened in 1936, and a new Maternity Hospital and a new Medical

School were to follow in the next two years. The most favourable conditions had been provided for co-ordination and co-operation, if not indeed for the integration of services[142].

The Second World War

As the end of the fourth decade of the century approached, the instability of the international situation became obvious, and the possibility of war with Nazi Germany loomed large. In that event, devastating air raids could be expected to bring heavy civilian casualties. Even an invasion of the Scottish east coast was not ruled out. A Sub-committee of the Committee of Imperial Defence, under the Chairmanship of Sir Arthur Mac-Nalty, reported to the Government in October 1937 on effective methods of casualty disposal. As a result the Secretary of State for Scotland was made responsible for the organisation of an Emergency Hospital Service in Scotland (Region No 11 for Civil Defence purposes)[143]. Under an aerial bombardment it would, it was believed, be impossible to differentiate between service and civilian casualties. Accordingly the Government directed that the ordinary hospital resources of Scotland should, in general, be used for all wartime needs, service and civilian alike. Looking towards the uncertain future, it could be expected that any major aerial assaults would be directed at the industrial concentrations of Glasgow and Clydeside, with the Forth and Tay estuaries and the Capital City of Edinburgh as other probable targets. In the Spring of 1938 a survey of the available resources in hospitals and sanatoria, and their disposition relative to each other and to the probable location of casualties, was conducted by officers of the Department. The survey extended to accommodation in public assistance institutions and in schools, hotels and other buildings which could be adapted for those purposes. In the course of the survey, 256 local authority hospitals and Poor Law institutions with 21,018 beds, and 219 voluntary hospitals with 14,076 beds came under review. Within the general shortage throughout Scotland of hospital beds for peacetime use, long recognised, gross deficiencies were discovered in particular areas as, for example, in Lanarkshire and Dumbartonshire, whose residents had been accustomed to taking advantage of Glasgow's great hospitals. In 1938 Lanarkshire, with a population of 508,112, had only 197 general hospital beds; Dumbartonshire, with a population of 155,243, had only 77 general hospital beds, if the 120 beds of the Royal Infirmary's Canniesburn branch on the western outskirts of Glasgow were excluded. It was not unimportant that the siting of any major new constructions should have regard to their potential contribution to the solution of problems of hospital provision in the post-war period. Yet at the same time the risks of locating them in areas vulnerable to enemy attack had to be avoided[144].

In each of the country's five regions (Civil Defence Districts) a Medical

Officer of the Department was put in charge of the emergency arrangements, involving consultations with the Medical Officers of Health, the
local authorities and the voluntary hospitals. Operational planning was
undertaken in three stages, the first being concerned with the use for
casualties of existing facilities, provisional arrangements being made for
the transfer of normal patients to second line hospitals. The second stage
concerned the fuller use of the existing accommodation through concentration and expansion. The third stage of planning involved the extension of the organisation into positions which were outwith the existing
hospital services, importantly including new construction, and generally,
for safety reasons, sited at some distance from centres of population[145].

The Civil Defence Act 1939 authorised the Emergency Hospital
Scheme to proceed throughout the United Kingdom[146]. In Scotland
16,574 additional beds were produced. Of these, 7,038 were in seven
specially built hospitals; 8,526 were in new annexes to 25 existing institutions; 910 were in two converted hotels; 100 were elsewhere. Also
provided were 3,953 auxiliary hospital beds for the less seriously ill and
convalescent cases. Of these, 3,426 were accommodated in over 60 large
country houses. The seven new hospitals were distributed throughout
Scotland: Raigmore (near Inverness), Stracathro (Brechin, Angus),
Bridge of Earn (near Perth), Killearn (Stirlingshire near the northern
boundary of Dumbartonshire), Law Junction (Carluke, Lanarkshire),
Ballochmyle (Ayrshire) and Peel (Selkirkshire). A standard type of
building devised by the Ministry of Health, the Department of Health
for Scotland and the Office of Works was used. The hotels converted were
those of the LMS Railway Company at Gleneagles and at
Turnberry[147]. To staff the additional hospitals, and to supplement the
staffs of adapted or extended hospitals, an Emergency Medical Service
and a Civil Nursing Reserve had been formed, the latter numbering by
March 1942 almost 5,000, including 3,000 nursing auxiliaries[148]. By the
summer of 1944 124 voluntary hospitals and 36 local authority hospitals
were participating in the Emergency Hospital Scheme, together with 73
hospitals (including the seven major constructions) which were managed
directly by the Department, assisted by an expert Hospitals Administration Advisory Committee[149].

It was a cardinal principle of the Emergency Hospital Scheme that
specialised treatment should be secured at the earliest possible stage for
patients whose condition required it. This might involve a transfer to
another institution more suitably equipped[150]. Seven specialist orthopaedic centres, with a total of 1,980 beds, were set up in different
areas[151]. In the six years 1940 to 1945, inclusive, these orthopaedic
centres treated over 40,000 cases, of whom a quarter were civilians[152].
A further 28 centres, with 1,290 beds at their disposal, catered for plastic
surgery, psychoneurosis, neurosurgery, eye injuries and other special
needs[153]. These centres provided a great stimulus to specialist practice

in Scotland, which in the pre-war period had been restricted by the heavy dependence of voluntary hospital doctors upon private practice. The requirements of other nationals were specially catered for in several instances. The Canadian Red Cross Society established the Canadian Orthopaedic Unit at Hairmyres Hospital in Lanarkshire[154]. In Edinburgh a Norwegian hospital occupied a section of the Southern General Hospital[155] and the Paderewski Hospital was opened at the Western General Hospital to care for Polish civilians and service personnel[156]. Parallel but independent was the establishment of a Polish Medical School in the University of Edinburgh. This had been suggested by Lt.Col. Professor F.A.E.Crew, then Commanding Officer of the Military Hospital at Edinburgh Castle, who had noticed the number of professors and lecturers in the Medical Corps of the Polish Army, and the number of medical students in the Polish forces whose studies had been interrupted by the war. The exiled Prime Minister of the Polish Government, General Sikorski, accepted the offer of the University. Accommodation was allocated and the wards, clinics and laboratories of the Edinburgh hospitals were opened to the Poles[157]. The Scottish National Blood Transfusion Association was formed with a view to co-ordinating and developing the existing blood transfusion services in Scotland, with local committees for each of the five regions[158]. To supplement existing laboratory facilities emergency clinical laboratories were provided. An Emergency Bacteriological Service had been organised before the start of hostilities to serve both the civil and military authorities in the event of war, and to be available for scientific investigation if the enemy introduced bacteriological warfare[159].

The heavy and widespread air raid casualties feared in Scotland did not materialise beyond the concentrated attacks on Glasgow and Clydebank in mid March 1941, when over 1,000 were killed and over 4,000 wounded[160]. The initial evacuation of less serious cases from hospitals in areas believed to be vulnerable, and the restriction of admissions to urgent cases, were adversely affecting clinical practice and medical and nursing education. The Department found it possible to ease this situation by stating specific numbers of beds to be held empty for emergencies. Thus the hospitals concerned, with bed complements totalling 7,229 beds, were asked to keep available reserved quotas totalling 3,321 beds, the remainder being freed for their normal uses[161]. It was also found desirable and possible to return several thousand beds in sanatoria to their original purpose and to open fully equipped sanatorium units in two of the newly built emergency hospitals. Up to June 1944 two-thirds of the beds in the Scheme, then 24,000 in hospitals equipped for surgical work and 4,500 in convalescent hospitals, had been devoted to the treatment of members and ex-members of the services, casualties and sick people of both sexes, including those invalided from overseas[162].

While some beds were left vacant or even unstaffed, valuable uses were found for the remainder. By arrangement with the voluntary hospitals, and particularly from early in 1942, both medical and surgical cases from the lengthy waiting lists of these hospitals were treated in Emergency Hospital Scheme beds, and up to the middle of 1945 the number of such patients had reached 32,826[163]. The maintenance of the health of workers in the war industries, especially young people without any experience of industrial work – with the pressures of long hours, changing shifts, erratic meal times and travel difficulties – became a matter of concern. In January 1942 a supervision scheme was introduced in the area of the Clyde Basin with the co-operation of general practitioners who were asked to report cases of debility to the Department's Regional Medical Officer who would arrange for a medical examination followed by admission to one of the Emergency Scheme hospitals or convalescent homes, if necessary[164]. Between 1942 and 1946 nearly 15,000 workers were referred to the Regional Medical Officers under this Supplementary Medical Service Scheme[165].

The Normandy invasion in June 1944, with the subsequent battles, produced new demands on the Emergency Hospital Scheme in Scotland. More than 13,000 British and Allied casualties, and more than 3,000 German prisoners of war from the North-West European area were admitted. A further 5,000 British and Allied casualties came from more distant theatres of war. In addition the 'V' weapon attacks on the South of England led to the evacuation from London hospitals to the Scottish hospitals of over 5,000 patients[164]. With the end of hostilities a rapid scaling down of the demands of the Scheme on the voluntary and local authority general hospitals was possible. Co-operating with the voluntary hospitals, the Departmental hospitals continued to operate many of their special units for neuro-surgery, plastic surgery, orthopaedics, etc., and many ordinary civilian patients benefited. The Department saw these hospitals as making a permanent contribution to the hospital services of the country and were planning accordingly[167]. The Emergency Scheme had indeed remarkably foreshadowed the national hospital service of the future.

Post-war Prospects

The voluntary hospitals were also looking to the future. Meeting in October 1940, representatives of voluntary hospitals in all parts of Scotland discussed how to accelerate the movement towards a co-ordinated regional system of hospital services. Mr Barclay, as Chairman of the Scottish Branch of the British Hospitals Association, told the representatives that 'after the war it would not be possible for hospitals to return to the *status quo ante*, either financially or otherwise, and there was every reason why they should consider what changes should and must be made rather than wait until a new organisation was forced upon them at the dictation of others who were not particularly interested in the continuation of the voluntary system'[168].

Early in its life the Wartime Coalition Government also began to consider post-war policies. On 9th October 1941 its Minister of Health, Mr Ernest Brown, announced in the House of Commons that it was the objective of the Government, as soon after the war as possible, to ensure that appropriate treatment should be readily available to any person in need of it, this by means of a comprehensive health service. The Government proposed to lay on the major local authorities the duty of securing, in close co-operation with the voluntary agencies, the provision of such a service. It was envisaged that, in general, patients should be called upon to make a reasonable contribution towards the cost, whether through contributory schemes or otherwise, but that a grant would be forthcoming from the Exchequer towards additional burdens which the scheme would put upon local authorities. The Minister added that his colleague, the Secretary of State for Scotland, associated himself in general with those aims with respect to hospital policy in Scotland[169].

Following this announcement Mr Tom Johnston, the Secretary of State for Scotland, appointed in January 1942 a Committee, chaired by Sir Hector Hetherington, to consider appropriate arrangements for the post-war administration of the new emergency hospitals, and for promoting co-operation between the emergency hospitals, the local authority hospitals and the voluntary hospitals. The Committee was also asked to advise regarding suitable financial arrangements between voluntary hospitals and local authorities and between voluntary hospitals and patients in the context of a comprehensive and co-ordinated service. The Report of the Committee was presented in August 1943, by which time Sir William Beveridge's Report on Social Security and subsequent Ministerial pronouncements on that Report had given further substance to the schemes envisaged by the Government. The Committee had wrestled with the problem of discovering a method which would enable the two parallel peacetime hospital services to collaborate as partners in one comprehensive system whose organisation, to fulfil its purpose, would necessarily extend beyond the boundaries of existing local authorities. The solution proposed by the Committee utilised the accepted division of Scotland into five regions, each region to have a Regional Council, with the special provision of a subregional organisation for the South Western Region on account of its size. Membership of the Councils would be representative of the local authorities concerned, of the voluntary hospitals (appointed by the divisional councils of the British Hospitals Association), of the medical profession (possibly appointed by the Secretary of State's Medical Advisory Committee), and of medical education interests (appointed by the University of the region). The Secretary of State had instructed the gathering of information about the existing hospital resources in each region and the potential contribution of each institution to a regionally organised hospital service. It would be the function of each Regional Council to study the surveyors' report on each region and to prepare a provisional but comprehensive scheme. The Regional Councils, however, would be no more than advisors since the responsibility for the provision of the service was to be placed on the local authorities. Each local authority would be required to prepare a scheme for its own area, taking account of the relevant section of the Regional Council scheme and subject to revision in the light of comment by interested parties and institutions. The Secretary of State would then be asked to approve the final local authority scheme, having before him both the Regional Council's first draft plan and any observations which that Council wished to make on the local authority scheme. These Regional Councils would also be in a position to encourage co-operation in a variety of daily activities of the services[170].

The Committee recognised that the direct administration of the new EMS hospitals by the Department of Health was working well in war-time, but were the Department to retain direct control over its own hospitals in the post-war scheme, the objectivity of its decisions might be questioned. In any case the insertion of a third hospital system, in view of the difficulty of co-ordinating the existing two systems, was not to be contemplated. It was therefore recommended that the emergency hospitals be transferred to local health authorities on favourable terms (or exceptionally to a voluntary hospital or to a voluntary hospital acting in combination with a local authority), the allocation to be made by the Secretary of State in the light of the Regional Council's proposal for each such institution[171].

The Committee's views on the inclusion of the voluntary hospitals in a comprehensive hospital service were radically influenced by a real-isation that the characteristic features of these hospitals were no longer valid. Traditionally 'the voluntary hospital' was an institution for the charitable care of the sick poor, founded and supported by voluntary gifts and subscriptions, managed by trustees or directors appointed by donors and subscribers, and staffed by honorary physicians who relied for their income on the fees which they were able to charge their private patients. By the 1930's the leading voluntary hospitals had become great concen-trations of medical skill and resources available nowhere else to all classes of society. Medical men were looking for payment from the institutions in which they spent an increasing amount of their time. Unlike similar institutions in England, the Scottish voluntary hospitals were not accus-tomed to seek to recover the cost of treatment from their patients. In this they were also unlike the local authority hospitals which were required by the 1929 Act to recover the expense of treatment (although in practice the amounts so recovered were small). The adequacy of financial support from customary sources, including industrial workers' contribution schemes, had been a serious cause for concern to voluntary hospital managements in the pre-war period. The Committee did not believe that this support could be expanded sufficiently in the post-war circumstances to cope with price increases, the cost of the medical advances, new standards of remuneration for nurses, and the payment of medical staff. An increase in costs of 50 *per cent* could be expected from those causes. The Committee's solution was a form of taxation, namely a compulsory contributory scheme co-extensive with the social security arrangements resulting from the Beveridge report, its rates of contribution to be such that 60 *per cent* of the aggregate cost of hospitals, voluntary and statutory, would be produced thereby. The deficit would be met in assumed proportions by interest on hospital endowments, by voluntary subscriptions and legacies, and by local authority or central government subventions. A formula for the distribution of finance to the hospitals was proposed which involved the division of the hospitals, whether voluntary or statutory, into three categories, teaching or key hospitals, non-teaching hospitals over a certain size, and the rest. Payments to the individual institutions would take account, according to an assumed ratio, of bed complement and occupancy rate as occasioning expense in differing degrees[172]. Even the Chairman of the Committee jibbed at the complexity of the rule of thumb methods envisaged for the collection and distribution of funds, but on one matter the Committee's view was clear and definite: that the compulsory hospital contribution should give title to free treatment including maintenance in hospital[173].

The principle of free medical advice and treatment was affirmed in the White Paper which the Health Departments published in February 1944 to promote thinking on the meaning and method of a comprehensive health service[174].

In a separate section of the White Paper devoted to 'The Service in Scotland' the pattern proposed for the administration in England and Wales of hospital and associated services of all kinds – a combination of local authorities covering a defined area of suitable size and resources – was rejected as likely to produce in Scotland unwieldy areas destructive of local government administration. Instead, the regional framework used by the successive earlier committees and during the wartime emergency was accepted as appropriate for the suggested establishment of five Regional Hospitals Advisory Councils whose membership would include in equal numbers the nominees of the voluntary hospitals in the region and the nominees of new Joint Hospital Boards to be set up to manage groups of local authority hospitals. Medical and medical-educational interests could be represented on the Councils in some degree. The Joint Hospital Boards would have the duty of preparing schemes for the hospital service of their areas after consultation with the voluntary hospitals and with their Regional Advisory Council, which would also be a source of advice for the Secretary of State when he was

approving or amending area schemes. Thus the suggestions contained in
the White Paper largely paralleled the proposals of the Hetherington
Committee in a less complex form. Such public health services as maternal and child health, school health and special clinics would be left with
the local health authorities. In England and Wales the provision and
maintenance of health centres, an emerging concept, would be the responsibility of local authorities, but in Scotland the smaller size of the
whole country and the distribution of its population pointed to its treatment as one area for these purposes. For an experimental period the
responsibilities might be placed with the Secretary of State[175].

The Hospital Survey

The groundwork in preparation for the organisation of a fully co-
ordinated and comprehensive hospital service in Scotland was undertaken on behalf of the Department of Health by seven prominent medical
men, Professors R.S. Aitken, C.F.W. Illingworth, J.M. Mackintosh, Mr
J.W. Struthers and Drs R.J. Peters, H.E. Seiler and H.Hyslop Thomson.
In twos or threes they surveyed the institutional resources of each of the
five regions, personally visiting most of the units concerned to assess the
quality, equipment, size and location of their buildings in relation to the
contribution which each, adapted or extended if need be, could make to
a comprehensive and up-to-date hospital service for the local or the
regional populations. Many of the premises were found to be structurally
defective; many old Poor Law institutions were quite unfit for hospital
purposes; many general units were overcrowded, a condition aggravated
by wartime precautionary measures in spite of the additional building for
emergency purposes; many small infectious disease units were condemned as obsolete in the light of current thinking about the treatment
of infectious disease[176]. The surveyors decided to set standards for their
own guidance in determining the extent of the deficiencies in bed numbers which all previous reports on the subject had pronounced to be
gross. They were particularly concerned about provision for the chronic
sick whose numbers would increase with the ageing of the population,
while distinguishing the 'aged and infirm', a term they would have
preferred to apply to those who might only require domestic assistance
and the attentions of a visiting district nurse. Accommodation for children's orthopaedics, rheumatic diseases and other long term conditions,
and, in district hospitals, for medical problems of adults, needed to be
substantially augmented. Thus it was decided that the standard provision of general hospital beds should be, in a closely knit industrial area,
at least 8 beds per 1,000 population, although in rural areas 4–5 beds per
1,000 might be permissible[177]. Such guidelines had in themselves no
absolute validity. Applied in the South Eastern Region, with ratios
ranging from 7 per 1,000 to 4 per 1,000 according to the nature of the

locality, an average of 6.5 per 1,000 resulted, which called for the addition of 1,374 beds to the existing 5,240 beds for general purposes. Yet the Mackenzie Committee's estimate of 1,040 additional beds needed in the voluntary hospitals of the region had in fact been met by 1938. The surveyors considered that the further increase which their formula called for could be justified by a host of uncertain factors: the present waiting lists (although not necessarily accurate evidence of demand), the benefits to patients from a longer stay in hospital which an increase in bed complement would allow, the opportunities which would be available for investigative admissions and preventive care, attention to cripples previously neglected, the expected increase in the proportion of Scotland's population aged over 65 from 84 per 1,000 in 1937 to 171 per 1,000 in 1971, the effect of the introduction of social insurance in diverting patients from private institutions to public general hospitals[178].

For maternity beds a standard of 4.5 beds per 100 births *per annum* was set. This figure allowed for 75 *per cent* of all confinements taking place in hospital, for an average stay of fourteen days, and for a 50 *per cent* reserve for fluctuations in demand, for antenatal and postnatal cases and for the isolation of suspects. Against this standard a serious deficiency in maternity beds was almost universal.

Other standards set were: for infectious diseases hospital beds 1.5 per 1,000 population and for pulmonary tuberculosis hospital beds 2 beds per death *per annum*. The importance of convalescent beds in relieving the problems of congestion in general hospitals was recognised and it was recommended that each larger hospital should aim in the first instance at having convalescent beds at its disposal equal to 20 *per cent* of the hospital's own beds[179].

The survey was conducted within the framework of five regions but the set boundaries of the regions were not hard and fast for all purposes. Thus while the surveyors decided to place the whole of Fife in their Lothian Region for administrative convenience, they recognised that a proportion of the population in East Fife were accustomed to seek their care in readily accessible Dundee and could be expected to continue so to do. It was indeed a matter of principle that medical practitioners and their patients should not be strictly circumscribed in their choice of hospital by administrative boundaries or other theoretical considerations[180]. Although the Western Isles north of Argyll were placed in the Northern Region, many islanders might wish to adhere to the traditional link between the Western Isles and Glasgow and this should be allowed. Similarly Orcadians might wish to preserve their long-standing association with Edinburgh, but the surveyors envisaged a strengthening of communications between Aberdeen and Orkney and Shetland, and on account of the shorter distance placed these groups of islands in their North-Eastern Region.

In proposing dispositions within regions, the surveyors were prepared on occasion to deny the priority of medical efficiency as they sought to meet what they believed would be the wishes of local residents. Thus in the arrangements proposed for infectious diseases in the Northern Region they modified their preference for centralisation to the extent of permitting the retention in the short term of a reduced number of beds in the small scattered infectious diseases hospitals, while recommending for the long term the provision of cubicle isolation blocks in two local general hospitals distant from the main infectious diseases hospital in Inverness[181].

Likewise in the North-Eastern Region they modified their advocacy of the concentration of general surgery in Aberdeen to the extent of approving the continuation by visiting surgeons of the more straightforward major surgery in the small country hospitals and even of surgery there, according to their expertise, by local general practitioners who had undertaken such work competently in the past[182].

In all regions, the new EMS hospitals, or annexes, were found to offer the possibility of a substantial reduction in the shortfall in bed numbers. Being situated outside, and usually at some distance from, urban centres they were classified as 'country general hospitals'. They seemed particularly valuable as housing for orthopaedic beds (as part of the organised orthopaedic service which the surveyors saw as mandatory for a region, the Princess Margaret Rose Hospital in the South-Eastern Region having set an example). Patients suffering from pulmonary tuberculosis and rheumatic diseases could also be so accommodated[183]. Raigmore for the Northern Region, Stracathro for the North-Eastern Region (although sited just beyond its southern boundary), Bridge of Earn for the Eastern Region, were earmarked for all three of these specialties, the beds for tuberculosis being in each case elements of a regional tuberculosis service headed by a Clinical Director.

The Northern, North-Eastern and Eastern Regions – with populations in 1938 of 185,000, 496,000 and 400,000 – could be administered as single undivided units and in the opinion of the surveyors each required a single co-ordinating body not only for initial planning but for the subsequent regulation of its hospital services[184].

In reviewing medical staffing the surveyors were concerned that high standards of quality should be maintained in all regions. To this end it was recommended that there should be University participation in the selection process for the more senior appointments. The importance of frequent contact between specialist and general practitioner was also stressed[185]. A further strengthening of specialist staffing in the Northern Region, beyond that already achieved by the Highlands and Islands Grants scheme, was recommended, also in the North-Eastern and Eastern Regions, particularly for the development of medical education in accordance with the recent report of the Inter-Departmental (Goodenough) Committee on Medical Schools[186]. One specialty inadequately represented in all three of those regions was paediatrics and in each case the appointment of a full-time paediatrician was recommended.

The South-Eastern Region and the Western Region, with populations in 1938 of 1,083,000 and 2,829,000 respectively, called for special solutions. It was decided to propose their division into sub-regions. The South Eastern Region should have four such sub-regions: Fife, Edinburgh, the Lothians, and the Border Counties (Berwick, Peebles, Roxburgh, Selkirk). The application of the standard ratios of bed requirements to the sub-regions exposed the degree of dependence of the surrounding counties on the Edinburgh hospitals in various respects. As an extreme case, the counties of East Lothian, Midlothian (excluding Edinburgh), and West Lothian should together, according to the formula, have had 196 maternity beds, but only 6 beds for maternity cases could be found! The surveyors considered that Edinburgh hospitals should serve the whole region for orthopaedic conditions in adults and children, for malignant disease, and for thoracic, neurological, and plastic surgery, etc. Apart from these special categories each sub-region should be expected to provide a complete hospital service for its patients. Relieved of these exceptional categories, Fife was still seriously short of beds to the extent of over 1,400[187]. It was suggested that Fife's needs should be met in the long term by two large district hospitals, each of over 1,000 beds, for general purposes, maternity and infectious diseases. These might be sited, one to serve the West of Fife, beside Dunfermline, and one to serve the East of Fife, at Cameron Bridge, with a further 150 beds at the latter site for pulmonary tuberculosis. In the short term temporary buildings might ease the situation[188].

The Lothian sub-region benefited from the EMS hutted annexe to Bangour Hospital, with an estimated peace-time complement of 1,100 beds, of which 450 were being used for tuberculosis patients. For the long term two new hospitals were proposed, one for the eastern area sited, say, at Haddington, and one for the western sited at Bangour, each to have some 700 beds for general purposes, maternity and infectious diseases, with the addition at one of these hospitals of 200 beds for pulmonary tuberculosis cases from both the Lothian and the Border counties[189]. In the Border sub-region the EMS Peel Hospital could provide in the immediate future 280 beds for general purposes and complicated maternity cases. As a long term policy a hospital of some 550 beds, with an adequate out-patient department staffed by specialists resident in the area, should be sited in the neighbourhood of St Boswells or Galashiels to serve the whole sub-region[190].

Edinburgh, with many hospitals of various categories, sizes and conditions presented a complex scene. The Royal Infirmary occupied a central position and could provide a maximum of 1,200 beds. There was a need for another major hospital of about 1,000 beds, especially if the recommendations of the Goodenough Committee regarding the size of the Edinburgh Medical School were to be followed. A site to the south-west of Edinburgh was suggested. The Princess Margaret Rose Hospital, linked with the major hospitals, would be the centre of orthopaedic treatment for the region, while on the other side of the city the Western General Hospital, substantially extended, and Leith Hospital as an accident centre and general practitioner hospital, could play important roles in their respective locations[191].

The Western Region exemplified to an even greater degree the pull on the surrounding populations exercised by great city infirmaries. The surveyors found it necessary to divide the Region into eight or even nine sub-regions: the Central (Glasgow) Sub-region, Dunbartonshire, Renfrewshire (possibly divided into East and West), Lanarkshire, Ayrshire, Stirling and Clackmannan, Dumfries, Wigtown and Kirkcudbright, and Argyll[192]. Of Dunbartonshire the surveyors remarked: 'the hospital provision in the county is meagre in extent and generally not of a high order'. In Renfrewshire, although the Royal Alexandra Hospital in Paisley was well equipped and the old Greenock Royal Infirmary was developing in a modern branch at Larkfield, 'hitherto a considerable number of Renfrewshire residents have gone to the [Glasgow] city hospitals for what may be regarded as district services'. As a result 'the Renfrewshire Sub-region as a whole is deficient in hospital accommodation of all types'. In Lanarkshire, before 1939, there had been a substantial deficiency of general and maternity hospital accommodation, although considerably reduced by the EMS Law Hospital and hutted annexes at Hairmyres which would eventually require replacement by more developed structures. Likewise, Ayrshire had received the Ballochmyle Hospital, and its new Central Hospital at Kilwinning had opened. The Dumfries and Galloway Sub-region was 'seriously deficient in hospital accommodation of all types' and the cramped site and awkward situation of the Dumfries and Galloway Royal Infirmary did not appear to permit the extensions which were desirable. In Stirlingshire the Stirling and Falkirk Infirmaries were modern but inadequate in size. Argyll and Bute lacked the more advanced facilities and would continue to send cases to Glasgow and Renfrewshire.

To remedy the deficiencies in these areas, which had been satellites of Glasgow, considerable reinforcement of medical staffs in respect of physicians, surgeons and pathologists was recommended. There was also a substantial building programme, of which the principal elements were a district hospital near Dumbarton with associated infectious disease and maternity hospitals; a new country general hospital in Renfrewshire; in Lanarkshire a new centrally placed hospital at Motherwell; new maternity units at Motherwell, Law Hospital and Bellshill, and a new infectious disease hospital, possibly near Hairmyres; a new district hospital and a new maternity hospital near Dumfries; in Stirlingshire a new central hospital catering for general medical and surgical cases (including the chronic sick, and with a special department for children), for maternity, for infectious diseases for the whole sub-region and for tuberculosis of the lung and other diseases of the chest[193].

During the 1930's Glasgow Corporation had been improving and expanding Stobhill, the Southern General, and other hospitals under their control, such that by 1941 the Corporation had obtained the approval of the Department of Health to a scheme, submitted in terms of Section 27 of the Local Government Act 1929, which included their 15 general and special hospitals, with 7,500 beds (excluding the mental hospitals), and which finally ended the association of the general hospitals with the Poor Law[194]. Accordingly the surveyors were able to classify the Western Infirmary, the Glasgow Royal Infirmary, the Victoria Infirmary, Stobhill Hospital and the Southern General Hospital as central hospitals, at the same time acting as hospitals of first reception for defined zones.

The population of Glasgow, put at 1,128,000, was augmented for the purpose of the calculation of demands on its institutions by 208,000 persons in respect of the estimated numbers of residents in Dunbartonshire, Renfrewshire, Lanarkshire, Stirling County and Argyll and Bute, who might look to the city for their hospital services[195]. Application of the standard ratios to a population of 1,300,000 produced a deficiency of 5,206 in beds for general purposes, maternity, pulmonary tuberculosis and infectious diseases, the first three of these categories being given high priority. Proposals for making some impact on this deficiency included a new hospital of 1,700 beds at Newton Mearns, extensions of 750 beds at Killearn and of 250 beds at Stobhill, and of 500–600 maternity beds at various locations[196].

The organisation of orthopaedic services in the Western Region was given special consideration. For Glasgow the use of Mearnskirk Hospital as a country hospital, working closely with the Royal Hospital for Sick Children, was recommended for the orthopaedic disorders of children. For wider needs three main sectors were suggested: towards the east, based upon the Royal Infirmary, in association with Hairmyres as the 'country hospital'; towards the south-west based upon the Victoria Infirmary, with Philipshill Annexe and possibly Ballochmyle Hospital; towards the north based upon the Western Infirmary, with Killearn Hospital. Special arrangements were thought to be appropriate for more distant Stirlingshire and Dumfriesshire[197].

The Secretary of State had asked the surveyors' advice as to how the arrangements in the Glasgow area for the treatment of cancer could be improved, the importance of the matter being indicated by the figures of mortality from cancer: 4,343 deaths in the West of Scotland in 1938. Although the surveyors had observed in Manchester and the Edinburgh Royal Infirmary the advantages of a single radio-therapy centre in a region, in the circumstances of Glasgow they thought it advisable to include the Royal and Western Infirmaries and Stobhill Hospital in the Cancer Service, but with a combination of the staffs of the three hospitals under a single head[198].

Part two: Towards an Integrated Health Service

A National Service

In July 1945 a Labour Government took office, with Mr Aneurin Bevan as Minister of Health and Mr J. Westwood as Secretary of State for Scotland, and new legislation was promoted on radical lines. The transfer of all hospitals, voluntary and municipal, to State ownership enabled the regional structure proposed in the White Paper for their administration to be further simplified, at the same time accommodating to the objections of the medical profession to local government control[192]. For Scotland it was proposed that Regional Hospital Boards appointed by and acting as the agents of the Secretary of State would have executive status extending beyond the merely advisory functions envisaged for the Regional Councils in the White Paper, while Boards of Management, appointed by and acting as the agents of the Regional Hospital Boards, would manage all the hospitals of the region, in groups which would include the former voluntary hospitals, this contrasting with the Joint Hospital Boards of the White Paper which were to be concerned with local authority hospitals only. English pragmatism and Scottish logic diverged in the treatment of the teaching hospitals in the two countries, for whereas the teaching hospitals in England were to be managed by Boards of Governors directly responsible to the Minister of Health (and were to see themselves as honoured islands of excellence), the teaching hospitals of Scotland were treated as an integral part of a fully comprehensive regional hospital service. Their essential role in such a service had been fully accepted by all the earlier investigators. Thus it would seem that an appreciation of this role, and not simply the importance of their bed complements, made their inclusion in a regional system inevitable[200]. At the same time the desirability of the representation of medicine, medical education and other important interests (specifically local health authority interests) in the membership of regional and group boards was acknowledged in the statutory requirements for their constitution, as was the claim of voluntary hospital interests to be considered in the making of the initial appointments[201].

In the Autumn of 1947 five Regional Hospital Boards were constituted by Order: for a Northern Region; for a North Eastern Region (including

Orkney and Shetland); for an Eastern Region; for a South Eastern Region (including Fife); and for a Western Region. Some 120 members in all were appointed to the five Boards, which ranged in size from 18 to 33 members. By the end of the year the Boards were engaged in appointing their senior officers – senior administrative medical officers, secretaries, treasurers – and in preparing their schemes, as provided by the Act, for grouping hospitals under Boards of Management and for the exercise of functions of these bodies[202]. Eighty-four Boards of Management were initially established, ranging in size from a six-hospital group in Glasgow (Glasgow Northern Hospitals) with a possible bed complement of nearly 4,000 beds, to a two-hospital group in Arran with 23 beds, or a unit with no official bed complement (Glasgow Dental Hospital and School). In general, grouping was made on a geographical basis (e.g. Oban and District Hospitals, Southern Ayrshire Hospitals); but usually mental illness and mental deficiency institutions, together or separately, were given their own Boards of Management. In the cities, grouping might have regard to the nature of the patients cared for, the Aberdeen Maternity Hospital and the Royal Aberdeen Hospital for Sick Children, although built alongside the Aberdeen Royal Infirmary at Foresterhill, being placed with other maternity units and an infectious diseases hospital in an Aberdeen Special Hospitals group; or the grouping might have regard to the nature of the treatment, as for the Glasgow Homeopathic Hospital; or of its function as the rehabilitative Astley Ainslie, Edenhall and Associated Hospitals group (constituted after the transfer of Edenhall Hospital from the Ministry of Pensions in 1953). Many groups included clinics of a specialist nature. The major teaching hospitals, with their ancillary institutions, could have constituted groups in themselves. In Glasgow, however, the opportunity was taken to link the infirmaries with local authority or EMS hospitals, the Western with Killearn (as the surveyors of 1946 had suggested), the Royal with the Belvidere and the Eastern District Hospital, the Victoria with Mearnskirk. Stobhill, Robroyston and Ruchill, three large local authority hospitals, were placed in the same Glasgow Northern Hospitals group. In Edinburgh the Northern Hospitals group comprised the municipal general hospitals, while the smaller voluntary institutions were shared between the Central and Southern groups (so named for convenience rather than geographical accuracy). Such groupings permitted the appointment to Boards of members, both lay and medical, who shared a common interest and a background of similar experience. As with Regional Boards, Boards of Management assembled together, in unpaid service, men and women from different walks of life who had an interest in hospitals and in the contribution which hospitals could make to the welfare of their local communities[203,204].

The wealthier voluntary hospitals brought to their Boards of Management their remaining endowment funds, the income from which could be used for research or amenity or other special projects. In accordance with the Act of 1947 and the subsequent Hospital Endowments (Scotland) Act 1953, a Hospital Endowments Commission reviewed the £13 million of such funds (which produced an annual income of nearly half a million pounds) and prepared reallocation schemes under which endowments, carrying some 16 *per cent* of the annual income, were transferred to Boards of Management which lacked such supplementary resources and to the Regional Boards. Endowments carrying 22 *per cent* (just over 100,000 *per annum*) of the annual income were given to a specially constituted Hospital Endowments Research Trust[205].

The Act provided that by an Order in Council His Majesty would name 'the appointed day' on which the voluntary and local authority hospitals would vest in the Secretary of State, and from which the Secretary of State would be responsible for providing 'throughout Scotland, to such an extent as he considered necessary to meet all reasonable requirements,' hospital accommodation, medical, nursing and other services required for the purposes of hospitals, and the services of medical specialists. The appointed day was the 5th July 1948. All but a few Scottish hospitals, of which some mental deficiency institutions run by the Roman Catholic Church were the more important, passed into State ownership. They contained nearly 64,000 beds as shown in the following table[206]:

Region	General Special & Children's Beds	Maternity Beds	Infectious Diseases & Sanatoria Beds	Mental Hospital Beds	Mental Deficiency Institutions Beds	Total Beds
Northern	986	91	442	1,082	—	2,601
North Eastern	1,781	266	905	2,374	32	5,358
Eastern	2,504	229	1,039	2,582	350	6,704
South Eastern	4,675	524	2,360	4,152	747	12,458
Western	12,832	1,588	7,494	11,775	3,070	36,759
Totals	22,778	2,698	12,240	21,965	4,199	63,880

The Regional Hospital Boards and the Boards of Management held initial meetings to take up their respective duties and to establish such structures of standing committees as they considered appropriate to their responsibilities. Monthly meetings of boards became the regular pattern at both levels, supplemented by the work of the standing committees. At both levels financial control called for its particular machinery. The Regional Boards, exercising a comprehensive supervision over the hospital and specialist services of their regions, had a responsibility for securing the effective disposition and efficient use of resources in which medical staff establishment, and buildings and equipment were key factors. As they identified deficiencies in services, newly emerging needs, and the potential of new technologies, the Regional Boards undertook the planning and costing of the necessary measures. Beyond the obligatory Finance Committee, Boards of Management suited their circumstances with respect to the distribution of functions among their members. Many appointed committees to handle general business or they might have committees for planning, property, and building work, for medical and nursing services or even for emergencies. They might accede to the personal interest of members in particular institutions or in sub-groups of institutions by establishing house committees or visiting arrangements in some form[207]. The business of Boards of Management was effected by a Secretary and Treasurer, appointed by the Regional Board (with provision for the views of the Board of Management in the selection process). Similarly appointed was the group Medical Superintendent, continuing the precedent set by the major teaching and local authority hospitals in the earlier period. In less than one third of the 84 hospital groups in 1957, however, the appointment of a full-time administrative medical superintendent had been considered appropriate[208]. For exchange of information about Government policies and the problems of the hospital service, the Chairmen of the five Regional Boards met regularly with the Secretary of State. The Senior Administrative Medical Officers of the Boards met likewise with the Chief Medical Officer of the Department[209]. Finance for the running costs of hospitals and for hospital capital expenditure was received by Regional Hospital Boards through the Department of Health from the Treasury, as an element in the budgeted moneys voted by Parliament on a cash basis for each financial year. The primary allocation was intended to maintain at their existing level the services provided in the preceding year. Proposals for the introduction of new developments were carefully screened by Regional Boards and, if need be, by the Department. Those which appeared justified were placed in order of priority as claimants for growth allocations. The approval of capital expenditure which would have maintenance consequences implied subsequent acceptance of the additional running costs involved. It was to prove more difficult to devise a system for the identification, scrutiny and eradication of activities which, in the disposition of limited resources, might no longer be justified[210].

In an inflationary era the maintenance of a level of service necessitated not only the meeting of rising prices of supplies and services but also the inevitable increase in salaries and wages awarded to hospital staffs. Since 1943 nurses in both local authority and voluntary hospitals had been receiving a substantial increase in pay (and an accompanying improvement in conditions of service) in accordance with the recommendations of the Nurses' Salaries Committee set up in 1941 under the Chairmanship of Professor Taylor. To assist the employing authorities in their straitened circumstances to meet the cost, the Government had contributed 50 *per cent* of the increase[211]. In spite of this improvement the competing opportunities of employment in other spheres, which had appeared for young women during the War, resulted in a shortage of some 6,000 nurses in Scottish hospitals by 1948[212]. As to medical staff the Government announced in June 1948 its acceptance, in principle, of the recommendations of the Interdepartmental (Spens) Committee on the remuneration of full-time and part-time consultants and specialists. In March 1949 a complete scheme for the payment of hospital medical and dental staff, in line with the Spens recommendations, was published and, after discussion between the Health Departments and a Joint Committee of the Royal Colleges, the Scottish Royal Incorporations and the Central Consultants and Specialists Committee, the Joint Committee recommended acceptance of these terms[213].

For other categories of staff interim arrangements were made, with protection of existing terms, until Whitley Council machinery could be established for the negotiation of rates of remuneration and conditions of service applicable to both sides of the Border. A clause in the Whitley Council Constitution provided for appropriate representation of Scottish interests in determining the membership of the General and the several Functional Councils. Provision was also made for a Scottish Advisory Committee whose opinion on the effect of decisions touching Scotland could be sought[214].

Rising Costs and their Control

Assured of financial support from the Central Government (which had coped with the cost of total war) hospital managements looked at their institutions with fresh eyes, abandoning the spartan make-do-and-mend methods of wartime, proceeding with repair work which had been postponed through the years of the emergency, and seeking to apply standards of accommodation and catering which would make residence in hospital acceptable to all the classes now entitled to use them. Medical staff were concerned to offer new diagnostic techniques, and new physical and chemical treatments developed before, during and after the War. General practitioners, newly responsible for the primary care of the total population, welcomed the availability of a specialist consultant service. The original estimates placed before Parliament, which had been based on information supplied by the hospitals, proved grossly inadequate. In the first nine months of the Service Scottish hospital running costs were at the rate of £19.7 million *per annum*, increasing in the first full year, 1949–50, to £24.4 million. By 1953–54, in spite of the Treasury's efforts to place a ceiling on the cost of the Health Service as a whole, Scottish hospital running costs had reached £32.7 million[215], and by 1959–60, £48.3 million[216]. The decline in the value of the pound continued relentlessly and the cost of the hospital and specialist services reached £110.7 million after a further ten years in 1969–70[217], and by 1973–74, the last year of the tripartite structure, had nearly doubled that figure at £208 million[218].

Steps to restrain the ever rising volume of expenditure were initiated early. To secure the benefits of bulk purchase of supplies central contracting was an obvious economy measure for a huge public service. Regional Boards and the Health Departments gradually extended the practice of inviting tenders for the supply of both medical and general items used by the hospitals in large quantities. Expert surveys of the radiological equipment in use throughout the country revealed much that was obsolete and special arrangements were made for the acquisition and distribution of up-to-date X-ray apparatus. Appreciating that the drug bill was an important constituent of its expenditure, the Western Regional Board had produced by 1959 a list of non-proprietary equivalents of proprietary drugs and chemical preparations, which it issued to the hospital doctors of the Region (and made available to other Regions) in the hope that the doctors would choose the cheaper alternatives[219].

Comparison of the accounting returns of the hospitals in the first years of the service revealed considerable variation in their expenditure under many heads. Apart from differences in function, in patients' needs and in their treatments, variations might arise from the characteristics or layout of buildings, different standards of equipment and staffing, and good and bad management practices. In 1952 the Secretary of State addressed a personal letter to the Chairmen of the Regional Boards asking that a review of staff establishments be undertaken to ensure that the minimum of personnel be employed[220]. A team of experts looked at selected hospitals, and the Department's Adviser on Domestic Administration visited 60 hospitals, either by invitation or where figures indicated the possibility of reduction or reorganisation. The findings in selected hospitals indicated a possible reduction in domestic staff of 7 *per cent* but overall the surveys produced a reduction of 0.7 *per cent* only[221].

The subjective analysis of each hospital's expenditure initially used, although improved in April 1954[222], failed to provide sufficiently meaningful data for management purposes. Experimental schemes of departmental costing were introduced in selected hospitals. A Working Party on Hospital Costing devised a practical method of analysis of hospital expenditure on functional principles so as to provide figures of cost, which could be related to appropriate units of achievement, of types of ward or specialty, of ancillary treatment departments and of such services as catering, heating, maintenance of grounds and nurse teaching. The new procedure, more straightforward than the perhaps overelaborate costing system being applied in England, was approved for introduction in April 1963[223]. During the same period the attention of the Department of Health had turned to the potential of the techniques of work study in the pursuit of economy and efficiency. Work study teams were established by the Department and by the Regional Boards and a wide variety of investigations were conducted during the following years[224].

The rising tide of hospital expenditure had been attributed in some quarters to extravagance and waste. In 1953 a Committee chaired by Mr C.W. Guillebaud was appointed by the Minister of Health and the Secretary of State for Scotland to review the financial situation of the Health Service, current and prospective. The moderate findings and modest recommendations emanating from the Committee after three years of investigation (which included occasional references to the Scottish situation) made its Report something of a non-event at the time. Its importance lay in the fact that the distinguished members set the seal of their authority on the acceptance that a National Health Service in the middle of the twentieth century required such levels of public expenditure, in 1953–4 about three and a quarter *per cent* of the gross national product. They had found 'no opportunity for making recommendations which would either produce new sources of income or reduce in a substantial degree the annual cost of the Service', while recommending in the interests of the future efficiency of the Service an increase in the level of hospital capital expenditure[225]. They were unwilling to forecast how the cost of the Service would vary over the next twenty years or so, dependent as this would be on the rate at which the country would be able to make good the deficiencies in the Service, the rate at which the hospital capital investment programme could be expanded, fluctuations in the levels of wages and prices and changes in medical techniques and in the incidence of disease and accidents. As to the effect of population changes, changes in age structure by themselves were calculated, 'on a number of drastically simplified assumptions', to increase the cost of the service by only three and half *per cent* between 1951–52 and 1971–72. (A further increase of four and a half *per cent* would be attributable to the rise in population projected for England and Wales by the Government Actuary.) It was noted that, looking forward to 1979 for the numbers of the single elderly, the biggest users of hospitals, the Actuary had calculated a negligible increase for men, and for women an actual decline. The Committee concluded that population changes by themselves were not likely to exert a very appreciable effect on the future cost of the National Health Service, a surprising opinion in view of later concern about the cost of caring for an ageing population[226].

The Hospital Plan and its Implementation

Inevitably during the first years of the Service little thought was given to new building. Attention was concentrated on deferred repair work, renovation, adaptation and the renewal of worn-out furnishings and obsolete equipment. Indeed in the year 1949–50 nearly half of the £1.6

million devoted to hospital capital expenditure, and in the following year over one-third of the slightly increased sum of £1.9 million, was spent on furnishing and equipment. By 1954–55 expenditure on buildings reached £2 million and, with the stimulus of the Guillebaud Committee's recommendation, reached £3 million by 1959–60[227]. Yet up to that time about 50 *per cent* of the building moneys had been devoted to schemes costing no more than £30,000[228]. The Vale of Leven Hospital, erected near the south end of Loch Lomond and partially opened in December 1955 and the only new hospital to be completed during the first ten years of the Service, was a Civil Defence project[229], although it filled a gap indicated in the hospital survey of 1946. Needs which necessitated new construction were, however, being identified and assessed, and by 1960 the Regional Boards and the Department had arrived at feasible programmes for the next five years with provisional forecasts covering a further five years to 1970[230]. Thus when the Minister of Health (Mr Enoch Powell) presented to Parliament in January 1962 a Hospital Plan for England and Wales for the ten years up to 1970–71[231], the Scottish Secretary of State was not behind-hand with his Hospital Plan for Scotland[232]. (Later in 1962, as from 1st June, an integrative measure was to take effect in the Scottish Office, when the Department of Health for Scotland was succeeded by the Scottish Home and Health Department[233]; but only in Northern Ireland was the integration of Social and Health Services later pursued at the operational level[234].)

The Scottish Plan declared its basic principles, the first of these being that since hospitals, local authority services and general practitioner services must offer a comprehensive range of services, each making its own peculiar contribution, the hospitals should confine their attention to patients requiring the treatment which only hospitals can provide, while general practitioners and community services must be capable of meeting the needs of their particular forms of care. Secondly, the regional organisation of the hospital services required that the central hospitals (which in all but one of the regions were teaching hospitals), must be reconstructed and modernised to enable them to offer high standards of care, effective medical education and progressive research. All hospitals in which the training of nurses and medical auxiliaries was undertaken must be in a position to offer satisfactory accommodation, facilities and variety of experience. Thirdly, the number and size of clinical units in major hospitals, and their distribution between hospitals, must have regard to economy and effectiveness in the distribution of consultants[235].

Studies in selected areas of the country, including those sponsored by the Nuffield Provincial Hospitals Trust, had aimed at establishing the number of beds required to meet effective demand under given conditions of occupancy[236,237]. For the purposes of the Plan it was considered that a ratio of 2.5 beds per 1,000 population, or over a region a ratio of

3 beds per 1,000 to allow for teaching and highly specialised facilities, might meet the need for acute beds (excluding general practitioner beds and beds for respiratory tuberculosis and other infectious diseases), as compared with the then current rate of 3.8 per 1,000. The lower ratio assumed efficient management of the acute units, accompanied by adequate provision of longer term care, particularly for old people, and of domiciliary care. This marked reduction on the ratios considered appropriate by the surveyors of the 1940s reflected not only changes in the dominant disease patterns but also a new attitude to the function of the hospital in the post-war era, when advances in technology were bringing more exact diagnosis and more effective treatment intensively applied. Outside the hospital home conditions for the reception of discharged patients were improving considerably. For maternity a ratio of 0.69 hospital beds per 1,000 of the population of the time was indicated. Other appropriate ratios were suggested for beds for old people, for the mentally defective, for respiratory tuberculosis, and for other infectious diseases[238].

The application of these ratios indicated for acute beds a surplus of 3,911 beds over the whole country[239], but the second principle of the Plan demanded the substantial rebuilding, renovation or expansion of eight key teaching hospitals, three in Glasgow, two in Edinburgh, two in Dundee and one in Aberdeen, whose obsolescent state could not be ignored. Also, as the earlier surveyors had discovered, the numerous population of many areas could secure the benefits of specialist care in hospital only by arduous journeys to the main centres. The remedy for this deficiency lay in the provision of suitably located district general hospitals; Dumfries, Ayr, Kilmarnock, Coatbridge, Motherwell, Greenock, Paisley, Kirkcaldy and West Lothian were chosen to receive them. Inverness, as the centre for the Northern Region, also required its special facilities. The advancing technology of certain specialties, branches of surgery and radiotherapy, necessitated the provision of highly specialised regional units. Progress had already been made with regard to thoracic surgery and, in new buildings in Edinburgh, to neurosurgery and radiotherapy. Major remaining deficiencies were now to be remedied: in respect of radiotherapy with units in Aberdeen and Dundee and two in Glasgow; in respect of neurosurgery with a unit in Glasgow to replace the wartime arrangements at Killearn; in respect of plastic surgery, with units in Glasgow and Edinburgh[240].

The application of the relative ratio produced a surplus of 3,675 beds for infectious diseases including respiratory tuberculosis, the Western Region contributing the bulk of these[239]. It was noted, however, that trends in infectious disease conditions pointed towards the disappearance of the specialist hospitals. Treatment of infectious diseases might instead be undertaken in annexes to major or district hospitals[241]. The Western and South Eastern Regions between them had a shortfall of 3,287 beds for the chronic sick. The possibility of continuing to adapt beds no longer required for tuberculosis or other functions offered one means of alleviating this serious situation. Most of the new district hospitals would include geriatric assessment units which would be linked with long-stay accommodation in the older hospitals in their areas. To meet shortages in maternity accommodation in and around Glasgow, the Queen Mother's Hospital at Yorkhill, and the Bellshill Maternity Hospital were under construction and several other units were projected. Other provisions were being made for the mentally ill and mentally deficient. Alongside this ambitious programme each Regional Board would be continuing with major and minor work to improve or adapt existing premises. Many hospitals not included in the reconstruction programme would require modernisation of X-ray and laboratory facilities[242]. In 1960, to facilitate minor schemes, the ceiling cost of a project which a Regional Board could incur without prior approval of the Department, increased from £10,000[243] to £30,000 in 1955, had been further increased to £60,000[244].

The formulation and execution of plans of this magnitude demanded technical and administrative expertise in substantial quantity. Because there had been no new hospital construction other than the hutted EMS hospitals since the 1930s, progress in the early years of the Service was handicapped by a dearth of persons with experience of modern hospital building in the many disciplines affected: health professionals and administrators; architects and contractors. The requirements of specialised departments were complex and continually developing. Many professionals, health authorities and statutory authorities had to be consulted and their demands reconciled. For major projects the range of contractors capable of undertaking such work was limited and in many areas the availability of an adequate labour force needed special attention[245]. For the co-ordination of the multiplicity of concurrent activities involved in the progressive stages of major schemes, network analysis was thankfully adopted as a valuable technique for planning the timetable, measuring progress and identifying causes of delay[246].

With experience, smoother and more rapid progress became possible, and by 1966 the Department could speak of four years as being the maximum time for the planning process of the normal major scheme up to the letting of the contract. The decision to rebuild on a restricted site, as in the case of the Edinburgh Royal Infirmary, was a self-imposed handicap[247]. The technique of work study, already making a contribution to operational efficiency, was called upon to explore the possibilities of improved design in new construction. Special attention was given to those units most directly concerned with patient care: wards, outpatient departments and casualty departments[248]. Developments in medical and nursing practice, such as early ambulation, intensive care and the increasing use of outpatient clinics for investigation and treatment, had to be catered for. The post-war period was seeing rising standards of living in the community, and the public expectation of amenity in hospitals was rising accordingly. A study of ward work sponsored by the Nuffield Provincial Hospitals Trust[249] had resulted in the construction in 1955 of an experimental unit at Larkfield Hospital, Greenock, a similar experimental unit being erected in Belfast[250]. The findings of an extensive examination by a multi-disciplinary team of hospital ward work in Scotland and elsewhere were published in a Hospital Planning Note on Ward Design[251]. Its recommendations were applied in the 120-bed extension at Falkirk Royal Infirmary whose new outpatient department was based on the advice of another Planning Note on the organisation and design of outpatient departments[252]. To offer a focal point for the collection and dissemination of information about hospital design, construction and management, the Scottish Hospital Centre (later to be called the Scottish Health Service Centre) was opened in Edinburgh in the grounds of the Western General Hospital, as a joint enterprise of the central Department and the Regional and group Boards, the construction cost being provided from Exchequer funds and the running costs from Board endowment funds. The Centre's facilities included an exhibition hall, a conference room, a lecture theatre, and a library which was to become extensive[253].

In 1964 the Hospital Plan for Scotland was updated in the light of progress and of newly recognised needs. The largest insertion into the programme was a new general hospital which was to be constructed at Gartnavel, Glasgow. As a consequence of this and of an increase in the scope of other schemes, the starting dates for the building of the hospitals at Ayr, Motherwell and Paisley were deferred[254]. Two years later a review of the Plan was undertaken. The programmes for the Western and South Eastern Regions had been disrupted by the emergency measures necessary to deal with the serious condition of the buildings of the two children's hospitals, that in Glasgow having developed structural defects, that in Edinburgh facing unacceptable maintenance costs. Rebuilding of both institutions seemed called for, the Glasgow Sick Children's Hospital remaining at Yorkhill, the Edinburgh Hospital to be transferred, it was proposed, to the north-west side of the city beside the Western General Hospital[255]. The 1966 Review abandoned the hope of making useful realistic projections for more than five years ahead, dependent as such projections were on the rate of growth of the economy and Government priorities of the time and circumstance, but it declared a new principle with a view to strengthening the links between general practitioners and hospital: that henceforth no new hospital would be built without the fullest consideration being given to the possibility of including in the scheme a health centre to enable general practitioner and community services of the locality to be functionally integrated with the hospital service. The possibility of the application of the same principle to existing smaller hospitals would also be explored. It was hinted that underlying this line of thought were larger questions relating to the administrative organisation necessary to secure integrated health services in local communities[256].

With the specific purpose of detailed comparison between the findings and recommendations of the surveyors of the 1940s and the situation twenty-four years later, a survey of all the hospitals in Scotland was undertaken in 1970 by the Scottish Hospital Centre. The change over the years in the hospital scene revealed by the survey was considerable. Many small units outside the main centres of population had either not been incorporated in the National Health Service or, having been taken over, had subsequently been disposed of. The functions of others had been changed and these had been adapted accordingly, e.g. to accommodate geriatric cases or to serve as general practitioner units. Many had been upgraded in varying degrees. Several small hospitals had been built to serve thinly populated areas, as, for example, at Lerwick, Fraserburgh, Fort William and Dunoon. The district general hospital at Kirkcaldy in Fife had been completed. Others were nearing completion, at Gartnavel in Glasgow, at Greenock, and on the site of the Crichton Royal Hospital at Dumfries. In these the design principles of the Falkirk ward had been applied. Also nearing completion was the vast teaching hospital complex at Ninewells, Dundee. Important specialist blocks had been added at Edinburgh's Western General Hospital and a main ward block at Aberdeen Royal Infirmary. The redevelopment of the Western Infirmary, Glasgow, was well advanced. Between July 1948 and December 1969 expenditure of £83.8 million on major schemes had provided over 9,000 beds, with associated facilities, in new or substantially altered hospitals[259].

In the ensuing years the growing concern to facilitate the association of general practitioners and the community services (and where appropriate the specialist services) was evidenced in the construction of health centres. The numbers of functioning health centres, in or adjacent to hospitals but more often independently sited, increased from 4 in 1966[258] to 170 in 1983[259]. During the same period the programme for the provision of district general hospitals was steadily pursued, with the completion of Gartnavel (1972), Dumfries (1974), Monklands (1976), Inverclyde Royal (1978)[260] and North Ayrshire (1981)[261]. Many ward units and departments were upgraded, many maternity units and geriatric units extended or added, engineering services modernised, and a number of staff residences and area board offices built.

Area Health Boards

The 1966 Plan Review had suggested the possible need for reorganisation of the Service. Ten years before, the Guillebaud Committee had recognized the imperfection of the tripartite structure, although rejecting a remedy which would separate domiciliary health from social services[262]. The administration of the respective arms of the Service had been designed to accord in the least disturbing guise with the historical experience and peculiar nature of each, appointed boards for the hospitals, councils of appointed members and professional representatives to supervise the contractual arrangements with general practitioners, and committees of elected councillors for the management of community services. The disparate nature of these bodies scarcely facilitated coordination. The vertical organisation of the hospital service, where boards composed of responsible men and women were subordinated to similarly constituted boards for the purpose of executing plans made for them by the superior boards within the controls exercised by the superior boards, was not one to promote co-operation. In general, however, friction was minimized through the good sense of board members and their officers. At the same time the proximity of Boards of Management to their hospitals, whilst being of some value, tended to impinge on the sphere of delegated responsibility which would attract able administrators to positions as hospital managers[263].

The establishment of a single board to take responsibility for all three branches of the health service operating within a defined area would be a means of ensuring that the development of co-operation between those working in the different branches would at least not be impeded by administrative segregation. At the same time the responsibilities for making plans and for their execution could be placed with one and the same body. Earlier, the geographical extent and population size of the two regions in the south of the country had been reasons for rejecting as impracticable the association of hospital management responsibilities with the supervision of local community services. Now the location of the new district general hospitals in areas distant from the city facilities was making these outlying areas self-sufficient in respect of the bulk of acute medical and surgical specialties, as indeed the surveyors of 1946 had desired. Administrative areas, smaller in size than the larger Regions, made more comprehensive responsibilities feasible.

Developments in the practice of medicine, both inside and outside the hospitals, were bringing their own pressures for change to bear on the established structures. A Joint Working Party of doctors and health service administrators, chaired by Dr J.H.F. (later Sir John) Brotherston, was appointed in December 1965 by the Secretary of State, 'To consider what developments in the hospital service are desirable in order to promote efficiency in medical work'. In its First Report of May 1967, '*Organisation of Medical Work in the Hospital Service in Scotland*', the Working Party advocated the organisation of hospital medical staff into broad specialty divisions which would permit flexibility in the allocation of beds and other resources, which the changing circumstances of specialisation and medical techniques called for, while at the same time allowing for specialties which cut across traditional boundaries. These divisions could encompass specialties which were definitely related to individual hospitals, such as medical and general surgery, and specialties for which an area or sector pattern was appropriate, such as ear, nose and throat surgery, obstetrics and geriatrics. For certain specialties – e.g. obstetrics, geriatrics and mental deficiency – resources outwith the hospital service might be of considerable importance. The divisional organisation of specialties of this nature should be linked with other branches of the health and welfare services in the community[264]. The Working Party declared, however, that the full attainment of the needed integration of the three branches of the service required legislation, which, having regard to the radical change involved, should be preceded by full consultation with all those concerned[265].

The Re-organisation of the Service

In December 1968, following the example of the Minister of Health in respect of England and Wales, the Secretary of State for Scotland, Mr William Ross, published a Green Paper which presented for public discussion a range of tentative proposals for the re-organisation of the Service[266]. After extensive discussions, a change of Government, and a Government White Paper of July 1971[267], the National Health Service (Scotland) Act of 1972 brought the establishment of fifteen single-tier health boards, responsible for the hospitals and community health services in areas whose boundaries coincided with those drawn up for reorganised (regional or district) local government. The areas designated corresponded to a remarkable degree with the regions or sub-regions of the 1946 survey, major differences being the amalgamation of parts of Dunbartonshire and Renfrewshire with Argyll to form the Argyll and Clyde area, and the union of Edinburgh with the greater part of the Lothian counties to form the Lothian area[268].

England had the advantage that its Act had been passed in advance of the Scottish Act. The necessity of meeting the common deadline of the appointed day, 1st April 1974, at which time the new administrations were to take responsibility for the health services, challenged the resources of the Scottish Department in a period of financial stringency. Chairmen of Health Boards had been appointed by January 1973 and it had been intended that they, together with chief officers of their Boards and a nucleus of Board members, should proceed to formulate administrative schemes for their Boards. The appointment of Board members and chief officers being delayed until the summer of 1973 or later, however, this task was undertaken by *ad hoc* area study groups constituted by the Board Chairmen[269]. The Department directed the study groups' attention towards the suitability of dividing their areas into geographical districts for management purposes [270]. The insertion of rigid divisions, fixed geographically into the internal administrative arrangements of area boards which were intended to function with a considerable degree of autonomy was surprising, although the device was useful in permitting the creation of standardised designated posts for which applications could be invited from members of the administrative staffs of the disbanding authorities and which would secure the continuity of the supervision of services at the stage of transfer to the new authorities. Indeed the concept of the geographical district as the basic management unit took so powerful a hold that it led to the five areas (Borders, Dumfries and Galloway and the three Island areas) which did not lend themselves to such division, being described as 'single-district areas'.

The re-organisation necessitated a fresh look at the Boards' top administrative appointments and respective responsibilities. In face of the complexity of the relationships between professionals in the administration of health services, the principle which initially prevailed was that of team management. This was given expression in the 'executive group', comprising medical, nursing, financial and lay administration. The Department prescribed the inclusion of area executive groups in the administrative schemes of the Health Boards and, since a district level was being established, of district executive groups on the same pattern[271]. The spheres of responsibility of those four officers were designated, but could frequently overlap. It was hoped that, by invoking co-operation and consensus, the common purpose of ensuring good patient care would override natural inter-professional sensitivity or rivalry. It was proposed that the district executive groups would enjoy the maximum possible delegation of powers consistent with the overall responsibility of the area executive group, but district officers were to be responsible to the chief officers of their professions; where a district executive group could not reach agreement on a matter within its delegated authority, the decision should be referred to the area executive group.

Inevitably the administrative posts at the area and district levels attracted the more experienced of the administrative staffs of the dissolving Boards of Management at the expense of the quality of administration at the institutional level[272]. As a consequence district administrators could find themselves involved in what was properly the function of unit administration. Similar influences were at work in the spheres of functional services, catering, etc. where the hierarchy of expertise made uncertain the level at which decisions should be taken[273].

Limited Resources: Unmet Needs

The launch of the re-organised Service coincided with the arrival of an adverse economic climate, and by 1976–77 a new system of control of expenditure by cash limits (except for family practitioner services) set at the beginning of each financial year had been introduced[274]. The policies appropriate to the circumstances of the remainder of the decade had been indicated in April 1976 by the Secretary of State, Mr Ross, in a memorandum suitably named '*The Way Ahead*'. The need to operate the Service within budgets which allowed for a lower degree of growth than formerly, was emphasised. Urgently needed developments could be provided only through the rationalising of existing services and cutting back on less essential aspects of care. In order to make resources available for the promotion of health in the community, particularly in areas of multiple deprivation, for the strengthening of preventive services, and for the improvement of hospital and community services for the elderly, the mentally ill, and the mentally and physically handicapped, the growth of the acute hospital sector must be curbed. This meant the limitation of acute beds (other than highly specialised beds provided on a regional or national basis) to 2.5 per 1,000 population, the ratio prescribed in the 1962 Plan. It was contended that, although in 1974 98.9 *per cent* of all births took place in hospital, a declining birth rate gave the opportunity for reductions in expenditure, including the closure of beds in under-used maternity units. For the elderly the provision of long-stay beds should not exceed 1.5 beds per 1,000 population aged 65 and over, but more day hospital facilities were needed, as also for the care of the physically handicapped[275].

The prescriptions of '*The Way Ahead*' were reinforced by the Planning Council's report '*Scottish Health Priorities for the Eighties*' with its pointers for a further six years up to 1986. Here maternity services were categorized as requiring a lower than average rate of growth, while acute hospital services were relegated to the group of programmes in which developments could be afforded only to the extent of savings secured in the operation of existing services[276]. The efforts of the Working Party on Revenue Resource Allocation, whose final report was issued in May 1977, had resulted in guidelines consistent with the priority document in putting a brake on the growth of expenditure in those areas which included the highly developed teaching centres in Glasgow, Edinburgh and Dundee, in favour of areas whose services of a more modest sort were under-developed[277].

The acute sector could hardly complain, for it had been particularly favoured in the phenomenal increase in expenditure on the National Health Service during its first thirty years. From an annual rate of £20 million in 1948–49[278], the running expenses of the hospital service were to exceed £500 million by 1978–79[279]. Much of this monetary increase must, of course, be attributed to inflation, but the underlying growth was remarkable. After the first year's jump, real growth over the whole service in the next six years was no more than 6 *per cent*[280]; yet in the ten years to 1965–66 it was around 52 *per cent*[281] and in the following ten years ending 1975–76 around 58 *per cent*[282]. Within that context the hospital, specialist and ancillary services (the acute sector predominating), which had been taking 61 *per cent* of the Service's money in 1960–61[283], were taking 72 *per cent* of its (increased) money by 1973–74[284]. As to expenditure on hospital services per head of population Scotland was spending more than any of the English Regions (as it was on health services as a whole) and was spending over 20 *per cent* more than Wales[285].

Expenditure on drugs and other medical supplies had risen with the enlargement of medical knowledge, but the hospital service being labour intensive, it was in the staffing of hospitals that the increased input of resources can be most plainly demonstrated. The cost of nursing is the largest single item of hospital expenditure and, in relating staff numbers to cost, allowances must be made – for changes in terms and conditions of service, in function and educational arrangements and standards, and in staff categories and their proportions. Yet the Scottish hospital service, which at the outset was employing the equivalent of about 19,000 full-time nurses[286], was by 1978 employing almost 50,000 such nurses[287], which, relative to the population, was about one-third more than the United Kingdom as a whole[288]. The full-time equivalent numbers for the next largest category, 'Ancillary and Other' (domestic staff, porter, tradesmen, etc), had roughly doubled at almost 28,000[287]. The full-time hospital doctors – 1,850 in 1953[288,289] – numbered over 4,000 by 1978[287]. Numbers of full-time 'Professional and Technical' staff, perhaps 1,000 in 1948, had reached 2,000 by 1953[290] and by 1978 exceeded 6,000[287]. Many of the 6,000 administrative and clerical staff employed in 1978[287] were engaged on secretarial and record work in medical departments. The achievements of the additional personnel are reflected numerically, for, although the number of staffed beds varied little, (in 1948, 58,000 and in 1978, 59,000), the numbers of in-patients treated almost doubled (in 1948, 383,000 discharges and in 1978, 749,000 discharges) and the numbers of new out-patients nearly trebled (in 1948, 1.26 million and in 1978, 3.23 million, with out-patient attendances rising from 4.55 million to 8.9 million)[291,292]. The remarkable increase in therapist and diagnostic staff is indicative of the revolution in medicine which had been taking place. But as old problems such as the chest diseases were brought under control, new demands were arising: for care of the growing numbers of the aged, for spare-part surgery, for abortion, for treatment of road casualties and the diseases of over-indulgence and compensatory addiction.

Exposed to these pressures health authorities were obliged to make painful choices between very desirable alternatives, dramatically instanced by the decision of the Secretary of State to override the decision of the Lothian Health Board to secure funds for the extension of geriatric accommodation by closing the small Bruntsfield Hospital with its long tradition of catering specially for women's needs[293]. After years of expansion, and aware of the possibilities of further technical advances, the professionals in the service were frustrated by the new financial handicaps. Among the sections of staff in which trade unionism had been a growing influence, attempts to secure economies, by work study or even contracting out certain services, ('privatisation'), were unwelcome and the establishment of some private institutions, for which Scottish conditions offered a relatively inhospitable climate, was regarded askance. It is not surprising that in face of the multiplicity of claims for attention, the Health Departments from their wider viewpoint began to lay greater emphasis on prevention, on education and on the exercise of greater personal responsibility for the preservation of health[294].

Management Responsibilities

The upheaval of the re-organisation in circumstances of financial stringency had resulted in much public and professional disquiet, particularly in England where the structural framework adapted to cope with the larger area and much greater population had brought a multiplicity of levels involved in decision-making which, associated with elaborate consultative machinery, produced delay and frustration[295]. The Government's response was to appoint a Royal Commission on the Health Services to consider the best use and management of the Services' (limited) resources of finance and manpower[296]. The theme of the re-organisation had been the association of hospital services and community services. Studies had underlined the importance for a patient's medical care of uninterrupted continuity between community and hospital[297,298] and it seemed logical to fashion the administrative structure to match this requirement. The establishment of districts had emphasised the geographical aspect of services (already catered for by the statutory areas) at the expense of the management of the institutions. Yet the major part of the resources of the Health Service, in the form of purpose-built accommodation, sophisticated apparatus, and assemblages of specialised skills, was concentrated in the hospitals. The Royal Commission acknowledged the need for expansion of hospital administration at unit (or sector) level; this was a practical proposition in accordance with the often stated principle that management decisions should be taken as close as possible to the level at which they are to be implemented[299]. In Scotland, in response to this recommendation, the Secretary of State, Mr George Younger, invited Health Boards to undertake a review of their management structures, which, involving the abolition of districts, would expand the responsibilities of managerial posts at unit or sector level[300]. The Royal Commission had declared that the chief administrator of a hospital should be clearly responsible for co-ordinating all services in the institution, which meant that staff who were part of a functional hierarchy (and the Commission identified more than twenty functional disciplines, such as works, engineering, catering, supplies and personnel), while remaining professionally answerable for their services, should be responsible to the administrator in charge for their daily work[299]. Thus staff engaged in non-clinical support functions should, in contrast to their previous semi-autonomous situation[301], be fully integrated into the unit operation, while the expertise of the functional officer at a higher level should normally be contributed in an advisory capacity[302].

In November 1983 the Secretary of State announced his decision that all Health Boards should dispense with district management systems, and in the following month Boards were instructed to base the administration of their local services on 'units of management', meaning 'coherent and discrete areas of management responsibility forming a distinct management level to which substantial decisions can be devolved'. The aim was to secure:

   (i)   *clear accountability and control;*
   (ii) *cost-effective management;*
   (iii) *observation of cost reduction targets;*
   (iv) *budgetary and resource efficiency,*

with a view to providing better health care through the better use of resources[303]. The Secretary of State had expressed his general agreement with the principles of the Report of the National Health Service Management Inquiry presented by Mr Roy Griffiths to the English Minister in October of the same year[304]. In accordance with that report he was soon to propose the appointment of General Managers in Health Boards[305] (whom Griffiths saw as sharpening up the decision taking of consensus management: the integration in one person of responsibility for planning, implementation and control of performance). Such general managers would, under the direction of their Chairmen and Boards, have overall responsibility for the effective discharge of Board business, existing senior officers reporting to them on matters relating to the management of the Service (although chief professional officers would remain the principal advisers to the Boards on matters within the area of their professional responsibility, with direct access to the Boards on such matters)[306]. General managers were to be appointed by Health Boards before the end of 1985; thereupon a further review of unit structure would presage the introduction of general managers at unit level[306]. The word 'unit', as used in the Scottish circulars and by Griffiths, no longer referred to an individual institution but to an administrative construct, the 'unit of management' mentioned above. Such units of management could be (a) a single hospital but were normally (b) a group of hospitals; or (c) being (a) or (b) together with community services; or (d) community services in part or whole of the Board's area;

or (e) a client care service or group of services as, for example, a mental illness hospital with psychiatric community services[300].

By mid 1984 the Health Boards had established their group units. Comparison can be made between the new patterns and the results of the similar operation conducted by Regional Hospital Boards 36 years earlier. Using the particular examples of the 1948 arrangements quoted previously, the then Oban and District Hospitals constituted the institutions of the new North Argyll Unit of the Argyll and Clyde Health Board; the former Southern Ayrshire Hospitals now constituted the institutions of Unit 2 of the Ayrshire and Arran Health Board, subject to the allocation of their maternity hospital to Unit 3, a maternity services group; the former Ayrshire Mental Hospitals constituted the institutions of Unit 4. Aberdeen General Hospitals constituted the institutions of Unit 1, (acute services) of the Grampian Health Board, subject to the allocation of Morningfield Hospital to that Board's Unit 3 (geriatric services). Aberdeen Special Hospitals, less the City Hospital, constituted Unit 2 (maternity and child health services).

Even had it so wished the wider compass of the Western Region was not available to the Greater Glasgow Health Board. Tighter local schemes were adopted for its eleven units. Edinburgh – with twelve units, including a Community Unit concerned with General Practice and Health Centres – provided parallels, with some modifications, with the grouping of hospitals of the earlier period[307].

Over the whole scene some contraction in areas and grouping compensated for the added responsibilities for community health services. Voluntary members had been eliminated at group management level. Otherwise was 1984 much more than a unitary re-arrangement of 1948? A new factor is the General Manager as a 'driving force seeking and accepting direct and personal responsibility for developing management plans, securing their implementation and monitoring their achievement'[306]. Can his leadership restore something of the optimism and excitement of the earlier date?

Also emerging is the Scottish Health Management Efficiency Group of Health Department and Health Service personnel (SCOT-MEG) constituted by the Secretary of State to devise and supervise national programmes of efficiency reviews to be conducted by health authorities, so providing overdrive and direction to Health Boards and General Managers[308]. It is expected to promulgate national standards. Standardisation has advantages. The efficient application of the high technology of the modern acute hospitals seems to call for rationalised systematisation and simplification, characteristics of the computerised assembly line. The review programme initially proposed by the Efficiency Group was directed at facility usage and the operation of support services. The extension of the search for effectiveness and economy into the organisation and management of clinical services awaits further research with which a Health Service Research Unit is being charged. At the beginning of the century, when this short history opened, sympathetic personal attention was a large component of medical practice. Such must surely remain an essential element in a medico-social service in the community, and in those institutions which are concerned as much with caring as with curing. Can SCOT-MEG integrate or co-ordinate, or at least reconcile, the two contrasting forms of service?

References

(1)   Turner, A.L., *Story of a Great Hospital*. Edinburgh, 1967, p.6.
(2)   Burdett, Sir H., *Burdett's Hospitals and Charities 1902*. London, 1902, pp.537, 559.
(3)   Hamilton, D, and Lamb, M., *Surgeons and Surgery*. In: Checkland, O., and Lamb, M., Health Care as Social History: the Glasgow Case. Aberdeen, 1982, p.76.
(4)   Turner, A.L., 1937, *op. cit.*, p.383.
(5)   Turner, A.L., 1937, *op. cit.*, p.212.
(6)   Gibson, H.J.C., *Dundee Royal Infirmary 1798–1948*. Dundee, 1948, pp.36–37.
(7)   Griffin, G.J., and Griffin, H.J.K., *Jensen's History and Trends of Professional Nursing, 5th Edition*. Saint Louis, 1968, p.451.
(8)   Burdett, Sir H., *Burdett's Hospitals and Charities 1913*. London, 1913, p.167.
(9)   Ferguson, T., *Scottish Social Welfare 1864–1914*. Edinburgh, 1958, p.485.
(10) Public Health (Scotland) Act 1897, Ch.38, 60 & 61 Vict., Sec.66(1).
(11) Philip, R.W., "An Address on Tuberculization and De-Tuberculization", *Brit. Med. J.*, 1912, 1, pp.873–77.
(12) Royal Commission on the Poor Law and Relief of Distress: Report on Scotland. Cd. 4922. London, 1909, Memorandum by Professor Smart, p.312.
(13) Bowman, A.K., *The Life and Teaching of Sir William Macewen*. Glasgow, 1942, pp.14–16.
(14) Lamb, M., *The Medical Profession*. In: Checkland, O., and Lamb, M., 1982, *op. cit.*, p.26.
(15) Ferguson, T., 1958, *op. cit.*, pp.303–05.
(16) Departmental Committee on Poor Law Medical Relief (Scotland). Cd.2008. Edinburgh, 1904, p.20.
(17) Gaffney, R., *Women as Doctors and Nurses*. In: Checkland, O., and Lamb, M., 1982, *op. cit.*, p.146.
(18) Ferguson, T., 1958, *op. cit.*, p.307.
(19) Macgregor, Sir A., *Public Health in Glasgow 1905–1946*. Edinburgh, 1967, p.135.
(20) Scottish Health Service Planning Unit, A Review of the Scottish Health Service, Edinburgh, 1979, App.E., p.216.
(21) Chalmers, A.K., *The Health of Glasgow 1818–1925*. Glasgow, 1930, pp.155, 156,(footnote).
(22) Chalmers, A.K., 1930, *ibid.*, p.155 (footnote).
(23) Dow, D.A., *The Rottenrow*. Carnforth, Lancs. 1984, pp.57, 61.
(24) Turner, A.L., 1937, *op. cit.*, p.70.
(25) Act for the Amendment and Better Administration of the Laws Relating to the Relief of the Poor in Scotland 1845, Sec.67.
(26) Departmental Committee on Poor Law Medical Relief (Scotland) Report, Cd. 2008. Edinburgh, 1904, p.85.
(27) *Ibid.*, pp.23–24.
(28) *Ibid.*, pp.26–27.
(29) *Ibid.*, p.57.
(30) Ferguson, T., 1958, *op. cit.*, pp.306–07.

(31) Macgregor, Sir A., 1967, *op. cit.*, p.136.
(32) Royal Commission on the Poor Laws and Relief of Distress: Report on Scotland. Cd. 4922. London, 1909, p.29.
(33) *Ibid.*, pp.150–51.
(34) *Ibid.*, pp.82–83.
(35) *Ibid.*, pp.50–51, 59–71.
(36) *Ibid.*, p.259 (Minority Report).
(37) *Ibid.*, p.260 (Minority Report).
(38) *Ibid.*, pp.269–70 (Minority Report).
(39) Ferguson, T., 1958, *op. cit.*, pp.343, 432.
(40) Gilbert, B.B., *The Evolution of National Insurance in Great Britain*. London, 1966, pp.390–97.
(41) Cohen, P., *The British System of Social Insurance*. London, 1932, pp.31–33.
(42) Scottish Board of Health: Hospital Services (Scotland) Committee. Report on the Hospital Services of Scotland. Edinburgh, 1926, p.41.
(43) Burdett, Sir H., *Burdett's Hospitals and Charities 1913*. London, 1913, p.96.
(44) Highlands and Islands Medical Service Board. First Report. Cd.7977. Edinburgh, 1915, p.4.
(45) Highlands and Islands Medical Service Committee. Report to the Lords Commissioners of His Majesty's Treasury. London, 1912, pp.25–28 & pp.51–52, (App.3).
(46) Highlands and Islands Medical Service Board, Third Report. Cd.8519. London, 1917, p.11.
(47) Turner, A.L., 1937, *op. cit.*, pp.318–20.
(48) MacQueen, L., and Kerr, A.B., *The Western Infirmary 1874–1974*. Glasgow, 1974, p.68.
(49) Macpherson, Maj. Gen. Sir W.G., *History of the Great War: Medical Services General History, Vol.I*. London, 1921, p.75.
(50) Robertson, E., *The Yorkhill Story*. Glasgow, 1972, pp.91,50.
(51) Craig, J., *A Short History of the Royal Aberdeen Hospital for Sick Children*. Aberdeen, 1968, p.11.
(52) Macpherson, Maj. Gen. Sir W.G., 1921, *op. cit.*, pp.80–81.
(53) Rae, H.J. *Public Health in the North-East*. In: Tocher, J.F., (Ed.), The Book of Buchan. Aberdeen, 1943, p.292.
(54) Chalmers, A.K., 1930, *op. cit.*, p.185.
(55) Macpherson, Maj. Gen. Sir W.G., 1921, *op. cit.*, p.77.
(56) Best, S.H., *The Story of the British Red Cross*. London, 1938, p.155.
(57) Calder, J., *The Vanishing Willows: The Story of Erskine Hospital*. Bishopton, 1982, pp.3,13,15.
(58) Best, S.H., 1938, *op. cit.*, pp.145,155.
(59) Mackenzie, T.C., *The Story of a Scottish Voluntary Hospital*. Inverness, 1946, p.211.
(60) Burdett, Sir H., *Burdett's Hospitals and Charities, 1920*. London, 1920, p.142.
(61) Macpherson, Maj. Gen. Sir W.G., 1921, *op. cit.*, p.86.
(62) Watson, W.N. Boog, *A Short History of Chalmers Hospital*. Edinburgh, 1964, p.15.
(63) McLaren, E.S., (Ed.), *A History of the Scottish Women's Hospitals*. London, 1919, pp.141–58, 195–213.
(64) *Ibid.*, p.56.
(65) Patrick, J., *A Short History of Glasgow Royal Infirmary*. Glasgow, 1940, pp.28,34.
(66) Smith, C., *Medical Radiology: Its Practical Application 1895–1914*. In: Checkland, O., and Lamb, M., 1982, *op. cit.*, pp.105–06.
(67) MacQueen, L. and Kerr, A.B., 1974, *op. cit.*, p.53.
(68) Ferrier, J., *The Greenock Royal Infirmary 1806–1968*. Greenock, 1968, p.108.
(69) Mackenzie, T.C., 1946, *op. cit.*, p.241.
(70) Murray, I., *The Victoria Infirmary of Glasgow*. Glasgow, 1967, pp.61–64.
(71) Scottish Board of Health. Third Annual Report 1921. Cmd.1697. Edinburgh, 1922, p.56.

(72) Scottish Board of Health. Eighth Annual Report 1926. Cmd.2881. Edinburgh, 1927, p.181.

(73) MacQueen, L., and Kerr, A.B., 1974, *op. cit.*, p.71.

(74) Ministry of Health, Department of Health for Scotland. Reports of the Committees on Medical Auxiliaries, Cmd.8188. London, 1951, p.101.

(75) Nurses Registration (Scotland) Act 1919, 9 & 10 Geo.V, Ch.95, Sec.1.

(76) Burdett, Sir H., (original editor), *How to Become a Nurse*, 12th Edition. London, 1933, pp.189–205, 278–82, 300–02.

(77) Dow, D.A., 1984, *op. cit.*, p.96.

(78) Turner, A.L., 1937, *op. cit.*, pp.349–56, 357 (footnote).

(79) Ministry of Health Consultative Council of Medical and Allied Services. Interim Report on the Future Provision of Medical and Allied Services. Cmd.693. London, 1920, p.5.

(80) *Ibid.*, p.6.

(81) *Ibid.*, pp.15–17.

(82) Spann, R.N., *The Use of Advisory Bodies by the Ministry of Health.* In: Vernon, R.V., and Mansergh, N., (Eds.), Advisory Bodies. London, 1940, pp.229–30.

(83) Scottish Board of Health: Hospital Services (Scotland) Committee, 1926, *op. cit.*, p.8.

(84) *Ibid.*, p.18.

(85) *Ibid.*, p.10.

(86) *Ibid.*, pp.18–20.

(87) *Ibid.*, pp.16–17.

(88) *Ibid.*, p.21.

(89) *Ibid.*, pp.27,30.

(90) *Ibid.*, p.53.

(91) *Ibid.*, p.15.

(92) *Ibid.*, p.16.

(93) *Ibid.*, p.45.

(94) *Ibid.*, pp.41–43.

(95) Scottish Board of Health, 1927, *op. cit.*, pp.155–56.

(96) *Ibid.*, p.158.

(97) Central Bureau of Hospital Information, *The Hospitals Year Book 1941.* London, 1941, pp.177–85.

(98) *The Glasgow Herald*, June 10, 1937, p.10.

(99) Whyte, W.E., *The Local Government (Scotland) Act 1929.* Edinburgh, 1929, pp.2–4.

(100) Macgregor, Sir A., 1967, *op. cit.*, pp.137–39.

(101) Department of Health for Scotland. Committee on Scottish Health Services. Report. Cmd.5204. Edinburgh, 1936a, pp.234–35.

(102) *Ibid.*, p.403, App.VI.

(103) Tait, H.P., *A Doctor and Two Policemen.* Edinburgh, 1974, p.158.

(104) Catford, E.F., *The Royal Infirmary of Edinburgh 1929–1979.* Edinburgh, 1984, pp.24–26.

(105) Department of Health of Scotland. Consultative Council on Medical and Allied Services. Report on Hospital Services. Edinburgh, 1933, pp.6–8.

(106) Scottish Board of Health. Consultative Council on Local Health Administration and General Health Questions. Report on a Reformed Local Authority for Health and Public Assistance. Edinburgh, 1923, p.7.

(107) D.H.S., 1933, *op. cit.*, pp.9–10.

(108) D.H.S., Third Annual Report 1931. Cmd.4080. Edinburgh, 1932, p.77.

(109) D.H.S., Sixth Annual Report 1934. Cmd.4837. Edinburgh, 1935, p.96.

(110) D.H.S., Ninth Annual Report 1937. Cmd.5713. Edinburgh, 1938, p.102.

(111) *Ibid.*, p.102.

(112) *Ibid.*, p.102.

(113) *Ibid.*, p.103.

(114) D.H.S., 1935, *op. cit.*, p.96.

(115) D.H.S., Tenth Annual Report 1938. Cmd.5969. Edinburgh, 1939, p.108.

(116) D.H.S., Eighth Annual Report 1936. Cmd.5407. Edinburgh, 1937, p.96.
(117) D.H.S., 1935, *op. cit.*, p.92.
(118) *Ibid.*, p.175.
(119) D.H.S., 1932, *op. cit.*, p.81.
(120) *Ibid.*, p.78.
(121) D.H.S., Seventh Annual Report 1935. Cmd.5123. Edinburgh, 1936b, p.97.
(122) D.H.S., 1936a, *op. cit.*, p.196.
(123) *Ibid.*, p.205.
(124) *Ibid.*, pp.233–236.
(125) *Ibid.*, pp.239–240.
(126) Robertson, E., 1972, *op. cit.*, pp.18–19.
(127) D.H.S., 1936a, *op. cit.*, pp.241–42.
(128) *Ibid.*, p.245.
(129) D.H.S., 1939, *op. cit.*, p.127.
(130) Robertson, E., 1972, *op. cit.*, p.111.
(131) Alexander, W.A., *John Thomson 1856–1926*. In: Guthrie, D., The Royal Edinburgh Hospital for Sick Children 1860–1960. Edinburgh, 1960, pp.39–42.
(132) Robertson, E., 1972, *op. cit.*, p.40.
(133) Henderson, J.L., *Charles McNeil (1881–)*. In: Guthrie, D., 1960, *op. cit.*, pp.42–45.
(134) D.H.S., 1939, *op. cit.*, p.75.
(135) Midwives and Maternity Homes (Scotland) Act 1927. 17 & 18 Geo 5, Ch.17.
(136) Nursing Homes Registration (Scotland) Act 1938. 1 & 2 Geo 6, Ch.73.
(137) D.H.S., 1939, *op. cit.*, pp.75–76.
(138) Catford, E.F., 1984, *op. cit.*, pp.34–35.
(139) Radium Commission. Second Annual Report 1930–1931. Cmd.3958. London, 1931, pp.17–21.
(140) Catford, E.F., 1984, *op. cit.*, pp.57–58.
(141) Dow, D.A., 1984, *op. cit.*, p.104.
(142) Rorie, D., (Ed.), *The Book of Aberdeen*. Aberdeen, 1939, various pages.
(143) Dunn, C.L., (Ed.), *The Emergency Medical Services Vol. II*. London, 1953, pp.5–6.
(144) *Ibid.*, pp.10–13.
(145) D.H.S., 1939, *op. cit.*, p.171.
(146) Civil Defence Act 1939, Part VII, 2 & 3 Geo 6, Ch.31.
(147) Dunn, C.L., (Ed.), 1953, *op. cit.*, p.25.
(148) *Ibid.*, p.57.
(149) D.H.S., Summary Report for the Year ended 30th June 1944. Cmd.6545. Edinburgh 1944, p.14.
(150) D.H.S., Circular No.310/1941.
(151) Dunn, C.L., (Ed.), 1953, *op. cit.*, p.27.
(152) *Ibid.*, p.39.
(153) *Ibid.*, p.27.
(154) *Ibid.*, p.32.
(155) Tait, H.P., 1974, *op. cit.*, p.160.
(156) Tomaszeski, W., (Ed.), The University of Edinburgh and Poland. Edinburgh 1968, pp.46–47.
(157) *Ibid.*, pp.42–45.
(158) Dunn, C.L., (Ed.), 1953, *op. cit.*, pp.68–69.
(159) *Ibid.*, pp.64–68.
(160) Macgregor, Sir A., 1967, *op. cit.*, pp.165–66.
(161) Dunn, C.L., (Ed.), 1953, *op. cit.*, p.99.
(162) D.H.S., 1944, *op. cit.*, pp.14–15.
(163) D.H.S., Summary Report. Year ended 30th June, 1945. Cmd.6661. Edinburgh, 1945, p.15.
(164) D.H.S., Summary Report. Year ended 30th June, 1942. Cmd.6372. Edinburgh, 1942, p.11.

(165) D.H.S., Summary Report. Period from July 1945 to December 1946. Cmd.7188. Edinburgh, 1947, p.38.
(166) D.H.S., 1945, *op. cit.,* p.15.
(167) D.H.S., 1947, *op. cit.,* p.38.
(168) *The Scotsman*, October 24th, 1940, p.3.
(169) D.H.S., Committee on Post-War Hospital Problems in Scotland, Report. Cmd.6472. Edinburgh, 1943, p.42.
(170) *Ibid.,* pp.9–17.
(171) *Ibid.,* pp.30–34.
(172) *Ibid.,* pp.18–30.
(173) *Ibid.,* pp.38–41.
(174) Ministry of Health. Department of Health for Scotland, A National Health Service. Cmd.6502. London, 1944., p.12.
(175) *Ibid.,* pp.42–45.
(176) D.H.S., Scottish Hospitals Survey. General Introduction to the Report. Edinburgh, 1946, pp.3–9.
(177) *Ibid.,* General Introduction, pp.10–12.
(178) *Ibid.,* Report on the South-Eastern Region, pp.19–21.
(179) *Ibid.,* General Introduction, pp.12–13.
(180) *Ibid.,* General Introduction, p.4.
(181) *Ibid.,* Report on the Northern Region, p.21.
(182) *Ibid.,* Report on the North-Eastern Region, p.13.
(183) *Ibid.,* General Introduction, p.6.
(184) *Ibid.,* Report on the Northern Region, p.7.
(185) *Ibid.,* Report on the North-Eastern Region, p.7.
(186) *Ibid.,* Report on the Northern Region, p.31.
(187) *Ibid.,* Report on the South-Eastern Region, pp.25–27.
(188) *Ibid.,* Report on the South-Eastern Region, pp.37–39.
(189) *Ibid.,* Report on the South-Eastern Region, p.40.
(190) *Ibid.,* Report on the South-Eastern Region, pp.42–43.
(191) *Ibid.,* Report on the South-Eastern Region, pp.31–32.
(192) *Ibid.,* Report on the Western Region, p.9.
(193) *Ibid.,* Report on the Western Region, pp.62–122.
(194) Macgregor, Sir A., 1967, *op. cit.,* pp.147–48.
(195) D.H.S., 1946, *op. cit.,* Report on the Western Region, p.35.
(196) *Ibid.,* Report on the Western Region, pp.58–60.
(197) *Ibid.,* Report on the Western Region, pp.25–28.
(198) *Ibid.,* Report on the Western Region, pp.13–18.
(199) Ross, J.S., The National Health Service in Great Britain. London, 1952, pp.101–04, 335.
(200) *Ibid.,* p.337.
(201) National Health Service (Scotland) Act 1947. 10 & 11 Geo 6, Ch.27, pp.64–66.
(202) D.H.S., Report for the Year 1948. Cmd.7659. Edinburgh, 1949, p.31.
(203) *Ibid.,* p.28.
(204) Milne, J.F., (Ed.), *The Hospitals Year Book 1949–50,* London, 1949, pp.519–86.
(205) D.H.S., Hospital Endowments Commission, Report: Hospital Endowments. Cmd.9516. Edinburgh, 1955, pp.1–9.
(206) D.H.S., 1949, *op. cit.,* p.27.
(207) S.H.H.D. Scottish Health Services Council. Report of a Committee (Chairman, W.M. Farquharson-Lang). Administrative Practice of Hospital Boards in Scotland, Edinburgh, 1966a, pp.33–35.
(208) D.H.S., Report by a Committee of the Standing Advisory Committee on Hospital and Specialist Services (Chairman Sir George Henderson). Medical Superintendents and Medical Staff Committees. Edinburgh, 1957a, p.7.
(209) D.H.S., 1949, *op. cit.,* p.29.

(210) Anderson, D.S., *Accounting and Hospital Finance*. In: Peters, R.J., and Kinnaird, J., (Eds.), Health Services Administration. Edinburgh, 1965, pp.427–28, 437–39.

(211) D.H.S., Report. Year ended 30th June, 1942. Cmd.6372. Edinburgh, 1942, p.16.

(212) D.H.S., 1949, *op. cit.*, p.36.

(213) Ross, J.S., 1952, *op. cit.*, pp.151–52.

(214) Milne, J.F., (Ed.), 1949, *op. cit.*, pp.660–61.

(215) Committee of Enquiry into the Cost of the National Health Service (Chairman Guillebaud, C.W.). Cmd.9663. London, 1956, p.290.

(216) D.H.S., Report 1960. Part I Health and Welfare Services. Cmnd.1320. Edinburgh, 1961, p.58.

(217) S.H.H.D., Health Services in Scotland. Report for 1970. Cmnd.4667. Edinburgh, 1971, p.102.

(218) S.H.H.D., Health Services in Scotland. Report for 1974. Cmnd.6052. Edinburgh, 1975, p.85.

(219) D.H.S., Report 1950. Cmd.8184. Edinburgh, 1951, p.35.

(220) D.H.S., Report 1952. Cmd.8799. Edinburgh, 1953, p.45.

(221) D.H.S., Report 1953. Cmd.9107. Edinburgh, 1954, pp.59, 64.

(222) D.H.S., Circular S.R.B. 54/18.

(223) S.H.H.D., Circular S.H.M. 62/68.

(224) D.H.S., Report 1959. Cmnd.983. Edinburgh, 1960, pp.64–65.

(225) Committee of Enquiry (Guilleband), 1956, *op. cit.*, p.268.

(226) *Ibid.*, pp.48–49.

(227) D.H.S., Hospital Plan for Scotland. Cmnd.1602. Edinburgh, 1962a, p.12.

(228) D.H.S., Hospital Building: Scotland. Progress Report 1. Edinburgh, 1962b, p.5.

(229) S.H.H.D., Hospital Design in Use 1. Vale of Leven Hospital, Edinburgh, 1963, p.3.

(230) D.H.S., 1961, *op. cit.*, p.59.

(231) Ministry of Health, Hospital Plan for England and Wales. Cmnd.1604. London, 1962.

(232) D.H.S., 1962a, *op. cit.*

(233) S.H.H.D., Health and Welfare Services in Scotland. Report for 1962. Cmnd.1996. Edinburgh, 1963, p.2.

(234) Brown, Sir T., *The Integration of Health and Social Services – The Northern Ireland Experience*. Hospital and Health Services Review, 75, 1979, pp.315–18.

(235) D.H.S., 1962a, *op. cit.*, pp.13–15.

(236) Nuffield Provincial Hospitals Trust and University of Bristol, *Studies in the Functions and Design of Hospitals*. London, 1955, pp.149–85.

(237) Airth, A.D., and Newell, D.J., *The Demand for Hospital Beds*. Newcastle-upon-Tyne, 1962.

(238) D.H.S., 1962a, *op. cit.*, pp.17–18.

(239) *Ibid.*, pp.24,28,30,32,34.

(240) *Ibid.*, pp.20–21.

(241) *Ibid.*, p.18.

(242) *Ibid.*, pp.21–22.

(243) D.H.S., Report 1956. Cmnd.140. Edinburgh, 1957b, p.9.

(244) D.H.S., 1961, *op. cit.*, p.63.

(245) D.H.S., 1962a, *op. cit.*, p.19.

(246) Watts, G., *Aids to Efficiency*. In: Milne, J.F., and Chaplin, N.W., (Eds.), Modern Hospital Management. London, 1969, pp.445–46.

(247) S.H.H.D., Review of the Hospital Plan for Scotland. Cmnd.2877. Edinburgh, 1966b, p.7.

(248) D.H.S., 1962a, *op. cit.*, pp.39–42.

(249) Nuffield Provincial Hospitals Trust and the University of Bristol, 1955, *op. cit.*, pp.19–20.

(250) The Nuffield Foundation. Nuffield House, Musgrave Park Hospital, Belfast. London, 1962, p.i.

(251) S.H.H.D., Hospital Planning Notes 1: Ward Design. Edinburgh, 1963.
(252) S.H.H.D., Hospital Planning Note 6: Organisation and Design of Outpatient Departments. Edinburgh, 1967a.
(253) S.H.H.D., Health and Welfare Services in Scotland. Report for 1965. Cmnd.2984. Edinburgh, 1966, p.64.
(254) S.H.H.D., Revision of Hospital Plan for Scotland. Edinburgh, 1964, p.3–4.
(255) S.H.H.D., 1966b, *op. cit.*, p.13.
(256) S.H.H.D., 1966b, *op. cit.*, p.4–5.
(257) Scottish Hospital Centre. Survey of Scottish Hospitals: Centre Note. Edinburgh, 1971a, pp.1–5.
(258) S.H.H.D., Health and Welfare Services in Scotland. Report for 1967. Cmnd.3608. Edinburgh, 1968a, p.101.
(259) S.H.H.D., Health in Scotland 1983. Report by the C.M.O. Edinburgh, 1984, p.18.
(260) S.H.H.D., Health Services in Scotland. Reports for respective years.
(261) S.H.H.D., Health in Scotland 1981. Report by the C.M.O. Edinburgh, 1982, p.59.
(262) Committee of Enquiry (Guillebaud). 1956, *op. cit.*, p.54.
(263) Scottish Health Services Council. Report (Farquharson-Lang). 1966a, *op. cit.*, pp.22–23.
(264) S.H.H.D., Organisation of Medical Work in the Hospital Service in Scotland. First Report of the Joint Working Party (Chairman Dr. J.H.F. Brotherston). Edinburgh, 1967b, pp.15–19.
(265) *Ibid.*, p.11.
(266) S.H.H.D., Administrative Reorganisation of the Scottish Health Services. Edinburgh, 1968b.
(267) S.H.H.D., Reorganisation of the Scottish Health Services. Cmnd.4734. Edinburgh, 1971b.
(268) National Health Service (Determination of Areas of Health Boards) (Scotland) Order 1974. SI No.266.
(269) S.H.H.D., Health Services in Scotland. Report for 1974. Cmnd.6052. Edinburgh, 1975, p.3.
(270) S.H.H.D., Circular HSR (73) C7. Health Board Districts. Edinburgh, 1973.
(271) S.H.H.D., Circular HSR (72) C3. The Administrative Structure of Health Boards. Edinburgh, 1972.
(272) Mitchell, R., The First Year of the Reorganised Scottish Health Service. *Hospital and Health Services Review*, 1975, 71, 5, p.159.
(273) Stevenson, Sir S., *Decision Making in the National Health Service in Scotland*, I.H.S.A Conference Address reported in Hospital and Health Services Review, 1979, 75, 3, p.96.
(274) S.H.H.D., Health Services in Scotland. Report for 1977. Cmnd.7237. Edinburgh, 1978, p.44.
(275) S.H.H.D., The Health Service in Scotland: The Way Ahead. Edinburgh, 1976, pp.7, 16–19.
(276) Scottish Health Service Planning Council. Report of a Working Party. Scottish Health Authorities Priorities for the Eighties. Edinburgh, 1980, p.73.
(277) S.H.H.D., Working Party on Revenue Resource Allocation. Report. Scottish Health Authorities Revenue Equalization. Edinburgh, 1977a, Table 7, p.94.
(278) Committee on Enquiry (Guillebaud) (1956), *op. cit.*, Table 56, p.290.
(279) S.H.H.D., Health Services in Scotland. Report for 1978. Cmnd.7607. Edinburgh, 1979, p.45.
(280) D.H.S., Scottish Health Statistics 1958. Edinburgh, 1959, p.188.
(281) S.H.H.D., Health and Welfare Services in Scotland. Report for 1966. Cmnd.3337. Edinburgh, 1967, p.1.
(282) S.H.H.D., Health Services in Scotland. Report for 1976. Cmnd.6812. Edinburgh, 1977b, p.64.
(283) D.H.S., Report 1961 Part I, Health and Welfare Services. Cmnd.1703. Edinburgh, 1962c, p.8.

(284) S.H.H.D., 1975, *op. cit.*, p.85.
(285) Royal Commission on the National Health Service. Report. Cmnd.7615. London, 1979, p.15.
(286) D.H.S., 1959, *op. cit.*, Sec.VIII, Table 8, p.153.
(287) Scottish Office. Scottish Statistical Abstracts No.9/1980. Edinburgh, 1980, Table 3.12, p.35.
(288) Royal Commission on the National Health Service. 1979, *op. cit.*, Table 13.1, p.187.
(289) D.H.S., 1959, *op. cit.*, Sec.VIII, Table 8a, p.154.
(290) Central Statistical Office. Annual Abstract of Statistics No.94. London, 1957, Table 60, p.61.
(291) D.H.S., 1959, *op. cit.*, Sec. VIII, Table 1, p.144.
(292) Scottish Office, 1980, *op. cit.*, Table 3.1, p.27.
(293) *The Scotsman*, June 26, 1985, p.18.
(294) D.H.S.S., (For the Health Departments of Great Britain and Northern Ireland), Prevention and Health: Everybody's Business. London, 1976, p.17.
(295) Royal Commission on the National Health Service, 1979, *op. cit.*, pp.28–34.
(296) *Ibid.*, p.1.
(297) Ferguson, T., and MacPhail, A.N., *Hospital and Community*. London, 1954, pp.143–44.
(298) King Edward's Hospital Fund for London, Working Together: A study of coordination and cooperation between general practitioner, public health and hospital services. London, 1968, pp.6,11,28–31.
(299) Royal Commission on the National Health Service, 1979, *op. cit.*, pp.318–19.
(300) S.H.H.D., NHS Circular 1981(GEN)14. Edinburgh, 1981.
(301) Beveridge, C., "Canny Scots keep options open." *Health and Social Services Journal*, April 5th, 1984, p.408.
(302) Savage, G.G., *Structure and Management of the National Health Service in Scotland*. I.H.S.A. (East of Scotland Branch) and Faculty of Community Medicine (Scottish Committee) Conference reported in Hospital and Health Services Review, 1980, 76, 5, p.184.
(303) S.H.H.D., NHS Circular 1983 (GEN)27. Edinburgh, 1983.
(304) Griffiths, R., (Leader of Inquiry). *NHS Management Inquiry Main Recommendations*. London, 1983.
(305) Scottish Office Circular 634/84. Edinburgh, 1984.
(306) S.H.H.D., NHS Circular 1985 (GEN)4. Edinburgh, 1985.
(307) Chaplin, N.W., (Ed.), *The Hospital and Health Services Year Book 1985*. London, 1985, p.424 *et seq.*
(308) S.H.H.D/DS (1985) 35., Efficiency in the National Health Service: Report of the NHS Efficiency Programme Group.

3. *The Public Health Services*

Scott Wilson

CONTENTS

About the Author

Dr THOMAS SCOTT WILSON MD, FRCP(G), FFCM.

After a distinguished career in Public Health in which he was the last
Medical Officer of Health of the City of Glasgow, Dr Thomas Scott
Wilson MD, FRCP(G), FFCM, is at present Community Medicine
Specialist, Greater Glasgow Health Board with remit in Environmental
Health, Infectious Disease Control and Health Education. He is the
author of a number of Papers on Public Health matters. He served as a
Major in the RAMC during World War II.

Author's Note

The chapter on Public Health traces the early origins of organised interest in the subject developing in mid and late Victorian times and proceeds to problems of the present day.

The triumphs are highlighted, such as the elimination of gross overcrowding and the progress made in housing the population. The Clean Air Act of 1956, one of the most important preventive measures of this century, is briefly dealt with. The changing situation in infectious disease and the triumphs of Immunisation are dealt with. Criticism is made about the slowness of development of immunisation programmes prior to the Second War. The slow progress towards the adoption of Fluoridation of Water is discussed. Modern problems such as Hepatitis B, Legionnaires Disease and Acquired Immune Deficiency Syndrome (AIDS) are touched on.

The hospital provision for Infectious Disease over the last 100 years is dealt with and the proportion of beds earmarked for this is compared with general hospital provision.

Sir John Brotherston came to be Chief Medical Officer of the Scottish Home and Health Department following a distinguished academic career, latterly as Professor of Public Health at Edinburgh University. He was known and liked by everyone in the medical field and he himself had great detailed knowledge of what was happening in the hospital scene and in the various Public Health Departments in Scotland. His influence spread far furth of Scotland. Sir John Brotherston continued the tradition set up by his predecessors of regular briefings of Medical Officers of Health at St Andrews House on contemporary issues.

The Public Health Services

Introduction

As the introductory chapter made clear, the nineteenth century witnessed a gradual but fundamentally important change in the community's approach towards public health. By the end of the century, the old negative approach, involving the isolation or banishment of obvious sources of infection and spasmodic attempts to abate nuisances, had been largely replaced by one based upon the recognition of the benefits of attacking systematically the conditions which promoted ill-health. This change in outlook was both reflected and stimulated by a number of late nineteenth century Acts of Parliament which may be said to have laid the foundations of the modern public health service in Scotland.

While the 1860s saw cities such as Glasgow and Edinburgh take the first steps along the road to a modern public health service, Scotland's smaller burghs and rural authorities displayed a marked reluctance to follow their example. By the 1870s it was becoming apparent, firstly, that many local authorities would not tackle necessary sanitary reforms of their own volition, and, secondly, that the parish, the basic unit of local government outside the burghs, was too small to administer efficient and modern public health services[1]. The Local Government (Scotland) Act of 1889 provided a solution to part of the problem. This Act enlarged the areas of rural public health administration through the creation of District Committees and County Councils (to whom the powers and duties of the old Parochial Boards were transferred), and required the new local authorities to employ both a medical officer of health and a sanitary inspector whose powers and responsibilities were to be prescribed by the Board of Supervisors[2]. The problem of public health provision in the smaller burghs was alleviated, if not solved, by the passage of the Burgh Police Act of 1892, which required all burghs to appoint medical officers of health and sanitary inspectors, and laid down regulations relating, among other things, to the laying out and cleansing of streets, stairs, and houses, the erection of new buildings, the height of ceilings, the lighting and ventilation of rooms, and the provision of water supplies and sewerage[3].

The Burgh Police Act of 1892 did not, however, tackle the administrative nonsense of small burghs, with populations numbered in hundreds, operating as separate, independent public health authorities. Indeed, the Act and its successor, the Burgh Police Act of 1893, encouraged the creation of more of these burghs. Under the earlier Act, seven or more inhabitants of a 'populous place' containing 700 or more people could apply to the Sheriff to determine whether their place of residence should be erected into a police burgh. If, upon inquiry, the population was found to exceed 2,000, the Sheriff was compelled to grant the application. These provisions were democratised by the latter Act which vested in householders the right to decide upon the question of erection into a burgh[4], but this much needed safeguard did not stem criticism from public health officials. For example, Dr John C. McVail, the Medical Officer of Health for Dunbartonshire, argued that, with the formation of large sanitary areas under the 1889 Local Government Act, the need for the formation of small burghs had disappeared, and that the public health responsibilities of all small burghs, both old and new should be transferred to the newly created district committees and county councils [5]. Unfortunately, the constructive criticisms of enlightened officials such as McVail were to go unheeded until 1929.

Nevertheless, despite the problems created by the continued existence of the small burghs, there can be no doubt that the 1889 Local Government Act and the 1892 Burgh Police Act facilitated improvements which justified Dr A.K. Chalmers, the Medical Officer of Health for Glasgow between 1898 and 1925, in claiming that 'the beginning of the 90s' ... marked the opening of a new era in public health administration in Scotland'[6]. Further advances were made possible by the Public Health (Scotland) Act of 1897, which confirmed the changes made in 1889 and 1892, and introduced two important innovations. The first of these authorised the Local Government Board for Scotland to instruct local authorities to provide hospital accommodation for those suffering from infectious diseases, while the second rendered mandatory the provisions of the Infectious Disease (Notification) Act of 1889, under which cases of smallpox, cholera, diphtheria, membranous croup, erysipelas, scarlet fever, and other fevers, including typhus, typhoid, enteric, relapsing, and puerperal, were to be notified immediately to the Medical Officer of Health in order that action might be taken to prevent the spread of the disease[7]. The importance of these provisions can hardly be exaggerated, for, as we shall see, the services which were subsequently developed by public health departments contributed significantly to the great reduction in the incidence of and mortality from infectious diseases in early twentieth century Scotland.

By 1900 sanitarians could look back with a sense of achievement and forward with optimism. Almost all the available evidence pointed to a considerable improvement in the nation's health since the mid nineteenth century, while the recent advances in the statutory provisions for public health administration, with the greatly expanding corpus of medical knowledge permitted confidence in the successors of Gairdner, Russell, and Littlejohn to contribute significantly to further improvements. However, while the annual reports of the medical officers of health testify to the advance being made at the turn of the century, they also supply copious evidence of the huge task which still lay ahead. These reports are filled with descriptions of and comments on the grossly overcrowded and insanitary state of much of Scotland's housing, both urban and rural; the inadequacy of many of the country's water supply and sewerage systems; the inefficiency of cleansing and scavenging services; the contamination of milk and food supplies; the pollution of the environment by industrial and domestic waste products; and the horrifying toll of human life and health, particularly that of children, exacted by diseases, many of which could be prevented or at least controlled by the application of current medical knowledge. How these problems were tackled is, in large part, the story of the public health service in twentieth century Scotland.

The Environmental Services

Water Supplies

The close connection between insanitary living conditions and the incidence of infectious disease was well recognised by Victorian sanitarians, and much of their effort was therefore directed at improving the quality of environmental services. Progress, however, was slow, largely because of the reluctance or inability of the smaller local authorities in particular to find the large sums of money necessary to fund wholesome water supply and efficient sewerage systems, the most essential but also expensive of environmental services. From about 1905 onwards the Local Government Board, tiring of this inactivity, began to apply steady pressure on the more recalcitrant authorities to provide healthy water supplies. Many of these authorities had to be threatened with prosecution before they were persuaded to take effective action, and in some cases it was found necessary to institute legal proceedings[8]. Nevertheless, despite the more interventionist role adopted by the central department, progress continued to be slow and problems remained. In 1936 the Cathcart Committee reported that there were 'areas whose supplies are either inadequate in quantity or fall below an acceptable standard of purity', and called for immediate Government action to remedy this situation[9]. The problem, the Committee believed, was largely an administrative one in origin. Outside the burghs water supplies were generally provided by so-called special districts which were set up specifically for that purpose. By the mid 1930s there were over 1700 special districts in Scotland, many of which were small in size and had correspondingly limited financial resources. The result was that not only were many of the special districts unable to make adequate provision on modern lines for the necessary service, but also the existence of a great number of small schemes rendered it difficult, in some cases, to provide a comprehensive and satisfactory scheme for the whole county or region[10]. The report recommended that special districts should be abolished and larger administrative areas formed, but the formidable difficulties associated with those proposals proved insurmountable at that time and administrative reform was delayed. The White Paper on *A National Water Policy*, which was published in April 1944, proved more successful in influencing Government policy. It proposed that Government should provide a substantial grant to assist local authorities in providing or improving water supplies, that amalgamation of water authorities should be encouraged and, if necessary, enforced, and that power should be vested in the Secretary of State for Scotland to require, where necessary, water authorities to transfer supplies to other needy authorities. These recommendations were adopted by the National Government as part of its post-war reconstruction policy, and incorporated into the Rural Water Supplies and Sewerage Act which received the Royal Assent in July 1944[11]. It was largely as a result of this Act that rural Scotland was finally provided with adequate and wholesome water supplies. Another wartime initiative which did much to improve the quality of water supplies was the installation of chlorination plants by urban water authorities on the instruction of government between 1939 and 1942[12]. At the end of the war attempts were made in some parts of Scotland, including Glasgow, to have chlorination discontinued, but its value in improving the level of protection against water-borne bacteriological infections was fortunately recognised and these attempts failed. All public water supplies are now treated by chlorination or alternative methods to ensure safety.

In the mid 1950s the central department initiated an investigation into the effects of the fluoridation of water supplies upon dental health. Kilmarnock and Ayr, two towns with very similar qualities of water supply, having been chosen as the loci of the investigation a research team was appointed to study the effects of fluoridated water upon caries rates in Kilmarnock and compare them with those recorded in Ayr where the water supply had not been treated. Although marked improvements took place in the teeth of the citizens and in particular the children of Kilmarnock, the town council decided to discontinue the experiment[13]. A few authorities such as Wigtonshire, subsequently agreed to add fluoride to their water supplies, but, despite Scotland's abysmal dental health record and the fact that there was no reliable evidence to suggest that fluoridation endangered health, there was widespread resistance to this prophylactic measure, and the 1960s saw the town councils of both Glasgow and Edinburgh reject proposals for fluoridation. By the 1970s, however, attitudes were beginning to change. Scotland's two largest cities agreed in principle to install fluoridation schemes, and, following local government re-organisation, Strathclyde Regional Council decided to fluoridate all its water supplies. Agreement had been reached between Strathclyde Region and the four health boards concerned on the financing of the venture and preliminary planning was well advanced, when proceedings initiated by anti-fluoride activists halted all work. When the case came to trial Lord Jauncey, the judge, found that, while the proposed concentration of fluoride carried no risk to health and would reduce the dental caries rate, local authorities were not permitted by the Water (Scotland) Act to add fluoride to water supplies[14]. This matter has been corrected by the passing of the Water (Fluoridation) Act 1985.

Although Sir Robert Christison, Professor of Medical Jurisprudence in the Unversity of Edinburgh, had established in the middle of the nineteenth century that lead pipes should not be used to conduct water over distances and that the risk of dangerous impregnation with lead is greatest in the purest water supplies[15], until relatively recently many of

Scotland's water supplies were highly plumbosolvent and were carried to homes in lead pipes and stored there in lead tanks. The problem was particularly marked in the west of Scotland where the 'softness' of the water increased its plumbosolvency. In the early 1970s Sir Abraham Goldberg, Regius Professor of the Practice of Medicine in the University of Glasgow, and a team of associates identified a number of families in rural areas suffering from lead poisoning caused by drinking lead contaminated water over a long period of time[16]. This work stimulated an investigation in Glasgow into water lead in houses and blood lead in their occupants. In some areas, particularly those where drinking water was stored in lead tanks, the levels of lead contamination were found to be unacceptably high. Responding to these findings, Glasgow City Council secured agreement with the Lower Clyde Water Board to remove lead pipes and add calcium to the city's water supply in order to reduce the plumbosolvency of Loch Katrine water. In addition, the Council decided in 1973 that all municipally owned houses undergoing refurbishment were to have their lead pipes and tanks removed, while in the early 1980s the Government began offering generous grants to enable private householders to remove the offending pipes and tanks. While the results of the grant scheme have proved rather disappointing, much has been achieved in the public sector where many tens of thousands of houses have been dealt with since 1973. Moreover, the addition of calcium or, in Castlemilk, phosphate has greatly reduced the plumbosolvency of Glasgow water, the ph value of which has risen from 6.3 in 1978 when the scheme was started to 9.0 in 1980 when the calcium dosage was increased. Nevertheless, Strathclyde Regional Council's Water Department estimate that between 5 and 15 *per cent* of dwellings in Glasgow may still have unacceptably high levels of lead in their water. Elsewhere too, much has been done in recent years to reduce lead contamination of water supplies. In Ayr, for example, an investigation in December 1980 revealed high lead concentrations in tap water collected from dwellings equipped with lead plumbing, and a very plumbosolvent water supply, the ph value of which varied between 4.5 and 5.5. The water supply was subsequently treated with lime, and a follow-up study, conducted between December 1982 and February 1983, found that the ph value of the water had been raised to around 9, and that there had been a large decrease in both water lead and blood lead levels[17].

Drainage, Sewerage, and Cleansing

The second half of the nineteenth century had seen remarkable sanitary progress in Scotland, but, especially in the smaller burghs and villages, there was still considerable room for improvement. Household refuse was no longer thrown out of windows and doors into the street, but the introduction of the ashpit and the privy midden had brought their own problems. Ashpits, which were generally located in a court or yard behind houses, formed receptacles for the contents of the privy middens and all manner of waste. They were generally emptied weekly or fortnightly, and their contents dumped in the street from where they were removed either by 'scaffies' employed by the local authority or by contractors who were usually local farmers[18]. In the burghs the introduction of efficient drainage systems was facilitated by the development of modern water supply schemes[19] and enforced by the Burgh Police Act of 1892 which provided that the local authority shall 'cause to be made under the streets to elsewhere such main and other sewers as shall be necessary for the effectual draining of the burgh.'[20]. Although there was no statutory requirement on local authorities to insist upon the provision of water closets, the sanitary advantages of such equipment over the abominable ashpits and middens which did so much to spread diarrhoeal diseases were becoming recognised by both public health officials and the more enlightened town councils. In Glasgow, for example, the 1890s marked the beginning of a long process whereby water closets were introduced in place of ashpits[21]. Throughout Scotland burgh authorities began to serve notice on owners to fit up sinks in well ventilated and well lighted places with suitable connections to the sewer, to remove ashpits and privy middens and provide water closets for themselves or their tenants, to equip their houses with rhones and downpipes, and to have their back courts properly paved and drained[22]. These measures highlighted the problem of sewage disposal. Many seaside authorities, such as Aberdeen, Dundee, and Edinburgh, discharged untreated sewage directly into the sea, but inland burghs were prevented by the Rivers Pollution Prevention Act of 1876 from discharging liquid or solid sewage into rivers or streams and were discovering that the favoured alternative, known as 'broad irrigation', was incapable of dealing with large quantities of sewage. Increasingly, such burghs turned to the filtration or chemical precipitation method of sewage purification[23]. In Glasgow, for example, the sewage works at Dalmarnock and Shieldhall, which opened in 1894 and 1910 respectively, both employed the chemical precipitation method[24]. In the counties, the situation in the early part of the century was less than satisfactory. The county councils and the special drainage districts, which had been set up following the passage of the Local Government (Scotland) Act of 1889, were not compelled to provide adequate drainage and sewerage for their inhabitants. The Public Health Act of 1897 only stipulated that the local authority 'shall have the power to construct within their district, and also, when necessary for the purpose of outfall or distribution or disposal or treatment of sewage, without their district, such sewers as they may think necessary for keeping their district properly cleansed and drained'[25]. Under no statutory obligation to provide adequate sewerage, and, in many cases, lacking the necessary financial resources for the expensive task of building and maintaining a modern sewerage system, many of Scotland's rural authorities did little or nothing. In 1936 the Sanitary Inspectors' Association of Scotland stated that

> "Progress in providing proper drainage facilities for the towns and villages in Scotland has not been so marked as is the case with water supplies. Many rural areas are without drainage due the heavy cost involved in providing it. In such areas sanitary progress is consequently at a standstill. In a number of towns and villages the sewers are inadequate to deal with the volume of sewage they are required to carry, and the sewage works are of antiquated design and incapable of dealing efficiently with the sewage. Here again the cost is the obstacle which prevents improvements being carried out."[26]

The sewage problems of rural areas were ultimately tackled by the Rural Water Supplies and Sewerage Act of 1944 which encouraged local authorities to combine to provide efficient sewerage schemes, introduced powers enabling the Department of Health for Scotland to compel recalcitrant authorities to co-operate in providing schemes, and provided central Government grants to assist local authorities to construct sewerage schemes or bring existing ones up to modern standards[27]. Just as the post-war years saw a great improvement in rural sewage disposal and treatment facilities, so they also witnessed some significant developments in urban sewage disposal schemes. In 1977 Edinburgh finally abandoned its old policy of directly discharging sewage into the Forth and introduced precipitation treatment, with the resultant sludge being taken aboard the appropriately named MV Gardyloo to a point well out in the North Sea for disposal. Fifteen years earlier the Corporation of Glasgow had decided to rebuild Dalmarnock sewage works and introduce a complete treatment activated sludge plant, which was opened in 1968. A further modern sewage works has since been opened at Shieldhall.

Housing

The central role played by bad housing conditions in promoting poverty and disease had been well recognised in the nineteenth century, and considerable efforts had been made to improve the quality of the country's housing stock. Nevertheless, despite these efforts, the scale of the problem remained daunting. The Census of 1911 revealed that of the 1,010,531 inhabited houses in Scotland, 12.8 *per cent* were one room 'single ends', while another 40.5 *per cent* were two apartment 'room and kitchen' dwellings. In Glasgow, Dundee, and Paisley rather more than 60 *per cent* of the population lived in one or two roomed houses, while in Aberdeen, Edinburgh and Perth the relevant figure was over 30 *per cent*[28]. Three years earlier one writer on housing had stated that 'present conditions are thoroughly bad', adding that 'not only are lives lost through insanitary housing, but, worse still, a chronic condition of low vitality and ill-health is fostered in our towns.'[29]

The crux of the problem, it was gradually coming to be realised, was the inability of private enterprise to build houses of suitable standards at a cost low enough to be borne by the working classes[30]. In an attempt to find a solution to this vexing problem, a Royal Commission was appointed in October 1912 to inquire into and report on the housing of the industrial population of Scotland rural and urban. The Royal Commission, which presented its report in October 1917, told a grim tale of appalling housing conditions in mining villages, crofting townships, farm workers' cottages, old burghs, industrial towns, and cities alike, and recommended that the State should accept some direct responsibility for the housing of the working classes[31]. This recommendation was accepted by the National Government, which declared its determination to build 'houses fit for heroes' returning from the first world war. The outcome was the Housing (Scotland) Act of 1919, which provided state subsidies for the construction of approved council housing, but proved to be a failure. The combination of local government inexperience in house building and the absence of properly trained advisory staff and effective cost controls resulted in the first generation of council houses being over priced and few in number[32]. Only 25,000 were built before the Government, disappointed at the lack of building activity and alarmed at the high costs of the Addison Act subsidies, decided to change policy. The Housing Act of 1923 offered a subsidy of £6 per house *per annum* for a period of twenty years, which was to be paid through local authorities to private builders[33]. This measure succeeded in stimulating house building, with over 50,000 houses being built under its provisions, but the housing provided was generally outwith the financial reach of lower income families. The Housing (Financial Provisions) Act of 1924, which was generally known as the Wheatley Act after John Wheatley, the Minister of Health in the first Labour government, shifted the emphasis back towards municipal housing, increased the level of subsidy to £9 per house *per annum*, and extended the length of the subsidy to forty years[34]. From 1924 until 1933, when the National Government's Housing (Financial Provisions) (Scotland) Act reduced the level of subsidy to £3, local authorities built on a large scale. Nevertheless, despite its undoubted success in increasing the rate of house construction, the Wheatley Act failed to deal with the problem of the slums. In 1930, the second Labour government's Housing (Scotland) Act shifted the emphasis of housing policy towards slum clearance. Under this measure slum clearance areas were defined and a subsidy of £2.50 per year for a period of forty years was awarded in respect of every person rehoused from a clearance area[35]. This new emphasis upon slum clearance was maintained by the Conservative government's Housing Act of 1935, which required local authorities to conduct surveys of over-crowding, established a minimum standard in respect of the number of persons to be accommodated within a given size of house, and introduced a state subsidy of £6.75 per house per annum over a period of forty years for houses built to reduce overcrowding[36].

The inter-war programme, which resulted in over 300,000 new houses being built in Scotland, succeeded in improving the quality of the housing stock and contributed to the improved health of the population. Nevertheless, serious problems remained. In 1935 a survey revealed that almost 50 *per cent* of the Scottish housing stock was sub-standard and that 22.5 *per cent* of Scottish houses were overcrowded[37], while the Cathcart Committee reported in 1936 that over 300,000 houses lacked their own water closets and that almost 30,000 were without any indoor water facilities[38]. The housing problem was exacerbated by the cessation of house building during the second world war and by the immediate post-war shortages of raw materials and manpower for building purposes, but by the late 1940s a massive house building programme had been initiated by government in an attempt to solve the nation's housing crisis. This programme, which in Scotland was directed at public sector housing, was continued by successive governments through the 1950s, 1960s, and early 1970s. It succeeded in clearing away almost all of the old slums, reducing greatly the number of one and two roomed houses, and providing many Scots with their first houses containing fixed baths and indoor water closets. In Glasgow the proportion of households without fixed baths and exclusive access to a water closet fell from 56 *per cent* and 37 *per cent* respectively in 1951 to 4.7 *per cent* and 0.8 *per cent* respectively in 1982, while the percentage of one and two apartment houses fell from 11 *per cent* and 36.3 *per cent* respectively in 1951 to 2.3 *per cent* and 16.1 *per cent* respectively in 1981[39]. Despite the achievements of the post-war housing programme, however, serious problems remained. The 1971 Census revealed that Scotland had 77.5 *per cent* of Britain's worst 5 *per cent* of socially deprived areas and that post-war housing estates figured notably in the statistics relating to overcrowding and other measurements of social deprivation[40]. Since then some important steps have been taken to remedy the situation. Vast sums of public money have been channelled through urban aid programmes into the most deprived areas. The most notable of these programmes, the Glasgow Eastern Area Renewal project, or GEAR for short, has attempted, with some apparent success, to revitalise one of the most depressed and depressing areas of Glasgow. Nevertheless, the huge scale of Scotland's contemporary housing problem is apparent to anyone who either lives in or visits the vast, poverty stricken, damp ridden, and culturally and socially impoverished proletarian ghettoes which ring too many of our towns and cities. The inhabitants of such areas tend to have more health problems than those of more salubrious districts, and, while many and various factors contribute to this situation, there can be little or no doubt that bad housing plays a still significant part in fostering disease among a section of our population.

Atmospheric Pollution and Clean Air

The nineteenth century industrial revolution, which was largely powered by steam and fuelled by coal, resulted in a great increase in the level of atmospheric pollution. Some attempts were made in the middle of last century to reduce that pollution, but they were largely ineffective, and it was only when evidence began to be collected towards the end of the Victorian epoch confirming the commonsense belief that polluted air damaged the health of those breathing it that some effective preliminary steps were taken to tackle the problem. The link between atmospheric pollution and the high incidence of respiratory diseases in our industrial areas was well expressed by Dr James B. Russell, the Medical Officer of Health for Glasgow, who stated in 1895:

"We are a catarrhal, expectorating people because we live in a huge industrial town, situated at the seaward end of the trough of a valley which from one end to the other is covered with smoke, drifting in wreaths and clouds with the wind, or is in a calm filling up the trough so that nothing is to be seen between the higher ground on either side but a sea of smoke. Living thus we live constantly on the edge of a catastrophe. Whenever the scavenging of the air is interrupted by calms so that the smoke product accumulates, the atmosphere of our streets thickens and the daylight becomes twilight."[41]

Faced with increasing demands for tighter controls upon smoke pollution, which in part were sponsored by the influential Smoke Abatement Association, Parliament decided to act. Section 384 of the Burgh Police (Scotland) Act of 1892 provided that every person who, in a burgh, used, caused, or permitted or suffered to be used, any furnace or fire so that smoke issued therefrom, was liable to a penalty unless he proved that he had used the best practicable means for preventing smoke, and had carefully attended to and managed the said furnace or fire so as to prevent, as far as possible, the escape of smoke therefrom[42]. Outside the burghs, the relevant legislation was the Public Health (Scotland) Act of 1897 Section 16 of which declared that any fireplace or furnace in any manufacturing or trade process which did not, so far as was practicable, consume its own smoke was to be deemed a nuisance within the meaning of the Act[43]. Thus, while the Burgh Police Act placed the onus on the person using the furnace to prove that he had used the best practicable means to prevent the emission of smoke, the Public Health Act placed the onus on the local authority to prove that the person using the furnace had not used the best practicable means to prevent the emission of smoke.

This was a serious drawback, and it rendered the Public Health Act of little value in the battle against smoke pollution. The Burgh Police Act was not without its own drawbacks. In the first place, it did not apply to domestic fires, which, burning at a lower temperature than industrial furnaces, tended to release vast quantities of unconsumed hydro-carbons into the atmosphere, and, in the second place, mines and iron and steel production processes were excluded from its provisions.

In Glasgow, the local authority secured, shortly after the passage of the Burgh Police (Scotland) Act of 1892, a local Act giving it additional powers to deal with smoke pollution resulting from mining and steel making processes. The Glasgow Police (Further Power) Act of 1892 symbolised the determination of the city fathers to clean up Glasgow's air. Classes were established for the instruction of boilermen in efficient methods of stoking, manufacturers and others were advised on methods of reducing smoke emissions, and firm action was taken against factory owners who persistently poured 'black smoke' into the atmosphere[44]. These activities led to a material improvement in the city's atmosphere. In 1900 the intimations of 'excess smoke' given to furnace users by the city's Smoke Inspectors amounted to 17.5 *per cent* of the chimneys observed, but by 1922 the proportion had fallen to 1.7 *per cent* despite the fact that in the interim the definition of 'excess smoke' had been tightened considerably[45]. Elsewhere too improvements were being made due to the efforts of the local authorities, the growing realisation among industrialists that only inefficient furnaces produced large quantities of smoke, and the increasing availability of cheap electrical power. In 1936 the Cathcart Committee reported that 'atmospheric pollution by industrial smoke has greatly lessened in recent years.'[46]

By the 1920s it was recognised that domestic fireplaces were responsible for more atmospheric pollution than industrial furnaces. In 1923 it was estimated that 35 million tons of raw coal were burnt annually in British domestic fireplaces as against 114.5 million tons of raw coal in industrial furnaces, but that the unconsumed combustible matter emitted as smoke from the former was 5 to 6 times greater than that escaping from the latter[47]. The solution to the problem, it was then believed, lay not in extending legislation to control smoke emissions from household chimneys, but rather in making available gas, electricity, and solid smokeless fuel to the public. In 1925, for example, the Corporation of Glasgow developed a solid smokeless fuel, known as *Kincole*, for use in domestic grates[48]. The difficulty with Kincole and other alternatives was expense. 'If smokeless fuel could be produced at a price both economically comparable and approximately as efficient (as coal)', the Cathcart Committee argued, 'there is no reason to think that the public would not use it.'[49] Little progress, however, was made during the next twenty years in producing cheaper alternative fuels, and the public continued to heat their homes with coal. In December 1952 much of

London was enveloped in a killer smog which resulted in bronchitis death rates rising by over 800 *per cent*. In the aftermath of this disaster, the Government appointed a committee under the chairmanship of Sir Hugh Beaver to examine the whole question of air pollution. The committee's recommendations were adopted by the Government and formed the basis for the Clean Air Act of 1956. One of the greatest preventive measures of this century, the Clean Air Act tightened controls upon industry's smoke emissions and authorised local authorities to issue orders declaring the whole or any part of their district a smoke control district in which the emission of smoke from a chimney of any building will be an offence. Its success has been dramatic. In Glasgow, for example, the smoke levels in the atmosphere had been more than halved by the mid 1960s, and by 1982 nearly 80 *per cent* of the city's houses were covered by smoke control orders[50]. Progress was even swifter in Coatbridge, where the eleventh and final smoke control order became operative on 30 November 1969, making what had formerly been one of Scotland's most polluted towns one of the first to be declared 'smoke free'[51]. Such indeed has been the progress throughout Scotland that it is necessary nowadays to travel to a seaside coastal town or to one of the remaining mining villages to observe the sort of smoky atmosphere that only thirty years ago enveloped much of urban Scotland.

Supervision of Food Supplies

Since at least as far back as the middle ages the sale of unwholesome foodstuffs had been treated as a criminal offence, but it was only with the great nineteenth century advance in medical knowledge that surveillance became anything more than rudimentary. The Public Health (Scotland) Act not only provided for local government officials to inspect animals and foodstuffs and seize and destroy any found unfit for human consumption, but also required slaughterhouses to obtain an annual licence from their local authority[52]. The effectiveness of these provisions clearly depended upon the enthusiasm with which local authorities utilised them, and in the early years of this century there were complaints that some authorities were less than strict in their system of inspection[53]. Standards, however, soon improved, and by 1936 the Department of Health for Scotland could state that a 'very great improvement has been effected within the last few years in the cleanliness and sanitary condition of slaughterhouses and on the whole it can be said that the supervision of slaughterhouses is now reasonably well carried out'[54].

The inter-war years witnessed growing demands for tighter regulations governing the preparation and sale of food, and for making food poisoning a notifiable disease. Public awareness of the dangers inherent in unhygienic food handling practices was growing, and was beginning to influence consumer choice and the behaviour of food manufacturers and traders. The pace of this progress, however, remained slow, and the Department of Health for Scotland reported in 1956 'there is still much need for education in these matters.'[55] Determined to force an acceleration in the pace of progress, Parliament passed the Food and Drugs (Scotland) Act in 1956. This measure authorised the issue, firstly, of hygiene regulations prescribing methods of preparing and handling food and, secondly, of orders requiring the registration of food manufacturers and traders with the local authority. It also assisted the control of food poisoning by introducing compulsory notification and by authorising Medical Officers of Health to seize and destroy suspected food[56]. In 1959 the Food Hygiene (Scotland) Regulations were issued by the Secretary of State under Section 13 of the Food and Drugs (Scotland) Act of 1956. These regulations provided for the hygienic handling of food by persons employed in the food industry, and regulated the construction, equipment, and maintenance of premises, vehicles, stalls, etc. in which food was handled. They required adequate washing facilities to be provided for food handlers and for the equipment and utensils used in food premises, specified precautions to be taken when reheating food or using vulnerable foodstuffs, and introduced compulsory notification of certain infections suffered by food handlers which were likely to cause food poisoning[57]. These regulations, and the food hygiene education programme which accompanied their introduction, had a considerable measure of success. By the mid 1970s, however, it had become apparent that new regulations would have to be drawn up to deal with the increasing number of cases of food poisoning attributable to the consumption of factory farmed poultry. The Poultry Meat (Hygiene) (Scotland) Regulations, which were issued in 1976, required poultry to be slaughtered and cut up in premises licensed for that purpose, and laid down regulations as to slaughter and evisceration procedures, ante and post mortem inspections, and hygiene controls in the slaughterhouse. Nevertheless, despite more stringent regulations and hygiene education campaigns, food poisoning remains a problem. Attention is now being focused on the development of techniques such as irradiation to eliminate bacteria from foodstuffs, the registration of food premises, and the abolition of Crown immunity from prosecution in regard to kitchens in National Health Service hospitals and other publicly owned premises.

The important place of milk in the diet of the nation, and particularly in that of children, and the fact that contaminated milk had been responsible for epidemics of diphtheria, scarlet fever, typhoid, paratyphoid, brucellosis, and tuberculosis, rendered the maintenance of the highest possible standards of surveillance a matter of some concern. The late nineteenth century saw in a series of Dairies, Cowsheds, and Milk Shops Orders issued by the central department, the development of a highly complex if inefficient system of surveillance. These Orders made provision for registering all persons carrying on the trade of cowkeeper, dairyman, or purveyor of milk with the local authority, for regulating the lighting, ventilation, cleansing, drainage, and water supply of dairies and cowsheds, for protecting milk against infection and contamination, and for authorising local authorities to issue their own regulations for these purposes[58]. The effectiveness of these Orders largely depended, however, on whether local authorities took their responsibilities seriously. Some authorities made considerable efforts to improve the quality of the milk supply in their areas, but others were less energetic, and some made no effort whatever. In 1909 only 221 of the 312 Scottish local authorities were enforcing dairy regulations, and demands began to arise both for an extension of local authority powers in regard to milk supplies and for measures to enforce their rigorous application[59]. These demands were answered in 1914 with the passing of the Milk and Dairies (Scotland) Act. Under this measure every dairy and the cattle in every dairy were to be inspected at least once every year by the Medical Officer of Health and the Veterinary Inspector respectively, every dairyman was, following a report from the Medical Officer of Health or the Sanitary Inspector, to be registered with the local authority, and every local authority was required to make bye-laws dealing with the inspection of cattle in dairies, the purity of milk, and the cleanliness of cows and of persons engaged and utensils used in the milk trade. The 1914 Act also required every case of cattle disease and every case of infectious disease amongst dairy employees to be reported to the Medical Officer of Health, permitted that official to issue an Order stopping milk supplies which had caused disease, and authorised the central department to take legal proceedings against local authorities who had failed to enforce the mandatory provisions of the Act or their own bye-laws[60].

The Milk and Dairies (Scotland) Act did not, however, come into operation until 1925, and, owing to the impoverished condition of the dairying industry in the later 1920s and early 1930s, little was accomplished in the succeeding decade. The Milk Act of 1934 radically altered the situation by providing central government subsidies to the dairy industry in the form of a bonus payment of 2.25d. per gallon to producers holding a licence for the sale of tuberculin tested milk, and 1.25d. per gallon to those in possession of a Standard (Grade A) licence. The pace of progress quickened during the second world war with an increase in the bonus payment to producers owning tuberculin tested herds and the introduction of the attested herds scheme. There were large increases in the numbers of tuberculin tested herds and licence holders under the Milk (Special Designation) Order (Scotland) of 1936 during the second world war, while the war years also witnessed a considerable tightening up of local authority supervision of dairies and a marked improvement in the efficiency of pasteurisation processes[61].

In the years following on the end of the second world war steady progress continued to be made towards the goal of a safe milk supply.

Between 1946 and 1956 the proportion of 'tuberculin tested' and 'certified' milk rose from 56.8 *per cent* of total milk sales to 96.4 *per cent*, while by the latter date 75 *per cent* of all milk sold in Scotland was pasteurised[62]. In 1959 the Department of Health for Scotland reported that for the first time all milk sold to the public came from cows which had passed the tuberculin test, and that 78.09 *per cent* of milk sold to the public was pasteurised[63]. This progress has been maintained in recent years, and in 1980 the Milk (Special Designation) (Scotland) Order made pasteurisation obligatory for all milk sold in Scotland after 1 August 1983. This radical measure which has still to be adopted in England and Wales, should go a long way to eradicating all milk borne diseases. The challenge of the future is to ensure, by thorough bacteriological testing and stringent quality control procedures at the dairies, that the highest standards are maintained.

The Control of Infectious Diseases

Many measures and developments have contributed to the control of infectious diseases. Improvements in the standards of housing, sanitation, water supply, and surveillance of meat and milk supplies, better living and working conditions, a better educated population, improved recreational facilities, and a generally higher standard of living have all contributed to rising standards of health and the falling incidence of and mortality from infectious diseases. This section will deal solely with the Infectious Disease Service which developed from a rudimentary beginning in the late nineteenth century and came to play a significant part in the control of diseases which, treated as a group, were the greatest cause of ill-health and death among the Scottish population in the early part of this century.

The foundations of the modern Infectious Disease Service were laid in the latter part of the nineteenth century. From the 1860s onwards the more progressive local authorities were appointing medical officers of health, building hospitals for the isolation and treatment of infectious diseases, and obtaining in the form of local Police Acts powers for the compulsory notification of infectious disease in order that epidemics might be checked through the timely removal of suspected cases to hospital, the disinfection of infected houses, furniture, and clothing, and the tracing and surveillance of contacts. The pace of progress noticeably quickened towards the end of the century. The Local Government (Scotland) Act of 1889 and the Burgh Police Act of 1892 required all Scottish local authorities to appoint medical officers of health, while the Public Health (Scotland) Act of 1897 made mandatory the provisions of the Infectious Disease (Notification) Act of 1889 (under which the more important infections were to be notified immediately to the appropriate medical officer of health), and empowered the central department to require recalcitrant local authorities to provide hospital accommodation for those suffering from infectious diseases. The 1897 Act also empowered the medical officer of health to enter and inspect any premises in which he suspected the presence of any infectious disease, and to examine any person found on such premises. Other important provisions of this great Act related to the disinfection of infected premises and furniture and clothing found therein and to prohibitions on infected persons acting in ways likely to facilitate the spread of infection.

By the turn of the century the service was developing apace. The newly established University departments of public health were training post-graduate medical students in the specialised epidemiological skills required of medical officers of health. Public health officials were gaining invaluable practical experience in the surveillance and control of infec-tious diseases. Bacteriological laboratory services were being established, most notably in Glasgow, Lanarkshire, and Aberdeen, and were render-ing valuable assistance in the diagnosis and control of diseases such as diphtheria, typhoid fever and tuberculosis[64]. In the public eye, how-ever, perhaps the most impressive evidence of development was to be seen in the construction of new fever hospitals. Some of these hospitals were relatively small affairs with three wards for the reception of diphtheria, scarlet fever, and enteric fever cases, but others were large imposing establishments built in accordance with the latest medical thinking on the treatment of infectious disease. Of this latter group, the largest were Ruchill Hospital in Glasgow with 408 beds and the City Hospital in Edinburgh with 600 beds, which were opened in 1900 and 1903 respectively[65]. Hospitals such as these played an important role not only in treating patients but in providing training for medical men and nurses intending to specialise in infectious diseases.

Tuberculosis

The early decades of the twentieth century witnessed a significant expansion of the Infectious Disease Service. In March 1906 the Local Government Board for Scotland issued a circular advising local author-ities that pulmonary tuberculosis was an infectious disease within the meaning of the Public Health (Scotland) Act of 1897, that the sections of that Act applicable to other infectious diseases were applicable to phthisis, and that the statutory obligation resting on local authorities to deal with and control infectious diseases therefore extended to pul-monary tuberculosis. The circular advised local authorities to model their schemes on that of the Edinburgh voluntary movement pioneered by Dr R.W. Philip and recommended measures including notification, disinfection, the provision of dispensaries and sanatoria for early cases, and the establishment of hospital accommodation for the isolation of advanced cases. By 1911 the provision for institutional treatment under tuberculosis schemes had been so far developed that there were available for the treatment of pulmonary tuberculosis 480 beds in hospitals and sanatoria belonging to local authorities and an additional 550 beds in voluntary institutions – a total provision equivalent to one bed per 4,622 of the population, exclusive of beds in Poor Law institutions[66]. At the same date compulsory notification of pulmonary tuberculosis was in force in the areas of local authorities representing 57.8 *per cent* of the population, while other local authorities had adopted systems of voluntary notification[67]. Subsequently, on 1 August 1912, notification of pulmonary tuberculosis became compulsory throughout Scotland under regulations issued by the Local Government Board, and then, on 1 July 1914, compulsory notification was extended to include all forms of tuberculosis.

The passage of the National Insurance Act of 1911, which provided among other benefits 'sanatorium benefit' for insured persons, gave a big impetus to the tuberculosis campaign. An immediate increase in sanatorium accommodation was called for to meet the requirements of the insured population, and a grant in aid of the capital cost of providing such accommodation was voted by Parliament. In 1912 Parliament voted for a further grant, subsequently known as the Hobhouse grant, which met one half of the local authorities net annual expenditure on the treatment of tuberculosis. When, in 1920, sanatorium benefit ceased to be one of the benefits provided under the National Insurance scheme, the responsibility for the treatment of insured and non-insured alike fell on the local authorities and a fixed annual compensatory grant was voted in support of the additional rate-borne expenditure thereby incurred[68].

Encouraged by the provision of Treasury grants and prompted both by statutory obligations and by the exhortations of the medical profession and mobilised public opinion, the tuberculosis service grew at a remarkable rate. By 31 December 1914 the Local Government Board had approved for the treatment of pulmonary tuberculosis 96 sanatoria, hospitals and other institutions with 2,114 beds[69], while by 1924, despite the interruption to progress occasioned by the demands of the first world war, the number of 'approved' hospitals and sanatoria had increased to 111 and the number of beds had risen to 4,154[70]. The inter-war years saw further growth in the service, with the city of Glasgow, for example, opening a new sanatorium at Mearnskirk with 464 beds in 1928[71], and by 1938 there were 115 'approved' hospitals with a total of over 5,000 beds in Scotland[72].

Venereal Disease

Another important area into which the Scottish public health service expanded in the early years of this century was that of the prevention and treatment of venereal diseases. Following the report in 1916 of the Royal

Commission on Venereal Diseases, which estimated that 10 *per cent* of the urban population might be infected with syphillis and recommended the establishment of local authority centres for the early diagnosis and treatment of venereal diseases, the Local Government Board for Scotland issued regulations in October of the same year requiring local authorities to provide free, convenient and confidential treatment for those suffering from the diseases in question. By 1924 there were forty-one treatment centres in Scotland, twelve of which were located in Glasgow and six in Edinburgh. A few were located in premises specially set apart for the purpose and administered directly by the local authority, some were situated in local authority infectious disease hospitals, a number were based in poorhouse hospitals, but the great majority were attached to or associated with voluntary hospitals or infirmaries. Whatever their location, these centres were established and maintained by the relevant local authorities who received a 75 *per cent* Treasury grant in support of their expenditure. A few local authorities, most notably Glasgow, provided their own treatment centres, but the usual practice, as in the provision of other infectious disease hospitals, was for local authorities to combine under the terms of Section 83 of the Public Health (Scotland) Act of 1897 to provide so-called combination treatment centres. Much had been achieved by the mid-1920s, but much still required to be done. The Scottish Board of Health argued that seventeen more treatment centres were required before provision could be considered 'fairly complete', while an unacceptably large, albeit declining, percentage of patients were failing to complete their course of treatment and were returning to the community to spread infection[73]. By the end of the inter-war period, however, the position had markedly improved. In 1938 the Department of Health for Scotland reported that the number of new cases had fallen significantly since the 1920s, and that the percentage of patients discharged as cured from the fifty-two 'approved' venereal disease treatment centres had increased since 1924 from 39 to 57 *per cent*[74].

The Expanding Role of the Infectious Disease Hospital Service

While the great majority of venereal disease patients were treated as out-patients, other categories of patients were increasingly admitted to local authority infectious disease hospitals. The Scottish Board of Health reported in 1925 that 'the demand for beds is growing on account of the increasing practice of giving hospital treatment to sufferers from pneumonia, encephalitis lethargica, etc., and of the policy of trying to control mortality in infants and young children from measles and whooping cough, by removal from unsuitable homes to hospital.'[75] This development had the support not only of general practitioners, who welcomed the 'relief afforded them by the treatment in hospital of cases to which it is difficult for the doctor in a busy practice to give adequate protection,' but also of local authorities who strove manfully to provide the additional beds, and of the general public who increasingly considered hospital treatment to be essential rather than merely desirable[76]. In 1926 the Scottish Board of Health reported that 'the hospitals for infectious diseases, originally designed to accommodate a limited class of infectious diseases only, have gradually become hospitals for the treatment of practically all acute diseases which in the light of modern knowledge are regarded as of an infectious nature.'[77]

While the decline in the incidence of diseases such as typhus, smallpox, and typhoid fever had released some hospital accommodation, it was clear that the growing demand for beds could only be met by an expansion in the infectious disease hospital service. In the urban areas in particular more beds were 'urgently required'[78], but the high cost of hospital construction and the financial stringency of the inter-war years placed severe limitations upon the pace at which Scottish authorities could move to solve the problem. Nevertheless, while the Department of Health for Scotland reported in 1935 that 'the rate of progress ... relative to needs has not been rapid and there is still a shortage of modern hospital facilities,' it added that a 'considerable amount of work has been done in recent years.'[79] Less than three months later, the Cathcart Committee found that of the 18,679 beds provided by the statutory hospitals in Scotland, 11,252 were set aside for the treatment of infectious disease. That the voluntary system, upon which Scotland had depended for its acute hospital provision until the later part of the nineteenth century, provided a total of 'only' 12,575 beds[80], is a fact which highlights the impressive rate of progress made by the local authority hospital service during the previous fifty or so years.

The need, however, was not simply to increase the number of beds available for the treatment of infectious diseases, but also to improve the quality of the hospital service provided. The Cathcart Committee, in that section of their report dealing with the institutional care of tuberculosis patients, argued that:

"Many of the beds are in small institutions and in parts of infectious disease and other hospitals that do not have adequate equipment or access to specialised treatment and supervision. In recent years there have developed special forms of treatment. ... It was submitted to us by the Department of Health for Scotland, the Society of Medical Officers of Health (Scottish branch) and leading medical authorities that these advances demand a greater degree of concentration than exists at present. The ideal should be to secure for every sufferer from tuberculosis in Scotland the advantage of the available resources of specialised skill and equipment, and we are satisfied that this ideal cannot be attained with the existing multiplicity of schemes operating in small areas. To secure the necessary degree of concentration, the pooling of resources over wider areas than at present is essential."[81]

The problem of small, financially inefficient, and medically inadequate hospitals applied to the general infectious disease service as well as to the special tuberculosis service. As early as 1924, the Scottish Board of Health was questioning the value of small infectious diseases hospitals, stating that 'the introduction of the motor ambulance has revolutionised the question of provision of infectious disease hospitals in the less densely populated areas, as patients can be removed to considerable distances from their homes without danger'. In future, the Board argued, these hospitals should 'be of a good size, adequately staffed and equipped to meet the needs of a wide area"[82]. The central department did much to encourage co-operation between local authorities in the provision of hospital services, but, while it could refuse to approve inappropriate hospital extension schemes, it could not enforce co-operation between unwilling councils. Thus, the progress which was made during the 1920s and 1930s was piecemeal in nature, and the absence of effective central power led to the perpetuation of some medical and administrative absurdities. In Motherwell, for example, the burgh infectious disease hospital was actually contiguous with that of the county council[83].

The Successes and Failures of the Pre-Second World War Infectious Disease Service

Despite its undoubted failings, however, the infectious disease service made a not insignificant contribution to the improvement in the health of the Scottish nation during the first part of this century. The system of notification, removal to hospital for isolation and treatment, and surveillance of contacts helped to limit the spread of highly infectious and deadly diseases. While many examples could be given, reasons of space dictate that one must suffice. In August 1935 a serious outbreak of typhoid fever occurred among a party of Scottish pilgrims who had just returned from Lourdes. Eighty-nine of the party fell victim to the disease of whom eight died. The prompt and thorough action taken by the Glasgow public health staff, in whose city the first case occurred, in tracing the other members of the party, communicating with the medical officers of the various local authorities throughout the British Isles in whose areas the pilgrims lived, and keeping all contacts under close supervision may well have prevented an epidemic of alarming proportions. In the event, the outbreak was checked so quickly and thoroughly that only four secondary cases were recorded, which was a remarkable achievement in view of the large number of primary cases and the wide area over which they were spread[84]. Another interesting point to emerge from this outbreak was that the case fatality rate was 9 *per cent*, a figure which corresponded well enough with that of 8 *per cent* for the disease over the whole year, but contrasted quite dramatically with the 15 *per cent* or so which was commonly recorded in the early 1920s[85]. Some of the credit for this reduction was probably owing to improved hospital treatment. Caution is required, for many factors may have contributed to a fall in case mortality rates, but most experts believed that the specialist skill of medical and nursing staff and the more favourable environment provided in hospitals (in contradistinction to that pertaining in many working class homes) played some part in reducing the case fatality rate of such infectious diseases as tuberculosis, whooping cough, measles, pneumonia, and diphtheria. The Cathcart Committee, for example, wrote of 'the supreme importance of skilled [hospital] treatment and nursing' in combating acute pneumonia[86], while the great epidemiologist Dr Peter McKinlay argued that 'in a disease such as diphtheria, during the course of which urgent and dangerous situations are liable to occur, it is conceivable, indeed likely, that admission to hospital would favourably influence case fatality'[87].

The Infectious Disease Service, however, could hardly claim the lion's share of the praise for the reduction which had taken place in the mortality from typhus, typhoid, smallpox, and tuberculosis since the late nineteenth century. Improvements in the housing, nutrition, and general standard of living of the nation were largely responsible for the virtual eradication of typhus and the dramatic decline of tuberculosis , while the marked fall in the number of cases of enteric fever was in large part attributable to the development of modern sewerage and water supply services. Moreover, the failures of the Infectious Disease Service, and of the Public Health Service as a whole, were as notable perhaps as the triumphs. Diseases such as diphtheria, whooping cough, measles, and scarlet fever remained unchecked, while tuberculosis continued to be a 'formidable disease' which was responsible, in the mid-1930s, for about one third of all deaths in the age group 15 to 24[88].

A Missed Opportunity: Diphtheria Immunisation in the 1920s and 1930s

The mid-1920s saw some early faltering steps taken in the direction of the preventive control of diphtheria, a major disease the incidence of which had been rising since at least as far back as the first decade of the century and had reached epidemic proportions during 1920 and 1921. In 1924 the Medical Officers of Health for Aberdeenshire and Edinburgh began limited immunisation programmes which involved giving injections of toxin-antitoxin mixture to children who had been Shick tested and found to have no immunity to the disease[89]. These local programmes were subsequently extended, but few local authorities followed the example set in the north east and the capital city. The seemingly inexorable rise in the incidence of the disease, it is true, persuaded some local authorities to encourage immunisation programmes by providing vaccine free of charge and paying general practitioners to administer it, but the Department of Health for Scotland could still lament in 1935 that, even in the aftermath of an epidemic which had seen notifications rise to an all time high of 11,824 cases in 1934, 'for the country as a whole little progress has been made towards the measure of immunisation that is necessary to influence the incidence of the disease'[90]. This failure was, to say the least of it, extremely disappointing. The vaccine was both effective and safe, and was highly recommended by the central department which as early as 1926 had confidently stated its belief that immunisation programmes would not only relieve local authorities of much expenditure on the hospital treatment of sufferers but also effect a 'considerable saving in life'[91]. Moreover, what evidence was then available suggested that parents were generally agreeable to the immunisation of their children. In Aberdeenshire, for example, more than 80 *per cent* of those parents applied to by the local authority in 1935 gave the necessary consent[92]. It is therefore difficult to accept that the statutory restriction preventing local authorities from adopting compulsory immunisation schemes represented much of a barrier to effective preventive measures. All this suggests that the blame for the lack of progress in the 1920s lies squarely on the shoulders of the local authorities. However, an explanation of why so many local authorities failed to develop immunisation programmes against diphtheria and also, incidentally, scarlet fever (a disease whose virulence was declining but was still capable of claiming over 100 deaths per annum in the early 1930s, and of which a partly effective vaccine had been available since the mid-1920s) must await a detailed study of the local government records of the period.

The Control of Diphtheria

It was the dramatic rise in the incidence of diphtheria between 1939 and 1940 from 9,922 to 15,069 confirmed cases which finally persuaded Scottish public health authorities of the need for a national immunisation programme[93]. The Department of Health distributed immunisation materials to local authorities free of charge and organised a massive publicity campaign involving the press, the broadcasting service, and public advertisement in an attempt to persuade parents of the wisdom of having their children protected against the disease. The campaign met with considerable success. By the end of June 1941 approximately 440,000 children of school age and under, representing about 40 *per cent* of the age-group population, had been immunised[94], while by 30 June 1942 some 792,000 children, or 69 *per cent* of the age group population, had been dealt with[95]. Much anxiety, however, was caused by the relative failure to persuade parents of pre-school children to have their children immunised, for it was in the pre-school years that diphtheria was most common and its fatality rate highest. Attempts to raise the acceptance rates for this age group met with no immediate success, and the percentage of immunised children under five years of age actually fell between 1942 and 1946 from 58 to 37 *per cent*. In March 1946 the Department of Health issued a circular to local authorities urging them to make intensive and sustained efforts to increase the number of immunised children throughout the country and to place special emphasis in their campaign on the immunisation of pre-school children[96]. Increased local authority efforts and greater public responsiveness led to the level of protection against diphtheria among the pre-school population rising to approximately 50 *per cent* in 1948[97] and about 70 *per cent* in 1957[98]. As the level of protection against the disease increased so its incidence and mortality fell. In 1939, a typical year before the immunisation campaign got underway, there were 9,922 notifications[99] and 395 deaths, while by 1944 the relevant figures were 6,835 and 183 respectively[100]. Progress continued to be made throughout the later 1940s and the 1950s, and in 1957 the Department of Health for Scotland noted with some satisfaction that only two deaths from the disease had been recorded in the previous year[101]. Since then the relatively high level of immunisation among the population has ensured that diphtheria has been effectively controlled. The last outbreak of the disease in Scotland occurred in Motherwell in 1968 when there were six cases with two deaths in non-immunised children[102].

The Immunisation Campaign against Whooping Cough

The dramatic results achieved by the immunisation campaign against diphtheria encouraged public health authorities to try out similar procedures in an attempt to bring other infectious diseases under control. The apparently successful field trials of whooping cough vaccines in the United States of America encouraged some Scottish local authorities to make arrangements for similar vaccines to be made available for their child populations, and by 1950 twenty-five such authorities were offering pertussis vaccines[103]. The Department of Health for Scotland, however, had serious doubts about the efficacy of the vaccines then available and did nothing to encourage the development of immunisation schemes. These doubts seem to have been shared by the public health staffs of local authorities, for in the early 1950s little was done beyond making various types of vaccine available to children whose parents had requested protection for their offspring[104]. In 1957, following on the Report of the Medical Research Council's Committee on Whooping Cough Vaccines, the central department's policy changed. Being satisfied that an effective pertussis vaccine could now be produced, it urged local authorities to offer vaccination against whooping cough, and to make arrangements for the purchase of suitable vaccines. The local authorities responded eagerly to this initiative and by the end of the year forty-three out of fifty-five had submitted proposals for whooping cough immunisation schemes[105]. The response of the general public was also enthusiastic and within two years the central department was reporting that the acceptance rate for pertussis vaccine was as high as that for diphtheria[106]. The introduction in the early 1960s of the triple antigen, giving protection against diphtheria and tetanus as well as pertussis, gave a boost to the immunisation campaign by reducing the level of parental inconvenience and infant distress, but while the improved immunisation rate of 70 *per cent* or so was sufficient to contribute substantially to a reduction in the incidence of the disease it proved incapable of eradicating it[107].

Virtually from the commencement of the whooping cough immunisation programme doubts were expressed about the efficacy and safety of the vaccine, but these had little or no effect until the mid-1970s when, following press publicity concerning the risk of serious adverse reactions to the vaccine, the acceptance rate began to decline. The fires of controversy were further stoked in February 1976 when an article appeared in *The Lancet* arguing that the fall in pertussis morbidity and mortality had been due to factors other than immunisation and that the use of the vaccine had given rise to an unacceptable level of adverse reactions[108]. Growing public apprehension was expressed in a marked decline in the vaccination acceptance rate which, from an encouraging 77.2 *per cent* in 1974 before the controversy broke, fell to 66.8 *per cent* in 1975 and to 55.6 *per cent* in 1976[109]. It was clearly important that the whole matter should be cleared up as quickly as possible, and to that end the Joint Committee on Vaccination and Immunisation asked a Sub-Committee on Complications of Vaccines to review all the evidence. Having studied the evidence forwarded by the Adverse Reactions Sub-Committee of the Committee on the Safety of Medicines, the sub-committee presented its report on 26 May 1977 maintaining that there was a low incidence of serious adverse reactions to the vaccine, stating that a full course of immunisation with a vaccine containing a pertussis component not only reduces the incidence of the disease but also diminishes its severity, and recommending that routine whooping cough vaccination should continue[110]. The public, however, remained unconvinced, and even the whooping cough epidemic of 1977–79 with its attendant mortality failed to persuade them of the benefits of vaccination[111]. Unless the public's confidence in whooping cough vaccine can be restored, there is good reason to believe that infant lives will continue to be lost to a disease which can be controlled by a high level of immunisation.

B.C.G. Vaccination

In 1949, one year after some local authorities began making arrangements for whooping cough vaccination of children, a limited scheme for B.C.G. vaccination against tuberculosis was introduced in Scotland. Perhaps because of the opposition of the enormously influential Sir Robert Philip, vaccination, which had been practised in France and elsewhere since the 1920s, was long delayed in Scotland and, when finally adopted, treated with great caution. Under the 1949 scheme local health authorities were invited to make arrangements for vaccinating contacts of persons suffering from the disease, and, for this purpose, the services of the tuberculosis physicians of the new Regional Hospital Boards, who were already working with the authorities on other preventive aspects of tuberculosis control, were made available to them[112]. The invitation was eagerly accepted and by 1951 fifty-two of the fifty-five local health authorities had taken powers under Section 27 of the National Health Service (Scotland) Act of 1947 to operate B.C.G. vaccination schemes[113]. In 1952 the scheme was greatly expanded when vaccination was offered to children approaching school leaving age[114], while subsequent extensions saw the service offered to infants, students, and all hospital workers. By 1956 fifty-three local health authorities offered B.C.G. vaccination to children aged between thirteen and fourteen years, and five had approved schemes for the vaccination of infants[115]. Infant vaccination was given up in the early 1970s except for immigrant children born in the Indian sub-continent, but the vaccination of older children aged between ten and thirteen years continues to this date.

While there is no doubt that B.C.G. vaccination has assisted greatly in bringing about a dramatic decline in the tuberculosis mortality rate per 100,000 of population from 64 in 1946, to 14 in 1956, 5 in 1966, and 2 in 1976[116], other factors have also played an important part in the post-war defeat of the disease. Just as the improvements in the standards of Scottish housing and nutrition which took place between the 1870s and 1930s did much to reduce mortality from tuberculosis, so the further improvements in the standard of living which have been such a marked feature of post-war Scotland have contributed to the disease's continuing decline. Advances in diagnosis and treatment, however, have probably been at least as important as improvements in the environment. The introduction of mass radiography programmes locally in the 1940s and nationally in the mid-1950s facilitated the early diagnosis and treatment of the disease and helped to prevent the spread of infection, while the discovery of streptomycin in 1944 and of other chemotherapeutic agents in subsequent years gave the well organised tuberculosis service an opportunity to attack the killer bacillus directly and successfully.

At a time when we are being continually bombarded with all sorts of depressing statistics suggestive of national decline, it is both refreshing and instructive to remind ourselves of the fact that the death rate per 100,000 of population from respiratory tuberculosis has fallen from 155 in 1901 to only 1 in 1982. The triumph over tuberculosis represents one of the great achievements in modern Scottish history, and it is a triumph in which the public health services have played not an unimportant part.

The Control of Poliomyelitis

Unlike many countries, such as the United States of America, pre-war Britain did not suffer from a high incidence of poliomyelitis. This picture, however, began to change in the immediate post-war years. There was a major epidemic in Scotland in 1947 which resulted in 1,434 cases and 131 deaths[117], while the number of notifications in non-epidemic years began to show a disturbing upward trend. By 1953 the Department of Health for Scotland could with justice state that 'poliomyelitis presents one of the most difficult and important problems in preventive medicine'[118]. Much attention was, by this time, focused on the vaccine which had been developed and was being tested in large scale trials in the USA and Canada. Following the successful outcome of these trials, the decision was taken in 1956 to introduce a Salk-type poliomyelitis vaccine in Scotland.[119]. At first the limited amount of British vaccine available severely restricted the scale of the programme, but within a relatively short period production difficulties were overcome and the programme was expanded. The government's decision in September 1957 to import Salk vaccine from Canada and the USA permitted a full scale programme to be contemplated, and an invitation was issued to local health authorities to make arrangements for offering vaccination to all children under the age of fifteen years[120]. This programme proved popular with a public anxious to protect its children, and the high immunisation acceptance rates, which in some localities reached 95 *per cent*[121], contributed greatly to what the Department of Health for Scotland described in 1960 as the 'dramatic' fall in the number of notifications[122]. A mini-epidemic in 1962 emphasised both the fact that the disease had not as yet been brought under control and the need for further efforts to secure the highest possible level of protection against poliomyelitis.

Progress towards the required goal was facilitated by the introduction in that same year of the live attenuated (Sabin) vaccine, which, being orally administered, proved especially popular[123]. Immunisation rates dropped in the mid-1970s as a result of the less well-informed public's worries about the safety of all vaccines, but fortunately they never fell far enough to endanger the control which had been won over the disease in the early 1960s.

The Immunisation Campaigns against Measles and Rubella

Encouraged by the success of the immunisation campaigns against

diphtheria, whooping cough, tuberculosis, and poliomyelitis, public
health officials were, by the mid-1960s, beginning to turn their attention
to the possibility of using vaccines to control measles and rubella. Neither
of these last named diseases could compare with the others as a killer, but
measles could cause considerable illness in children, requiring the use of
expensive hospital facilities and resulting in upset to families, while
rubella contracted by unprotected pregnant women could cause serious
foetal abnormalities. In 1966 the Joint Committee on Vaccination and
Immunisation, while declining to recommend a programme of general
measles vaccination until full information was obtained on the duration
of the protection afforded by the vaccine, agreed that the vaccine should
be made available to individual doctors requesting it for their
patients[124]. Two years later, with the efficacy of the vaccine established,
the Scottish Home and Health Department accepted the new advice of
the Joint Committee on Vaccination and Immunisation that measles
vaccine should be offered to all children under sixteen years of age, and
issued regulations making cases of the disease notifiable under the terms
of the Infectious Diseases (Notification) Act of 1889 as from 1 October
1968[125]. The campaign encountered some early difficulties. Supplies of
vaccine from one manufacturer had to be withdrawn in 1969 after they
were found to cause some cases of measles, and the resultant shortage of
vaccine severely restricted the campaign[126]. With the help of imports
from the USA vaccine supplies were soon restored to the required level,
but the acceptance rate, despite advertising campaigns utilising the
press, television, and posters, proved disappointing[127]. Throughout the
1970s the acceptance rate among children under three years of age (at
whom the campaign was primarily aimed) hovered around the 50 *per cent*
mark. Possibly because of greater efforts on the part of the Scottish
Health Education Group and some Health Boards in recent years, acceptance rates for measles immunisation have risen between 1982 and
1984 from 57 *per cent* to 64 *per cent*[128], but even these improved levels of
protection are incapable of controlling a highly infectious disease such as
measles. Other countries, most notably the USA and Sweden, have
shown not only what a thorough, scientifically organised immunisation
campaign against measles can achieve but also how much farther we in
Britain still have to go. It is, or rather should be, a matter of some
embarrassment and perhaps even shame that in 1981 there were fewer
reported cases of measles in the USA with a population of well over 200
million than in Scotland with a population of only five million[129].
There are not only good humanitarian but also excellent economic
reasons for following the example set in America and Scandinavia, as the
cost of a full immunisation scheme would be more than offset by savings
to the National Health Service in terms of general practitioners' time,
hospital admissions, and prescribed medicines.

The success of other countries, again most notably the USA and

Sweden, in bringing rubella under control in recent years is likewise a source of some embarrassment in Britain where the immunisation programme has achieved less than totally satisfactory results. In July 1970, following advice from the Joint Committee on Vaccination and Immunisation the central department recommended that girls between the age of eleven and fourteen should be immunised with live attenuated rubella virus vaccine, and from September of the same year supplies of this vaccine were issued free to local health authorities[130]. The campaign got off to a slow start, with only 37.2 *per cent* of girls in the target age group being immunised by the end of 1971[131], but it soon began to pick up momentum, and by 1975 the acceptance rate among eleven to fourteen years olds had risen to over 80 *per cent*[132]. Since then, however, the acceptance rate has remained fairly static, and, while there is some evidence that the immunisation campaign is having some effect in reducing the number of rubella cases in females over the age of fourteen, we still have some way to go before we can eradicate rubella as a source of congenital infection[133].

Present Day Problems of Control

There are, quite apart from the need for improved immunisation programmes against whooping cough, rubella, and measles, some important problems in infectious disease control which remain to be solved. Some of these problems are of long standing, while others have only come to prominence in recent years. Bacillary dysentery and salmonellosis, for example, have been a source of some anxiety since the 1940s and 1950s respectively, while Legionnaire's Disease and AIDS have only been identified in the last ten years. Bacillary dysentery, mostly of the milder Sh.Sonnei type, began to attract serious attention in the 1940s when, almost certainly as a result of improved methods of diagnosis, notifications of the disease began to rise appreciably[134]. No evidence was uncovered of the disease being spread by communal food handling or by flies, and by the mid-1950s suspicion began to fall on the communal lavatories, which were then a common feature of working class tenement life, as the most likely method by which dysentery was spread[135]. The substantial reduction in the numbers of such lavatories and, in all likelihood, an increasing public awareness of the value of higher standards of personal hygiene, contributed to the decline in the prevalence of the disease during the later 1960s and 1970s, but dysentery still remains a problem albeit a much diminished one. No decline, however, has been noticeable in the incidence of salmonellosis, the reported number of cases of which more than trebled between 1972 and 1982[136]. Hygiene education campaigns and stricter regulations governing the preparation and handling of food seem to have had little effect, although the Milk

(Special Designation) (Scotland) Order of 1980 which required all milk sold in Scotland after 1 August 1983 to be heat treated has been successful in eliminating the general community outbreaks of salmonellosis which had been relatively frequent in previous years[137]. Irradiation treatment of foodstuffs, if widely adopted, should reduce substantially the number of outbreaks associated with salmonella contaminated foods and in particular factory farmed poultry, but it can do nothing to reduce the growing number of cases contracted by Scots travelling or holidaying in foreign countries.

The great expansion in the amount of foreign travel which has taken place in the post-war years and in particular since the 1960s has created new problems in infectious disease control. A growing number of cases of salmonellosis and bacillary dysentery are contracted abroad, while Scots are more likely nowadays to be infected with typhoid and paratyphoid fever on holiday in the Mediterranean than at home. Moreover, the increasing frequency of travel to and from tropical and sub-tropical countries where malaria is endemic has led to the recrudescence of a problem which had given little trouble since the immediate post first world war period when soldiers had returned home from the Middle-East suffering from the disease. The relatively high levels of notification of this disease recorded throughout the 1970s and early 1980s strongly suggests that many travellers, and in particular Asian immigrants revisiting India and Pakistan, are either badly advised as to the importance of taking prophylactic medication during their visit and for six weeks afterwards or choose not to comply with that advice. No prophylactic measures exist, as yet, to combat deadly haemorrhagic viral fevers such as Marburg Disease, Ebola Fever, and Lassa Fever which began to attract attention in Britain when a patient returned from West Africa to England suffering from Lassa Fever in 1976. The possibility of a similar case arising in Scotland and the consequent advisability of providing protection for both the community and health service staff treating such a case led swiftly to the issue of regulations making these diseases notifiable and to the establishment of a special isolation unit at Ruchhill Hospital (Glasgow) for their treatment[138].

Legionnaire's Disease, Hepatitis B, and Acquired Immune Deficiency Syndrome (AIDS) are perhaps the most important of the infectious diseases which have begun to cause serious concern in recent years. The organism Legionnella Pneumophila was first isolated in 1977 following an investigation into an outbreak of a pneumonic type of illness among a group of American ex-servicemen who had been attending a convention in Philadelphia. This discovery allowed work to proceed in Scotland, and elsewhere, on the diagnosis of cases of pneumonia of previously unknown aetiology, and it was soon ascertained that Legionnaire's Disease had been responsible for a mysterious outbreak of a pneumonic type of illness among a party of holidaymakers who had returned to Glasgow from Benidorm in July 1973[139]. Legionnaire's Disease is probably a disease of some vintage which has in the past been mistakenly diagnosed as pneumonia, and it is neither exotic nor, in normal circumstances, a major threat to public health. Infection is normally spread through the air by small droplets of contaminated water, and can be prevented by the regular cleaning and chlorination of cooling towers, evaporative condensers, humidifiers, shower heads, etc. No such confidence can be expressed with regard to AIDS which, like Legionnaire's Disease, has attracted a great deal of frequently ill-informed attention from the mass media. This condition, which was first described in 1981, is generally believed to be caused by a retrovirus known as HTLV III which is spread by means of intimate sexual contact, transfusion of contaminated blood and blood products, and the repeated insertion of contaminated objects (usually drug abusers' needles) into the bloodstream. New blood screening procedures have been adopted to prevent the infection of those, most notably haemophiliacs, who require transfusions, but practising homosexuals and intravenous drug abusers remain seriously at risk from a condition which shows some signs of rapidly increasing in incidence and may assume epidemic proportions. Just as the spread of AIDS has been facilitated by an increased level of drug abuse in recent years, so too has the growing incidence of Hepatitis B been largely attributable to increased drug addiction. A vaccine affording protection against this blood-borne disease has been developed and made available to health service staff most at risk of contracting Hepatitis B from patients, but it is extremely unlikely that an immunisation campaign to protect drug abusers would prove practicable. The success of campaigns to discourage drug misuse offers the best chance of lowering the incidence of the disease.

The Achievement of the Infectious Disease Service

Despite the appearance of new problems, the continuation of some older ones, the re-emergence of others such as the venereal diseases (the number of new cases of which has been rising annually since the later 1950s and shows as yet no sign of declining), the record of the infectious disease service is deserving of some praise. The dramatic decline in morbidity and mortality from infectious disease since the late nineteenth century testifies to not only the massive improvement which has taken place in the standards of living of the community and in the quality of medical treatment but also the value of the public health service in general and of the infectious disease service in particular. Whereas 50 *per cent* of all deaths a century or so ago were caused by infectious disease the figure nowadays is less than 1 *per cent*[140]. Diseases, whose very names used to strike fear into whole communities, are now little more than memories. Typhus, a common cause of death in nineteenth century working class areas, has been eradicated, as has smallpox, while typhoid fever and tuberculosis, which formerly struck so frequently, are now comparative rarities. Poliomyelitis and diphtheria have been brought under control in a way which would probably have astonished pioneers like William Gairdner and James Russell, and, although the immunisation campaign against whooping cough has been less than totally successful, the incidence of and mortality from the disease have been greatly reduced. The extent of the triumph over infectious diseases may be measured by the falling proportion of hospital beds allocated to the treatment of patients suffering from this category of illness. While there were 11,262 beds, representing over one third of total hospital accommodation, devoted to the treatment of infectious disease in 1934[141], by 1983 there were only 744 beds for Respiratory Medicine and 662 for Communicable Diseases out of a total hospital establishment of 60,174 beds[142].

The consequences of the advances made against infectious disease have been many and varied. One of the most significant has been the great reduction in infant and child mortality which has undoubtedly contributed to the decline in average family size and to a profound change in the perception of women's role in society. Equally significant, perhaps, has been the large reduction in the number of men and women in the prime of life who have been killed or disabled by infectious diseases such as tuberculosis. The social and medical consequences of this advance can hardly be overstated. Fewer orphans have to be provided for, fewer widows have to struggle in poverty to bring up their children, and fewer families are reduced to penury by the illnesses contracted by their 'bread winners'. From a medical point of view, however, the most important consequence has been the steadily growing proportion of our population who live on into old age and fall victim to those diseases, frequently chronic and therefore expensive to treat, which are associated with advancing years. The ageing of the population which has necessitated the transfer of health service resources into geriatric and psycho-geriatric medicine is, in large part, owing to the progress made against infectious disease since the late nineteenth century.

Health Education

The radical shift which has taken place during the course of this century in the nature of the health problems facing the peoples of Scotland and other Western countries has called for a profound change in the strategy of those organisations concerned with the public health. The elaborate machinery which was developed to control infectious disease has little relevance to the control of cardio-vascular disease, cancer, strokes, and the degenerative diseases of old age which have become the major causes of death in our society. If we wish to reduce the heavy toll of life exacted by lung cancer, bronchitis, heart disease, etc. (and a comparison of Scotland's record in respect of mortality from those diseases with those of similar industrialised countries suggests that there is massive scope for such a reduction) then we are probably only going to achieve progress if we persuade our fellow citizens to abandon many of their habits and change their life-styles.

There is nothing novel about health education. Medical men have been attempting since time immemorial to persuade their patients, with varying degrees of success, to adopt more healthy modes of living. The State, however, played no part in health education until relatively recently, and the propagation of information on healthy living was for a long time left to voluntary agencies like the British Social Hygiene Council and the National Association for the Prevention of Tuberculosis, and to the endeavours of individual enthusiasts like Dr Roger McNeil, the Medical Officer of Health for Argyllshire, who at the turn of the century was urging that domestic science should be incorporated into the school curriculum[143]. The entry of the State, on a somewhat tentative and limited basis, into the field of health education was heralded by the establishment of the National Health Insurance scheme in 1913 and the development of the maternity and child welfare service in the early years of this century. The National Insurance Act empowered the Insurance Committees which were set up to administer medical benefit to spend money on health education, and, in time, some of these organisations began to issue pamphlets to the public and organise lectures, while much of the work of the maternity and child welfare clinics and health visitors was educational in its nature. There can be no doubt that the efforts of the early health educators contributed significantly to the improvements which medical observers of the 1930s remarked upon as having taken place since the turn of the century in the standards of personal cleanliness, food hygiene, and child care, and in the public's attitude towards the expectation of health. Nevertheless, despite improvements, expert opinion in the 1930s was seemingly unanimous in the view that there was an 'urgent need for further improvements in health standards' and that the gap 'between what is known and what is practised' remained unacceptably large[144]. In the opinion of the Cathcart Committee:

"no great improvement can be expected in the general health of the nation unless an organised attempt is made to convince each person of the necessity of observing fundamental rules and of developing such habits, attitudes, and ideals as will promote physical, mental and emotional well-being. For these reasons, we consider that health education should be placed in the forefront of national health policy"[145].

The Committee, believing that the key to the success of a health education system lay in directing its efforts towards influencing the development of children's attitudes towards health rather than in attempting to alter the established life-style of adults, recommended that health education should begin in the nursery school and continue throughout the years spent in primary and secondary schools, and that the role of the school medical service should be expanded to provide the necessary supervision. The Cathcart Report also urged that the role of the general practitioner as the family adviser on health should be strengthened and emphasised, and that the Department of Health for Scotland should, in co-operation with the Scottish Education Department and local authorities, initiate measures for health education and assist appropriate organisations working in that field. A body similar to the English Central Council for Health Education, it was recommended, should be established to co-ordinate policy by ensuring that the varied activities of the central departments of health and education, local authorities, and voluntary agencies did not conflict[146].

The Cathcart Report plotted a masterly course for the future development of health education in Scotland, but for a long time the navigator's expert advice was largely ignored. Although the Scottish Council for Health Education was formed in 1943 to promote education in the science and art of healthy living[147], health education was given a relatively low priority within the Health Service until the 1960s. However, the steadily rising mortality from cigarette smoking related diseases like lung cancer and bronchitis throughout the 1950s helped to change attitudes towards the value of health education. In May 1964 a Joint Committee of the Central and Scottish Health Services Councils under the chairmanship of Lord Cohen of Birkenhead published a report which stressed the need for a stronger impetus to be given to health education within the National Health Service. The Cohen Report recommended that expenditure on health education should be increased substantially, arguing that the injection of additional funds into an improved health education programme was more likely to produce worthwhile results than a similar increase in funding for the therapeutic services. Crucial to any improvement in health education, the Report maintained, was a strengthening of its formal organisation. This could be achieved, it was argued, by the establishment of a new body with responsibility for developing health education policies and programmes at a national level, which would take over the health education functions of the Scottish Home and Health Department and the Scottish Council for Health Education[148]. The Cohen Report was favourably received by government, and, in April 1968, the Scottish Health Education Unit was set up in the Scottish Home and Health Department to develop effective national health education programmes. Stress was laid upon the need for the Unit to improve educational methods and techniques as it had been worryingly clear since the late 1950s that, while the general public were aware of the health risks associated with such habits as cigarette smoking, there was a marked 'consumer resistance' to health propaganda urging the abandonment of those habits[149]. The new Scottish Health Education Unit therefore initiated research projects to evaluate the effectiveness of particular campaigns and to assist in the planning of future programmes. Much of this research was aimed at discovering ways of increasing the impact of health education campaigns designed to improve the country's appalling record in respect of cardiovascular disease and dental health, but some effort was also directed at improving the effectiveness of those campaigns which sought to promote the immunisation programme, family planning services, and a responsible attitude towards alcohol use. This research undoubtedly improved what might be termed the marketing skills of the Unit and other organisations involved in health education. By the early 1970s, for example, anti-smoking propaganda was being focused on 'target groups' such as expectant mothers who had been identified as potentially highly responsive to the message of the health educators[150]. Progress, however, remained slow, – painfully and frustratingly slow – and the central department's annual reports of the 1970s echoed those of the early 1960s both in their remarks about the relative unresponsiveness of the public to health education campaigns and in their bitter references to the 'heavy expenditure ... incurred in convincing the young and impressionable that the use of tobacco or alcohol is a mark of maturity, sociability or virility'[151].

The re-organisation of the National Health Service in 1974 seemed to promise greater opportunities for the advance of health education. The Scottish Health Education Unit ceased to be a part of the Scottish Home and Health Department and became a separate division of the new Common Services Agency, assuming responsibility, in both an advisory and executive capacity, for those aspects of health education best managed at a national level. Health board representation on the management committee of the CSA was intended to ensure that the future activities of the Unit were developed in close association with those undertaken by the health boards in their own localities. Other administrative alterations were also expected to bring benefits. It was hoped that the unification of the administrative structure of the National Health Service would remove old barriers, make the resources and expertise of the health educators more readily accessible to the hospital and general practitioner services, and enable health campaigns to be organised on a broader basis and in a more co-ordinated way than had been possible in the past. Equally importantly, re-organisation was intended to encourage and facilitate co-ordination of local initiatives in health education. The Scottish Home and Health Department recommended that each health board should establish a health education department headed by an Area Health Education Officer and staffed on the minimum basis of one health education officer for every 50,000 of population[152].

The mid-1970s witnessed not only important organisational changes but also a profoundly significant shift in official government policy which was marked by the publication in 1976 of *Prevention and Health: Everybody's Business*[153] and *The Way Ahead*[154], both of which stressed the need to give health education a more prominent role than it had formerly enjoyed in the National Health Service. That it was not the Government's intention to place health education in the forefront of national health policy, as the Cathcart Committee had urged forty years previously, was apparently confirmed by the publication of the White Paper on *Prevention and Health* in 1977[155]. The future prospects of health education were further brightened at this time by the growing willingness of television, radio, and other mass media organisations to give wider coverage of social, community, and health education topics, and by the development of University and College courses in health education designed both for those intending to make a career in health education and for those whose work involved or might involve a health education component[156].

Despite the advances of the mid-1970s, some important problems remained. The division of responsibility between the Scottish Health Education Unit and the Scottish Council for Health Education, which had existed since the Unit's foundation in 1968, was highly unsatisfactory, but the necessary solution was somehow avoided until April 1980 when the two organisations were at last merged to form the Scottish Health Education Group[157]. This merger facilitated a long overdue review of health education training which led in turn to a more coordinated and better planned system of in-service training[158]. However, the task of organising health education in the health board areas and of providing local support to other professions in this field continued to fall on an unacceptably small number of Health Education Officers. At the end of 1982 there were only forty-six full-time Health Education Officers at various grades employed by the health boards[159], a staffing level less than half the minimum of one officer per 50,000 of population recommended by the Scottish Home and Health Department at the time of reorganisation. (The Greater Glasgow Health Board has nearly met this target of one in 50,000.)

Health education does not as yet have the high priority and funding which were envisaged in the mid-1970s. This had hindered progress over the last decade or so, and will in all probability continue to do so. There is still a great deal to be done. Scotland, as in the 1950s, has one of the worst records in the world for lung cancer, heart disease, and bronchitis. Far too many of our citizens still smoke cigarettes, consume alcohol to excess, eat unbalanced diets containing too much fat and not enough fibre, and take little or no exercise. Nevertheless, there have been some pleasing developments in recent years which have eased the disappointments. Cigarette smoking is now a minority habit, the benefits of a healthy diet are more generally appreciated and acted upon, and the expansion of interest in sporting activities such as jogging bears witness to the greater interest in physical fitness. We undoubtedly live in a more health and fitness conscious country than formerly, but whether that consciousness can be raised quickly and highly enough to improve our abysmal health record significantly in the years to come is a question to which no confident answer can be given.

Conclusion: from Public Health to Community Medicine

Community Medicine is not a new specialism, but rather a new and more appropriate title for that branch of medicine which is basically concerned with the study of health and disease in populations. It is still recognisable as the discipline pioneered in nineteenth century Scotland by Gairdner and Littlejohn. Nevertheless, the last century or so has seen some significant changes in the role of those working in this branch of medicine. Some of these changes have been referred to obliquely in the story which has been recounted on previous pages, but their importance to a fuller understanding of the history of the public health services in twentieth century Scotland is such that they must be narrated more directly, if of necessity somewhat succinctly, here[160].

The Medical Officers of Health of late nineteenth century Scotland concentrated their attention upon understanding the relationship between the environment and the infectious diseases which were then so prevalent, and upon securing such improvements in the environment as were found necessary to obtain a measure of control over those diseases. The role of the Medical Officer of Health, however, was not limited to that of environmental health, for from the beginning he was responsible for and closely involved in the work of the local authority infectious diseases hospitals which began to be erected in the second half of the nineteenth century. The first four decades of this century saw an immense expansion in the responsibilities of the Medical Officer of Health. The development of the maternity and child welfare service, the school medical service, and the tuberculosis service[161], the expansion of the infectious diseases hospital system, and the transfer of the Poor Law hospitals to the local authorities left the Medical Officer of Health in control of a very sizeable empire indeed by the mid-1930s. Such was the scale and pace of this expansion that the Cathcart Committee stated in 1936 that 'unless a policy is framed and developments are guided by it, the local authority services are bound to extend further into general medical practice, and ... influence if not determine the future medical organisation of the country'[162].

The progress towards a municipally based medical service was abruptly halted in 1947. With the passage of the National Health Service (Scotland) Act the sun appeared to set on the empire which the Medical Officers of Health had built up over the preceding half of the century or so. The infectious disease, tuberculosis, and general (ex Poor Law) hospitals were taken away and placed under the control of the new Regional

Hospital Boards. Deprived of their invaluable clinical contacts and reduced considerably in status, public health specialists faced something close to a crisis. While the development of the immunisation campaigns in the 1940s and 1950s and the growing emphasis on the importance of preventing disease and promoting health from the mid-1960s onwards helped to restore the specialism's self-confidence, the tripartite structure of the National Health Service, by cutting public health off from any close involvement with the general medical and hospital service, prevented the Medical Officer of Health from contributing as fully as he might have done to the Health Service.

The integration of health services brought about by the reorganisation of the National Health Service in 1974 radically altered the role of the public health or community medicine specialist, as he was now called, and restored him to his place in the forefront of Scottish medicine. Charged with investigating and assessing the health needs of the population and establishing health care priorities, community medicine specialists were required to involve themselves in the full range of services relevant to their redefined function. In addition to their traditional responsibilities for communicable disease control and health information, they were expected to strengthen their links with local authority departments concerned with social work, education, and environmental services, and to develop a new relationship with the various clinical divisions of the Health Service, including general practice. There was no intention to manage or supervise the clinical specialisms, but rather to provide information from data supplied by the information services, and thus to create an essentially collaborative relationship which would assist in bringing about improvements in the services provided[163]. It is as yet perhaps too soon to judge whether community medicine has achieved all the goals set for it in 1974, but it seems clear that the development over the last decade or so of a better planned and organised health service which knows its priorities and tries, with little public understanding and less financial support, to meet them is owing in no small part to the efforts of Scotland's community medicine specialists.

References

(1) Ferguson, T., *Scottish Social Welfare 1864–1914*, (Edinburgh & London, 1958), pp.165–68.
(2) *Ibid*, pp.168–70.
(3) Whyte, Sir W.E., *Local Government in Scotland. With complete statutory references.* Second Edition. (London, Edinburgh, & Glasgow, 1936), pp.52, 81, 98–193.
(4) *Ibid*, pp.53–54.
(5) Reports of the Medical Officer of Health for Dunbartonshire. These are available from Mitchell Library, Glasgow.
(6) Chalmers, A.K. The Health of Glasgow 1818–1925. An outline. (Glasgow, 1930), p.12. Corporation of Glasgow, 1930.
(7) Ferguson, T. *op. cit.*, pp.175, 405, 494.
(8) *Ibid*, pp.182, 188.

(9)   Department of Health for Scotland. *Committee on Scottish Health Services Report.* Cmd. 5204, (Edinburgh, 1936), p.121.

(10)   *Ibid*, pp.117–21.

(11)   Macnalty, Sir A.S., Ed., *History of the Second World War. United Kingdom Medical Series. The Civilian Health and Medical Services.* Volume II. (London, 1955), p.274.

(12)   *Ibid*, pp.273.

(13)   *Reports of the Department of Health for Scotland and the Scottish Health Services Council 1955.* Cmd. 9742. (Edinburgh, 1956), p.50; Scottish Home and Health Department. *Health and Welfare Services in Scotland Report for 1962.* Cmd. 1996. (Edinburgh, 1963), pp.24–25.

(14)   Scottish Home and Health Department. *Health in Scotland 1983.* (Edinburgh, 1984), p.36.

(15)   Goldberg, Sir A., Why did Glasgow not consult Christison of Edinburgh in 1854? *Edinburgh Medicine* No.22. (September/October 1983), p.9.

(16)   *Ibid*, p.10.

(17)   Sherlock, J.C., Ashby, D., Delves, H.T., Forbes, G.I., Moore, M.R., Patterson, W.J., Pocock, S.J., Quinn, M.J., Richards, W.N., and Wilson, T.S., *Human Toxicology* (1984), III, pp.383–92. Sherlock, J., Smart, G., Forbes, G., Moore, M.R., Patterson, W.J., Richards, W.N., and Wilson, T.S., *Human Toxicology* (1982), I, pp.115–22.

(18)   Department of Health for Scotland. *Committee on Scottish Health Services Report.* Cmd. 5204. (Edinburgh, 1936), p.40.

(19)   Ferguson, T., *op. cit.,* p.191.

(20)   An Act for regulating the Police and Sanitary Administration of towns and populous places, and for facilitating the union of Police and Municipal Administration in burghs in Scotland. [henceforth cited as Burgh Police (Scotland) Act, 1892]. *55& 56 Vict. Ch.55.* Section 219.

(21)   Chalmers, A.K., *op. cit.,* p.281.

(22)   Ferguson, T., *op. cit.,* p.196.

(23)   *Ibid*, p.197.

(24)   Greer, W.T., Dalmarnock Sewage Treatment Works, Glasgow. *Institute of Water Pollution Control,* Annual Conference, Edinbugh 25/29 September 1972; and Greer, W.T., The Design and Construction of Shieldhall Sewage Treatment Works, Glasgow. *Institute of Water Pollution Control.* Annual Conference, Buxton 8/11 September 1980.

(25)   An Act to consolidate and amend the Laws relating to the Public Health in Scotland [henceforth cited as Public Health (Scotland) Act, 1897]. *50&61. Vict. Ch.38.* Section 103.

(26)   Department of Health for Scotland. *Committee on Scottish Health Services Report.* Cmd. 5204, (Edinburgh, 1936), p.122.

(27)   An Act to make provision as to water supplies, sewerage and sewage disposal in rural localities, and to make expenses incurred by rural district councils in connection with water supply, sewerage and sewage general expenses. *7&8.Geog.VI.Ch.26.*

(28)   Ferguson, T., *op. cit.,* p.86.

(29)   Chalmers, A.K., *op. cit.,* p.22

(30)   Ferguson, T., *op. cit.,* p.153.

(31)   *Ibid*, p.154.

(32)   Harvie, C., *No Gods and Precious Few Heroes. Scotland 1914–1980,* (London, 1981), p.71.

(33)   Whyte, Sir W.E., *op. cit.,* p.431.

(34)   *Ibid*, p.432.

(35)   *Ibid*, pp.433–45.

(36)   *Ibid*, p.435.

(37)   Harvie, C., *op. cit.,* p.70.

(38)   Department of Health for Scotland. *Committee on Scottish Health Services Report,* Cmd. 5204, (Edinburgh, 1936). p.124.

(39) *City of Glasgow District Council, Environmental Health Reports, 1981,* Report.

(40) Adams, I.H., *The Making of Urban Scotland,* (London, 1978), p.231; Harvie, C., *op. cit.,* p.155.

(41) James B. Russell Papers, Mitchell Library, Glasgow. Russell had many pamphlets published in 1895.

(42) Burgh Police (Scotland) Act, 1892. 55&56 Vict. Ch.55. Section 384.

(43) Public Health (Scotland) Act, 1897. 60&61. Vict. Ch.38. Section 16(9).

(44) Chalmers, A.K., *op. cit.,* pp.450–52; Ferguson, T., *op. cit.,* p.203.

(45) Chalmers, A.K., *op. cit.,* p.449.

(46) Department of Health for Scotland. Committee on Scottish Health Services Report. Cmd. 5204. (Edinburgh, 1936), p.133

(47) Chalmers, A.K., *op. cit.,* p.448.

(48) *Ibid,* p.452,

(49) Department of Health for Scotland. Committee on Scottish Health Services Report. Cmd. 5204. (Edinburgh, 1936), p.135.

(50) City of Glasgow District Council *Annual Report of the Environmental Health Department for 1982.* p.40.

(51) Private communication from Mr C.A. Thomson, Director of Environmental Services, Monklands District Council.

(52) Public Health (Scotland) Act, 1897. 60&61.Vict.Ch.38, Sections 33(1) and 43.

(53) Ferguson, T., *op. cit.,* p.243.

(54) Department of Health for Scotland. *Committee on Scottish Health Services Report.* Cmd. 5204. (Edinburgh, 1936), p.99.

(55) *Report of the Department of Health for Scotland 1956.* Cmd. 140. (Edinburgh, 1957), p.86.

(56) *Ibid,* p.84.

(57) *Report of the Department of Health for Scotland 1959.* Cmd. 983. (Edinburgh, 1960), p.94.

(58) Whyte, Sir W.E., *op. cit.,* pp.403–4.

(59) Ferguson, T., *op. cit.,* p.240.

(60) Whyte, Sir W.E., *op. cit.,* pp.405–7.

(61) Macnalty, Sir A.S., Ed., *History of the Second World War. United Kingdom Medical Series. The Civilian Health and Medical Services.* Volume II. (London, 1955), pp.277–81.

(62) *Report of the Department of Health for Scotland 1956.* Cmd. 140. (Edinburgh, 1957), p.86–7.

(63) *Report of the Department of Health for Scotland 1959.* Cmd. 983. (Edinburgh, 1960), p.92.

(64) Ferguson, T., *op. cit.,* pp.419–20.

(65) *Ibid,* pp.480–82.

(66) *Sixth Annual Report of the Scottish Board of Health 1924.* Cmd. 2416. (Edinburgh, 1925), p.54.

(67) Ferguson, T., *op. cit.,* p.431.

(68) *Sixth Annual Report of the Scottish Board of Health 1924.* Cmd. 2416. (Edinburgh, 1925), p.54–5.

(69) Ferguson, T., *op. cit.,* p.432.

(70) *Sixth Annual Report of the Scottish Board of Health 1924.* Cmd. 2416. (Edinburgh, 1925), p.56.

(71) *First Annual Report of the Department of Health for Scotland 1929.* Cmd. 3529. (Edinburgh, 1930), p.95.

(72) *Tenth Annual Report of the Department of Health for Scotland 1938.* Cmd. 5969. (Edinburgh, 1939), p.95.

(73) *Sixth Annual Report of the Scottish Board of Health 1924.* Cmd. 2416. (Edinburgh, 1925), pp.62–8, 227.

(74) *Tenth Annual Report of the Department of Health for Scotland 1938.* Cmd. 5969. (Edinburgh, 1939), pp.96, 206.

(75) *Sixth Annual Report of the Scottish Board of Health 1924.* Cmd. 2416. (Edinburgh, 1925), p.80.

(76) *Ibid,* pp.71, 80.

(77) *Seventh Annual Report of the Scottish Board of Health 1925.* Cmd. 2674. (Edinburgh, 1926), p.92.

(78) *Sixth Annual Report of the Scottish Board of Health 1924.* Cmd. 2416. (Edinburgh, 1925), p.80.

(79) *Seventh Annual Report of the Department of Health for Scotland 1935.* Cmd. 5123. (Edinburgh, 1936), p.95.

(80) Department of Health for Scotland. *Committee on Scottish Health Services Report.* Cmd. 5204. (Edinburgh, 1936), pp.399–400.

(81) *Ibid*, p.204.

(82) *Sixth Annual Report of the Scottish Board of Health 1924.* Cmd. 2416. (Edinburgh, 1925), p.81.

(83) *Seventh Annual Report of the Department of Health for Scotland 1936.* Cmd. 5123. (Edinburgh, 1936), p.96.

(84) *Ibid*, pp.89–90.

(85) *Sixth Annual Report of the Scottish Board of Health 1924.* Cmd. 2416. (Edinburgh, 1925), p.74.

(86) Department of Health for Scotland. *Committee on Scottish Health Services Report.* Cmd. 5204. (Edinburgh, 1936), p.195.

(87) McKinlay, P.L., The Trend of Diphtheria in Relation to the Immunisation Campaign, *Health Bulletin*, Vol. V, No.5, (November, 1947).

(88) Department of Health for Scotland. *Committee on Scottish Health Services Report.* Cmd. 5204. (Edinburgh, 1936), pp.203.

(89) *Sixth Annual Report of the Scottish Board of Health 1924.* Cmd. 2416. (Edinburgh, 1925), pp.72–3.

(90) *Seventh Annual Report of the Department of Health for Scotland 1935.* Cmd. 5123. (Edinburgh, 1936), p.88.

(91) *Seventh Annual Report of the Scottish Board of Health 1925.* Cmd. 2674. (Edinburgh, 1926), p.97.

(92) *Seventh Annual Report of the Department of Health for Scotland 1935.* Cmd. 5123. (Edinburgh, 1936), p.89.

(93) Macnalty, Sir A.S., Ed., *History of the Second World War. United Kingdom Medical Series. The Civilian Health and Medical Services.* Volume II. (London, 1955), p.264.

(94) *Summary Report by the Department of Health for Scotland for the period from 1st January 1939 to 30th June 1941.* Cmd. 6308. (Edinburgh, 1941), p.16.

(95) *Summary Report by the Department of Health for Scotland for the year ended 30th June 1942.* Cmd. 6372. (Edinburgh, 1942), p.14.

(96) *Report of the Department of Health for Scotland for the period July 1945 to December 1946.* Cmd. 7188. (Edinburgh, 1947), p.32.

(97) *Report of the Department of Health for Scotland for the year 1948.* Cmd. 7659. (Edinburgh, 1949), p.25.

(98) *Report of the Department of Health for Scotland 1957.* Cmd. 385. (Edinburgh, 1958), p.60.

(99) *Summary Report by the Department of Health for Scotland for the period from 1st January 1939 to 30th June 1941.* Cmd. 6308. (Edinburgh, 1941), p.16.

(100) Macnalty, Sir, A.S., Ed., *op. cit.,* p.264.

(101) *Report of the Department of Health for Scotland 1956.* Cmd. 140. (Edinburgh, 1957), p.24.

(102) Scottish Home and Health Department. *Health and Welfare Services in Scotland. Report for 1968.* Cmd. 4012. (Edinburgh, 1969), p.7.

(103) *Report of the Department of Health for Scotland and the Scottish Health Services Council 1949.* Cmd. 7921. (Edinburgh, 1950), p.27.

(104) *Report of the Department of Health for Scotland and the Scottish Health Services Council 1952.* Cmd. 8799. (Edinburgh, 1953), p.28.

(105) *Report of the Department of Health for Scotland 1957.* Cmd. 385. (Edinburgh, 1958), p.60.

(106) *Report of the Department of Health for Scotland 1959.* Cmd. 983. (Edinburgh, 1960), p.23.

(107) Scottish Home and Health Department. *Health and Welfare Services in Scotland. Report for 1964.* Cmd. 2700. (Edinburgh, 1965), p.22.

(108) Bassili, W.R., and Stewart, G.T., Epidemiological Evaluation of Immunisation and other factors in the control of Whooping Cough, in *The Lancet*, 28th February, 1976. volume I, pp.471–73.

(109) Scottish Home and Health Department. *Health and Welfare Services in Scotland. Report for 1976.* Cmd. 6812. (Edinburgh, 1977), p.51.

(110) Department of Health and Social Security. *Whooping Cough Vaccination. Review of the Evidence on Whooping Cough Vaccination by the Joint Committee on Vaccination and Immunisation.* (London, 1977), pp.33–4.

(111) Scottish Home and Health Department. *Health in Scotland 1980.* (Edinburgh, 1981), p.22.

(112) *Report of the Department of Health for Scotland and of the Scottish Health Services Council 1949.* Cmd. 7921. (Edinburgh, 1950), p.27.

(113) *Reports of the Department of Health for Scotland and the Scottish Health Services Council 1951.* Cmd. 8496. (Edinburgh, 1952), p.15.

(114) *Reports of the Department of Health for Scotland and the Scottish Health Services Council 1952.* Cmd. 8799. (Edinburgh, 1953), p.16.

(115) *Report of the Department of Health for Scotland 1956.* Cmd. 140. (Edinburgh, 1957), p.30.

(116) Scottish Home and Health Department. *Health Services in Scotland. Report for 1976.* Cmd. 6812. (Edinburgh, 1977), p.46.

(117) *Report of the Department of Health for Scotland for the year 1947.* Cmd. 7453. (Edinburgh, 1948), p.24.

(118) *Reports of the Department of Health for Scotland and the Scottish Health Services Council 1953.* Cmd. 9107. (Edinburgh, 1954), p.27.

(119) *Report of the Department of Health for Scotland 1956.* Cmd. 140. (Edinburgh, 1957), p.22.

(120) *Report of the Department of Health for Scotland 1959.* Cmd. 385. (Edinburgh, 1958), p.59.

(121) *Report of the Department of Health for Scotland 1959.* Cmd. 983. (Edinburgh, 1960), p.24.

(122) *Report of the Department of Health for Scotland 1960. Part 1. Health and Welfare Services.* Cmd. 1320. (Edinburgh, 1961), p.25.

(123) Scottish Home and Health Department. *Health and Welfare Services in Scotland. Report for 1962.* Cmd. 1996. (Edinburgh, 1963), pp.12–13, 16.

(124) Scottish Home and Health Department. *Health and Welfare Services in Scotland. Report for 1966.* Cmd. 3337. (Edinburgh, 1967), p.14.

(125) Scottish Home and Health Department. *Health and Welfare Services in Scotland. Report for 1968.* Cmd. 4012. (Edinburgh, 1969), pp.9–11.

(126) Scottish Home and Health Department. Scottish Health Services Council. *Health Services in Scotland. Reports for 1970.* Cmd. 4667. (Edinburgh, 1971), p.12.

(127) Scottish Home and Health Department. Scottish Health Services Council. *Health Services in Scotland. Reports for 1971.* Cmd. 4970. (Edinburgh, 1972), p.13.

(128) Scottish Home and Health Department. *Health in Scotland 1984.* (Edinburgh, 1985), p.28.

(129) Campbell, A.G.M., "Measles Immunisation: why have we failed?" in *Archives of Disease in Childhood.* (1983), Vol. 58, pp.3–5.

(130) Scottish Home and Health Department. Scottish Health Services Council. *Health Services in Scotland. Reports for 1970.* Cmd. 4667. (Edinburgh, 1971), p.13–4.

(131) Scottish Home and Health Department. Scottish Health Services Council. *Health Services in Scotland. Reports for 1971.* Cmd. 4970. (Edinburgh, 1972), p.14.

(132) Scottish Home and Health Department. *Health Services in Scotland. Report for 1976.* Cmd. 6812. (Edinburgh, 1977), p.45.

(133) Scottish Home and Health Department. *Health in Scotland 1984.* (Edinburgh, 1985), p.28.

(134) Macnalty, Sir A.S., Ed., *History of the Second World War. United Kingdom Medical Series. The Civilian Health and Medical Services.* Volume II. (London, 1955), p.265.

(135) *Report of the Department of Health for Scotland 1957.* Cmd. 385. (Edinburgh, 1958), p.26.

(136) There were 867 notified cases in 1972 and 2,621 in 1982.

(137) Scottish Home and Health Department. *Health in Scotland 1984*. (Edinburgh, 1985), pp.29–30.

(138) Scottish Home and Health Department. *Health Services in Scotland. Report for 1976*. Cmd. 6812. (Edinburgh, 1977), pp.5, 86–7.

(139) Scottish Home and Health Department. *Health Services in Scotland. Report for 1977*. Cmd. 7237. (Edinburgh, 1978), p.5.

(140) *Ibid*, p.11.

(141) Department of Health for Scotland. *Committee on Scottish Health Services Report*. Cmd. 5204. (Edinburgh, 1936), pp.399.

(142) *Scottish Health Statistics 1983*. (Edinburgh, 1984), p.60.

(143) Ferguson, T. *Scottish Social Welfare 1864–1914*. (Edinburgh & London, 1958), p.227.

(144) Department of Health for Scotland. *Committee on Scottish Health Services Report*. Cmd. 5204. (Edinburgh, 1936), pp.103–4.

(145) *Ibid*, p.106.

(146) *Ibid*, pp.107–13.

(147) Macnalty, Sir A.S., Ed., *History of the Second World War. United Kingdom Medical Series. The Civilian Health and Medical Services*. Volume II. (London, 1955), p.321–2.

(148) Ministry of Health. The Central Health Services Council and the Scottish Health Services Council. *Health Education Report of a Joint Committee of the Central and Scottish Health Services Councils*. (London, 1964), pp.58–61.

(149) *Report of the Department of Health for Scotland 1959*. Cmd. 983. (Edinburgh, 1960), p.60.

(150) Scottish Home and Health Department. *Health Services in Scotland. Report for 1974*. Cmd. 6052. (Edinburgh, 1975), p.37.

(151) Scottish Home and Health Department. Scottish Health Services Council. *Health Services in Scotland. Reports for 1972*. Cmd. 5323. (Edinburgh, 1973), p.55. The Annual Report for 1960 quoted one Medical Officer of Health remarking ruefully that "Efforts to bring to the notice of school children and youths the dangers of smoking have continued, but in view of the high pressure salesmanship directed to the opposite viewpoint by means of billboards, glossy magazine advertisements and T.V. presentations portraying the romance and joy of smoking particular brands of cigarettes, local anti-smoking propaganda is of little avail". *Report of the Department of Health for Scotland 1960. Part 1. Health and Welfare Services*. Cmd. 1320. (Edinburgh, 1961), p.21.

(152) Scottish Home and Health Department. *Health Services in Scotland. Report for 1977*. Cmd. 7237. (Edinburgh, 1978), p.20.

(153) Department of Health and Social Security. *Prevention and Health: everybody's business. A reassessment of public and personal health*. (London, 1976).

(154) Scottish Home and Health Department. *The Health Service in Scotland: the Way Ahead*. (Edinburgh, 1976).

(155) Department of Health and Social Security. Department of Education and Science. Scottish Office. Welsh Office. *Prevention and Health*. Cmd. 7047. (London, 1977)

(156) Scottish Home and Health Department. *Health Services in Scotland. Report for 1977*. Cmd. 7237. (Edinburgh, 1978), pp.21–3.

(157) Scottish Home and Health Department. *Health in Scotland 1980*. (Edinburgh, 1981), p.27.

(158) Scottish Home and Health Department. *Health in Scotland 1982*. (Edinburgh, 1982), p.33.

(159) *Ibid*, p.34.

(160) This part of the story is treated more fully in the introductory chapters.

(161) The importance of these services is such that they have been treated separately in the chapters written by Drs Tait and Clayson.

(162) Department of Health for Scotland. *Committee on Scottish Health Services Report*. Cmd. 5204. (Edinburgh, 1936), pp.162.

(163) Scottish Home and Health Department. *Community Medicine in Scotland*. (Edinburgh, 1973).

PART III:
Some Services etc. of Special Note

CONTENTS

1. *Mental Health and Mental Handicap*

A new look at old Patterns of Care

Drummond Hunter

CONTENTS

About the Author

T. DRUMMOND HUNTER, LL.B., F.H.S.M.

Educated at Edinburgh University (History and Law). After the Second World War, practised law in Ayrshire and in Edinburgh until 1955. From 1955 to 1974, he was Group Secretary and Treasurer of the Royal Edinburgh and Associated Hospitals; he was a member of the Scottish Health Services Council from 1958 to 1962. Member of Farquharson-Lang Committee on the Administrative Practice of Hospital Boards from 1962 to 1966. From 1974 to 1984 Secretary of the Scottish Health Service Planning Council. Presently Chairman of the Scottish Institute of Human Relations (since 1977) and Chairman of the Scottish Council on Disability (1985). Also since 1985, Chairman of Penumbra Limited – a company formed to promote supported accommodation for mentally ill young people who would otherwise have to be accommodated in mental hospitals.

Author's Note

An academic doctor who had a deep rooted aversion to 'standing hyp-
notised in front of the status quo', and who was determined not merely
to observe the world, but to change it, John Brotherston had three major
preoccupations: first, only if it acquired a strategic planning dimension
could the National Health Service function 'with integrated therapeutic
purpose', secondly, the 'powerhouse of the hospital' achieved maximum
effectiveness when it was able to share its resources with the community
service and, thirdly, public participation in the health care system was
the pre-condition of high professional standards, as well as of effective
services for priority groups like the elderly, the mentally ill, the mentally
handicapped and the disabled.

That the following paper (without that ever having been the intention) is an oblique commentary on these three preoccupations is a
testimony to their robustness and centrality.

'A New Look at Old Patterns of Care' describes how the mental health
and mental handicap services have moved, in this century, from the
particularist – concentrating on one part of the mind or of the body – first
to the whole person, and then to the whole person in his or her situation
in the whole community. Only the last section of the paper goes further
than Sir John might have been prepared to go; but he would have
applauded my right to stand on his shoulders.

Towards the end of his life, John Brotherston came to believe that
much of his struggle had been vain, as if some hidden spring had snapped
and things were whirling back to the very circumstances that he had
sought to change. Nothing ever turns out as one had hoped it would, but
it was difficult to convince Sir John (so imbued with scepticism had his
normally sanguine temperament become) that progress was a zig-zag
affair, with its own subtle dialectic, and that the most accurate motto for
the years which had followed his departure from the Scottish Office, in
1977, might yet turn out to be *'reculer pour mieux sauter'*.

Certainly, joint planning strategies, care in the community and public
participation have all quite suddenly acquired new momentum. If it has
sometimes seemed that 'consumerism' might be taking the place of genuine public participation, or that community care might have attractions
as a device for cutting back on the statutory services, the underlying
trend has been positive; and this is a more significant phenomenon than
the much acclaimed move (which Sir John distrusted) towards
Griffiths-type general managers.

William Morris wrote about 'how men fight and . . . the thing that they
fought for . . . when it comes, turns out to be not what they meant, and
other men have to fight for what they meant under another name'. It is
good to know that the goals in pursuit of which John Brotherston spent
his life are already being fought for all over again, with renewed fervour
and commitment.

Mental Health and Mental Handicap

A new look at old Patterns of Care

Past and Present

In Scotland, as in other civilised countries, perspectives on the mentally
ill changed dramatically at the end of the eighteenth century. This
wide-ranging development (its roots can be traced back to the humanism
of the Renaissance) has been called the First Psychiatric Revolution[1].
The Second Revolution, which stressed individual therapy rather than
social control and humane containment, took place at the beginning of
this century. Whether or not, or to what extent, it is correct to claim that
a Third Revolution has been in progress since the 1950s – a claim that
will be discussed in the last section of this paper – there can be no doubt
that, in the important advances which have characterised mental health
care since the last decades of the eighteenth century and right up to the
present time, the part played by Scotland has not been an insignificant
one.

The so-called First Psychiatric Revolution, and subsequent developments in the twentieth century, can be properly understood only if it
is recalled that, in medieval times, superstitious fears so abounded that
insanity, madness, lunacy – call it what you will – was associated with
witchcraft. This meant that, when healing wells (like the one at St Fillans
in Perthshire, referred to by Scott in 'Marmion') and other mystical
devices had failed to achieve a cure, there was the probability that
madness would end, not merely in cruelty and persecution, but actually
in death, as society purged itself of those whom it regarded as being
possessed by the Devil.

As the modern nation-states struggled into being in the seventeenth
and early eighteenth centuries, madness was secularised, so to speak, and
the emphasis was placed on social control, the means of such control
being the methods used for criminals, namely, the stocks, prisons, etc,
with the addition, for the mentally ill, of workhouses, and madhouses,
where these were available[2].

In 1785 Jean Colombier, Inspector General of French Hospitals and

Prisons, summed up the situation of the mentally ill, in Europe in the eighteenth century, in succinct and devastating terms:–

> "Thousands of lunatics are locked up in prisons without anyone even thinking of administering the slightest remedy. The half-mad are mingled with those who are totally deranged, those who rage with those who are quiet; some are in chains while others are free in their prison. Finally, unless nature comes to their aid by curing them, the duration of their misery is lifelong, for unfortunately the illness does not improve but only grows worse"[2].

Humane care of the insane was a consequence of the European Enlightenment. In tune with the humanitarian movement, which swept through the new nations of the West in the years before, and immediately after, the French Revolution, a new era was inaugurated for the mentally ill, when, in 1793, Dr Philippe Pinel (the first bust of whom, outside France, was to be placed above the arched entrance to the new Royal Edinburgh Asylum for Lunatics,which admitted its first patients in 1813) struck the shackles from the insane in the Bicêtre in Paris. It has been suggested that Pinel may have been influenced by the example of William Perfect, who, in England in 1776, had liberated a maniacal patient, confined in a work-house, from his chains[3]; and it is worthy of note that the charter for the first mental hospital, or asylum, in Scotland, namely, the Royal Asylum at Montrose (which was eventually opened in 1781) had been granted in that self-same year.

Scottish doctors, like Sir William Morrison (who instituted, in Edinburgh, in 1823, a course of lectures in mental diseases), Dr Andrew Combe and Sir Robert Christison, kept in close touch with the work of Pinel and his pupil Esquirol; and, in addition to the Montrose Royal Asylum, the following pioneer mental hospitals constituted by Charter and Act of Parliament, were established between 1800 and 1839:–

1781 Montrose Royal Asylum (now Sunnyside Hospital);

1800 Aberdeen Royal Asylum (now the Royal Cornhill Hospital);

1813 Royal Edinburgh Asylum (now the Royal Edinburgh Hospital);

1814 Glasgow Royal Asylum (now Gartnavel Royal Hospital);

1820 Dundee Royal Asylum (now Liff Royal Hospital);

1820 Perth Royal Asylum (now the Murray Royal Hospital);

1839 Crichton Royal Asylum (now the Crichton Royal Hospital).

Scotland's Royal Asylums set a model for the humane care of the mentally ill. This model was based on the psychological concept of 'moral management' of the insane, and it has been claimed that Dr W.A.F. Browne, the first Medical Superintendent of Sunnyside Hospital, who became Medical Superintendent of the Crichton Royal Hospital in 1838, and a Commissioner in Lunacy in 1857, anticipated modern techniques of group therapy with his realisation of the importance of the 'association of lunatics in groups'[4]. Perhaps, however, what was important at that time about the model was the fact that it was a medical model, rather than a model based on the belief that, where they were not possessed by the Devil, the mentally ill were criminals.

Although it is clear that Scotland was in close touch with progressive psychiatric thinking, the Royal Asylums were mainly for private patients, i.e. they were mainly for the respectable ladies and gentlemen of Scotland, who had fallen prey to 'mental maladies', and for whom there had to be provided a serene and well ordered environment in which they could be maintained at the level of comfort to which they had become accustomed[5].

A very different story prevailed with regard to pauper lunatics, who could be found, in workhouses and poorhouses, lying naked on straw in the most miserable circumstances conceivable; and it is well-known that it was the spectacle of the poet Fergusson, lying at death's door under such conditions, that inspired Dr Andrew Duncan, President of the Royal College of Physicians of Edinburgh, to found the Royal Edinburgh Hospital. This sordid and deplorable situation was not put to rights until Dorothea Lynde Dix, pioneer, as she was, of asylum reform in America, intervened personally with the British Government in 1855, after a visit to Scotland, which had filled her with indignation and horror[3].

This intervention led to the Lunacy (Scotland) Act 1857, and, in due course, to the provision of district asylums for the poor throughout the country. The Act also set up the General Board of Commissioners in Lunacy for Scotland.

The new asylums represented a substantial investment of resources; but what the House of Commons Select Committee on Social Welfare, referring, in its recent report on Community Care, to the growth of asylums throughout Britain in the nineteenth century, called 'an astonishing commitment of money on staff and buildings'[6] is less astonishing than it seems when it is appreciated that it was a wholly characteristic nineteenth century development, since the commitment was not so much to health care as to social control and, in effect, to a legalistic, as well as to a medical, solution of the problem of mental illness. Viewed from an eighteenth century perspective, the transferring of mental illness from the witch-hunting, or criminal, to the medical, arena was an important gain. The use of doctors as an instrument of State control, i.e. chiefly for the protection of the public, seems less acceptable when viewed from the standpoint of the twentieth century[7].

In the last analysis, just as the first public health department in Edinburgh consisted of a doctor and two policemen[8], so the nineteenth century asylums were medico-legal, rather than purely medical institutions[9].

Clearly, Bentham's notion that law was collective medicine also meant that, in the nineteenth century, medicine (and in particular psychiatric medicine) was dangerously close to being an agency of the law (note *(a)*).

This became more apparent as the nineteenth century progressed, and we can now see that, in the same way as superstitious beliefs in lunacy-healing wells rapidly degenerated into torture and burning at the stake, and in the same way as crude notions about social control quickly became synonymous in the seventeenth and eighteenth centuries with the brutal repression of the insane, so moral management regimes equally rapidly degenerated into the legalistic custodialism, which increasingly typified Scottish asylums as the nineteenth century wore on – this custodialism involving a return to those methods of restraint and seclusion, which had largely been abandoned during the 'moral management' era, as this era was best defined, perhaps, by Amariah Brigham in 1847:–

> "The removal of the insane from home and former associations, with respectful and kind treatment under all circumstances, and in most cases manual labour, attendance on religious worship on Sunday, the establishment of regular habits and of self-control, diversion of the mind from morbid trains of thought, are now generally considered as essential in the Moral treatment of the Insane"[2].

If the therapeutic pessimism, and the organic or hereditary concepts of mental illness which accompanied custodialism, were to be overcome, there had to be a break with the past; and, although the Kraepelinian system of classification (note *(b)*), and the search for an organic basis for mental illness continued to be prominent in the early part of this century, much more significant in the event was the parallel work on motivation, which focused on the search for underlying psychological and emotional factors in the genesis of abnormal reactions and called in question, therefore, institutional methods and treatment. Also beginning to be stressed, even at this early date, was the need for a thorough study of the social factors involved in mental illness[10]. This trend towards a primary emphasis on the patients' personality, and on the dynamics of his life history, led in the years immediately before and after the First World War, to such a complete reorientation of the psychiatric approach and point of view that it is not an exaggeration to refer to the changes which took place in these years as the Second Psychiatric Revolution[1]. We shall see presently what the fruits of this revolution were, and how it led, later in the century, to claims that a Third Psychiatric Revolution[1] was under way.

Unaffected by humanitarian considerations until the middle of the nineteenth century, the services for the mentally handicapped in Scotland have become progressively more linked with the mental health services, a process which was first given formal recognition in the Mental Deficiency and Lunacy (Scotland) Act 1913. The seal was set on this rapprochement by the Mental Health (Scotland) Act 1960, which bracketed mental illness and mental handicap together under the term 'mental disorder'. This grouping together of the two services was not altered by the Mental Health (Scotland) Act 1984.

Simultaneously (and somewhat paradoxically) the social and educational aspects of mental handicap, which were well recognised in the nineteenth century and earlier this century, have begun in Scotland, as elsewhere[11], to assume importance all over again.

As indicated above, institutional care of the mentally handicapped developed later in Scotland than institutional care for the mentally ill. This was due to a general belief in this country in the early years of the nineteenth century (in spite of enlightened developments, at that time, in France and Switzerland) that special services were not needed for idiots, imbeciles and other mentally subnormal people[12]. In the past, in rural communities, handicapped people had been treated with a high degree of tolerance; and it was only as the twin processes of industrialisation and urbanisation accelerated that the level of social and other skills required of people, if they were to survive in, and not impede the functioning of, the open society which was now coming into existence, was raised to such an extent that institutional care for the mentally handicapped became an imperative need.

The provision of such care in Scotland, on a country-wide basis, did not get properly under way until after the First World War, as the reports of the Board of Control between 1914 and 1930 clearly reveal[13].

As the whole question of institutional (rather than community) care for the mentally handicapped has recently become even more problematic than the question of such care for the mentally ill, it is ironical that the programme of institutional provision initiated by the 1913 Act, but not activated until the 1920s and 1930s because of the First World War, is only now reaching completion. This 'time lag' has ensured for Scotland's most recently completed hospitals for the mentally handicapped a somewhat ambivalent reception. This was only to be expected, since it had become increasingly clear, in the 60's and 70's, that jointly planned and community-based local services were the best way of meeting the needs of people with mental handicap[14].

A brief and impressionistic glance at the history of the mental health and mental handicap services in Scotland cannot do justice to the complex issues involved, but it is important to take some account of the ways in which these services have developed, because more, perhaps, than is the case in regard to any other form of medical or social care in Scotland, the present pattern of services for the mentally disordered is not only a product, it is also a prisoner, of the past. Paradoxically, our nineteenth century forebears, in their deeply concerned search for order, stability and permanence, may, in some respects, have presented the generations succeeding them with patterns of care which have proved difficult to adapt to the turbulent environment of the twentieth century. In relation to the mental health services, the difficulties involved in moving out from the old mental hospitals towards new patterns of provision have been well-expressed in a recent writer's concern 'to recognise the extent of past investment – both human and financial – in the mental hospitals and the need to use these resources creatively in the gradual movement towards alternative forms of provision'[15]. Both in the mental health field and in that of mental handicap, the central question is how best to manage the major transition involved in developing new patterns of care so that, rather than clinging tenaciously to their traditional functions (or becoming increasingly abandoned as new resources are established) the great institutions inherited from the past, and representing, in their day, a dramatic advance in the care and treatment of the mentally ill and the mentally handicapped, are so transformed in their role that they are able to make their own distinctive contribution to the progressive development of that integrated range of local services (involving a new emphasis on day care) which is now seen to be the way forward[11, 16].

The Mental Health Services

1900–1948: De-Asylumising the Asylum

Whereas the First Psychiatric Revolution revolved round the name of Pinel, the Second Revolution revolved round that of Freud[1]. Taking place, as it did, at the turn of this century, this second wave of development was sparked off by the therapeutic pessimism characteristic of the 'tranquil and orderly' custodialism, to which institutional psychiatry had regressed in the later years of the nineteenth century, when the causes of insanity 'in order of their influence' were considered to be 'heredity, orginal mental constitution, original physical constitution and physical disease'[17].

Freud, of course, had his predecessors, such as Dubois, Janet, Breuer and many others, and he had contemporaries in Jung and Adler, who diverged in opposite directions, but it was he (although psychologists like William James were moving in the same direction) who became the symbol of the distinctive contribution of this period, namely, the exploration of the psycho-dynamic aspects of psychiatric disorders.

As Macfie Campbell, the Scottish psychiatrist, who went to America from the Royal Edinburgh Hospital towards the end of the 20's, and some years later became Professor of Psychiatry at Harvard, so cogently expressed it:–

> "The problem of the psychiatrist was no longer to identify a clinical picture but to get to grips with the actual dynamic situation, to reconstruct in detail the life history, with atten-

tion to the sensitizing or conditioning influence of environmental factors and with due appreciation of the nature of
emotional disturbances, of substitutes and evasive reactions,
of symbolic expressions, of the various modes of getting satisfaction for the complicated needs of the individual"[18].

If Pinel had opened the door to the humane treatment of the mentally
ill, he had done so in what was still a social control context. Freud opened
the door to the treatment of mentally ill people as individual human
beings, in whom inner motivation was more important than pressure
from without and who, in their psychological evolution, had encountered
problems of living, with which they could be helped to cope.

The movement pioneered by Freud (but soon going beyond his
biological determinism, as, for example, in the internationally recognised
work of the Scottish psycho-analyst, W.R.D. Fairbairn, who, with his
emphasis on human, or object, relations, has been credited [19] with
turning Freud the right way up) initiated an era of therapeutic optimism
and brought psychiatry, as 'medicine's other half', into that condition of
parity with physical medicine,which had eluded the nineteenth century
asylum psychiatrists, or 'alienists'.

As infectious diseases began to be brought under control, the demand
for psychiatric treatment grew. Although, in its first flush of proselytising
zeal, psycho-analysis had sometimes worn an aspect of 'psychiatry unlimited'[20], this had been followed by a period of disillusionment and
cynicism, since a psycho-analytically orientated approach could never
have coped with the total burden of psychiatric illness (not to speak of
alcohol problems, drug abuse and social pathologies like war and crime).
Nevertheless, in order to forestall criticisms in regard to the 'medica-
lisation' of human problems, like the criticisms later to be levelled at
doctors by Ivan Ilich and others, this reaction went too far; and, whether
it was a question of taking issue with, or fervently advocating, psycho-
analysis, it is hardly in doubt that the emphasis on the psycho-dynamics
of individual growth and development was the yeast which created the
remarkable ferment in the mental health services at the beginning of this
century, and which still, as it continues to acquire new insights, leavens
the eclectic approach of most Scottish psychiatrists.

The reaction against legalism and custodialism, described by Dr
George Robertson, Physician Superintendent of the Royal Edinburgh
Hospital from 1908–1932, as 'the de-asylumising of the asylum', had
already begun to make itself felt in the last decades of the nineteenth
century. As early as 1869, indeed, the revolutionary policy of 'open
doors' for asylums was recommended; but, although 'this system (note
(c)) was another example of the commendable attempt to assimilate the
conditions of asylum life to ordinary life'[21], this proposal was premature
– so premature, in fact, 'that open doors' began to be widely adopted in
Scottish mental hospitals only in the 1950s and 1960s.

By the turn of the century, however, and even if only in a limited way as yet, the policy of 'de-asylumising the asylum' finally entered the realm of the practicable and the possible.

A significant development at this time was the progressive diminution in the use of restraint and seclusion in Scottish asylums. Between 1896 and 1911 there was 'a remarkable falling off' in the use of these methods, as shown in the following table[17]:–

	Average yearly no. of patients	Average yearly no. of patients restrained			Average yearly no. restrained per 100 resident	Average yearly no. subjected to seclusion	Average yearly no. secluded per 100 resident
		For surgical	For other reasons	Total			
1896–1901	10,805	8.4	50.8	59.2	0.55	114.0	1.05
1902–1906	12,360	9.2	27.2	36.4	0.29	72.4	0.59
1907–1911	13,812	11.2	21.4	32.6	0.24	30.6	0.22

In the Mental Deficiency and Lunacy (Scotland) Act 1913[22], there was an important mental health provision which simplified the practice of voluntary admission, long favoured by the Commissioners in Lunacy, by making it possible for a person to avoid the need for certification and to enter an asylum 'as a voluntary boarder', on his or her own written application.

From this time on the proportion of voluntary boarders to certified admissions steadily increased; and, in one of the Royal Hospitals, the number of voluntary admissions in 1923 actually exceeded the number admitted compulsorily[23].

The 1913 Act was also important in the administration of the mental health services in Scotland, since it abolished the General Board of Commissioners in Lunacy set up by the 1857 Act, and replaced it by the General Board of Control for Scotland. This Board, which was invested with responsibility for overseeing the mental handicap, as well as the mental illness, services, survived until the Mental Health (Scotland) Act 1960, when it was replaced by The Mental Welfare Commission, which is less concerned with control than with the rights of individual patients.

The system of voluntary admissions, as simplified by the 1913 Act, was highly relevant to the process of assimilating the asylum to the general hospital. Other important developments in this direction were, first, the practice, which, by 1914, had been accepted in a number of the larger Scottish asylums, of appointing lady matrons to be in charge of the whole asylum under the Medical Superintendent (with night matrons in charge of both male and female staff), secondly, the appointment of trained hospital nurses designated as 'Assistant Matrons' to control and supervise each division of the asylum under the matron; and, thirdly, the employment of a greatly increased staff of female nurses on the male side of the institution[22].

A further significant bridge between psychiatry and general medicine came into being, in the early years of the twentieth century, when observation wards were established in many of the large general hospitals. Pressure for the establishment of special wards for the mentally ill in general hospitals had been building up throughout the latter part of the nineteenth century, because psychiatrists like Mitchell, Sibbald, Skae, Clouston and Macpherson believed that such an arrangement, apart from its advantage from the teaching point of view, would create a more optimistic outlook and would expedite recovery; and, in 1887, Dr John Carswell, Certifying Physician in Lunacy and Lecturer in Mental Diseases, Anderson College, Glasgow, who believed that 'all recent cases of mental disease should be treated in hospital reception homes before being sent to asylums', had been the first person in Scotland to make arrangements for the treatment, in two wards of Barnhill Parochial Hospital, of temporary, non-certified patients[12].

It was not until 1904, however, that the Corporation of the City of Glasgow, impressed by the success of the Barnhill policy, provided wards to accommodate 50 patients at Duke Street General Hospital, where Carswell took charge until he was succeeded by Dr Ivy Mackenzie. In 1922 another 120 observation beds were established at Stobhill. Thus were the first steps taken in an important new development in the psychiatric services, which probably did more than anything else, at that time, 'to dissipate the mysticism which surrounded the treatment of mental disorder'[12].

When, in 1932, he was appointed Consultant Psychiatrist to the Royal Infirmary of Edinburgh, Dr David (later Sir David) Henderson, who had also been appointed in that year Physician Superintendent of the Royal Edinburgh Hospital and Professor of Psychiatry at Edinburgh University, was permitted to supplement the clinical instruction of students and postgraduates by demonstrating psychiatric syndromes which were seldom seen in mental hospitals but were a frequent occurrence in general practice. 'Their rapid and successful treatment' he was to write later, 'did more to educate the medical profession, and to break down prejudice, than years of talking'[12]. Professor Henderson's experience is particularly interesting, because it shows how, out of these early observation wards for the treatment of psychiatric emergencies, there grew the more sophisticated psychiatric units in general hospitals, which are now accepted policy and which deal with all those manifestations of mental illness that call for in-patient treatment, but not for admission to a mental hospital.

Sometimes such clinics were established at the mental hospital, as when Dr Robertson, conscious of the fact that officers and men returning from the 1914–18 war in severe states of mental and nervous breakdown should not be admitted to the asylum, and impatient with the out-of-date legal statutes that governed the admission and treatment of patients, persuaded the managers of the Royal Edinburgh Hospital, in the 1920s, not only to build a new wall so that one wing of West House (now Mackinnon House) would be left outside the asylum and could thus be designated the Jordanburn Nerve Hospital and Psychological Institute, but also to establish a number of Nursing Homes, principally in the vicinity of Craig House (opened as a private hospital by Sir Thomas Clouston in 1894) in which, as in Jordanburn Hospital, treatment could be given informally.

The establishment of psychiatric out-patient departments at general hospitals was a further development, in the early years of this century, which helped to consolidate the links between the psychiatric and the acute services. The first out-patient psychiatric clinic of this kind in Scotland was set up, in 1910, at the Western Infirmary in Glasgow by Dr L.R. Oswald, Physician Superintendent, at that time, of Gartnavel Royal Hospital[12].

Dr Robertson also took another initiative, in the preventive field, when he established in 1929 a Psychiatric Out-Patient Clinic for Children (like the clinics for adults already established at the Royal Infirmary and at Jordanburn Hospital). This was a manifestation, in Scotland, of the concern for all phases of child development, which characterised the psychiatric services of many countries in the early twentieth century.

Dr Robertson had also been responsible for instituting, in 1912, a postgraduate course for the Diploma in Psychiatry – the first of its kind in Scotland. His own appointment, in 1918, as the first Professor of Psychiatry in Scotland, and his election, in 1925, as President of the Royal College of Physicians, constituted notable landmarks in the struggle of Scottish psychiatry to gain its proper place in the medical firmament; and it is worth noting that Sir David Henderson, Robertson's successor, both as Physician Superintendent of the Royal Edinburgh Hospital and as Professor of Psychiatry at Edinburgh University, was also, in due course, elected President of the Royal College of Physicians.

Although there had been a Lectureship of Psychiatry at Glasgow University since 1880 (the Lecturer, however, *not* being a member of the Faculty of Medicine) and although a similar Lectureship was established at Aberdeen in 1927, Chairs in Psychiatry, or Mental Health, were not established at Glasgow, Aberdeen and Dundee until 1944, 1940 and 1962 respectively (note *(d)*). Thus it came about that the teaching of psychiatry gradually, but none the less perceptibly, began to bulk more largely in the medical curriculum, the overall tendency being to cut loose from Kraepelinian descriptions of psychotic syndromes and to utilise psychological principles and reaction types[12].

Important advances were also made, during the early years of the century, in the education and training of mental nurses; and one of the effects of the Great War of 1914–18 was that it quickened the pace of psychiatric advance, just as it quickened the pace of technological and social advance. The same was true, but at a deeper level, perhaps, of the Second World War. This war finally put an end to many of the enthusiasms and illusions of the Freudian years, in particular the illusion that psychiatry could prevent war. At the same time, however, it gave an immense fillip to the importance of psychiatric skills, not only in the assessment and selection of officers, for example[24], but also in rehabilitation, the group therapy work carried out at Northfield with returned prisoners of war being particularly important for the future[25,26].

So what was the position in the years immediately following the Second World War? The formal link with general medicine and the genuine acceptance of psychiatry as 'medicine's other half' were all but accomplished. It was a crucial achievement. On the other hand, it was only the end of the beginning. The policy of de-asylumising the asylum had focused mainly on medicalising psychiatry and had actually left the asylum system more or less intact, with patients still occupying unnacceptably large wards, in buildings that went back to the middle or late years of the nineteenth century, and with some fairly formidable Physician Superintendents in charge of the major hospitals, who had not been able wholly to rid themselves of paternalism, and of the custodial ethos (note*(e)*). If anything, indeed, the whole system of caring for the mentally ill in Scotland was under greater pressure than ever before, at this time, because of the overcrowding which had inevitably taken place during the War and which was still unalleviated in the late 1950s. How this problem was tackled is the subject of the next section of this chapter.

The Mental Health Services

1948–1985: Medicine's Other Half

Since it brought them into the same political, administrative and financial arena as the general medical services, the coming into being, in 1948 of the National Health Service was an important milestone in the development of Scotland's mental health services.

All the earlier illusions about the unlimited potential of psychiatry having been abandoned, their place was taken by a new awareness of the problems of Scotland's mental hospitals which were largely, as we have seen, a legacy of the nineteenth century. Now it had become a question, not merely of psychiatrists being trained and practising their art like other doctors – and thereby ensuring great improvements in the *physical* health of their patients[27] – but, above all, of the mental hospitals, where these psychiatrists were based, throwing off their aura of custodialism and taking their place alongside other hospitals as centres of active treatment and rehabilitation. Nineteenth century concepts of legalism and custodialism had to be overcome, not only at the *professional*, but also at the *institutional* level.

This meant the development of new medical and rehabilitative techniques for dealing with mental illness. In Scotland some of these techniques may have stemmed, directly or indirectly, from the research into the pathology of mental illness carried out in the laboratory of the Scottish Asylums, which had been set up in Edinburgh in 1897, under the direction of Dr W. Forbes Robertson, and which had survived until 1932.

One of the most important techniques, however, was electroconvulsive therapy (ECT) pioneered by Cerletti and Bini in 1938[28] and brought into extensive, and much more sophisticated, use in the 1950s. On occasion, after the Second World War, lobotomies were performed; and insulin, or deep coma therapy, which had raised hopes before the war, was still in use in one or two Scottish hospitals in the 1960s, although its chief value seems to have resided in the 'placebo' effect which any intensive approach tends to produce.

The most effective technological advance was the revolution in chemotherapy, which began to get under way in the mid 1950s, and which, in the next three decades, produced a whole range of new, powerful and highly effective, drugs, whose side-effects, if they are administered for the wrong reasons, can be damaging.

If, in this account, strictly medical techniques have been referred to first, it is not because these techniques were necessarily first in order of significance from a strictly therapeutic point of view. Indeed, from a Freudian perspective (Freud had distrusted the 'medical model') such techniques could be held to have marked a regression (in modern, hidden form) to those methods of physical restraint to which the 'moral management' regimes of the early nineteenth century had ultimately returned. Paradoxically, however, the new techniques of 'restraint' were also liberating in important ways, since they could be seen as the essential preliminaries which made the patient accessible (first) to more fundamental psychotherapeutic, sociotherapeutic and behavioural approaches and (secondly) to care in the community.

The burgeoning of this wide range of new therapies and rehabilitative techniques involved doctors and nurses in acquiring new skills. In particular the therapeutic role of the nurse was accorded proper recognition, as was that of the social worker. Clinical psychologists began to make an increasingly important contribution, both in an investigatory and in a therapeutic role[29]. Creative arts therapies appeared on the scene; and occupational, recreational and industrial therapy were developed in more therapeutically purposive ways.

The most striking immediate change in the mental hospital, as a result of these advances in treatment, was the addition of a short-stay function to its traditional 'asylum', or long-stay, function. Admissions to such hospitals have increased steadily over the years since 1948, but because many conditions can now be treated on a short-term, or even on an out-patient or day-patient basis, this change has been accompanied by a decrease in bed numbers[30].

The Mental Health (Scotland) Act 1960, which recognised the legal implications of these clinical developments, and, in effect, equated mental hospitals with general hospitals, gave further impetus to the liberalisation of the mental health services. Today, some 90 *per cent* of all admissions are informal, ('voluntary' admission having been abolished by the Act) and only a small minority of patients are admitted comulsorily.

The initial reduction in bed numbers in mental hospitals, which resulted, in large measure, from these advances in treatment, led in England to forecasts of a dramatic reduction in the need for mental hospital, in-patient provision. These forecasts were not accepted in Scotland; and, in fact, they were disproved, in due course, by events south of the Border[6].

The truth is that the new, short-stay units frequently functioned on the 'revolving door' principle, and on the basis of a heavy re-admission rate. Moreover, it was clear that hospital facilities would continue to be required for functional and organic illness, personality disorders, and increasingly for some problems of misuse of alcohol and drugs[16]. It was also clear that there would be a growing need for in-patient services for the elderly with mental disability[31].

The suspicion that, by means of the 'revolving door', the symptoms were being alleviated, while the problems remained, led to a new emphasis on rehabilitation techniques which by tackling the 'hard core' opened up a 'Second Front' and thereby reduced the existing overcrowding in mental hospitals. In this respect the 'social therapies', to which patients were now accessible, assumed a special significance. The great value of these therapies was that they could liberate long-stay patients from institutional care and make it possible for them to resume their place in the community.

The pressing need to overcome institutionalisation (note *(f)*) had already led to the concept of the 'open door' hospital, which was pioneered at Dingleton Hospital, Melrose, by Dr George Bell, who reported that the process of opening the doors of all the wards at Dingleton had been completed as early as 1949[32]. Dr Bell was a shrewd and enlightened Scottish psychiatrist, whose long experience in mental hospitals had led him to the view that the first essential of all further advance in mental hospital treatment depended on an 'open door' approach. He was also well aware of the negative consequences of stigma and 'labelling' (and, therefore, of the key role of public relations) long before these topics became the subject of important studies by Goffman[33], R.D. Laing[34], Szasz[35], Scheff[36] and others.

Unsparing in his efforts to prepare the local community for the action which he was about to take, Dr Bell was convinced that only in a mental hospital with open doors could there be released these psychodynamic forces within the individual patients (and within the members of the nursing and medical staff) which were the basis of good patient/staff relationships and which 'kindled a flame of hope leading ultimately to discharge after many years of residence'[32].

Not everyone in Scotland agreed with this diagnosis; but, while freedom was not the only therapeutic measure employed at Dingleton, Dr Bell took the determined view that it was the essential first step and that the alternative to freedom was no longer acceptable:

> "The ultimate fate of almost any chronic mental patient under the locked door system is dementia. This is not so in the milieu of the open door; the disease, if not cured, can be alleviated and there is evidence that the process of mental deterioration can be reversed. If widely adopted, the system will inevitably lead to a steadily diminishing number of patients in mental hospitals and effect a substantial saving in the National Health Service"[32].

These developments at Dingleton (one of the first mental hospitals in the world – if not the first – to open *all* its doors) led in due course (although misgivings about the possible over-use of drugs, in the process of liberating patients, continued to be expressed in some quarters) to a general acceptance of the 'open door' philosophy. 'The success which Bell has attained', wrote Sir D.K. Henderson, 'is extremely gratifying; he has put his beliefs and methods to a severe test, but with the aid of splendid community relationships, and to a lesser extent by the use of modern physical and pharmacological treatment he can be proud of his achievements'[12].

It was left to another Scottish psychiatrist, Dr Maxwell Jones (internationally known for his use of 'social psychiatry' concepts at the Henderson Hospital) who came to Dingleton as Physical Superintendent in 1962 (remaining there until 1969), to carry forward Dr Bell's work by developing the hospital into a 'therapeutic community', in which everyone involved (including the patients themselves) 'became the doctor', the essence of therapy being the development of responsible and mutually supportive relationships within the traditional hierarchical structure of the hospital[37].

These group therapy and therapeutic community concepts, which were derived from the work of sociologists and social anthropologists, as well as of psychiatrists, and which were central to the approach of the now growing number of 'social psychiatrists', had clear affinities with the 'whole person' approach. This had played a significant part in Scottish psychiatry ever since at different times earlier in the century, Sir David Henderson and Dr R.D. Gillespie, co-authors, in 1928, of the still widely used *Textbook of Psychiatry*, had worked with Adolf Meyer at the 'psycho-biologically' orientated Phipps Clinic, which is attached to the Johns Hopkins Hospital in Baltimore.[38]

Himself a protegé of Sir David Henderson, Maxwell Jones extended the concept of the whole person to the whole ward and to the whole hospital; and in his last years at Dingleton, he was already beginning to extend it to the whole community outside the hospital[39], in what was effectively an extension of psychiatric concepts into the wider, political arena. This, as we have seen, had sometimes led to burnt fingers in the past, but however tentatively it was now being embarked upon, it could hardly be regarded as not having a unique and highly significant con-tribution to make to these wider issues; and it is worth noting that Maxwell Jones has made this the central theme of his work in America over the last fifteen years.

Coinciding with these profound changes in mental hospital régimes, which were aimed at helping them to throw off their inherited mantle of legalism, a great many practical steps were taken to improve the rehabil-itation and resettlement services by developing industrial therapy, as we have seen, along more purposive lines, by setting up social skills and aids-to-daily living units in the hospital and by establishing links with rehabilitative and social facilities in the community. Through this special emphasis on rehabilitation, both occupational therapists and social workers, whose contribution in this field had always been a key one, acquired a greatly enlarged importance in the mental health team, which has not diminished now that it is increasingly a question of 'alter-natives to employment' for many of those who have been mentally ill.

Because of these developments, mental hospitals in Scotland gradually began to reach out into the communities which they served[40]. Some long-stay patients were able to return to their own homes, others were provided with different forms of accommodation in the community, whether what was involved was a hostel or half-way house, some form of supported accommodation, a group home, sheltered housing, ordinary housing, guardianship or whatever. It was, and still is, a valid criticism that these facilities tended (and still tend) to be provided in a piecemeal and unco-ordinated fashion[16] without their necessarily having access to appropriate day services, like those which are now provided in day hospitals and, to a minuscule extent, in local authority or voluntary day centres.

This emphasis on care in the community had received its first explicit formulation in the Report of the Royal Commission on the 'Law relating to Mental Illness and Mental Deficiency' which had been published as long ago as 1957[41].

Highly critical of the inappropriate confinement of patients for long periods in institutions in which they were inevitably cut off from normal life, the Commission made its position clear in the following passage:–

"The recommendations of our witnesses are generally in favour of a shift of emphasis from hospital care to community care. In relation to almost all forms of mental disorder there is increasing medical emphasis on forms of treatment and training and social services which can be given without bringing patients into hospitals as in-patients or make it possible to discharge them from hospital sooner than was usual in the past".

The Commission's Report applied only to England and Wales, but its recommendation that there should be a shift of emphasis from hospital to community care was also specifically endorsed, so far as Scotland was concerned, by the 1958 and 1959 reports of the Dunlop Committee[42,43].

The main task, therefore, of the mental health services in the 1950s and 1960s was to reduce the number of beds required for mental illness by:

(1) Providing alternative systems of support in the community and getting as many as possible long-term patients back into the community;

(2) Avoiding hospital stay and reducing it to a minimum through the provision of treatment on a short-term basis;

(3) Developing the primary mental health services.

Rehabilitation psychiatry, as we have seen, is that special area of psychiatry which is concerned with the problem of returning long-stay patients to the community, from what might have become (had there been an exclusive focus on short-term treatment) the dangerously neglected 'back wards' of the hospital. In important respects, as we have seen, rehabilitation, or tertiary prevention, with some 41 *per cent* of National Health Service hospital beds occupied by mental patients, was the strategic factor in the 1950s and 1960s.

There was also a rapid development in Scotland between 1948 and 1986 of special interests within the psychiatry of secondary prevention, for example, child and adolescent psychiatry, forensic psychiatry, liaison psychiatry, drug addiction, the psychiatry of old age, alcohol-related problems, crisis intervention, and community psychiatry. It is a strength of Scottish psychiatry, however, that these special interests have all tended to develop *within* general psychiatry and have not involved psychiatrists in 'splitting off' into separate specialisms[16].

The invaluable contribution made to secondary prevention by this growth of specialist skills, and by the development of short-stay facilities within the mental hospital, has already been emphasised.

In the field of primary prevention, Scottish psychiatrists also took important initiatives, between 1948 and 1986, in developing out-patient clinics in the community, and in beginning to work more closely than in the past both with the primary health care team and with voluntary agencies. At the same time steps were taken to foster mental health education, both nationally and locally, and voluntary participation in the mental health services was encouraged, as never before, in Scotland.

These were developments of key significance, because it had already become clear, in the late 1960s and early 1970s, that the bulk of mild to less mild mental illness could best be treated or managed in the community, and that the next phase for the mental health services should be care in the community, not merely as an extension of, but essentially as an alternative to, hospital care, and as a method not so much of 'turning on the tap of hospital discharges' (tertiary prevention) as of 'turning off the tap of admissions' (primary prevention)[44].

The reorganisation of the National Health Service, in 1974, when taken in conjunction with the re-organisation of local authorities a year later, was particularly significant for the mental health services, since it reinforced the trend towards shared care in the community, with the hospital becoming an alternative to community care.

In the 1950s and 1960s, because of the outward pressure exerted by overcrowded mental hospitals as they tried to extend the care of their patients into the community, it had sometimes seemed that the mental health services radiated outwards from the mental hospital. After the 1974 reorganisation of the National Health Service, this view gradually changed. Mental health was increasingly seen to be something which was best provided for in the community, and which became a matter for the mental hospital only when day care and other community based strategies had failed. Community psychiatrists began to have an active role, the first appointment of such a specialist having been made at Craigmillar in Edinburgh several years before the 1974 reorganisation. As indicated above, it was particularly emphasised, in regard to this special interest, that it, too, should not be divorced from general psychiatry. Indeed, instead of the community psychiatrist being a special kind of psychiatrist, every psychiatrist should, perhaps, be a special kind of community psychiatrist, with an increasingly significant consultative (as distinct from treatment) role in a wide variety of community settings[16].

Similarly, with the growing emphasis on sectorisation[16], with mental hospitals sub-dividing themselves into smaller living units, (which would ideally be provided in the localities which they served) and with nursing staff uniforms becoming less formal, or going out of use altogether in some wards, it was almost beginning to be possible to look upon the mental hospital, in its increasingly *supportive* role, as a special facet of a community based pattern of care, and upon mental hospital nurses as special instances of the nurses employed in the community psychiatric nursing services, which had first come into existence in the late 1960s and early 1970s and were now, in the 1980s, developing important links with the primary health care team.

Given the renewed emphasis, after 1974, on community based patterns of care, there were important developments in the general practitioner services, which recognised the key contribution of the general practitioner, who, with one third to one half of his work-load being mental-health-related, was calculated to be coping with the vast bulk of relatively straightforward mental health problems.

Among these developments were vocational training in mental health, closer contacts with the specialist mental health services, and a growing tendency to work in wider networks, involving other agencies, both statutory and voluntary.[16]

There were also important developments after 1974 in the involvement of the re-organised local authorities, particularly the new regional social work departments, in the mental health services[45]. At first it was thought that the absorption of National Health Service psychiatric social workers into the new social work departments would be a retrogressive step. In fact, this structural change opened up an indispensable channel of communication with these departments. Fears that psychiatric social workers would lose their specialist skills, and simply become generic social workers, proved to be ill-founded; and, in due course, with the passing of the Mental Health (Scotland) Act 1984, Mental Health Officers were scheduled to reappear on the scene in a new role.

Valuable developments also took place in the voluntary sector, both through the restructuring of the Scottish Association for Mental Health (and the setting up of energetic local associations, like Link in Glasgow) and through the growth of self-help groups, which was still in progress, when this paper was being written, with the setting up of a group on Alzheimer's Disease and of Scottish Action on Dementia (SAD).

Although all three of these new agencies had done little more than establish contact with each other, 'at the coal face', in the years between 1974 and 1986, and had not yet succeeded *pace* in the Joint Liaison Committees recommended in 1977 by the Mitchell Report[46], in realising their full potential in a properly integrated mental health service, this should not be allowed to obscure the fact that, in spite of financial difficulties and the difficulties involved in settling into their new roles, these agencies *had* established positive contacts at the individual level and were, therefore, ready in the mid 1980s for the more ambitious task of planning and delivering services in that co-ordinated way, which is now seen to be the *sine qua non* of an effective mental health service.

The years between 1948 and 1985 saw many promising changes in the mental health services in Scotland, not least in significant moves towards integrated mental health services for children and young people[47]; but these changes were still mainly on the periphery of an inherited pattern of services, which remained stubbornly in place. Local changes, which pointed in the direction of community care, could not realise their full potential because they were not replicated by those changes at the centre which are essential if innovative approaches are not to wither on the bough[45].

In consequence, if there was good reason to applaud change and innovation during these years, there was also good reason to be frustrated by the apparent inertia of local authorities, health boards and the central government, as if all progress in this field had seized up and the iron law of the *status quo* had taken over.

No doubt the statistical projections of Tooth and Brooke were rejected in Scotland[16], not simply on technical grounds, but also because it was instinctively (and realistically) concluded that it would not be easy to escape from the country's traditional reliance on institutional forms of provision. But there is always the danger that realism of this kind will also become a self-fulfilling prophecy.

In Scotland, at the end of 1961, there were 19,672 mentally ill patients occupying hospital in-patient places, corresponding to 3.8 per thousand population, or 15 *per cent* more proportionately than England and Wales[48]. This heavy dependence on hospital care went hand in hand with a very low level of activity in the local health and welfare services. Indeed, between 1951 and 1962, local authority expenditure on mental health services remained constant, which means that it actually declined very substantially in real terms. Such provision as was made seems to have been in the field of mental handicap, and the expansion of local authority services in the 1960s hardly touched on the mentally ill.

The Scottish psychiatric in-patient population remained remarkably stable during the 1950s and 1960s and changes in subsequent years were marginal rather than substantial. Up to and including 1973 the total resident population fluctuated between 19,000 and 20,000. This prevalence rate has to be compared with the contemporary English occupancy rate of 1.9. Scotland, with little more than one-tenth of the population of England and Wales, had one-fifth of their number of psychiatric in-patients.

Although the annual rate of admission to mental hospitals rose from 17,000 *per annum* in the mid 1960s to 23,714 in 1982, the hospital population did begin to fall and in 1982 stood at 15,678, with a projected figure of 16,410 for 1991, which allows for 3,500 additional cases of senile dementia. By this time, of course, however it may have been achieved, the corresponding English figure was approximately 76,000; north of the Border there remained proportionately *twice* as many people under in-patient care as in England. There was also, in Scotland, a relative lack of expansion in general hospital provision for the mentally ill, although this relative lack is now less than it was ten years ago, when only one eighth of all psychiatric admissions were to general hospitals, this being half the English figure.

The heavy Scottish emphasis on in-patient care was not affected by the expansion of out-patient services (from 109,308 attendances in 1965 to 227,994 in 1983) which, instead of providing an alternative service for those who would otherwise have been admitted to a psychiatric ward, seem to have been required in order to cope with rising expectations in the community for treatment for mental illness[48].

Again, in comparison with England, day hospital facilities developed slowly in Scotland. In March 1983, there were three day centres (making a total of 160 places available) for the mentally ill, provided by local authorities and voluntary organisations. At that date, there were 485 places available in hostels and support accommodation for those who had been discharged from mental hospitals[16]. If the levels of provision in Scotland had matched those prevailing in England (which were generally held to be seriously inadequate), there should have been between seven and eight times as many day-centre places, and between two and three times as many residential places.

In 1975 and 1976, a modestly successful 'joint finance' initiative had been launched by the Department of Health and Social Security in England, whereby the National Health Service (in cases where it would be to the benefit of the health service to do so) was empowered to make available, on certain terms and conditions, financial help to social service departments (social work departments in Scotland). In England and Wales the total funds available have been steadily increased since 1976, to an estimated £104.6 million in 1985/86[6]. In relation to the total problem this is still a modest sum, but 'joint finance' is intended to stimulate *additional* joint planning initiatives.

In Scotland, a similar 'support finance' scheme was not launched until 1980; and it met with little enthusiasm particularly among local authorities[48]. In 1985/86 the total sum expected to be disbursed on support finance schemes in Scotland was only £3½ million. Following on a Consultative document on 'Care in the Community', which was issued in 1982[49], the Minister in England made certain improvements in 'Joint finance' provision. In addition to making more money available, he extended the scope of the scheme to include housing, education and voluntary bodies. In Scotland, in 1985, the Scottish Home and Health Department issued a circular which had the same general thrust, but which, possibly with questionable wisdom in view of their budgetary difficulties, delegated the provision of support finance to Health Boards[50].

It could be argued that joint planning and support finance are also symbolic gestures (given existing financial constraints) rather than real attempts to initiate care in the community. On the other hand, it has been postulated that, although, initially, they make joint planning unattractive, straitened finances could still, in the long run, actually *promote* joint working *at every level*, between Health Boards, local authorities and voluntary organisations, with support finance providing some initial stimulus in a number of key areas[59]. It could be a significant confirmation of this view that the Secretary of State, in the circular referred to above, has now requested (note *(g)*) Health Boards and local authorities to prepare, in conjunction with the appropriate voluntary bodies, joint plans for the mental health and mental handicap services by the end of 1986. But, of course, joint plans aimed merely at saving resources are not the same as joint plans aimed at making the best use of resources.

Clearly 'support finance' in Scotland has lagged behind the English arrangements for 'joint finance', and the amount involved has been proportionately much less than it should have been on a straight comparative basis, never mind the backlog of neglect, in Scotland, in regard to community care. This was partly due to the fact that local authorities, faced by intractable problems of poverty and multiple deprivation, had other more pressing priorities. Partly, it was due to fears in Scotland that support finance might reduce the National Health Service budget and slow down upgrading work on the country's legacy of nineteenth century hospitals.

Whether Scotland has been dragging its feet, because the real health priorities of the Department lie elsewhere, or whether a more cautious and realistic view has been taken of the politics of the situation, must remain an open question for the time being.

In a recent study, the late Professor Martin came to the following conclusion:

"It would no doubt be unreasonable, especially in recent and current economic circumstances, to expect Departments of State to be intensely active in promoting innovation in the public services, but it is hard to shake off the impression that in Scotland there has, in this field of work, been an excess of complacency and a lack of self-examination both in the central department and in the relevant professions"[48].

Before this verdict could be reckoned to be a just one, it would be necessary to establish that Health Boards and local authorities, as well as the central government, were indeed guilty of an excess of complacency, and a lack of self-examination. It would also be necessary to take into account these basic problems of poverty and multiple deprivation which beset local authorities in Scotland, and to which Professor Martin himself makes reference. Given the Scottish Health Authorities Priorities for the Eighties (SHAPE) guidelines, it may also be a little harsh to say that 'whereas in England a policy of community care has been promulgated, but only very incompletely and imperfectly carried through, in Scotland nothing has been promised and virtually nothing achieved'. The Scottish position is precisely the position now being recommended in the Short Report[6]; and, in spite of a noticeable lack of public pressure in this area of concern[48], the tortoise may yet overtake the hare. At the same time, it is undoubtedly true that Scotland's sluggish progress towards community care has been widely perceived, within Scotland, as being due to the factors specified by Professor Martin; and that perception is, in itself, an important aspect of the problem. There may even be a suspicion that the 'excess of complacency' to which Professor Martin refers, is a policy of calculated neglect that is designed to block any change in a pattern of expenditure which favours the acute services. Is the real, as distinct from the manifest, policy of the Government, to stabilise provision for the mentally ill (and the mentally handicapped) at current levels (allowing for some *modest* improvements here and there) with the crucial help (first) of a Mental Welfare Commission skilled at 'absorbing pressures' (note *(h)*), and cautiously strengthened in the direction of patients' rights by the 1984 Act; and (secondly) of the Scottish Hospital Advisory Service (SHAS), which was set up in 1972, after the Elie Hospital scandal in Wales, to keep a weather eye on conditions in long-stay hospitals in Scotland, and (since, unlike the English Health Advisory Service (HAS), it includes mental handicap hospitals in its remit) to carry out, in respect of these hospitals, the functions carried out, south of the Border, by the Development Team for the Mentally Handicapped. In regard to the elderly with mental disability, the top priority in SHAPE, where it is not a question of community care so much as of the provision of Continuing Care Units, it certainly seems that the low status of this sector and its lack of a powerful lobby, either within or outwith the National Health Service, have played a major part in delaying progress[51].

Services for the Mentally Handicapped 1948–1985

Although the demand for community care for the mentally handicapped is now even more pressing than the demand for such care in relation to the mentally ill, the opposite was the case until the late 1960s and early 1970s.

In a book published as recently as 1964, the late Sir David Henderson expressed the traditional view:–

"While the Minister of Health has talked hopefully about the depopulation and ultimate closure of certain of our mental hospitals no one has been reckless enough to suggest that in the near future the hospitals for the subnormal will become similarly redundant. These hospitals have a much more lively air about them, the spirit of clinical and scientific research is taking root in them, and biochemistry geneticists and educational (*sic*) psychologists are bringing light and knowledge into dark places. In the community the establishment of special schools, of occupational centres for children and adults of sheltered workshops and of facilities for employment in the open market have proved highly successful. They have not only contributed to the happiness and welfare of the patients but have also created an incentive and stimulus to teachers and trainees – and by so doing less necessity has arisen for hospital accommodation. We must, however, not delude ourselves about the progress which has been made. It has been great but not nearly enough to make any real impression on the increasing number of subnormal persons in the population and the waiting lists of patients who are in urgent need of indoor treatment; some require to wait for months or even years. Segregation, sterilisation, contraception, spacing of pregnancies, family allowances and other eugenic measures only help so far; our knowledge has not advanced to the stage whereby social, cultural, medical and genetic measures can out-weigh the constitutional anomalies which represent our ancestral inheritance"[12].

Sir David was writing shortly after Lord Adrian had said: 'We have arrived, and must continue to aim, at keeping alive every child that is born, but we have succeeded so well in diminishing early mortality that we are constantly preserving many unfavourable genes which would otherwise have died out. If we set out to save the unfit, we must expect more unfitness in the world, and the inheritance of factors that promote it'[12].

In these circumstances it was natural that Sir David, as a spokesman for what we would have to call 'the old school', should have taken a pessimistic, or as he put it, a 'realistic', view of the human race and of man's ability to 'breed out defects and thus improve the human stock'[14].

All this changed within a few short years; and, to a dramatic extent, as the 1960s progressed, pessimism, or 'realism', was replaced by optimism, and by purposive attempts to employ non-institutional, or 'normalising', strategies in the field of mental handicap. Partly this optimism was due to advances in genetics which held out new hope for the future and, in effect, counteracted the black picture painted by Lord Adrian. It was also due to the 1960 Mental Health (Scotland) Act, and to the subsequent rapprochement between the mental handicap and the mental health services, which now began to get under way on a significant scale. There may also have been some realisation, already apparent in the Fyfe Report of 1957[52] that through processes of 'labelling', 'stigmatising' and 'institutionalising', society itself 'manufactured' mental handicap (in the same way as it 'manufactured' mental illness) and that the situation, therefore, might be more under control than had been thought. Additional pressures arose from the sense of outrage which followed the discovery that people had often been confined in mental handicap hospitals quite unnecessarily, and in some instances for moral, rather than for medical, reasons.

The upshot of all these converging factors was the growth in the 1970s, and 1980s of a powerful drive in Scotland, as elsewhere, to reintegrate the mentally handicapped into the community.

In spite of efforts initiated in 1828 at the Bicêtre in Paris 'to train and educate "idiots" '[53], it was not until much later that the training and education of the mentally handicapped became a matter of active concern in Scotland. Until the middle years of the nineteenth century, special care for people thus afflicted was actually considered useless and unnecessary and they drifted into workhouses, asylums, prisons, or wherever they could find shelter, thereby adding to the overcrowding of such institutions and 'complicating' whatever medical and nursing services were available[12].

At last, in 1852, as a result of active campaigning by, among others, Dr John Coldstream of Edinburgh[53], Sir John and Lady Ogilvy founded the Baldovan Institution for the treatment and education of defectives on their estate near Dundee. Baldovan provided for 30 orphaned and 'imbecile' children, but was later, in 1855, confined to mentally handicapped children, with life in the fresh air, exercise, and good food being combined with education and training. The first institution of its kind in Scotland, it was licensed in 1904 for the care of 160 children. It is now, as Strathmartine Hospital, associated with the Royal Liff Hospital and with the Department of Psychiatry at Dundee Medical School. By a coincidence, it was also in 1855 that a few friends joined together in taking a house in Gayfield Square in Edinburgh, which a certain Dr Brodie and his wife undertook to conduct as 'a training school for idiots'[53].

In her report to the Home Office after her visit to Scotland in 1855, Dorothea Dix commented adversely on the treatment of the mentally handicapped. The Royal Commission, in its subsequent report, recorded that there were 2,603 idiots and imbeciles in Scotland (i.e. 2 per 1,000 of the population), with 15 of them being in Baldovan and in the house at Gayfield Square.

Gayfield Square being an unsuitable location, the Society for Education of Imbecile Youth in Scotland was formed in 1859, to gather funds and provide facilities 'to train Imbecile Children so as to qualify them, as far as possible, for the duties and enjoyments of life'[53].

By 1861 ground had been purchased at Larbert and the building of the Royal Scottish National Hospital commenced. Dr Brodie was appointed Medical Superintendent as from Whitsunday 1862, and, in May 1863, 9 patients were transferred from the house (Hope Park) in Gayfield Square. In 1863 Dr Brodie also found time to visit institutions in America. He retired in 1867 and thereafter took pupils privately at his home at Liberton. He was succeeded first by Dr Adamson of Montrose (who followed the methods established by Voisin in Switzerland in 1837) and then in 1871 by Dr Ireland who published, in 1877, one of the first text-books in the UK on mental deficiency. On his retiral early in 1881, Dr Ireland also took imbecile children into his house at Prestonpans.

Tuke published figures for 1881 showing 195 imbeciles in Training Schools for Imbeciles in Scotland. This would presumably include Larbert (124), Baldovan (47), Dr Brodie (10), with the balance being with Dr Ireland.

The next voluntary body to provide facilities was the Glasgow Association for the Care of Defective and Feeble-minded Children, which in 1906, founded the Waverley Park Home at Kirkintilloch for the protection, elementary education and industrial training of mental defectives.

These early beginnings were aimed at the training of children in the hope that they could return home to do useful work, but those who were unable to do so had, on reaching the age of 16 years, either to be transferred to a lunatic asylum or discharged into the community, where they were liable to be neglected and exploited. There was an increasing demand that the law should be changed to allow public funds to be used so that adults could stay in mental deficiency institutions. The Royal Commission, which was set up in 1904, found an incidence of mental deficiency of 0.46 *per cent* of population and felt that 44.45 *per cent* of this (i.e. 2 per 1,000) required provision in institutions either in their own interest or for the public safety. The findings of the 1904 Commission led to the Mental Deficiency and Lunacy Acts of 1913, which were anticipated in the provision for adults by Glasgow Parish Council Stoneyetts Hospital for Mental Defectives being opened in 1913. The First World War stopped further local authority development until 1925, when the District Board of Control started a small unit for females at Gogarburn, Edinburgh, with a unit for males being provided in the following year. In 1925 an estate beside Larbert Institution was purchased to develop as a permanent home (or colony) for the feeble-minded, and four years later the Colony for adults was developed at Baldovan. In 1929, the first part of Lennox Castle was opened as a Colony for mental defectives, and with the transfer to Lennox Castle, in 1936, of the last of the mental defectives from Stoneyetts the latter then became a hospital for mental illness.

Developments at Baldovan, Gogarburn, Larbert and Lennox Castle continued until they were stopped by the outbreak of war in 1939. After the war, with the setting up of the National Health Service, they, along with Waverley Park, were taken over as hospitals for mental defectives.

Under the National Health Service further provision was made for mental defectives, not only in these hospitals, but by the development of other hospitals which were no longer required for their original purpose, e.g. Glen Lomond at Kinross, Ladysbridge at Banff, and Kirklands at Bothwell. The first completely new mental deficiency hospital built under the National Health Service was Lynebank, Dunfermline in 1968, and this was followed in 1969 by Craig Phadrig at Inverness and, in 1975, by Merchiston Hospital, Renfrewshire.

The original institutions were provided on a voluntary and charitable basis, and there are still some voluntary institutions in existence such as those run by the Roman Catholics at Rosewell, Carstairs and Barrhead. The first of these, St Joseph's Hospital at Rosewell, was opened in 1924 by the Sisters of Charity. This Order, founded by St Vincent de Paul, has for centuries been concerned with caring for the handicapped in many countries. Later developments have been the Rudolf Steiner schools and Algrade School at Humbie Village, whilst Hansel Village near Kilmarnock is run as a sheltered workshop for the adult handicapped.

In Scotland, education authorities became responsible, in 1947, for the education of children who were described as 'ineducable but trainable'. These children were placed in junior occupational centres and trained by instructors; but, following the Report of the Melville Committee[54] and subsequent provisions in the Education (Mentally Handicapped Children) (Scotland) Act 1974, the centres were renamed schools, and teachers were appointed in addition to the instructors. The 1974 Act also gave education authorities responsibility for the education of children who had previously been described as 'ineducable and untrainable'.

After 1968, the new Social Work Departments were responsible for those in social need in the community; and care in the community first recommended in Scotland by the Fyfe Committee in 1957, was the central issue at an important conference which was held in Dublin in 1970, and which was attended by a substantial contingent from Scotland. Up to the late 1960s, therefore, changes in the care of the mentally handicapped people had taken place. It was only after the decade had ended, however, that the institutional base of the services for the mentally handicapped began to be called in question[55].

The Batchelor Report on The Staffing of Mental Handicap Hospitals, for example, had been concerned to improve the efficiency and effectiveness of hospital care: it was not within its remit to question the central role that was still accorded to the hospital in the care of the mentally handicapped[56].

Nevertheless, the rapprochement between mental handicap, and mental, hospitals, which had been given a significant fillip by the Mental Health (Scotland) Act 1960, and by the Batchelor Report, did eventually bring mental handicap hospitals into the mainstream of medicine, with all that this meant in terms of the investment in them of professional and administrative skills and other resources, thereby achieving for these hospitals some of that incentive to 'catch up' with, and, in some respects, surpass those improvements in the psychiatric field, which psychiatric hospitals had achieved through their links with (and, in terms of community care, their ability to 'leap-frog') general hospitals.

These changes in the status of mental handicap hospitals, and the interest which they now developed in community care, were accelerated and intensified by a growing conviction that the Jay Committee[57] was correct in saying that mentally handicapped people were not ill and that, accordingly, medical and nursing care in hospital was even less appropriate for the mentally handicapped than it was for the mentally ill. In particular, the Committee's views on the right of mentally handicapped people to be treated as individuals and to enjoy normal patterns of life within the community, met with general acceptance; and the transfer of responsibility for the education of mentally handicapped children in Scotland in 1975 to the 'normal' education authorities, following the report of the Melville Committee, has already been mentioned.

Other changes in Scotland which were designed, either to re-house mentally handicapped patients in the community, or to bring the mental handicap hospital itself, so far as possible, into the community, also took place in the 70s and 80s; and *two* Scottish reports[58,59] which had preceded Jay, were important, although cautious, milestones on the road to a new approach to people with mental handicap, based, not on institutional care, but on local (and local authority) services, i.e. on a community pattern of care, involving group homes, group tenancies, supported accommodation, hostel or hospital-annexe type provision, adult training centres, day centres and care at home[60], with opportunities for sheltered work, work in 'enclaves' or even work in the open market, and, equally, of course, with opportunities for social and leisure activities at least as rewarding as the kind of activities traditionally available in hospital settings.

Behind all these moves was the 'normalisation' philosophy pioneered by Dr Grunewald in Sweden in the late 1960s but taken up, with alacrity, in Britain, and in America. This philosophy, defined quite simply[61] as 'making available to the mentally retarded patterns and conditions of every day life,' had influenced Jay, but the Jay Report was over-ambitious in its attempt to create (at a cost which could not be afforded) a single category of care staff for the mentally handicapped; and, in Scotland, the emphasis continues to be laid on interdisciplinary team-work and shared training, with the qualifications involved in this shared training remaining discrete[62].

By the mid 1980s there was considerable disillusionment in community groups, as well as in doctors, nurses, social workers, psychologists, occupational therapists and others working in the field of mental handicap. It was felt that, in spite of the priorities set out in SHAPE, and in spite of 'a general trend towards developing the full individual potential of the mentally handicapped, enhancing their human dignity, integrating them into the community and giving them as normal and independent life style as possible'[63], provision for the mentally handicapped was still lagging seriously behind the needs of the community and, on the basis of the available evidence, was beginning to lag embarrassingly behind what was happening in the rest of Britain.

What was needed was a major shift from reliance on institutions to reliance on personnel and on the community itself. The fact remained, however, that residential care for the mentally handicapped in Scotland continued to be provided mainly by the Health Service; and this was likely to be the case for the foreseeable future[60].

The following table gives a clear picture of the position with regard to services for the mentally handicapped in Scotland in the mid-80s:–

	Recommended levels of provision, as places per 100,000 total population:		
	1972 Report	*A Better Life – 1978*	*England DHSS*
Hospital	120	120	67
Community	43	60	87

In 1985 Scotland's actual rate of hospital residence (129 per 100,000 total population) was still higher than the recommended figure of 120. The position on community provision was equally discouraging – out of a conservatively estimated requirement of 3,090 places only 1,200 community places had been provided.

There was particular criticism of the Scottish Home and Health Department for allegedly abdicating its responsibilities in this field. While it is recognised that services were actually delivered by health boards, local authorities and voluntary agencies, it was also strongly believed that, without political will at the centre, backed by additional resources, the local agencies would go on working within existing (and largely inherited) patterns of care. *Circular National Health Service (GEN) (85) 18*, with its request for joint plans to be prepared by the end of 1986, was a valuable step forward, but no more than a step, since additional resources were still being withheld. The Department's policy of monitoring the implementation of the SHAPE priorities was also thought to be an important step in the right direction; but it was viewed, at the same time, with a measure of scepticism. Would symbolic policy-making be followed by symbolic monitoring? Behind all the rhetoric, had the Scottish Office even come round to the view that, all in all, the least costly option for the mentally handicapped was institutional care?

Towards an Integrated Community

Both the mental health and the mental handicap services were top priorities in the Scottish Home and Health Department's 1976 Memorandum *The Way Ahead* and in its 1980 policy document *Scottish Health Authorities Priorities for the Eighties* (SHAPE)[64]; and, for both of these services, the overriding priority, as we have seen, was the all-important shift of emphasis to care in, and by, the community, a policy which had been high on the mental health agenda since the 1950s, and which had become the single most important consideration in the mental handicap services a decade or so later.

What has been achieved? An over-sluggish move to care in the community has been accompanied by a continuous, but also over-sluggish process of de-institutionalisation, which has involved a succession of attempts to 'de-asylumise the asylum', either by providing small-scale living units within mental and mental handicap hospitals or by creating such units in ordinary community settings, with all new institutional provision being planned in such a way that, while a genuine 'asylum' element would be retained, provision would, so far as possible, be both decentralised and integrated into the community.[16]

This process of change and adaptation has profound implications for the specialist mental health and mental handicap teams. Although these teams may continue to have institutional bases for some time yet, there is little doubt that they will find themselves working increasingly in community settings, with the members of the teams directly intervening in treatment less and less, as they begin to act chiefly in a consultative capacity to their front-line colleagues and to workers from other relevant 'hands on' organisations, these workers, in turn, directing their efforts more and more through self-help, and community development groups[16]. Unfortunately, however, the switch to community care is still a very long way from being an accomplished fact.

In Scotland, as we have seen, there has always been considerable scepticism about moving away from institutional care until alternative forms of care have been made available in the community. The consequence of the premature discharge of patients in England (chiefly, it has always been suspected, in order to cut costs) are now regarded, north of the Border, as a grave warning of what can happen when the shift to community care is not properly planned, and when it starts from the *hospital*, rather than from the *community*, end of the spectrum; in England, of course, a re-think is now taking place, with community care no longer being seen as an easy, or less costly, option[6].

On the other hand, the Welsh approach to community care of the mentally handicapped is being held up, (although it has not been without its problems) as an example of what *can* be achieved, and as convincing evidence for the view that the difficulties inherent in changing priorities in the National Health Service, and in getting off the ground joint planning initiatives on the part of health boards and local authorities, do not need to be insuperable, given a proper awareness of the possibilities, a real sense of urgency on the part of all concerned, and a genuine willingness, as is now beginning to be apparent in some parts of Scotland (and not only in consequence of *Circular National Health Service (GEN) (85) 18*) to set up the communication links, which are called for at the clinical, managerial and planning levels[16].

There is still considerable suspicion, in many quarters, that all the difficulties about implementing policies of care in the community stem from the fact that there is no real will (on the part of the politicians and the officials) to see these policies through, and that they are, as has been suggested above, nothing more than 'symbolic policies', which are designed to allay unrest while actually changing nothing.

In England the Select Committee on Social Welfare, in its report on Community Care[6], took the view that joint finance had exhausted its potential for development. It recommended the setting up of a 'Central Bridging Fund' to help authorities over the expenditure 'hump' that inevitably arises when new facilities are superimposed on an existing service, which cannot be run down until the new arrangements are fully in place. At the time of writing, the likelihood of such a fund being set up is remote, although 'earmarking' of this kind was also recommended in *Mental Health in Focus*[16].

An important feature of the last two or three decades in Scotland has been the systematic (and officially supported) development, both nationally and locally, of the voluntary sector, in relation to mental health and mental handicap, whether through the Scottish Association for Mental Health, the Scottish Society for the Mentally Handicapped, and the Scottish Council on Disability (and their local counterparts), or through specific self-help groups, like, for example, the National Schizophrenia Fellowship and the Down's Syndrome Association (and their local counterparts).

The Scottish Society for the Mentally Handicapped was formed in 1954 to campaign for this client group. With 79 branches throughout Scotland, the Society has been instrumental, *inter alia*, in getting Regional Housing Associations set up to build small family homes for adult mentally handicapped people (note *(i)*). One of the most valuable of these community-orientated initiatives may well prove to be the funding from April 1986 of a Chair of Learning Difficulties at St Andrews University, which will be taken over by the University in five years' time. This chair, it is hoped, will lead to a better understanding of mental handicap in Scotland, and, at the same time, accelerate the development of community care.

The Scottish Association for Mental Health has also been instrumental in developing, with the help of Link Housing Association, and the co-operation of the National Schizophrenia Fellowship (Scottish Branch), important pilot projects, by means of which mentally ill people, who would otherwise have had to remain in hospital, are able to live more normal lives in supported accommodation in the community.

It has sometimes been suggested that the Government's interest in mobilising community resources in this way is merely a backdoor way of reducing the statutory services, and, in effect, getting community care 'on the cheap'.

If this is the case, it is a policy which will almost certainly fail of its purpose. For there is little doubt that community care, involving as it must do an increase in *both* the statutory and voluntary services (which, as they expand, will need increased support) is likely to be a *more* costly option, at least for many years to come, even if one is thinking of cost not in terms of the whole social cost, but purely in terms of National Health Service and Local Authority budgets.

This can only mean that the struggle for community care will continue to be an uphill struggle, with attention focusing less and less on the merits of the policy and more and more on the problems of the implementation[65]. If the logic inherent in the wide range of developments which have taken place in the field of mental disorder during this century is not to be wholly frustrated, this struggle cannot be allowed to fail. To succeed, however, it will have to become a struggle for nothing less than community care, and community self-help, in the widest and most positive sense.

Dreikurs has described these developments in group therapy, and in social and community psychiatry, as the Third Psychiatric Revolution[1]: Bierer, in more fulsome vein, claimed that community care was the greatest psychiatric revolution ever[66]. Certainly the move to care in the community marks a new era, not only in regard to the mental illness and mental handicap services as such, but, above all, in regard to the basic attitudes of people to mental illness and mental handicap.

It is important to appreciate, however, that although in recent years there have been promising developments, particularly, perhaps, in regard to the provision of special needs housing, the Third Revolution is still the revolution that never was, or the revolution that, as yet, has manifested itself only to a limited extent. Today, community care, involving the development of locally based services, is still a peripheral, rather than *the central* aspect of the mental disorder services; and successive attempts over the last thirty years or so, to change this emphasis have met with only limited success as yet.

To some extent, this could be because care in and by the community represents a revolution in the care of the mentally ill and the mentally handicapped which is associated, to an uncomfortable extent, with the 'anti-psychiatric' view that 'society itself is the real patient', in that 'mental illness' and 'mental handicap' are, in some sense, 'invented' by human society and then used as a mechanism of social control, in much the same way as crime is 'invented' and then used for social control purposes[67].

As long ago as the early 60s, Dr George Bell, with characteristic shrewdness and humanity, asserted that the real patient was a highly legalistic, bureaucratically organised, and deeply divisive society that found it necessary to protect its own conventional set of values by making laws which labelled as criminal, or mentally ill, those for whom that particular society's 'way of seeing' was a way of *not* seeing[68].

As we have already seen, Dr Bell's successor at Dingleton, Dr Maxwell Jones also reached the conclusion that society itself would have to become a therapeutic community before the therapeutic community in the hospital could be effective.

Other indications of the importance which must be attached to the social origins of mental illness and to the view that the patient is best understood as the manifestation of a deep-seated social malaise, can be detected in the work of Glasgow-born, and Glasgow-trained, R.D. Laing, whose questioning of the community's over-dependence on, and collusion with, the statutory mental disorder services has been echoed, but in a less extravagant and more constructive way, by Dr J.D. Sutherland, a former Medical Director of the Tavistock Clinic, who, in 1967, became a consultant psychotherapist and community psychiatrist at the Royal Edinburgh Hospital, and who, in the early 1970s, was responsible for setting up the Scottish Institute of Human Relations, in order to further preventive psycho-therapeutic and counselling services in Scotland and, at the same time, advance knowledge about group dynamics and the functioning of organisations.

Like Lawrence Frank, who wrote of the trend towards a society which was no longer monolithic, but in which 'the parts were greater than the whole,' and which needed to reflect this development in 'a new politics'[69], Dr Sutherland sees 'the self', rather than society (with its consequential need for social control), as the starting point[20]. In terms of this perspective, the integrity of the self and the basic right of a person to develop his, or her, potential are rapidly becoming the paramount considerations, both in mental health and in mental handicap. This involves us in a totally new orientation to human existence, with inner motivation, *for the first time*, being given priority over external pressures, (and with people, as an inevitable corollary, being confronted with the awesome task of shaping their future instead of being shaped by it).

In a society where the centre of gravity has shifted away from social control concepts and external pressures, Bion's accusation that people have a 'hatred' of knowing about themselves, which leads them to reject and stigmatise mental illness (and mental handicap), will no longer be applicable. At the same time, no longer dependent on the statutory services to adjust them to society's norms, but on the contrary making active use of these services to reinforce their own self-initiated efforts to use their problems of living in order to develop their full potential, the mentally disordered may yet come to be regarded as a significant additional resource for the enrichment and development of society, rather than as people to be feared and rejected.

That this is not a far-fetched scenario is confirmed by what Ernest Becker wrote, as long ago as 1964, on the subject of schizophrenia:

"Even though schizophrenia becomes crippling in its extreme forms, one has only to glance down a list of historical figures to see how creative even seriously 'schizoid' individuals have been. 'Schizoid' is perhaps a better word than schizophrenic, but it also has a pejorative valuation. There is no way to dodge the issue. Schizophrenia refers to variations on the distinctively human mode, *with all that this entails*: namely, the immense enrichment of human life precisely because of and by means of human variation. Certainly if history had eliminated, or changed, individuals from among those we now call 'schizophrenic', mankind would be immeasurably poorer in art, science, and religion than it is now; our world would be unrecognizable. Karl Mannheim, addressing himself to this very problem, wondered whether society would indeed be able to get along without utilizing the historical contributions of its introverted members[70]".

Dexter has written in similar vein about the positive aspects of mental handicap as a necessary corrective to a society suffering from what Nietzsche called the 'inverse handicap' of normality[71]. Taking the services for the mentally ill and the mentally handicapped into the realm of care in the community i.e. into the realm of new and as yet unimagined forms (given the restricted social control forms with which we are familiar) of self-initiated care and self-healing (whereby mental illness and mental handicap could actually be used to help people redirect their lives into creative, self-actualising and self-fulfilling channels) is a highly significant new development, which could as easily be pioneered in Scotland as elsewhere. Indeed, a small country like Scotland, which has lagged behind England and Wales in the development of community facilities, but which has both a strong sense of community and its own Scottish Office in Edinburgh, should be well placed to 'leap frog' advances in the South (as it has successfully done, for example, in some aspects of penal policy, and, above all, in its system of juvenile justice) and to embark, wholeheartedly on the Third Psychiatric Revolution. Whether it will now do so clearly depends not only on its ability to deploy adequate resources for community care (with having a key role of the political will of Ministers and of those at the centre of power) but, above all, on its ability to adapt its political institutions and organisational structures, (which, with their emphasis on outmoded concepts of hierarchy and status, appear to have seized up at the prospect of the radical challenge to the *status quo* now confronting them), so that these institutions and organisational structures are geared not to stand in the way of, but actually to meet, the needs of individuals and of the community, in the post-industrial society which is now emerging from current confusions and upheavals[72].

As the technique by which the minority in society have achieved their identities at the expense of the majority, social control, which has been substantially modified over the centuries, is now finally under notice to quit. It is being realised that men and nations are globally interdependent, that national and international integration is the aim and that people (and nations) must therefore achieve their identities, not at each other's expense, but through each other, i.e. through the development of empathic relationships, or, in W.R.D. Fairbairn's terminology, relationships of 'mature dependence'[73].

In this situation, the likelihood is that labels like 'mental illness' and 'mental handicap' will no longer be relevant, since it will increasingly be a question not of social control work, with the psychiatrist acting in the role of a 'soft policeman', but rather of what Goffman called 'people work', with the community itself properly supported by psychiatrists and other professionals, who are prepared to blur and humanise their roles, becoming the key resource. The Third Psychiatric Revolution, which is taking an unconscionable time to materialise precisely because it has such far-reaching implications for the whole society, could thus turn out to be the last purely *psychiatric* revolution. This would mean that the true measure of the problem of mental disorder, which is a problem of society itself, a problem of social disorganisation that now exists on a world-wide scale[74], had at last been taken. Then there would dawn upon us a proper appreciation of the opportunities afforded by the solution of this problem for the development of a mature and fully integrated world-order, in which we would find it possible, for the first time, to put 'respect for others before self-interest'[75], and alongside which all previous world-orders, or partial world-orders, would be seen to have belonged to the prehistory of man.

Notes

(a) The humane impact of psychiatry on the nineteenth century legal system (as to which see Walker, N., *Crime and Punishment in Britain*. Edinburgh, 1965. University Press) must also be given due recognition. The 1857 Act, for example, laid it down that, in criminal cases, if the plea of insanity was successfully sustained, the lunatic should be detained 'during her Majesty's pleasure'. Hence the existence, in Scotland, of the State Hospital at Carstairs, the future of which, particularly in respect of its relationships with the other Scottish mental hospitals, has recently been questioned in Parliament and elsewhere[16].

(b) In an interesting, unpublished, dissertation, *The Mad, the Bad and the Sad: Psychiatric Care in the Royal Edinburgh Asylum (Morningside) 1813–1894* (Boston, 1984. University Graduate School). M.S. Thompson suggests that Scottish psychiatrists had, from an early date, adopted a social approach to mental illness, which contrasted sharply with the German medical, or 'physiological', approach.

(c) Like the Scottish system of 'boarding out'.

(d) In 1969, a chair of Forensic Psychiatry was established at Edinburgh, which is at present unfilled. An increase in the number of posts in this field in Scotland is now being urged upon the Government.

(e) The archetypal figure in this regard was Edinburgh's Sir Thomas Clouston, a towering figure in Scottish psychiatry between 1873 and 1907, whose son, not without irony,

wrote: 'I say "ruled" [the institution] because his word – even his nod – was law; a not uncommon characteristic of advanced Liberals holding strongly democratic theories'. (Clouston, J. Storer, *The Family of Clouston*. Kirkwell, 1948. Orcadian Press).

(f) In the 1880s, long before Dr Russell Barton invented the term 'institutional neurosis', Dr Urquhart, Physician Superintendent of the Murray Royal Hospital, in Perthshire, had written about 'asylum-made lunatics'.

(g) A request which the Minister has now indicated will be made mandatory if health boards and local authorities do not respond in a positive way. (*Hansard*, 11th April 1986.)

(h) An article on this theme, among others, appeared in *The Scotsman* of July 11th, 1984.

(i) In Dumfries, Annan, Stranraer, Stenhousmuir, Fort William, Gourock, Stirling, Helensburgh, Cumbernauld and Glasgow.

References

(1) Dreikurs, R., Group Psychotherapy and the Third Revolution in Psychiatry. *Int. J. Soc. Psych.*, 1955, 1, 3, pp.23–32. See also Bella, L. (Ed.) Handbook of Community Psychiatry and Community Mental Health. New York, 1964. Grune and Stratton.

(2) Rosen, G., *Madness in Society*. Chapters in the Historical Sociology of Mental Illness. London, 1967. Routledge and Kegan Paul.

(3) Tuke, D.H., *Chapters in the History of the Insane in the British Isles*. London, 198?. Kegan Paul, Trench & Co.

(4) Browne, W.A.F., What Asylums Were Are and Ought to Be: being the substance of five lectures delivered before the Managers of the Montrose Royal Asylum. Edinburgh, 1837. Adam and Charles Black.

(5) General Board of Commissioners in Lunacy: *Annual Reports passim*. Edinburgh, 1857–1900. HMSO. See also Asylum Reports *passim* 1823–1900.

(6) House of Commons Social Services Committee: Community Care with special reference to adult mentally ill and mentally handicapped people. *Second Report of the Committee*. Vol. 1. London, 1985. HMSO.

(7) Szasz, T., Personal communication, and see Ideology and Insanity. *Essays in the Psychiatric Dehumanisation of Man*. London, 1973. Calder and Boyers.

(8) Tait, H.P., A Doctor and Two Policemen. *A History of Edinburgh Health Department 1862–1974*. Edinburgh, 1974. Environmental Health Department of Edinburgh District Council.

(9) Jones, K., *A History of the Mental Health Services*. London, 1972. Routledge and Kegan Paul. For a more philosophical account, see Foucault, M., Madness and Civilisation. *A History of Insanity in the Age of Reason*. London, 1967. Tavistock.

(10) Adler, A., Social Interest. *A Challenge to Mankind*. London, 1938. Faber and Faber, and for a more epidemiological approach cf Sutherland, J.F., *Geographical Distribution of Lunacy in Scotland*. Glasgow, 1901. British Association for the Advancement of Science, and more recently Brown, G.W., and Harris, T., *Social Origins of Depression: A Study of Psychiatric Disorders in Women*. London, 1978. Tavistock.

(11) Independent Council for People with Mental Handicap: *Elements of a Comprehensive Local Service for People with Mental Handicap*. London, 1982. King's Fund Centre.

(12) Henderson, D.K., *The Evolution of Psychiatry in Scotland*. Edinburgh, 1964. E. and S. Livingstone.

(13) General Board of Control for Scotland: *Second Annual Report*. Edinburgh, 1916. HMSO, and see also *Fifth Annual Report*. Edinburgh, 1919. HMSO.

(14) Scottish Home and Health Department/Scottish Education Department: *A Better Life*. Report by the Sub-Committee on Mental Handicap of the Mental Disorder Programme Planning Group of the Scottish Health Service Planning Council. Edinburgh, 1979. HMSO.

(15) The late Professor Gerald Timbury: *Personal Communication*.

(16) Scottish Home and Health Department/Scottish Education Department: *Mental Health in Focus*. Report of the Mental Illness Sub-Committee of the Mental Disorder Programme Planning Group of the Scottish Health Service Planning Council. Edinburgh, 1985. HMSO.

(17) General Board of Commissioners in Lunacy: *Fifty Sixth Annual Report*. Edinburgh, 1914. HMSO.

(18) Campbell, C.M., *Destiny and Disease in Mental Disorders with special reference to the schizophrenic psychoses*. London, 1935. Thomas W. Salmon Memorial Lectures.

(19) Guntrip, H., *Personality Structure and Human Interaction*. London, 1961. Hogarth.

(20) Dr Sutherland, J.D., *Personal Communication*, and see Kessel, H., 'Who Ought to See a Psychiatrist?', *Lancet*, 1963, 1, p.1092. See also Sutherland, J.D. The Changing Role of the Psychotherapist in 'Towards Community Mental Health' by Sutherland, J.D. (Ed.). London 1971, Tavistock.

(21) General Board of Commissioners in Lunacy: *41st Annual Report*. Edinburgh, 1899. HMSO.

(22) General Board of Control for Commissioners in Lunacy: *53rd Annual Report*. Edinburgh, 1911. HMSO.

(23) General Board of Control for Scotland:*Tenth Annual Report*. Edinburgh, 1923. HMSO.

(24) Morris, B.S., Officer Selection in the British Army. *Occ. Psychol.*, 1949, 23, pp.219–34.

(25) Sutherland, J.D., and Fitzpatrick, G.A., *Some Approaches to Group Problems in the British Army*. 1945.

(26) Bion, W.R., The Leaderless Group Project. *Bull. Menninger Clinic*, 1946, 10, pp.77–81; and see Bridger, H., The Northfield Experiment. *Bull. Menninger Clinic*, 1946, 10, pp.71–6.

(27) General Board of Control for Scotland: *Seventeenth Annual Report*. Edinburgh, 1930. HMSO.

(28) Kennedy, R.I., *Physical Methods of Treatment*. In: Forrest, A.D., Affleck, J.W., and Zealley, A., (eds). Companion to Psychiatric Studies. *Second Edition*. Edinburgh, 1978. Churchill Livingstone; and see for misuse of drugs Miles, A., *The Mentally Ill in Contemporary Society*. Oxford, 1981. Martin Robertson.

(29) Scottish Home and Health Department/Scottish Health Service Planning Council: *Clinical Psychology in the Scottish Health Service*. Edinburgh, 1984. HMSO.

(30) Carstairs, V., and Redpath, A., In-patient care for mental illness in Scotland: past trends and the future prospect. *Community Medicine*, 1984, 6, pp.95–108.

(31) Scottish Home and Health Department/Scottish Education Department: *Services for the Elderly with Mental Disorder*. A Report by a Programme Planning Group of The Scottish Health Service Planning Council and the Advisory Council on Social Work. Edinburgh, 1978. HMSO.

(32) Bell, G.M., A Mental Hospital with Open Doors. *Int. J. Soc, Psych.*, 1955, 1:1, pp.42–8, and see Jones, D.M.H. *et al.*, Dingleton 1872–1922, 1972. Melrose. Dingleton Hospital.

(33) Goffman, E., *Asylums*. London, 1968. Penguin. See also his *Stigma: Notes on the management of Spoiled Identity*. New York, 1963. Prentice Hall.

(34) Laing, R.D., and Esterson, A., *Sanity, Madness and the Family*. London, 1964. Tavistock. See also Laing, R.D., *The Politics of Experience*. London, 1967. Penguin.

(35) Szasz, T., *The Myth of Mental Illness*. New York, 1960. Harper.

(36) Scheff, T.J., *Being Mentally Ill*. London, 1966. Weidenfield and Nicolson.

(37) Rapoport, R.N., *The Community as Doctor*. London, 1960. Tavistock. See also Jones,

M., *The Therapeutic Community*. New York, 1953. Basic Books.

(38) Batchelor, I.R.C. (Ed.), Henderson, D.K., and Gillespie, R.D., *Textbook of Psychiatry*. Tenth Edition, London, 1969. Oxford University Press. See also Henderson, Sir D.K., The 'doyen of British psychiatrists' in the mid 1950s: *personal communication*.

(39) Jones, M., *Beyond the Therapeutic Community*. New Haven, Connecticut, 1968. Yale University Press. See also Clark, D.H., *Social Therapy in Psychiatry*. 1974. See also Jones, M., *Maturation of the Therapeutic Community*. New York, 1976. Human Sciences Press.

(40) Hunter, T.D., New View of the Hospital, Lancet, Nov. 1962, p.933–935.

(41) Department of Health and Social Security: *Report of the Royal Commission on the Law relating to Mental Illness and Mental Deficiency*. London, 1957. HMSO.

(42) Department of Health for Scotland: *First Report by a Committee on Mental Health Legislation*. Edinburgh, 1958. HMSO.

(43) Department of Health for Scotland: *Second Report by a Committee on Mental Health Legislation*. Edinburgh, 1959. HMSO.

(44) Bennet, D., The Chronic Psychiatric Patient Today. *Journal of the Royal Society of Medicine*, 1980, 73, pp.301–3.

(45) See also Social Work Services Group of Scottish Education Department and Scottish Home and Health Department: *Social Work Services in the Scottish Health Social Service*. Edinburgh, 1976. HMSO.

(46) Scottish Home and Health Department/Scottish Education Department: *Report on Relationships between Health Boards and Local Authorities*. Edinburgh, 1977. HMSO.

(47) Scottish Home and Health Department/Scottish Education Department: *Crossing the Boundaries*. Report on Mental Health Services for Children and Young People. Edinburgh, 1983. HMSO.

(48) Martin, F.M., *Between the Acts. Community Mental Health Services 1959–1983*. London, 1984. Nuffield Provincial Hospitals Trust.

(49) Department of Health and Social Security: *Care in the Community*. A Consultative Document on Moving Resources for Care in England. London, 1981. DHSS.

(50) Scottish Home and Health Department: Circular NHS (GEN) (85) 18. 1985.

(51) Hunter, D.J., Cantley, C., and MacPherson, I., *Psychogeriatric Provision in Scotland*. Review of the Research Needs. Aberdeen University, 1984. Unit for the Study of the Elderly.

(52) Department of Health for Scotland: *Mental Deficiency in Scotland*. Edinburgh, 1957. HMSO.

(53) Primrose, D.A., The Development of Mental Deficiency Hospitals in Scotland. *Health Bulletin*, 1977, 35, 2. See also discussion on Mental Deficiency Bill. *RMPA*, 1912; Macgregor, A., *Public Health in Glasgow 1905–1946*, 1967., and the Annual Reports of the Scottish National Institution from 1862.

(54) Scottish Education Department (1973). The Training of Staff for Centres for the Mentally Handicapped. Report of the Committee appointed by the Secretary of State for Scotland. Edinburgh HMSO.

(55) Francklin, S., and Shearer, A., *Future Services for the Mentally Handicapped*, Memorandum sent to DHSS in May, 1971. London, 1971. 26 Lambolle Place, NW3.

(56) Scottish Home and Health Department: *The Staffing of Mental Deficiency Hospitals*. Edinburgh, 1970. HMSO.

(57) DHSS: Report of the Committee of Enquiry into Mental Handicap Nursing and Care. London, 1979. HMSO.

(58) Scottish Home and Health Department: *Services for the Mentally Handicapped*. Edinburgh, 1972. HMSO.

(59) Farquharson, R., Mentally Handicapped People in Scotland. A Case of Political Neglect. Action Group. Edinburgh, 1984.

(60) Scottish Home and Health Department: *Mental Subnormality in North-East Scotland*. A Multidisciplinary Study of Total Population. Scottish Health Service Studies 38.

Edinburgh, 1978. SHHD.

(61) Nirje, B., Ombudsman Riksrofbundet FUB *in Changing Patterns in Residential Services for the Mentally Retarded*. President's Committee. See also Scottish Health Education Group: *School Health Education, Sexuality and Mental Handicap*: 1985, this being an important aspect of normalisation.

(62) North of Scotland Social Work and Nursing Project (SWAN) (1985): *Report on Cooperation in Training*.

(63) Ward, A., *Scots Law and Mentally Handicapped*. Glasgow, 1984. Scottish Society for the Mentally Handicapped.

(64) Scottish Home and Health Department: *Scottish Health Authorities Priorities for the Eighties (SHAPE)*. Edinburgh, 1980. HMSO. SHAPE contained a more detailed statement of priorities than it had been possible to prepare in time for *The Way Ahead*, issued by the Department in 1976. It may be significant that in its Report for 1976 (Edinburgh, HMSO) the Department merely refers to 'some shift of emphasis as between the acute services, and the services for the elderly, the mentally ill, the mentally handicapped and the physically disabled.'

(65) Welsh Office: *Report of All-Wales Working Party on Services for Mentally Handicapped People*. Cardiff, 1982.

(66) Bierer, J., Past, Present and Future. *Int. J. Soc. Psych.*, 1960, Vol. VI, p.165.

(67) Barrat, S., and Fudge, C., *Policy and Action*. Essays on the Implementation of Public Policy. London, 1981. See also Smythe, T., *Political Constraints to the Development of Alternatives in Alternatives to Mental Hospitals*. Report on a European Workshop. National Association for Mental Health, Belgium and World Federation of Mental Health, 1980.

(68) The late Dr G.M. Bell: *personal communication*.

(69) Frank, L.K., The Need for a New Political Theory. *J. Am. Acad. Arts & Sci.*, 1967, 96, pp.809–16.

(70) Becker, E., *The Revolution in Psychiatry*. London, 1964. Free Press of Glencoe. For Bion's comment see Bion, W.R., Learning from Experience, London, 1962. Heinemann.

(71) Hunter, T.D., *New Patterns of Management and Organisation*. In: Forrest, A.D., Ritson, E.B., and Zealley, A. (Eds.). *New Perspectives in Mental Handicap*. Edinburgh, 1973. Churchill-Livingstone.

(72) Hunter, T.D., *New Perspectives on Mental Health and Mental Illness*. Edinburgh, 1985. National Schizophrenia Fellowship (Scotland).

(73) Fairbairn, W.R.D., *Psychoanalytic Studies of the Personality*. London, 1952. Routledge.

(74) Hunter, T.D., Resurrecting the Arena. *Sociology of Health and Illness*, 1981, 3:2, pp.220–38, and for the impact of social disorganisation on mental health, see Carstairs, G.M., Attitudes to Death and Suicide in an Indian Cultural Setting. *Int. J. Soc. Psych.*, 1955, 1:3, pp.33–46.

(75) Levi-Strauss, C., The Origin of Table Manners. *Introduction to a Science of Mythology: 3*. London, 1978. Jonathan Cape.

2. *Geriatrics*

Sir Ferguson Anderson

CONTENTS

About the Author

SIR FERGUSON ANDERSON O.B.E., K.St.J., M.D., F.R.C.P., Hon.F.A.C.P.

Sir Ferguson Anderson was formerly Professor of Geriatric Medicine at the University of Glasgow. He was also Advisor in Diseases of Old Age and Chronic Sickness for the Western Regional Board, Scotland, and Consultant Physician in Geriatric Medicine, Stobhill General Hospital, Glasgow.

Author's Note

This review of the development of Geriatric Medicine in Scotland traces the care of the elderly from the creation of the poorhouses, through the facilities provided by Parochial Boards, Parish Councils, Public Assistance Committees, to the changes produced by the National Health Service.

The concepts of accurate diagnosis, rehabilitation, and continuity of care remain the essential elements, while assessment, in its widest sense, ensures correct placement. As the service developed, the importance of efforts to improve the morale and motivation of the elderly was recognised as necessary to achieve the ideal of a healthy old age; no one can deny the intertwining of medical, mental and social problems in older people.

The steady progress in Scotland since then was greatly encouraged by Sir John Brotherston, who believed that this new service could not function properly until provision for the elderly in our society was adequate. Teaching of the changes associated with ageing and with the development of illness has become widespread, and here again, Sir John, with remarkable foresight, was among the first to recognise the importance of this aspect.

Geriatrics is now a recognised academic discipline, due to the efforts and enthusiasm of many individuals from the initial inspiration of Dr. Marjory Warren, of the West Middlesex Hospital

---

Geriatrics

Introduction

From the sixteenth century to within living memory legal provision for the care of the elderly was bound up with that for the poor. Our Jacobean ancestors believed that society had a Christian duty to maintain those whom the 1574 Scottish Poor Law referred to as 'the puyr, aigit and impotent [ie, infirm]'[1]. Such maintenance was based upon the domiciliary system whereby the poor received relief in their own homes. It was not until 1672 that the Scottish Parliament authorised the erection of poorhouses[2], and for a long time this statutory provision, which was intended to suppress vagrancy, remained a dead letter. In Scotland, the poorhouse was, by and large, a nineteenth century development. The old Scottish Poor Law made no explicit reference to the provision of medical relief, but some kirk sessions took, at least on occasion, a constructive view of the law and appointed surgeon apothecaries to treat the sick poor, including the elderly, under their charge[3]. The position was regularised in 1845 with the passing of the Poor Law (Scotland) Amendment Act which stipulated, firstly, that 'there shall be proper and sufficient arrangements made for dispensing and supplying medicines to the sick poor' lodged in poorhouses, secondly, that 'there shall be provided by the Parochial Board proper medical attendance for the inmates of every such poorhouse', and, thirdly, that Parochial Boards shall provide 'medicines, medical attendance, nutritious diet, cordials, and clothing' for the 'out-door' poor 'in such manner, and to such extent as may seem equitable and expedient'[4]. The reformed Scottish Poor Law followed the example of the English in making the conditions of residence within the poorhouse so unpleasant as to test rigorously the alleged disability or destitution of those seeking relief. The natural consequence of the 'poorhouse test' was, as one contemporary commentator explained, 'that many aged couples will struggle on to the end, and succeed, somehow or other, in maintaining themselves without rate-aid'. Few of those desperate enough to submit themselves to the 'test' ended up inside the poorhouse, for, as the same commentator observed in 1870, 'it has hitherto been almost universally the practice to give out-door relief' to the aged poor. In Glasgow, for example, there were only six elderly couples in the parish poorhouse in 1869[5].

This peculiarly Scottish emphasis upon domiciliary relief (which was, in part, to be explained by the fact that outdoor relief was considerably cheaper to provide than indoor) was doubtless welcomed by the aged sick, for the hospital facilities available in nineteenth century Scottish poorhouses were hopelessly inadequate. The sick were generally accommodated in the same dormitories as those which were inhabited by other categories of pauper; nursing services were invariably provided by untrained inmates; and facilities for diagnosis and treatment were rudimentary or non-existent. Towards the end of the century, however, advances in medical knowledge and the growing recognition that many conditions could not be successfully treated in the insanitary dwellings of the poor, led to demands for the expansion and improvement of hospital facilities. The pressure on the Poor Law authorities to provide modern hospital accommodation and services could not be ignored, for voluntary hospitals would not normally admit patients suffering from many of the conditions associated with the elderly, while the municipal hospitals only treated fever cases. The last two decades of the Victorian period witnessed a considerable improvement in the standard of medical care provided in poorhouses, but the Departmental Committee appointed by the Local Government Board for Scotland to inquire into Poor Law medical relief and the Royal Commission on the Poor Laws, which reported in 1904 and 1909 respectively, found that much still required to be done to bring the standard of care up to an acceptable level. The Royal Commission found that only in Glasgow had Poor Law hospitals been erected on sites detached from the general poorhouse and placed under the management of a medical superintendent, and that elsewhere poorhouse hospitals were 'managed under conditions which militate against their success as hospitals for the treatment of the sick'[6]. Since the introduction of a Treasury grant in 1885, there had been great progress in providing trained nurses for Poor Law hospital work, but the Royal Commission regretted that out of 68 poorhouses in Scotland there were still 26 without trained nurses and that in the other 42 staff numbers were generally maintained at the minimum level necessary to qualify for the grant[7]. Similarly, while the Departmental Committee found that diagnostic and therapeutic facilities had been greatly improved in recent years, observing that the best Poor Law hospitals were 'supplied with medical and surgical equipment, staff, and accommodation on a scale almost equal to that of the best general infirmaries'[8], the Royal Commission discovered that in many hospitals the medical staff were insufficient to undertake the work required of them. Dr Leslie Mackenzie informed the Commission that

"in most poorhouses the medical and nursing service is kept at the minimum necessary [to secure the grant]. In one poorhouse hospital, a single lady resident physician (with a visiting physician) has some 350 patients to attend to, and does her own dispensing as well. Her 'morning' round takes some five hours. In another poorhouse hospital, a lady resident has about the same number of patients to manage practically single-handed"[9].

The inadequacies of the service, which the 1904 and 1909 reports had drawn attention to, could only have been remedied if vast sums of public money had been made available, but the demands of rearmament and the First World War, and the economic difficulties associated with the post-war depression, meant that such sums were not forthcoming. Steps were, however, taken to improve the quality of the service. The Scottish Board of Health observed in its annual report for 1924 that 'during the last twenty or twenty five years, and especially in the latter half of that period, there has been a substantial improvement in the arrangements made for the medical attendance, nursing and general welfare of the sick in many poorhouses'[10]. The improvement was perhaps most evident in respect of the nursing service. Except where the number of sick was too small to justify the employment of trained nurses, the use of untrained inmates had been eliminated. Nonetheless, despite these improvements, certain serious difficulties remained; most notably the structural inadequacies of many older poorhouse buildings, which prevented 'any possibility of keeping pace with advancing medical knowledge and standards'[11].

The Local Government (Scotland) Act of 1929 effected a radical change in the system of local government. The Parish Councils (popularly elected bodies which had replaced the oligarchical Parochial Boards following the Local Government Act of 1889) were abolished, and their poorhouses, Poor Law hospitals, and 'outdoor' medical services for the sick poor were transferred to the thirty one reconstructed county councils and the town councils of the twenty four large burghs with populations over 20,000. In the city of Glasgow, for example, the Health Department became responsible for not only seventeen hospitals with approximately 10,000 beds, including four Poor Law and three mental deficiency hospitals with 2,400 and 1,300 beds respectively, but also the 'outdoor' Poor Law medical service which was conducted by part-time medical officers who treated mainly elderly patients either in local dispensaries or in their own homes. The two city poorhouses were transferred to the Corporation's new Public Assistance Committee and were managed by the Director of Public Assistance.

Some of the best equipped hospitals for the poor were turned into municipal hospitals. With the raising of the standards of these hospitals went a degree of exclusiveness in the choice of patient. The Relieving Officer could not admit a patient to a public health hospital, and the statutory right of admission of the destitute – the best feature of the Poor Law – began to be lost. Professor (later Sir John) Brotherston stated

"The legislation in this country in 1929–1930 which enabled the old 'Poor Law' hospitals to be taken over and made into acute hospitals, resulted frequently in their elderly population, previously cared for perhaps in a rather primitive way, being edged out. In some localities there has been a deficiency in geriatric accommodation ever since. Yet the policy was adopted with the best intentions and in the interest of modern medicine"[12].

The Origin of the Municipal Hospitals

Some Parish Councils built their own general hospitals: in Glasgow, in 1899, it was resolved to construct a large general hospital with 1,200 beds and two smaller district hospitals. As long as the Poor Law hospitals continued in this way, admission of a patient had to be preceded by, or if the case was urgent succeeded by, an application for poor relief by the patient or his or her next of kin, whether they were poor or well-off. This procedure meant that the patient acquired the legal status of pauper. Under the Local Government Act, local authorities were enabled to make a beginning with 'the break up of the Poor Law'. The Act allowed a local authority:

(a) to reorganise its hospital facilities with a view to the provision of treatment of sick people residing within its area and

(b) to increase its accommodation for the sick if necessary.

In both cases the Department of Health for Scotland must be satisfied that the hospital accommodation at the disposal of the Council, together with that provided by the voluntary hospitals or other institutions, was not reasonably adequate for the needs of the area. It was also made clear that before a local authority could administer the transferred hospitals the standards of treatment must be such as to commend themselves to the government. Thus the old mixed poorhouses would not qualify under any such scheme for the treatment of the sick. In the transferred general hospitals the poorhouse section housed a variety of inmates including old people who were gradually transferred to the poorhouse proper.

In 1936 the status of the hospitals run by the Public Health Department in Glasgow was such that the University established a professional teaching unit in Stobhill General Hospital for the professor of materia medica and therapeutics (Noah Morris), who started work in 1937. Alstead[13], who succeeded Professor Morris, has said of this event, 'in 1937 the channelling of academic enterprise through the wards of a Glasgow Municipal Hospital produced an alteration of attitude which anticipated by twelve years the revolutionary changes effected by the National Health Service'.

The Growth of Geriatric Medicine

In 1939 conditions for the destitute deteriorated because of the upgrading of many of the still existing public assistance infirmaries into Emergency Medical Service hospitals, and the overcrowding of the remaining infirmaries by evacuated patients from danger zones. In July 1948 the remaining Poor Law infirmaries, still housing deprived children, the aged, the infirm and destitute of all ages and the chronic sick, were transferred to the Regional Hospital Boards. The responsibility of the new authorities was limited by an Act of Parliament to 'hospital care'. By the Act of 1948 it was the duty of the local authority to provide residential accommodation for those persons who by reason of age, infirmity, or other circumstances needed care and attention not otherwise available to them. Provision could be made for residents suffering from minor ailments or illnesses usually nursed at home.

The Secretary of State for Scotland, through the Regional Hospital Boards, had to provide hospital accommodation to such an extent as he considered necessary to meet all reasonable requirements.

The following definitions were given for the sick and infirm:-

Sick (Responsibility of Regional Hospital Boards). Patients requiring continued medical treatment also supervision and nursing care including very old people who though not suffering from any particular illness are confined to bed on account of extreme weakness.

Infirm (Responsibility of the local authority). People who are normally able to get up and who could attend meals in the dining room or nearby day room including those who need a certain amount of help in dressing, toilet or moving from room to room and who from time to time may need to spend a few days in bed.

At that stage the category of older people classified medically as frail but ambulant proved difficult to accommodate and was often considered unsuitable by the local authority. Their institutions were initially loath to accept such individuals but with continued dialogue, and the passage of considerable time, homes for the frail elderly were eventually built by some authorities, while others accepted them in special wards set aside for this purpose. During this period of discussion many beds in hospitals were occupied by ill old people, often incorrectly diagnosed and unclassified. With the further increase in the numbers of the very old those who were mentally frail began to constitute another even more difficult problem. It must be noted that the outdoor medical service, which in cities like Glasgow had expanded from 1931 onwards, and which was running from many clinics a geriatric service providing old people with special care and keeping them under observation, was abolished under the National Health Service. Coupled with this setback was the fact that all hospitals, especially perhaps the former municipal ones, regarded themselves as 'acute', and thus difficulties now began to be experienced in obtaining the admission of an ill old person.

The Emergence of Geriatric Medicine

In 1881 Charcot[14] wrote 'The importance of a special study of diseases of old age would not be contested at the present day' and, in 1909, Nascher defined the word 'geriatrics' as the subdivision of medicine which is concerned with old age and its diseases[15]. Nascher was stimulated by seeing one of his teachers present an old woman with some minor complaint to his class saying 'she is suffering from old age, nothing can be done for her'. He eventually collected enough material to write a textbook on *Diseases of Old Age* in 1914, and according to Howell[16] the production of this work marked the beginning of the serious study of the care of the elderly.

British geriatric medicine started in 1935 with the appointment of Marjory Warren to the West Middlesex Hospital, when the adjacent Poor Law infirmary was taken over, and she developed in that infirmary a special geriatric unit, in which accurate diagnosis and her own outstanding gift of personal rehabilitation was practised[17]. Geriatric medicine (clinical gerontology) has since been defined as the branch of general medicine concerned with the health and the clinical, social, preventive and remedial aspects of illness in the elderly. The concepts of this subject were that old age is not a disease, that accurate diagnosis was essential, that many illnesses of elderly people were remediable, and that prolonged rest in bed without reason was dangerous. Marjory Warren's place in the history of geriatric medicine was made by her ability to inspire and teach the future teachers of this subject. George Adams stated in his memorial address that her unit had become widely recognised as the pioneer centre of medical care in these islands, and that men and women from medical and other services concerned with the care of the elderly were attracted from all corners of the earth to study her methods[18]. Marjory Warren[19], writing on the evolution of geriatric medicine, recalls that it was from a study of patients found in hospitals for the chronic sick that her system was formed. She continued 'The geriatric unit should ideally and whenever possible be an integral part of a general hospital and should there influence medical and public opinion in the care of the old. Much information and practical advice in the care of old people can be given by physicians practising geriatric medicine in helping patients who are under treatment in general wards'.

In 1942 Morris[20] wrote an article in a students' journal revealing the essential elements of a geriatric service with remarkable insight into the future. When he took over wards in Stobhill General Hospital in 1937, the routine was for the Chief to proceed up the ward to about the tenth bed, then wave to the other eight old patients lying on either side of the ward, cross the ward and pay attention to the other ten patients going down on the other side of the ward. The older patients were greeted and perhaps the only proper examination they had was on admission, the rest of their care being left to a devoted and excellent nursing staff; bed rest was the order of the day. Changes, however, were in the air.

In 1947 Lord Amulree and Trevor Howell encouraged progress further by founding the Medical Society for the Care of the Elderly, which became the British Geriatrics Society. Also in that year the Nuffield Foundation formed a committee, under the chairmanship of Mr Seebohn Rowntree, which carried out a sociological survey of old people in several localities and, in 1947, published an important work entitled *Old People*. In 1948 Sheldon[21] followed this with a review of part of the same sample in Wolverhampton which focused more on the medical aspects of ageing; it was called *The Social Medicine of Old Age*. Unfortunately no medical examinations of the subjects were possible.

In Scotland Oswald Taylor Brown and Nanette Nisbet were first-rate teachers of geriatric medicine and were infected by the enthusiasm of Marjory Warren. In 1951 Taylor Brown was appointed as a consultant to organise a geriatric service in the Eastern Region of Scotland based in Dundee. This post carried with it an honorary lectureship in clinical medicine at the University of Dundee, and from that time teaching of geriatric medicine started in Scotland. The first session granted was a two-hour meeting on a Saturday morning and attendance was voluntary. Such was the clinical acumen and skill of Taylor Brown that by 1955 geriatric medicine was taught regularly within normal teaching hours.

In Glasgow where there were a large number of elderly ill people awaiting admission to hospital a similar appointment to that in Dundee was made in 1952. It became obvious that if these old people were ever to be admitted to acute hospitals they must not stand in line with the younger sick: as in a time of bed shortage, there will always be an acute emergency case among the young. With constant pressure on beds it thus seemed essential, as Marjory Warren had recommended, to set aside beds in the acute hospital which would be for the exclusive use of the elderly. When these people are ill they require the diagnostic apparatus of the acute hospital, as accurate diagnosis, or more commonly a list of diagnoses, is particularly difficult to make in the elderly. Glasgow was therefore divided up into five sectors with each based on a teaching hospital. This reduced the waiting lists in each sector to more manageable proportions.

In spite of this it seemed at this stage that the problem of caring for elderly people when ill in ever increasing numbers was almost insoluble. So many of them were being admitted to hospital at a late stage in their illness because of the long waiting list. It was also clear that there was inadequate knowledge of the physiological changes associated with ageing. Ways of obtaining this information and of detecting illness at an earlier stage seemed essential.

In 1953, as a result of the initiative and drive of Dr Nairn Cowan, the Medical Officer of Health of Rutherglen, a Consultative Clinic for older people was established at the health centre in that Royal burgh. This particular site was chosen because the town was densely populated around the health centre and there was an excellent relationship with the local general practitioners. The name of the clinic was chosen with care as all are subject to growing older, and it was felt that this description would not inhibit individuals from attending. Drs Cowan and Anderson opened a dialogue with the general practitioners, who were asked to refer to the centre for clinical examination individuals who were 55 years and over and who had no complaints; or those with minor illness or difficulties and with housing or similar problems. In return for this action the doctors would receive a full report giving the results of the detailed clinical examination. No person was seen at the Clinic who had not been referred by their own doctor. On this understanding the local general practitioners gave their complete co-operation.

Attempts were thus made to obtain information about some of the changing attributes of 'normal' ageing, in the belief that it was nigh impossible to determine abnormality in the elderly if there was no comparison with fit older individuals. It was also felt that if illness could be diagnosed at an early stage treatment was more likely to be successful.

Useful facts did emerge from this experiment[22], but it was evident that at the Clinic only the individuals who could be brought there were being seen. Perhaps the most important finding was the realisation that there was the need for a health care team which should include a general practitioner, a district nurse, a health visitor, a social worker and paramedical staff, especially the chiropodist. The value of chiropody in the care of the elderly, especially those living at home, was obvious from the start. From the experience at the Rutherglen Consultative Clinic, when general practitioner health centres began to appear, consultants in geriatric medicine in the Glasgow area were required to run out-patient clinics at these centres. This was a source of help and stimulation to the general practitioners and encouraged them to initiate schemes of ascertainment of their own.

By 1964 Williamson and his colleagues[23] in Edinburgh were undertaking their fundamental research into the 'iceberg of unreported illness', demonstrating that even in excellent practices the general practitioner was, certainly in the urban setting, often unaware of significant illness among older patients. This brought into doubt the value of the self-reporting of illness in older individuals. From this excellent work there emerged various ways of seeking out disease by routine visiting of selected age groups, and making use of the age/sex register of the general practitioner, by members of the health care team (e.g. the health visitor[24]). These visits could only be undertaken with the consent and co-operation of the general practitioner. In later years Hamish Barber and his co-workers[25] in Glasgow continued to investigate the various options of ascertaining early illness.

In 1959 the Glasgow (now the Scottish) Retirement Council was established: a voluntary body which endeavours to improve the health of those in retirement and to spread the concept of prevention of illness by health education.

The Council, which is still in being, undertook three main tasks:
(a) Training for men and women before they retire, with particular stress on the preservation of physical, mental and social health.
(b) The setting up of hobbies and crafts centres where retired men could undertake, under instruction, woodwork or work in metal and women had sewing classes and instruction in callisthenics and dancing. A senior citizens orchestra was formed which still plays regularly at functions in the Glasgow area.
(c) The establishment of a *bureau* where part-time employment could be found for retired people who desired work.

The office is open in the afternoons every weekday and is staffed by knowledgeable volunteers.

Stress has been laid on these methods of trying to maintain the morale and stimulate the mental health of older people. This is an essential part of any attempt to preserve the independence of the elderly.

During this time the waiting list for admission to hospital for older people in Scotland had been drastically reduced. The widespread adoption of the principle of the geriatric assessment unit in teaching and district hospitals, and the steady build up of consultant appointments in geriatric medicine with appropriate senior registrar posts had transformed the picture. In Glasgow there were now 16 consultant appointments in this speciality and there had been a comprehensive building programme of 'Continuing Treatment Hospital Units'. The improvement in hospital services and in the ascertainment of early illness had, however, to be matched by a corresponding increase in the range and variety of domiciliary provision; and this in turn had to be assisted by ever-increasing numbers of places in old peoples' homes. Co-operation between local authority services and hospital provision has gradually improved but difficulties remain, even between different departments within the local authority e.g. social work departments and housing.

In recent years the belated appearance of 'sheltered housing' in Scotland has added a new and promising development to the care of older people. This is true also of the modern methods of personal intercommunication systems. Due respect must be paid to the number of voluntary organisations concerned with the welfare of older people. Selected examples are Age Concern, the British Red Cross, the Women's Royal Voluntary Services, the Crossroads Care Attendant Scheme and, in more recent times, those who administer and staff hospices.

The Academic Development of Geriatric Medicine

The fundamental importance of teaching has already been stressed, and one great advantage that Scotland possesses is the long established and well recognised university medical faculties. Instruction in this subject is essential to a wide variety of people and the only possible solution to this problem was the establishment of an academic department of geriatric medicine. In 1965 the first clinical chair of geriatric medicine in the world was endowed at the University of Glasgow, and research work was started at various health centres in co-operation with this department. One example was the survey of older people living at home based on the Kilsyth health centre[26]. This was followed by a study by Akhtar *et al*[27] of individuals 65 years and over living at home. Undergraduate and postgraduate teaching of medical students, with regular sessions for general practitioners, became the routine business of the department.

Courses were arranged for nurses and paramedical staff, and an active part was taken in the courses for preparation for retirement. Williamson's work in health surveillance, and his proven ability as a clinical teacher, was of such high quality that when a chair of geriatric medicine was established in Edinburgh he was the obvious choice.

The results of the research on nutrition[28] and the accumulated experience in teaching were demonstrated by the various textbooks which now appeared[29,30]. From this academic beginning fourteen chairs of geriatric medicine have been established in the United Kingdom and this subject has been widely recognised as an academic discipline[31].

Great assistance in the earlier development of geriatric medicine was given by the Royal College of Physicians of Edinburgh[32,33], and there is now a strict control by all the Royal Colleges of Physicians of the training of consultants in this speciality.

The World Health Organization has also played an important part by sponsoring month long courses for physicians from European countries as a stimulus to their training in geriatric medicine. The first was held in Glasgow in 1964 and was followed by one in Kiev in 1965, in Paris in 1966 and again in Glasgow in 1967. In 1974 a report was published on the organization of geriatric care[34], while in 1982 there was a special conference of the United Nations on Ageing which was held in Vienna.

In recent years consultant physicians from Scotland have travelled to almost every country in the world to give advice and instruction on planning and on the clinical care of the elderly.

Throughout the development of the medical services for the elderly in Scotland a strong lead, and constant support, was given by the Chief Medical Officer, Sir John Brotherston. Reviewing changes in the National Health Service in 1969, Brotherston[35] concluded:

> "Nothing will really flow smoothly in the National Health Service until we reach an adequate state of provision in our society for the elderly. This means many things apart from hospital beds. A major phenomenon of the elderly vis-a-vis the Health Service is under-demand, not over-demand. Later generations of the elderly may benefit in health in earlier years in a better environment but they will not be so stoic in the face of disability or so unwisely sparing of the medical service as are our contemporary veterans'.

In the future[36] there will require to be much more co-operation in the care of the elderly between the different providers of care and the health care professionals, with even greater diversity of services. Old people in time to come will, as has been suggested above, be much more demanding and will wish for higher standards in the services which are provided for them. More units in hospitals will be run jointly by physicians in geriatric medicine with orthopaedic surgeons, urologists and psychiatrists. Improved methods of communication will enable elderly people to remain for a longer time in their own homes. Hopefully, health education will ensure that individuals reach old age in a much healthier state than at present. To live long should be regarded as a prize and therefore rewards should be available for those obtaining this goal. It can be seen that much still remains to be done.

References

(1)   *The Acts of the Parliaments of Scotland,* III (Edinburgh, 1814), p.88.
(2)   *The Acts of the Parliament of Scotland,* VIII (Edinburgh, 1820), pp.89–91.
(3)   Hamilton, D. *The Healers, A history of medicine in Scotland* (Edinburgh, 1981), pp.51–52.
(4)   8 and 9 *Victoria,* cap.83. Sections 66 and 69.
(5)   Scotus, *The Scottish Poor Laws: Examination of their policy, history and practical action* (Edinburgh, 1870), p.264.
(6)   Royal Commission on the Poor Laws and Relief of Distress. *Report on Scotland,* (1909), Cd.4922, p.146.
(7)   *Ibid,* p.148.
(8)   *Report of the Department Committee appointed by the Local Government Board for Scotland to inquire into the system of Poor Law Medical Relief and into the rules and regulations for the Management of Poorhouses; together with supplement,* (1904), Cd.2008, p.23.
(9)   *Royal Commissions on the Poor Laws, op. cit.,* p.147.
(10) *Sixth Annual Report of the Scottish Board of Health.* (Edinburgh, H.M.S.O., 1925), Cmd.2416, p.189.
(11) *Ibid.* p.189.
(12) Brotherston, Sir J. 'Policies for the care of the elderly (i) an overview', in Kinnaird, J., Brotherston, Sir J. and Williamson, J., *The Provision of Care for the Elderly,* (Edinburgh, 1981), pp.17–23.
(13) Alstead, S. 'The effect of the National Health Service on medical education', Scott. Med. J., 7, (1962), p.375.
(14) Charcot, J.M., Clinical Lectures on Senile and Chronic Diseases. (London, 1881).
(15) Freeman, J.T., *Ageing: Its History and Literature.* (New York, 1979).
(16) Howell, T.H., *A Student's Guide to Geriatrics.* (London, 1970).
(17) Anderson, Sir F. 'The evolution of services in the United Kingdom', in Kinnaird, J., Brotherston, Sir. J. and Williamson, J., *The Provision of Care for the Elderly,* (Edinburgh, 1981), pp.117–123.
(18) Adams, G.F., 'Memorial Address for Dr. Marjory Warren, C.B.E.'. Geront. clin., *3,* (1961), p.1.
(19) Warren, Marjory, 'The evolution of geriatric medicine', Geront. clin., *2,* (1960), p.1.
(20) Morris, N., 'De Senectute', Surgo, *8,* (1942), p.28.
(21) Sheldon, J.H., *The Social Medicine of Old Age.* (London, 1948).
(22) Anderson, W.F., 'Research on ageing', *Health Bulletin,* 27, (1970), p.1.
(23) Williamson, J., Stokoe, I.H., Gray, S., Fisher, M., Smith, A., McGhee, A., and Stephenson, E., 'Old people at home – their unreported needs', *Lancet,* 1, (1964), p.1117.
(24) Anderson, Sir F., 'The affect of screening on the quality of life after seventy'. *J. Roy. Coll. Phycns.,* 10, (1976), p.161.
(25) Barber, J.H., and Wallis, Joan B., 'Assessment of the elderly in general practice'. *J. Roy. Coll. Gen. Pract.,* 26, (1976), p.106.
(26) Andrews, G.R., Cowan, N.R., and Anderson, W.F., 'The practice of geriatric medicine in the community: an evaluation of the place of health centres', in McLachlan, G., *Problems and Progress in Medical Care.* Essays on Current Research, 5th Series, (London, 1971), pp.58–86.

(27) Akhtar, A.J., Broe, G.A., Crombie, Agnes, McLean, W.M.R., Andrews, G.R., and Caird, F.I., 'Disability and dependence in the elderly at home', *Age and Ageing*, 2 (1973), p.102.

(28) Macleod, C.C., Judge, T.G., and Caird, F.I., 'Nutrition of the elderly at home: I. Intakes of energy, protein, carbohydrate and fat', *Age and Ageing*, 3, (1974), p.158. II. Intakes of vitamins', *Age and Ageing*, 3, (1974), p.209. III. Intakes of minerals', *Age and Ageing*, 4, (1975), p.49.

(29) Anderson, F., *Practical Management of the Elderly*. (Oxford, 1967).

(30) Caird, F.I., Dall, J.L.C., and Kennedy, R.D., *Cardiology in Old Age* (New York, 1976).

(31) Anderson, Sir F., 'Geriatric medicine: an academic discipline', *Age and Ageing*, 5, (1976), p.193.

(32) *The Care of the Elderly in Scotland*, Royal College of Physicians of Edinburgh. Publication No.22. (Edinburgh, 1963).

(33) *The Care of the Elderly in Scotland: A Follow-up Report*. Royal College of Physicians of Edinburgh. Publication No.37. (Edinburgh, 1970).

(34) World Health Organization Technical Report Series. No.548. (Geneva, 1974).

(35) Brotherston, Sir J., 'Change and the National Health Service', *Scott. Med. J.*, 14, (1969), p.130.

(36) Anderson, Sir F., 'Future developments in the U.K.', in Wood, C., *Health and the Family*, (London, 1979), pp.209–216.

3. *Tuberculosis*

Christopher Clayson

CONTENTS

About the Author

Dr CHRISTOPHER CLAYSON C.B.E., M.B., Ch.B., D.P.H., M.D.(Gold Medal), P.R.C.P.E., F.R.C.P.

Dr Christopher Clayson graduated in Medicine at Edinburgh University in 1926. An early personal encounter with the tubercular bacillus led him to the study of chest medicine, and he became lecturer in the University Department of Tuberculosis from 1939–1944. He became Consultant Chest Physician to Dumfries and Galloway Hospitals in 1944, and later President of the Royal College of Physicians of Edinburgh from 1966–1970, and was the first chairman of the Scottish Council for Postgraduate Medical Education from 1970–1974.

One unique distinction for a doctor was his chairing of the Departmental Committee on Scottish Licensing Law (1971–1973), which led to the Licensing (Scotland) Act 1976.

Author's Note

In 1882, it was finally proved that tuberculosis was an infective disease. The health services of the time were incapable of dealing with the situation. Charitable organisations began their devoted anti-tuberculosis work, and in time attracted the support and co-operation of official departments. What became known as the Co-ordinated Edinburgh Scheme for the Control of Tuberculosis was finally adopted as the model for Scotland in 1908, and for the whole country in 1913.

Progress was made difficult by two world wars, but one effect of the second conflict was that of more rapid improvements. These included mass radiography, specific immunisation, and the development and rational use of effective chemotherapeutic agents. The disease which was once captain of the men of death was rapidly reduced to a minor instrument of mortality.

John Brotherston's interest in preventive medicine began in 1940, when he worked with me for a time in the tuberculosis field – then beginning an enduring friendship. In the wider area of public health his influence and devotion remained with him throughout his life, and he liked to think that in many ways Scotland led the way in community health.

Tuberculosis

Prelude to the Twentieth Century

In the spring of 1882 a Scottish doctor, 25 years of age, packed his bags and hurried home to Edinburgh from Vienna, his mind filled with excitement and foreboding. Robert William Philip had seen the *tubercle bacillus* for the first time. His excitement arose from his profound appreciation of Koch's admirably scientific demonstration: his foreboding stemmed from its implication, namely that the hospitals in Great Britain, even when they had annexes for the treatment of fevers, were totally incapable of dealing with another vast infective disease.

At that time tuberculous patients were treated at the major general hospitals on a short term basis. Where general medical dispensaries existed they provided advice and medicines. Philip himself was appointed to the New Town Dispensary in Edinburgh in 1885, and this only served to increase his forebodings that no machinery existed which was capable of dealing with the enormous problem presented by tuberculosis. Not only was the prevalence of the disease extremely formidable, but it rapidly became clear that once *tubercle bacilli* had appeared in the sputum the great majority of patients died within two or three years. The recorded death rate from tuberculosis in all its forms in Scotland in 1882 was 308 per 100,000 of the population.

Philip propounded to his teachers a new doctrine. Clinical examination and what passed for treatment was not enough. All relevant information should be gathered in what he called a 'directory of tuberculosis'. An account of the patient's environment should be written down and, where possible, defects corrected. The patient should be instructed, since he was the subject of an infective disease, how to prevent infection spreading to others. All those in contact with the patient should be examined, and advice for the guidance of the whole family should be issued. The *bacillus* should be attacked in its breeding place, namely the home of the patient, and all these preventive measures should be co-ordinated from a new type of dispensary specially devoted to this work, with trained medical and nursing staff.

These novel ideas did not commend themselves to his teachers and Philip met with passive and even active discouragement. Nevertheless in 1887 he 'succeeded with the help of a few kind friends in establishing the Victoria Dispensary for Consumption in the heart of Edinburgh'[1].

The next step in the development of a co-ordinated scheme was the founding of a sanatorium. The 'few kind friends' emerged as the Victoria Hospital Tuberculosis Trust, which continued its fund raising efforts to this end. The idea was to create a hospital as near to the centre of the city as possible, not only for the convenience of patients and visitors, but also to afford a wider object lesson to the population, by identifying an urban site where fresh air treatment was clearly practicable. This was achieved in a charming Georgian mansion set in seven acres of ground a mile or so to the north of the city centre. In August 1894 the Victoria Hospital for Consumption received its first 14 patients, and in that year 297 cases were treated[2].

In England the challenge was taken up more slowly. On 20 December 1898 however, there was a famous meeting at Marlborough House, the London home of the Prince of Wales. The meeting was chaired by His Royal Highness in his own drawing room, and a crusade against tuberculosis was discussed. Having listened to the proposition that tuberculosis was a preventable disease the Prince asked in an immortal phrase: 'if preventable why not prevented?'. The result of this meeting was the formation of what ultimately became known as the National Association for the Prevention of Tuberculosis. Nevertheless it was not until 1909 that another charitable organisation opened the first of the English dispensaries on the Edinburgh model at Paddington.

1900–1910

The first decade of the twentieth century was a formative period in the Scottish tuberculosis campaign. By the year 1900 there were established in Edinburgh, for the first time anywhere, a dispensary and a hospital which were under the same clinical chief, R.W. Philip, and were supported by the voluntary endeavours of the Victoria Hospital Trust, which was devoted to the co-ordinated care and prevention of consumption. The death rate at that time was 224 per 100,000 of the population.

In July 1900 a notable development took place in the conclusion of important negotiations with the City of Edinburgh[3]. It had long been Philip's wish to separate the early curable cases from the more advanced type of patient for whom both medical and nursing requirements were different. The new arrangements with the city authorities enabled this to be achieved. Henceforth the Victoria Hospital was to be used as a sanatorium for early cases, and 50 beds in the New City Hopsital, Colinton Mains, were to be available as a refuge for the continuing care of sufferers from the advanced disease.

Philip pressed ahead with the development of the Victoria Hospital. Three modern pavilions were added in 1903 and were opened by Lord Salisbury. King Edward VII became the Hospital's Patron and the title 'Royal' was added to the Dispensary, the Hospital, and the Trust. Events followed rapidly. In 1905 the open air school was established at the hospital to take care of the children's education. In 1907 two more pavilions were added, and the last development in a busy decade was the opening of the Royal Victoria Hospital's farm colony at Polton near Lasswade. The planned object of this advance was to allow more purposeful training of men likely to have to earn their living in the open air, or who would require longer medical supervision than the sanatorium could provide. Meanwhile the demands on the Royal Victoria Dispensary were increasing rapidly, and in 1911 much larger premises were opened in Spittal Street in the city centre.

Although Philip's professional position, which he had done so much to create in the voluntary organisation, was uniquely personal, he laid great stress on co-ordination in any such scheme with local health departments. His general view[4] was that an anti-tuberculosis organisation should be more or less completely under the direction of the Medical Officer of Health, but as a separate and well defined department of public health activity. There should be close links between the Medical Officer of Health, the dispensary and the hospital. His connection with the sanatorium and the colony might be less distinct. Such arrangements would obviously assist in the problems of notification, and could be of enormous importance in securing the vital help of trained district nursing.

Developments were, of course, taking place elsewhere in Scotland. In the Glasgow area[5], apparently reversing the Edinburgh chronology, it seems that events gave precedence to sanatorium provision over dispensary needs. Nevertheless the same co-operation between charitable individuals, voluntary agencies and the local health authority was much in evidence. The Consumptive Homes at Bridge of Weir were founded in 1897 through the magnificent generosity of William Quarrier. The Glasgow and Western Scotland Branch of the National Association for the Prevention of Tuberculosis opened a sanatorium of 52 beds at Bellefield near Lanark. In both endeavours assistance by grants-in-aid was given by the Corporation of the City of Glasgow. Lanfine House for 14 patients, later increased to 44, was built by a charitable donor, near Kirkintilloch and served for the care of patients with advanced disease.

In 1910 the organised tuberculosis dispensary service began in Glasgow. The scheme comprised four district dispensaries in premises loaned by parish councils, relying for inpatient treatment on the voluntary sanatoria or Poor Law authorities[6].

Voluntary bodies were not always so successful, however good their intentions. A salute could nevertheless be paid to a charitably disposed individual who assembled a committee in Dumfriesshire in 1903, and appealed for funds to make practical provision for consumption[7]. The sum raised was generous for a country area but was found to be insufficient to build, equip and maintain a sanatorium. On attending his first meeting, a new member of the committee, possibly better informed than the rest, said that since pulmonary tuberculosis was an infectious disease, provision for its treatment should be made at the cost of the public health rates.

This opinion startled the committee and on 2nd September 1904 it was communicated to the Local Government Board for Scotland. In May 1905 the Board inquired of local authorities as to the incidence of pulmonary phthisis and whether any provision had been made for its notification and treatment. There followed on 10 March 1906 a general circular, written in fact by Philip, expressing the Board's opinion that pulmonary phthisis must be regarded as an infective disease under the Public Health (Scotland) Act and that provision must be made for its control, notification and hospital treatment. The generous Dumfriesshire subscribers to their own voluntary scheme, be it noted, did not desire their money to be refunded. Their committee administered its resources for the alleviation of suffering pending the inauguration of the statutory ventures to follow, and creating an atmosphere favourable to them. These statutory undertakings were notification and the National Health Insurance Act.

Notification

Ever since Philip had conceived his idea of a directory of tuberculosis recording all relevant facts, the thoughts of many responsible workers had been directed towards notification of sufferers from tuberculosis to the medical officer of health.

This was indeed a controversial issue. There were those who believed that any breach of the confidential doctor-patient relationship should be opposed. Others felt that while notification was right and proper, in acute infective fevers where the danger to the community was obvious and immediate, such a step was unnecessary and indeed without value in a chronic protracted illness like tuberculosis. Yet others felt that notification should be confined to the poorer classes, especially those in Poor Law institutions.

These arguments faded in the face of the Local Government Board's circular of March 1906. Edinburgh had adopted a voluntary system of notification in 1903, but since authorities had now been reminded that notification was necessary to meet the provisions of the Public Health (Scotland) Act events moved more speedily. Edinburgh accepted compulsory notification in 1907, Glasgow in 1910; and other authorities followed. Non-respiratory tuberculosis became notifiable on 1 July 1914.

Given compulsory notification in order to promote effective treatment and prevention, the logical next step was to consider whether compulsory notification should be reinforced by compulsory isolation where a refractory but infective patient refused treatment. Such a step was recommended by the Astor Committee in 1913, but in Scotland it was another precaution already provided for by the Public Health Act of 1897.

In England and Wales progress was slower. In 1911 the Public Health (Tuberculosis in Hospital) Regulations provided for limited notification of patients in institutions. In 1912 this was made of general application. Compulsory isolation was later possible under the Public Health Act of 1925. The procedure was complicated (as indeed it was in Scotland) but the fact that the power existed was found to be enough to exact co-operation from obstinate patients. In one step only England was slightly ahead of Scotland at that time: namely all forms of tuberculosis became notifiable in 1913. In both countries however, a certain professional perversity was observable in that notification was not uncommonly postponed till death or after, causing difficulties which are not unknown even today.

The National Insurance Act

Thus far the campaign against tuberculosis was a splendid example of co-operation between voluntary and official agencies. It is worth recalling that the death rate from all forms of tuberculosis had fallen to 178 per 100,000 of the population by 1911; and to 115 per 100,000 from respiratory tuberculosis.

Further progress was stimulated by the National Insurance Act of

1911. The Act of course had wide implications for all insured persons, but was of especial relevance to the tuberculous patient for whom the important provision of sanatorium benefit was defined. This meant sanatorium treatment, dispensary supervision and treatment by private practitioners for insured persons. Administration was in the hands of Insurance Committees, which could, if they thought fit, extend the sanatorium benefits to the dependants of any insured person.

In Scotland some of this was already possible under the Public Health Act of 1897. For instance, domiciliary treatment by nursing attendance and 'medicine' could be provided. Medicine in this context was held to include extra nutrition and 'comforts'. The Local Government Board had approved the expenditure of 5s. (25p) per week for these purposes out of what was then the tuberculosis maintenance grant.

Despite the fact that the Finance Act of 1911 made available £1½ million for the construction of sanatoria, the development of the concept of sanatorium benefit was necessarily slow.

The Local Government Board had adopted the Edinburgh scheme as a model for the administration of the campaign against tuberculosis in 1908. Nevertheless, Philip's concept[8] that the dispensary should be the uniting point for all other agencies in every considerable community had by no means been universally adopted. It seemed therefore that the wider implementation of the National Insurance Act on a United Kingdom basis would clearly take a long time, and on 22 February 1912 the Government appointed a Departmental Committee to advise it as speedily as possible on how to proceed.

The Astor Committee

The Departmental Committee was chaired by Mr Waldorf Astor MP (later Viscount Astor). The terms of reference were:

> "To report at an early date upon the consideration of general policy in respect of the problems of tuberculosis in the United Kingdom, in its preventive, curative and other aspects, which should guide the government and local bodies in making or aiding provision for the treatment of tuberculosis in sanatoria or other institutions or otherwise".

The world 'otherwise' was later taken to imply domiciliary treatment.

Not surprisingly R.W. Philip was a member of the Committee, and the interim report[9] which was presented to Parliament later the same year followed closely the co-ordinated scheme which had already been in full operation for about fifteen years in Edinburgh.

The report stated that the first unit of the proposed scheme should be the tuberculosis dispensary. The functions were precisely defined as:

> "(1) Receiving house and centre for diagnosis.
> (2) Clearing house and centre for observation.

(3) Centre for curative treatment.
(4) Centre for examination of 'contacts'.
(5) Centre for 'after care'.
(6) Information bureau and educational centre."

In some large units, and in many rural areas, branch dispensaries would be required. As a broad indication, one dispensary would be needed for 150,000 of the population in urban areas, but in rural areas would serve a smaller population.

The second unit of the scheme should be the institutional provision. The sanatorium was intended for patients where working capacity was likely to be restored. It could be situated close to a city but on account of cost a more isolated site was usually preferable. One bed per 5,000 of the population would be immediately necessary. The hospital for advanced cases was not required to be of a special type. Parts of ordinary hospitals or even of Poor Law institutions would serve. The number of hospital beds needed was not determined by the Committee.

These recommendations had certain unfortunate consequences, arising from the acceptance of the idea that sanatoria could be built in sites remote from the related dispensaries. This led to the Committee's recognition of two separate types of tuberculosis specialist, the medical superintendent for the former and the tuberculosis officer for the latter. For the same reason the split service became divorced from the mainstream of medicine. Neither of these developments was in accord with the original Edinburgh scheme, where it was fundamental that the service was in charge of one clinical chief who was not only in close contact with the Medical Officer of Health but also with the general medical field: Philip himself was a physician at Edinburgh Royal Infirmary. In practice the tuberculosis officer was usually a senior member of the staff of the Medical Officer of Health. This separation of tuberculosis from clinical medicine was not healed till the National Health Service Act became operative 35 years later.

The Astor Committee also recommended that provision for the treatment of tuberculosis should go further than that provided under the National Insurance Act of 1911. The Committee stated that 'no single case of tuberculosis should remain uncared for in the community, and whatever services the scheme provides should be available to all cases of the disease'[10].

In the government's acceptance of the interim report of the Astor Committee, Philip witnessed his co-ordinated scheme receive the national recognition which it had already been accorded by the Local Government Board in Scotland. The honour of knighthood was conferred upon him in 1913.

Immediate Results

The immediate results of Parliament's acceptance of the Astor Report was that the Local Government Board invited local health authorities to submit schemes for the control of tuberculosis.

The Royal Victoria Hospital Tuberculosis Trust gave to the City of Edinburgh its institutions, namely the Royal Victoria Hospital, with its associated farm colony, and the Royal Victoria Dispensary. Henceforth the management of the tuberculosis problem was in the hands of the Corporation as the public health authority. Similarly, the West of Scotland Branch of the National Association for the Prevention of Tuberculosis transferred Bellefield Sanatorium to Glasgow Corporation. It was a notable accomplishment that by the time war broke out in August 1914, Glasgow had six district dispensaries operative and 880 hospital beds available[11].

Small health authorities could not of course develop rapidly complete schemes of their own, especially as regards institutional provision. This led to the establishment of Joint Sanatorium Boards, a number of which had received their constitutions from the Local Government Board by the spring of 1914. In these undertakings beds were normally shared by the combining authorities in proportion to population. The medical superintendents of such sanatoria would naturally co-operate with several medical officers of health and their tuberculosis officers.

Before the official schemes could proceed very far the first world war broke out in August 1914. Inevitably this retarded the implementation of many local developments, but it did not have that effect on the Royal Victoria Hospital Tuberculosis Trust. It is therefore convenient at this point in the historical account of tuberculosis in Scotland to recall further contributions made by the Trust.

The Royal Victoria Hospital Tuberculosis Trust

After handing over its institutions to the City of Edinburgh, the Trust was confirmed in the possession of considerable funds which were utilised to great effect in a variety of ways.

In 1917 it endowed a Chair of Tuberculosis in the University of Edinburgh, and with notable prescience made it possible, when appropriate, to include allied diseases within the scope of the new department. Sir Robert Philip was appointed the first Professor of Tuberculosis. The health authorities of the City of Edinburgh agreed to an arrangement whereby the University staff in the Department of Tuberculosis should have a formal share in the full range of work at the Royal Victoria Dispensary and should have clinical charge of two pavilions at the Royal Victoria Hospital and 25 beds in the City Hospital, all of which was vital for undergraduate and postgraduate teaching in the department.

In 1921 the Trust founded a new establishment, Southfield Sanatorium, on the southern outskirts of Edinburgh. This institution was administratively outside the official service, and was not specifically related to the needs of Edinburgh. For some years, however, it did afford valuable facilities for certain local health authorities, as for example in the Highlands and Islands, which did not at that time have sufficient resources of their own. Furthermore one activity of the sanatorium was to seek out patients presenting some feature of special interest, thereby providing additional clinical teaching opportunities for the new university department.

One of the charitable functions which the Trust had carried out ever since 1887 was to grant material, or even financial, support to needy tuberculous patients and their families. This work covered extra nourishment, clothing and perhaps contributions to holidays. The activity was not confined to the City of Edinburgh and was intended to help those whom the Scottish Official Service, for one reason or another, could not assist. From 1968 onwards the identification of need in this connection was gradually transferred to the Scottish Branch of the Chest and Heart Association (now the Chest, Heart and Stroke Association) which continues to operate the service on behalf of the Trust.

For many years, and particularly since the endowment of the Chair of Tuberculosis, the Trust was able and anxious to assist in the promotion of research. From about 1950 onwards it devoted an increasing proportion of its resources to this end. Undoubtedly the Trust's most fruitful endeavours in the field were in support of signal advances in treatment made possible by a later incumbent of the Chair of Tuberculosis, Professor (later Sir) John W. Crofton, and by his colleagues in the Edinburgh school.

War and Peace

The effects of the country-wide campaign against tuberculosis could of course only appear after the whole national scheme became fully operational, which was not till some years after the 1914–1918 war. Yet the mortality from the disease had been falling for almost as long as returns had been collected. In 1887, as has been observed, the death rate for all forms of the disease was 308 per 100,000 of the population. In 1914 the figure was 162.

The causes of this decline were various and largely stemmed from the establishment of the Local Government Board in 1894, since when there followed slow improvement in national housing, nutrition, and in environmental and educational conditions generally. In part, probably a significant part, progress was also due to the long-term heightening of national resistance following the gradual elimination of susceptible strains in the population.

In this broad context the effects of the first world war on mortality from tuberculosis were negligible. The death rate remained virtually static for three years and the pre-war curve of improvement was fully re-established as early as 1919. In England by comparison there was an actual rise in mortality of 17 *per cent*: but this too dropped to below the pre-war level by 1919.

Nevertheless the available facilities at that time had to attempt to cope not only with the morbidity problems of the civil population, but also with large numbers of ex-service personnel whose disease was held to be attributable to the conditions of service. It was in this field that Tor-na-Dee Sanatorium, near Aberdeen, came into prominence in 1918 under the auspices of the British Red Cross Society. As the demand for service beds declined with the passage of time the sanatorium became a private institution until it was taken over by the official service in 1948.

In 1919 an Inter-departmental Committee under Sir Montague Barlow[12] examined the wider national problem of ex-service personnel, and made it clear that the responsibility for treating service patients was that of the area to which they belonged, and that they should be given priority in treatment and in training for work in civilian life.

This was a difficult task for which fully adequate facilities did not yet exist in the developing service. Nevertheless great efforts were being made. Whereas the Astor Committee had stated that one sanatorium bed per 5,000 of the population was required for immediate needs together with an unspecified number of hospital beds, Sir Leslie Mackenzie[13] was able to report in 1919 that 2,250 beds were already available (or one bed per 2,116 of the population), and that the planned total of 3,950 beds could equal one bed per 1,205 of the population. These developments were taking place widely, and various Joint Sanatorium Boards, postponed in 1914, were allowed to proceed with their arrangements. In Scotland as a whole the tuberculosis service, delayed as it was by the war, was in effective operation early in the 1920s and was still expanding, as for instance in the special provision being made for children at Mearnskirk Hospital near Glasgow.

Treatment was as yet largely conservative and was based on the traditional practice of fresh air, rest, graduated exercise and work. For most patients the stay in hospital was about a year, and for many much longer. Despite the introduction of diversional and occupational therapy, prolonged in-patient treatment was found by many patients to be wearisome and tedious.

The idea that so far as pulmonary tuberculosis was concerned, the period of treatment could be shortened and healing expedited by means of collapse therapy, was introduced from the continent via England. It began to gain pace in the 1920s and for the next 30 years or so, in one form or another, was to be a mainstay of treatment. The simplest, and therefore the commonest, method was artificial pneumothorax. If the patient was fortunate and good lung collapse was achieved without the limitation of intra-pleural adhesions, or if such adhesions when present could be easily divided, excellent results were obtained. If, however, treatment was persisted in despite indivisible adhesions, as it commonly was, disaster could and often did ensue. The wise physician was he who knew when to abandon the pneumothorax and seek another remedy. An alternative was to promote elevation of the appropriate leaf of the diaphragm by interruption of the phrenic nerve, reinforced if necessary by artificial pneumoperitoneum. If these devices were inappropriate the operation of extra-pleural pneumothorax or even thoracoplasty was possible in carefully selected cases. These last were major interventions only to be carried out in the larger regional centres. In 1954 the Department of Health for Scotland[14] was able to report that 12 such centres were in use for various thoracic disorders amenable to surgery.

There is no doubt that many patients who otherwise would have succumbed achieved arrest of the disease through one or more of these surgical procedures. Likewise there is no doubt that many patients merely attained a stable state of chronic disease and so survived to infect others. In both groups, whether arrested or chronically active, the penalty of survival was all too often permanently impaired lung function, a handicap which was one of the factors which led to the more careful and refined evaluation of respiratory physiology in sanatoria and chest clinics in the years which followed.

To a great extent, the difficulties of collapse therapy were overcome as a consequence of remarkable improvements in the art of anaesthesia, which allowed the newer resectional surgery to replace the older forms of collapse treatment, and so to extirpate the local disease. Similarly, the scope and safety of resection was increased by the later advent of chemotherapy, and eventually the surgical chapter in the treatment of respiratory tuberculosis was closed when chemotherapy by itself virtually replaced all other methods.

Between the wars the mortality from respiratory tuberculosis diminished rapidly. The average annual death rate during the quinquennium 1919–23 showed a drop of 21.4 *per cent* as compared with the previous five years. Thereafter, till 1939, the quinquennial drop was a steady 13 *per cent*, and in 1939 the death rate for 100,000 of the population was 54. For non-pulmonary tuberculosis the figures were even more striking during the period, the death rate dropping from 54 to 18.

The outbreak of the second world war in September 1939 confronted sanatorium superintendents and tuberculosis officers with an alarming situation. In the expectation of large scale bombing raids and enormous numbers of civilian casualties, sanatoria were evacuated as far as possible. This meant that many infective or potentially infective patients had to be cared for at home where fresh air therapy and the prevention of the spread of infection were impossible under 'black out' conditions at night. The situation necessitated a government organised evacuation of nearly 175,000 children[15] and others from the large cities and conurbations where they had become accustomed to drinking pasteurised milk, to country areas where at that time there was still a risk of bovine infection. Happily these dangers proved to be transient. In the absence of bombing raids on the scale expected there was a drift back to the towns, and by 1943[16] only 4,500 persons remained evacuated.

The mortality from tuberculosis associated with the second world war was very different from that related to the earlier conflict. The effects of the second war were serious and prolonged. The death rate from respiratory tuberculosis rose from 54 per 100,000 in 1939 to 63 per 100,000 in 1941. In 1945 it dropped to 60 per 100,000 but rose again to 66 per 100,000 in 1947 and 1948, and the actual pre-war level was not again achieved till 1950. Expressed in quinquennial figures the increase in mortality for the five years centred on 1941 showed a rise of 10.9 *per cent* as compared with the previous quinquennium, and a still further rise of 6.5 *per cent* took place during the five years centred on 1946. It was not until the quinquennium centred on 1951 that a modest drop in mortality of 3.9 *per cent* was recorded. The deaths from non-respiratory tuberculosis broadly followed this pattern, but by 1951 they constituted a much smaller proportion of the total deaths from tuberculosis as compared with pre-war years.

The number of notifications of respiratory tuberculosis gave an even more sombre picture than the death rate. They rose continuously from 4,567 in 1939 to 7,215 in 1943. This increase of nearly 37 *per cent* in four years seemingly suggested that the problem was out of control. After 1943 the rise in notifications continued but was capable of a different interpretation, since it was partly due to the use of mass radiography which was being developed at that time. Whatever the contributory factors were, the stark facts remained that between 1945 and 1948 the number of patients awaiting treatment in hospital increased by 57 *per cent* but the staffed beds to provide for them increased by only 5 *per cent*[17]. It was becoming very clear to those involved in dealing with the difficulties of the time that a reorganised tuberculosis service under the National Health Service (Scotland) Act 1947, would be severely tested.

Tuberculosis Under the National Health Service

As early as 1944 a government White Paper[18] stated that the tuberculosis service 'tends to be administered as a separate entity, perhaps not enough related to the diagnosis and treatment of other chest and respiratory conditions, or to the work of general hospitals, because it has come into being as a separately organised service.'

The National Health Service (Scotland) Act 1947 facilitated the remedy foreseen in the White Paper. The tuberculosis service was placed under regional control, and therefore had no longer to rely on funding by local authorities. Sanatorium superintendents and tuberculosis officers became known as chest physicians. A Departmental Circular[19] sought to promote clear links between the tuberculosis service and general medicine. It recommended the establishment of chest clinics and also in-patient facilities in general hospitals, including teaching hospitals, where this had not already been done. The medical staff should be organised to cover out-patients, in-patient duties, and domiciliary consultations at the request of general practitioners.

While the discharge of clinical duties was clearly a matter for Regional Hospital Boards, section 27 of the Act defined the continuing part to be played by the Medical Officer of Health. This included the work of health visitors, the supply of beds and bedding at home, the boarding out of child contacts where necessary, rehousing, and resettlement of tuberculosis persons in employment. Advice in these matters was to be conveyed by the chest physician to the Medical Officer of Health. Identifications of need in these and other ways was greatly eased by the attendance of health visitors and medical social workers at chest clinics and associated staff conferences.

Thus it came about that the original defect in the Astor type of organisation, which has already been commented on, was being repaired and the essence of the Edinburgh system of the 1900s was being restored. Another echo of that system was heard in 1943 when a scheme of financial allowances was instituted, as part of the official service, designed to encourage sufferers to take early treatment without incurring hardship which would affect the family. The procedure was administered by local authorities as agents for the Department of Health for Scotland. In 1948[17] when nearly 3,000 families were being helped in this way, further operations were transferred to the National Assistance Board.

The purposeful development of chest clinics, as distinct from tuberculosis dispensaries, broadened the interests and training of the old chest physician in relation to all chest disorders, but narrowed them in another field, since chest physicians were henceforth gradually relieved of their traditional control of the non-respiratory manifestations of tuberculosis. Whereas formerly they were clearly responsible for the hospital care and follow-up of the non-respiratory forms of the disease, with advice from appropriate specialists as necessary, under the evolution of the new service the appropriate specialists gradually assumed the clinical care of non-respiratory tuberculosis with advice from chest physicians, which was to become of the greatest importance in the developing and complex problems of chemotherapy. Such advice was always available, if not always sought.

In assessing the needs of the tuberculosis service in 1949 it was found that the original estimate of the Astor Committee in 1912, namely one dispensary for 150,000 to 200,000 of the population, was still remarkably accurate. A report[20] prepared jointly by the Central Consultants and

Specialists Committee (Scotland) and the Tuberculosis Society of Scotland demonstrated how conveniently the population figure of 200,000 could be reproduced, singly or in multiples, in relation to the population distribution of Scotland. Thus five urban sector clinics were appropriate for Glasgow, two for Edinburgh and one each for Dundee and Aberdeen. In sparsely populated areas more branch clinics were developed serving many specialities. These areas were defined in all regions, and the functions of the former tuberculosis officers and sanatorium superintendents were combined in the responsibilities of senior chest physicians with appropriate staff; and continuity of care was assured.

The Astor Committee's estimate of one bed for 5,000 of the population in 1912 was only for immediate needs and gave no identification of what would ultimately be required. In 1949 the figure was one bed per 1,000 of the population, and amid the pressing and continuing difficulties of the post-war period this was still not enough. Beds in fever hospitals, and also in some general hospitals, were brought into service, but beds required staffing and there were too few nurses. The Departmental Circular[19] referred to regretted that tuberculosis nursing had been carried out quite separately from general nursing. Staffing of tuberculosis beds was maintained either by nurses training for the infectious diseases part of the register or for the certificate in tuberculosis nursing offered by the British Tuberculosis Association. Steps were taken in 1950–51 to promote secondment of nurses from general training for a period of tuberculosis nursing. This experiment succeeded in the south-eastern and north-eastern regions but not to any extent elsewhere[21]. At that time also the state enrolled assistant nurse was beginning to make a significant contribution to the problem. In due course the reintegration of tuberculosis with respiratory disease and general medicine overcame these nursing difficulties, but not in 1950. Nevertheless the steps taken enabled substantial numbers of extra beds to be brought into service, not only in fever hospitals but in some general hospitals as well. As a result of the expanded service there was a welcome drop in waiting lists, but even so the resources of the time were still insufficient to solve an urgent problem.

Consequently in 1951 a unique experiment began. Under powers conferred by the National Health Service Act, 1951, 180 beds were made available in certain Swiss sanatoria selected on the advice of visiting specialists and officers of the Department of Health for Scotland[22]. Suitable patients were selected by Scottish consultants and flown out in monthly groups of 36. The Scottish Branch of the British Red Cross Society gave invaluable help by stationing two officers in Switzerland to look after the welfare of the patients. The experiment continued successfully till the end of 1955, and in April 1956 the contractual arrangements with the Swiss sanatoria were terminated. In all, 1,043 patients had been treated, with great relief on the pressure at home[23].

So effective had progress been during the ten year expansion of the service that at the end of the Swiss experience the number of staffed beds in Scotland actually exceeded the number of patients on the waiting list. Scotland was thus well placed to meet still further demands occasioned by the continuing development of mass radiography, and in particular by the massive two year campaign against tuberculosis which began in 1957.

Mass Radiography

It had long been taught that if the clinician waits for the appearance of physical signs in the chest, or for the discharge of *tubercle bacilli* in the sputum in order to diagnose pulmonary tuberculosis he waits too long, and that the diagnosis must be concluded before these things occur. This could most effectively be done by radiography. Naturally, the X-raying of family contacts and of hospital nurses engaged in tuberculosis work had been practised for years. To these groups were added pre-employment X-rays of those whose duties would entail care of children, and where practicable, work contacts as well. But to extend the system to large communities of apparently healthy people in order to discover unsuspected tuberculosis would have been prohibitively expensive, employing conventional techniques.

The development of preliminary screening by 70 mm photo-fluorography changed all that, and mass radiography became a workable procedure which began in Scotland in 1944, and became a function of Regional Hospital Boards in 1948. By 1952 major mobile units had been installed in all the four large cities and in Lanark county. At the same time static units began to be established in chest clinics. The former were designed especially for community surveys, and the latter for high prevalence groups such as symptom groups, contacts, professions and trades known to be at risk, and in due course immigrants. Those working with children were also a specially selected group.

In the first ten years of mass radiography 2,013,728 examinations were carried out; 10,461 previously unsuspected cases were discovered (or 0.05 *per cent*) of the total[24]. This underestimated the problem.

In 1957 a major two year campaign was begun involving Glasgow, the other cities and 18 or so additional community surveys. In total[25], including routine mass radiography, half the adult population of Scotland was examined by X-ray. The active cases detected numbered 2.3 per 1,000 examinations, while another 4.2 per 1,000 required a period of observation. In rural areas the incidence was much lower. In mid and upper Annandale[26] when 95 *per cent* of the adult population were X-rayed in a research project the incidence of new cases was 0.5 per 1,000. In Scotland as a whole, by the conclusion of the two year survey, the number of beds available was, as planned, sufficient to meet the increased demands.

From 1960 onwards mass radiography was again conducted on a more selective basis, with special attention to the high risk groups. By 1965[27] the return of active cases had dropped to 1 per 1,000 of those examined as compared with 5 per 1,000 ten years earlier. This favourable trend continued and was one of the matters considered in 1973 in the Report on 'The Future of the Chest Services in Scotland'[28] by a committee under the chairmanship of Professor John W. Crofton. The committee submitted proposals for the re-organisation of the mass radiography service. These became operative in 1977[29] when mobile units were reduced from eight to four, three in Glasgow and one in Edinburgh, with a Director to promote their national use to best advantage. The major static units remain.

Events proved this to have been a wise decision. The proportion of newly notified cases discovered by mass radiography in 1950 was 10.8 *per cent*. It reached its peak of 48.2 *per cent* in the campaign of 1957 and thereafter dropped to 17 *per cent* in 1960 and 5.1 *per cent* in 1981. Throughout this entire period the time-honoured method of tracing patients by contact examination yielded an almost constant figure of 11 *per cent* of new cases, which remained the figure for 1981[30].

Chemotherapy

It is one of the fortunate coincidences of medical history that while the number of notifications of respiratory tuberculosis continued to rise for 10 years after the end of the second world war, and while many previously unsuspected cases were being discovered by mass radiography, the direct attack on the *tubercle bacillus* was being successfully mounted for the first time.

The search for chemotherapeutic agents had been going on for many years. The greatest advances were the discovery of streptomycin (1944) followed by *p* amino-salicyclic acid and isoniazid. In due course a wide variety of less helpful 'reserve' drugs came into supportive use. In the late 1960s two new and very effective drugs, namely rifampicin and ethambutol, became available either as a combination, or each with one of the other major agents.

The developing use of the earlier remedies corresponded in time with the appointment in 1952 of Dr John W. Crofton to the Chair of Tuberculosis in the University of Edinburgh. As with so many new advances, early use had led to early problems. Divers difficulties were encountered by all workers in the field, and a variety of questions had to be answered. How do the different drugs work and what are their best combination? How long should treatment be continued? How often do patients relapse and why? What is the best treatment for patients whose progress has been complicated by bacterial resistance? Need patients be off work? How can the recent important advances in resectional surgery be developed to even better advantage by means of chemotherapeutic cover? How far can the introduction of steroids in chemotherapy help? How can new drugs be tested?

In order to secure answers to these questions coalitions of many workers were essential. Crofton sought the co-operation of the Tuberculosis Society of Scotland (now the Scottish Thoracic Society) and with a series of planned investigations on a nation-wide basis, in addition to work in his own department, answers were sought and found to all these questions. As the solutions emerged Crofton and his co-workers, as early as 1958[31,32], were encouraged to take the view that provided patients followed rigidly the treatment prescribed and were continuously supervised by experts, 100 *per cent* success in the treatment of respiratory tuberculosis was a reasonable aim.

One of the more serious obstacles to the accomplishment of this feat was the development of bacterial resistance to the drugs employed. In the early days of chemotherapy this was in part due to unwise or even inept prescribing, but that phase was dealt with as the importance of proper drug combinations became fully appreciated. A more lasting difficulty was that patients themselves all too often did not comply with the instructions given, or even defaulted on treatment.

The bacterial resistance which resulted was recognised as a serious menace, and in 1963 the Scottish Home and Health Department[33] nominated two Glasgow laboratories as reference laboratories for the investigation of the extent of the problem. Initial results[34] showed that of 566 patients in Scotland known to be discharging *tubercle bacilli* resistant to one or more drugs, 94 *per cent* were from those areas of Scotland which at that time comprised the Western hospital region. This geographical preponderance of bacterial resistance in the west reflected the magnitude of the problem in that part of Scotland. As long ago as 1947[35] it had been noted that the City of Glasgow contributed 36 *per cent* of all Scottish deaths from respiratory tuberculosis. Not surprisingly, therefore, ease of access to laboratories for the study of bacterial resistance led in turn to the discovery of a high proportion of patients discharging resistant organisms. More formal arrangements followed for the establishment of the Scottish Mycobacteria Reference Laboratory at Mearnskirk Hospital, which operated till 1980, when it was transferred to Edinburgh City Hospital.

In the 20 years which followed the alarming revelations of 1963, great progress was made in diminishing the problem. In 1983 31 cultures of mycobacterium tuberculosis from 419 new patients showed resistance to one or more drugs[34], (a percentage of 7). Of the 74 old (previously treated) cases 11 still gave positive cultures resistant to one or more drugs. The total number of patients discharging resistant *bacilli* had dropped from 566 in 1963 to 42 in 1983.

Even more important is that in 1983 of these 42 patients only one showed resistance to rifampicin and none to ethambutol. Clearly the lessons of the past have been learned, and various effective combinations of drugs are still available to form the basis of standard treatment.

The question may now be asked how near have Crofton and his colleagues come to the 100 *per cent* success which they thought to be a reasonable aim? In the Lothian region and health board area (population 749,395) only one man and two women died of respiratory tuberculosis in 1982, equivalent to a death rate of 0.4 per 100,000 of the population. In Scotland as a whole, for the same year, the death rate was 1 per 100,000. Compared with the Scottish death rate of 155 per 100,000 in the year 1901 this is an historic achievement. During the chemotherapeutic era there was a truly accelerating fall from 48 per 100,000 in 1950 to the present figure.

In Scotland organised chemotherapy could be grafted on to the existing tuberculosis service, and, as in all developed countries, this was an enormous advantage. In developing countries, however, circumstances were different and very difficult. Crofton's contributions in this regard are outside the scope of this history. Suffice it to observe that in 1977 his national and international work was recognised by the honour of knighthood.

Chemoprophylaxis

In 1913 the final report of the Astor Committee referred to the desirable aim of preventing active disease developing in persons into whose system the *tubercle bacillus* had entered. The committee did not go so far as to suggest how this highly desirable purpose could be achieved, apart from a general observation on diminishing the existing amount of infective material.

In 1925 Sir Robert Philip[37] argued that children with a strongly positive tuberculin reaction, but without clinical lesions and therefore not notifiable, should be treated with tuberculin, the only agent then available, preferably in a sanatorium. The idea was logical enough, and Philip with characteristic elegance of phrase, called the procedure 'anticipatory detuberculisation'. No great success was ever proved for the method, which is not surprising since even as late as 1931 Philip himself[38] estimated that 75 *per cent* of children reacted to tuberculin by the age of 14 years.

When the number of positive reactors diminished, and potent chemotherapeutic agents were made available, the same concept of anticipating trouble under the rather prosaic name 'chemoprophylaxis' became a more practical proposition. Opinions as to its value have varied between being fundamental to the eradication of tuberculosis, and having only a minor part to play in the strategy of prevention.

The current attitude to chemoprophylaxis was summarised in 1983 by the Joint Tuberculosis Committee of the British Thoracic Society[39]. The procedure should be considered in all children up to the age of 15 years with strongly positive tuberculin reactions, and even up to the age of 5 years with lesser grades of reaction. It is justifiable also in all Asian children whatever the degree of reaction. In general, however, the field for chemoprophylaxis is becoming limited, largely due to the remarkable progress in prevention made possible by specific immunisation.

BCG

The discovery of some special process of immunisation was another possibility referred to in the final report of the Astor Committee in 1913. Presumably at that time the medical members of the committee must have known that Calmette and Guerin had started their experiments in 1908, aimed at attenuating a bovine strain of the *bacillus* with specific immunisation in view. The bacteriological and experimental work was completed by 1921. The clinical application began in France in 1922, where for the next ten years immunisation was increasingly practised.

Philip was always very cautious over BCG despite his friendship with 'mon cher Calmette', who was deeply disappointed at his famous colleague's guarded attitude. Philip's caution was intensified when Petroff and others[40] claimed in 1929 to have dissociated BCG into virulent and avirulent colonies in culture. When Begbie[41], of the bacteriology department of the University of Edinburgh, did the same thing in 1930 with cultures freshly obtained from the Pasteur Institute, Philip's[42] caution turned into opposition and he expressed the opinion 'as to the ultimate protection against tuberculosis which is said to be conferred, we remain a good deal in the dark regarding the certainty of its occurrence, and regarding the extent and duration of protection ... and ... we must remain in the dark for a considerable time yet'. A few years later, when on some ceremonial occasion he planted a young tree in the grounds of Southfield Sanatorium, he said to a favoured pupil (the author) 'Dear boy, when you and I can smoke a cigar together in the shade of this tree we can talk again about BCG'.

Sir Robert Philip died in 1939. His influence was enormous, has lasted, and may have been one of the reasons why Scotland, and indeed the United Kingdom, was slower than many other countries in commencing schemes of specific immunisation.

In the year 1949, BCG was finally made available in Scotland[43]. It was reserved for use by physicians with experience of tuberculosis for the protection of nurses, medical students and contacts. By 1951 fifty-two of the fifty-five local health authorities had taken powers under section 27 of the National Health Service (Scotland) Act to operate BCG schemes. In 1952[44] school leavers aged 13 or thereby were added to the list of persons suitable for vaccination in order to achieve protection before the expected peak of morbidity was reached. Over the years vaccination was also offered to other groups, namely all hospital workers, all students and all new-born infants. By 1969[45] it was considered doubtful if vaccination of the last group was still necessary as a routine, though all children of immigrants were offered BCG at birth, and all incoming children as soon as possible.

The general policy for vaccination, as adopted in 1952, is in its essentials the same as is maintained today and has therefore been practised for about 30 years. The results have been impressive. An analysis was carried out in 1978[46] by the Research Committee of the British Thoracic Association which included data for Scotland as well as for England and Wales. The Scottish notification rates for tuberculosis in the age groups 15–19 years, among subjects who were previously vaccinated with BCG at the age of 10–13 years, was one quarter of the rate for tuberculin negative unvaccinated subjects. In the later age group of 20–24 years the corresponding figure was one eighth. The protective effectiveness of vaccination in these two age groups was estimated at 77 *per cent* and 88 *per cent* respectively. 'The special process of immunisation' which Astor had only hinted at in 1913, and which Philip had so seriously doubted in 1930, had actually come to pass and was clearly a triumphant factor in the control of tuberculosis.

Human Tuberculosis of Bovine Origin

In the same year that saw the interim report of the Astor Committee, John Fraser, (later Sir John Fraser Bt) published his famous investigation[47] showing that 60 *per cent* of cases of bone and joint tuberculosis in children were caused by the bovine *tubercle bacillus*. Appropriately the final Astor report in 1913 dealt largely with the question of bovine tuberculosis in humans. Indeed the only time the entire report contained the word 'eradication' was in relation to tuberculosis in cattle. For such an important aim the proposals were remarkably tentative. They were based on the idea of general legislation with local regulatory powers. The committee referred to pasteurisation of milk, but only with reservations. It also suggested measures towards reducing tuberculosis in cattle, including tuberculin testing and possibly the slaughter of animals with tuberculosis of the udder.

These cautiously expressed ideas received timely support in January 1914 when Mitchell[48] demonstrated that 90 *per cent* of cases of tuberculous cervical adenitis in Edinburgh and district were caused by the bovine type of *bacillus*.

With all this evidence it was to be expected that the government would take action, and the Milk and Dairies Acts were passed later in 1914. There were separate acts for Scotland and for England and Wales. In general, the sale of milk from tuberculous cows was prohibited, and samples of milk from the udder, or from any particular teat, could be taken. A local authority might, and if required by the Local Government Board must, appoint a veterinary surgeon for the purposes of inspection. It was perhaps to be expected that the Milk and Dairies (Scotland) Act would be more comprehensive than the English measure[49]. All dairies and milk shops had to be registered and inspected once a year by the Medical Officer of Health, and every cow had to be inspected annually by a veterinary surgeon.

The exigencies of the first world war made the practical operation of these measures impossible, and they were formally postponed *sine die* by further legislation in 1915, and again in 1922. Under the latter Act, however, it was possible for the Scottish Board of Health to produce in 1923 the Milk (Special Designation) Order. This order aimed at improving the purity and quality of milk, and four grades of milk were defined as: Certified (tuberculin tested and bottled on the farm); Grade A (tuberculin tested); Grade A; and Pasteurised. Despite the ambiguous nomenclature, which was widely misunderstood, the establishment of a graded milk scheme was a significant step forward, since at that time almost half the milk consumed came from infected cows.

One of the first herds to produce the highest grade of milk was at Gracemount Farm, and adjacent to Southfield Sanatorium near Edinburgh. This was yet another enterprise of the Royal Victoria Hospital Tuberculosis Trust. It was, in fact, an experimental farm, and the purpose of the experiment was to demonstrate that certified milk could be successfully marketed as a commercial concern without a subsidy. In this the Trust achieved its purpose.

The importance of the graded milk scheme was emphasised by growing evidence that not only were the common manifestations of tuberculosis in children frequently due to the bovine *bacillus*, but adult respiratory tuberculosis was involved as well. Clarke[50], quoting Griffith's 1937 figures, suggested that the *bacillus* accounted for 1 *per cent* of respiratory tuberculosis in England and Wales and 4.5 to 8.5 *per cent* in Scotland; Francis provided evidence that in the north of Scotland the figure was even higher[51].

The graded milk scheme was followed in 1937 by the attested herds scheme in which powers were made available for assisting the attestation of herds on the basis of negative tuberculin tests, with provision subject to satisfactory progress, for the slaughter of animals showing positive reaction in an attested area. In 1938 there were 134 certified herds and 1,251 tuberculin tested herds in Scotland. By 1960 the Department of Health for Scotland was able to report that all milk sold to the public came from cows which had passed the tuberculin test; and in 1970, it could be reported that 82 *per cent* of the milk had been pasteurised.

Nevertheless a cautionary note must still be sounded. In 1983[52] of 419 patients discharging *bacilli* from pulmonary lesions, 1.8 *per cent* were infected with the bovine strain. Of 90 patients discharging *bacilli* from non-pulmonary lesions, 8.9 *per cent* were infected with mycobacterium bovis. Since it is now generally accepted that tuberculosis has been eliminated from cattle in Scotland, it seems that recently discovered bovine infections in humans are most likely to be the result of late reactivation of old lesions in elderly subjects.

Control or Eradication

So far as human tuberculosis is concerned the Astor Committee's reports do not contain the word 'eradication'. The final report did suggest, however, that it was idle to hope that infection could be entirely 'eliminated'. That was over 70 years ago and it may well be asked whether the opinion is still valid.

Sir John Crofton's assertion that in the purposeful treatment of patients, subject to his prescribed conditions, 100 *per cent* success was a reasonable aim remains true, and this of itself in prey to time might well lead to eradication. But can it be hastened, since an obstinate residue remains? As recently as 1981 Crofton and Douglas[56] still felt that control was a more appropriate term than eradication.

By definition eradiction would imply that the death rate from tuberculosis, the notification rate and the tuberculin conversion rate among school leavers would all be zero. The first of these indices, on a national basis, has been 1 per 100,000 of the population for some years (though less than half that in the Lothian Health Board area). The Scottish notification rate for 1984 was 11.1 per 100,000 for respiratory tuberculosis and 3 per 100,000 for non-respiratory forms. This represents a decline of about 50 *per cent* in the last six years.

The most significant index of progress, has now become the tuberculin conversion rate. In 1952 the percentage of school leavers reacting positively to tuberculin was 56. In 1956 the figure was 18[53], appearing to indicate encouraging progress in tuberculosis control. Such confidence suffered a sharp shock when it became known that after a further 16 years the figure for 1973 was still 16 *per cent*, suggesting that the reservoir of infection had not diminished materially in that time[54]. There was still less satisfaction in the knowledge that the comparable figure for England and Wales was 8 *per cent* despite the much higher immigrant population south of the Border. The exact significance of this remarkable finding is necessarily obscure, since the positive tuberculin reactors included those with a very mild response (Heaf grade 1) where interpretation is open to doubt.

Nevertheless these observations were among the factors which led to the establishment of the Scottish Repiratory Tuberculosis Surveillance Programme, which began work in July 1977 under the chairmanship of

Sir John Crofton, and continues under that of Dr Norman W. Horne. The programme is based on detailed analysis year by year of data supplied by specialists in community medicine to whom patients have been notified, and by clinicians who have carried out the necessary treatment.

Whatever the actual differences in the tuberculin conversion rates between Scotland and England may prove to be, the Working Party is in no doubt that there is a difference in the incidence of respiratory tuberculosis north and south of the border. As their tenth report[55] succinctly states, 'it would appear that the incidence in the indigenous Scotsman is on average twice that of the indigenous Englishman.' Furthermore, the report indicates that the notification system of the two countries does not materially affect the recorded difference.

There are other reasons for caution which will operate increasingly, later in the twentieth century. They have been described by Horne[57] as 'problems of Tuberculosis in Decline'. For instance, respiratory tuberculosis is increasingly a disease of the elderly, particularly of old men. Diagnosis is made no easier by the frequency with which they fail to react to tuberculin; and treatment is no easier due to faulty memory and poor compliance. Again, even today, medical students may qualify without ever having seen a patient with respiratory tuberculosis, and many of their teachers may be relatively inexperienced.

The Crofton Report on the Future of Chest Services in Scotland in 1973 recommended *inter alia* two types of chest consultant. One would work in the district general hospital as a general physician with a special interest in chest medicine including respiratory tuberculosis. The other would work exclusively in respiratory medicine in teaching hospitals and become especially exprienced in the field.

Horne now appears to develop this idea a stage further in order to meet the problem of the obstinate residue. He suggests that there is a case for establishing tuberculosis reference centres where skills in diagnosis and management could be maintained, and which could advise in all aspects of the disease, not least control measures and regular surveillance of the problem. This additional development in the service would seem to be a soundly based conception,and may well become the chart and compass for the future. If notifications continue to decline, as in recent years, eradication of tuberculosis may yet be achieved by the end of the century.

Postscript

When Thomas Babington Macaulay wrote that history progresses by steps rather than by leaps he was perhaps oversimplifying the theme. So far as the story of tuberculosis in Scotland is concerned there were indeed many steps but there were also two great leaps. The first was the organisation of a planned and co-ordinated tuberculosis service. The second was the organisation and practice of rational chemotherapy. The latter could not have succeeded so dramatically as it did without the former. It is through such propitious chronological relationships that advancing history is made.

References

(1) Philip, Sir R.W., *Collected Papers on Tuberculosis*, p.22. Oxford University Press, 1937.
(2) Williams, H., *A Century of Public Health in Britain*, p.134. A. and C. Black, London, 1932.
(3) Philip, Sir R.W., *op. cit.*, p.51.
(4) *Ibid*, pp.59–60.
(5) Macgregor, Sir A. *Public Health in Glasgow*, 1905–1946. p.84. E. and S. Livingstone, Edinburgh and London, 1967.
(6) *Ibid*, p.86.
(7) Robson, J., *The Gallovidians* 1926, VII, p.54.
(8) Philip, Sir R.W., *op. cit.*, p.48.
(9) *Interim Report of the Departmental Committee of Tuberculosis*. London, H.M.S.O. 1912 (Cd. 6164).
(10) *Final Report of the Departmental Committee on Tuberculosis*. London, H.M.S.O., 1913 (Cd. 6641).
(11) Macgregor, Sir A., *op. cit.*, pp.92–93.
(12) *Report of the Inter-departmental Committee on Tuberculosis* (Sanatoria for Soldiers). London, H.M.S.O., 1919 (Cmd. 317).
(13) *Ibid*, Appendix 13.
(14) *Department of Health for Scotland, Annual Report*, 1954. (Cmd. 9417).
(15) *Department of Health for Scotland, Summary Report*, 1939–41. (Cmd. 6308).
(16) *Department of Health for Scotland, Summary Report*, 1943. (Cmd. 6462).
(17) *Department of Health for Scotland, Annual Report*, 1948. (Cmd. 7659).
(18) Ministry of Health: Department of Health for Scotland, 1944: A National Health Service. (Cmd. 6502).
(19) *Department of Health for Scotland, Circular RHB* (S)(50) 27.
(20) Tuberculosis Service in Scotland under the National Health Service. Central Consultants and Specialists Committee (Scotland) and the Tuberculosis Society of Scotland. *Brit. Med. J.*, 1950, 11, p.61.
(21) *Annual Report of the Department of Health for Scotland*, 1953. (Cmd. 9107).
(22) *Annual Report of the Department of Health for Scotland*, 1951. (Cmd. 8496).
(23) *Annual Report of the Department of Health for Scotland*, 1956. (Cmd. 140).
(24) *Annual Report of the Department of Health for Scotland*, 1955. (Cmd. 9742).
(25) *Annual Report of the Department of Health for Scotland*, 1958. (Cmd. 697).
(26) Cochran, J.B., Clayson, C., and Fletcher, W.B., *The Annandale Survey. Brit. Med. J.*, 1957, 11, p.185.
(27) *Annual Report of the Scottish Home and Health Department*. 1966 (Cmd. 3337).
(28) *Report on the Future of the Chest Services in Scotland* (The Crofton Report) 1977. Scottish Home and Health Department, H.M.S.O., 1973.
(29) *Annual Report of the Scottish Home and Health Department*, 1977. (Cmnd. 7237).
(30) Howie, U.K., Forbes, G.I., and Urquhart, J., *Scottish Respiratory Tuberculosis Survey. Report No.9.*, p.23. Edinburgh Scottish Health Service Common Service Agency, 1983.
(31) Ross, J.D., *et al.* Hospital Treatment of Pulmonary Tuberculosis. *Brit. Med. J.*, 1958, 1, p.237.
(32) Crofton, J., Chemotherapy of Pulmonary Tuberculosis. *Brit. Med. J.*, 1959, 1, 1610.
(33) *Annual Report of the Department of Health for Scotland*, 1963. (Cmnd. 2359).
(34) *Annual Report of the Department of Health for Scotland*, 1964. (Cmnd. 2700).

(35) *Annual Report of the Department of Health for Scotland,* 1947. (Cmnd. 7453).

(36) Calder, M.A., *Annual Report of the Scottish Mycobacteria Reference Laboratory,* 1983.

(37) Philip, Sir R.W., *op. cit.,* p.307.

(38) Philip, Sir R.W., *op. cit.,* p.390.

(39) Joint Tuberculosis Committee of the British Thoracic Society, Control and Prevention of Tuberculosis: a code of practice. *Brit. Med. J.,* 1983, 287, p.1118.

(40) Petroff, S.A., Branch, A., and Steenken, W., A study of Bacillus Calmette Guerin (BCG). *Amer., Rev. Tuberc.* 1929, 19, p.9.

(41) Begbie, R.S., Microbic Dissociation with Special Reference to Certain Acid Fast Bacilli. *Ed. Brit. Med. J.,* 1930, XXXVII, p.187.

(42) Philip Sir R.W., *op. cit.,* p.395.

(43) *Annual Report of the Department of Health for Scotland,* 1949. (Cmnd. 7921).

(44) *Annual Report of the Department of Health for Scotland,* 1952. (Cmnd. 8799).

(45) *Annual Report of the Scottish Home and Health Department,* 1969. (Cmnd. 4392).

(46) The Effectiveness of BCG Vaccination in Great Britain in 1978. Research Committee of the British Thoracic Association. *Brit. J. Dis. Chest.,* 1980, 74, p.215.

(47) Fraser, J., The Relative Prevalence of Human and Bovine Types of Tubercle Bacilli in Bone and Joint Tuberculosis occurring in Children. *J. Exp. Med.,* 1912, XVI, p.432.

(48) Mitchell, A. Philip, The Infections of Children with the Bovine Tubercle Bacillus. *Brit. Med. J.,* 1914, I, p.125.

(49) Williams, H., *op. cit.,* pp.176–77.

(50) Clarke, B.R., *Causes and Prevention of Tuberculosis,* p.190. E. And S. Livingstone, Edinburgh and London, 1952.

(51) Francis, J., *Tuberculosis in Animals. Symposium of Tuberculosis,* Ed. F.R.G. Heaf, p.299 Cassell, London, 1957.

(52) Calder, M.A., *op. cit.*

(53) *Annual Report of the Department of Health for Scotland,* 1957. (Cmnd. 385).

(54) *Annual Report of the Scottish Home and Health Department,* 1977. (Cmnd. 7237).

(55) Howie, V.K., Forbes, G.I., Urquhart, J., *Scottish Respiratory Tuberculosis Survey,* Report No. 10. p.74. Edinburgh, Scottish Health Service, Common Services Agency, 1983.

(56) Crofton, Sir J., and Douglas, A.C., *Respiratory Diseases,* Third Edition, p.239. London, Blackwell, 1981.

(57) Horne, N.W., Problems of Tuberculosis in Decline. *Brit. Med. J.,* 1984, 288, p.1249.

4. *Maternity and Child Welfare*
The Origins and Progress of the Maternal and Child Health Services

Haldane Tait

CONTENTS

About the Author

HALDANE P. TAIT M.D., F.R.C.P.Edin., F.F.C.M., D.P.H.

Haldane P. Tait was formally Principal Medical Officer of Child Health for the City of Edinburgh; Senior Medical Officer for the Community Child Health Service, Lothian Health Board. He is also Honorary President for the Scottish Society of the History of Medicine.

Author's Note

The Maternity and Child Welfare movement sprang chiefly from deep public concern at the continued high maternal and infant mortality rates at the beginning of the present century in contrast to the evident decline in the general death rate, brought about by the success of the sanitary reforms of the later nineteenth century. The movement, predominantly voluntary, was at first fragmentary, but soon combined together and powerfully compelled governmental action by legislative means. Progress was slow at first, but has steadily gained in strength and effectiveness as knowledge has increased and new measures adopted. The School Medical Service was, by contrast, initiated by governmental action, following the revelation by a Royal Commission of a general state of physical unfitness among the youth of the country. Since its inception in 1908, the service has shown three stages in its development. The first stage was largely devoted to routine inspection for detecting defects. In the second stage, i.e., during the inter-war years, progress was characterised by the establishment of treatment clinics for defects and the provision of special schools and classes for the handicapped. In the third stage – the present – the emphasis is on the early identification of abnormalities and of handicaps, and their amelioration.

This last stage brought the pre-school and school health services closer together. The Brotherston Report, masterminded by Sir John, is the blueprint for the promotion of an integrated child health service under the 1974 reorganised health service.

Maternity and Child Welfare
The Origins and Progress of the Maternal and Child Health Services

The origins of these services can be traced to a series of attempts, usually voluntary, and independent of each other, to improve various adverse influences acting on the health of the mother and her child. In time governmental recognition was achieved and legislative measures introduced, establishing the State's responsibility for the protection of the health of mother and child.

The environmental sanitary reform movement of the second half of the nineteenth century achieved a considerable measure of success by the beginning of the present century, as represented by a decline in the general death rate. Two death rates, however, did not share in this decline, the infant and the maternal mortality rates. There was, too, a decline in the birth rate, a feature shared with other Western European countries especially France, where pioneer maternal and infant welfare work greatly influenced subsequent developments in Britain.

The School Medical Service, as it was originally designated, developed from the findings of a Royal Commission appointed to advise on the place of physical education in Scottish schools and other educational establishments[1]. Its investigations revealed disturbing information on the health of many school children, a disquiet accentuated by the reported high rejection rate of army recruits in the Boer War[2]. The Commission, and a subsequent Interdepartmental Committee[3] covering the whole of the United Kingdom, both strongly recommended the routine medical inspection of scholars and students. Subsequent legislation established the School Medical Service, the first of the statutory child health services.

These enquiries were essentially related to health improvement and differed from the concurrent movement concerned with the protection of the child from neglect, exploitation and cruelty which culminated in the Children's Act, 1908. This placed important obligations on parish councils, the forerunners of children's and social work departments. The care of the unmarried mother and her child was a major concern for both health and poor law authorities, and voluntary organisations were active in this sphere providing mother and baby homes. The adverse effect of illegitimacy on infant death rates was obvious and immense. Illegitimacy was a frequent finding among uncertified infant deaths in Glasgow in 1874[4].

Maternal and Child Welfare Services

The attack on infant mortality was of multiple origin. Early interest was focused on epidemic diarrhoea which annually claimed hundreds of victims. During the 1890s progressive medical officers of health had arranged with registrars for leaflets on feeding and management of infants being issued to parents on the registration of a birth. The success attendant on Budin's *Consultations des Nourrissons* (Paris, 1892), and the infant milk depots or *Gouttes de Lait* of Variot (Paris, 1893) and Dufour (Fecámp, 1894) had their repercussions here. These French organisations had three main objectives – regular medical supervision and weighing of infants, encouragement of breast feeding, and where necessary, provision of sterilised cow's milk for artificially fed infants. Leith (1903), Dundee and Glasgow (both 1904) established milk depots[5].

Chalmers[6] describes subsequent developments at the Glasgow depot. A natural sequel to the work of these depots was renewed agitation for a pure public milk supply. A development at some depots or at continuation classes was the giving of systematic courses in infant hygiene, often spoken of as schools for mothers, again continental in origin.

Dundee Social Union (1906) pioneered a scheme of dinners for expectant and nursing mothers, another French contribution. So successful was this feature that the provision of meals for mothers, and milk for children on medical grounds, became an integral part of subsequent local authority schemes and was the prelude to the present day milk and vitamin scheme.

The official Glasgow delegation of Bailie Anderson and Dr Chalmers, medical officer of health, in company with Drs John Thomson and Dingwall Fordyce of Edinburgh, independent delegates, were prominent figures at the First International Congress of Infant Milk Depots (Paris, 1905). This event led directly to the First National Conference on Infant Mortality in Britain (London, 1906) from which originated the successful plea for the adoptive Notification of Births Act, 1907, giving official recognition to the infant welfare movement in Britain. Widely adopted in Scotland, covering some 60 *per cent* of the population, the Act required notification of all births to the medical officer of health within 36 hours of the event. Early home visitation of newborns by officially appointed health visitors often assisted by voluntary health visitor associations such as those formed in Edinburgh and Glasgow (1908) came into being. Health visiting became established and was soon recognised as being indispensable in any such scheme.

J.W. Ballantyne's initial pre-occupation with foetal pathology gradually gave way, under the influence of his colleague, Haig Ferguson, to a realisation that ante-natal care of the mother *for her own sake* was equally important. He started the first out-door ante-natal clinic in Britain at the Royal Maternity Hospital, Edinburgh in 1915[7].

Control over the education and practice of midwives was still lacking however. For many years the maternity hospitals of the four cities had granted certificates to women trained there, and their medical staffs formed a Scottish Examination Board for Obstetric Nurses in 1903[8]. But a high proportion of midwives were still untrained 'handywomen', the ignorance of many of whom was graphically demonstrated by Chalmers[9]. The Society of Medical Officers of Health for Scotland failed to get legislation passed but finally representations by a group of prominent Scottish medical men succeeded in securing the passage of the Midwives (Scotland) Act in 1915 which set up the Central Midwives Board for Scotland.

Conditions created by World War I and the employment of large numbers of women directed attention increasingly to their welfare and that of their children. The success of the Notification of Births Act, was such that its provisions were made obligatory by the Extension Act of 1915[10] and local authorities were further empowered to make provision either themselves or by arrangement with voluntary organisations for the health of expectant and nursing mothers and children under five years of age, a government grant being available for approved expenditure. The powers included the provision of maternity centres for advice to and treatment of expectant and nursing mothers, ensuring skilled attention for mothers and hospital provision for difficult or dangerous cases, home helps, convalescent and holiday homes; establishment of child welfare centres for advice and treatment of children under 5 years, hospital and convalescent facilities, day nurseries and nursery schools, and, for both mothers and children, home visitation by health visitors, and meals and milk on medical certification. By the end of 1915 extensive powers were now in the hands of local authorities to care for the health and well-being of mothers and children.

The background to these events and developments may be summarised in the following table:–

Year	Birth Rate (per 1,000 pop.)	Death Rate (per 1,000 pop.)	Infant Mortality Rate (per 1,000 live births)	Maternal Mortality Rate (per 1,000 live births)
1855–60	34.0	21.0	120.0	4.73 (1856–60)
1896–1900	30.0	18.0	130.0	4.32
1901–1905	29.0	17.0	120.0	5.1
1906–1910	28.0	16.0	112.0	5.8
1911–1915	25.0	16.0	113.0	5.8
1915	24.0	17.0	127.0	6.1

Schemes prepared by local authorities differed from each other in completeness and in character. Not all local authorities, varying so much in size and population, could be expected to make provision for a full range of activities, and joint action by two or more authorities was encouraged. By 1920 over 83 *per cent* of the population were covered by schemes. The Carnegie United Kingdom Trust sponsored reports on existing provision for the care of mothers and young children in Britain (1917), volume 3 referring to Scotland[11].

Progress

Among the early benefits of the Notification of Births Acts was the recognition of the widespread occurrence and seriousness of ophthalmia neonatorum, predominantly gonococcal in origin. To ensure prompt treatment Glasgow (1911) and Edinburgh (1913) had introduced notification before this was nationally secured in 1918. Midwives were required to call in medical aid in suspected cases and, under their rules, to instill 1 *per cent* silver nitrate or other silver salt into the eyes of the newborn routinely. Authorities were required to report centrally all cases of impairment or loss of sight. Between 1922–31, an average of 6 cases of impairment or loss of vision were reported yearly[12]. The sulphonamides and antibiotics dramatically altered the effectiveness and rapidity of treatment.

During the early 1920s severe outbreaks of measles and whooping cough took a heavy toll on child life and grants were made available to improve the efficiency of treatment and control measures. Work on the Schick and Dick tests was largely confined to the cities, and immunisation against both scarlet fever and diphtheria was increasingly practised. Combined prophylactic of scarlet fever and diphtheria gave encouraging results in Aberdeen[13]. The widespread occurrence of rickets caused concern at this time too, and Motherwell pioneered the prophylactic and curative use of artificial ultraviolet light therapy in 1924; two years later a report on its uses appeared[14]. The reappearance of rickets during the 1950s and 1960s served to emphasise the constant vigilance required in matters of education in nutritional principles in both indigenous and immigrant populations.

Under local government reorganisation in 1930, county councils became responsible for schemes formerly provided by their constituent small burghs and county districts. The large burghs remained responsible for their schemes. Increasingly, following reorganisation, erection of centres for joint use by maternity and child welfare and school medical services was undertaken. Children's medical and surgical units were developed in some of the larger municipal hospitals.

In 1936 the Cathcart Report[15] strongly endorsed the provision of maternity and child welfare schemes but pleaded that the general practitioner should play a larger part in them and that the two services for children under 5 years and for all other school children should be developed together to form one continuous service.

Stillbirths became registrable in 1939. Among the preparations for emergencies in the event of war was the Government Evacuation Scheme which came into operation on 1 September. From the five sending areas, pre-school and school children formed the first priority, the former being accompanied by parents or guardians as necessary. Some 135,000 children were evacuated. Other priorities followed including expectant mothers and a total of 175,000 persons were evacuated. But a drift back home set in almost immediately the scheme was launched, and by January 1940 only 41,000 remained in evacuation areas[16]. A revised plan, affecting school children, is discussed later.

The Orr Committee[17] led local authorities to re-appraise their schemes of child welfare and improve and extend them. With the advent of the National Health Service in 1948 all curative work at local authority child welfare centres ceased and activities became progressively more clearly preventive and educative with provision for inoculations. The name of the service gradually changed to 'child health' from 'child welfare', a term rather more appropriately applied then to the work of children's departments.

Increasing attention was paid to the early diagnosis of defects and to their treatment and management. There was already increasing emphasis on ascertainment, assessment and training of the handicapped school child as medical and educational methods of dealing with such children steadily advanced. This naturally led to a progressive shifting of emphasis towards the pre-school child and was an important step towards the integration of the two child health services. The need for the study of child development was consequently imperative, and courses of instruction were instituted by the Society of Medical Officers of Health in 1964 in London, and four years later the first course in Scotland was organised by the University of Edinburgh. Screening tests to detect defects became more refined and predisposing factors to the development of handicap more clearly defined. Retrolental fibroplasia and thalidomide deformities served to emphasise this latter point. Registers of handicapped and 'at risk' infants and children were therefore kept. These developments naturally pointed to the need for comprehensive assessment centres in association with paediatric departments of hospitals, and these were developed in some of the larger authorities.

While most of the health visitor's work was concerned with maternal and child health, her widened scope of activity under the National Health Service brought her into closer relationship with general practitioners and thus promoted systems of attachment of health visitors to general practices, many of which were already holding child health care sessions. Local authorities were urged to develop general practitioner/authority co-operation[18], including attachment of health visitors, district nurses, midwives and other authority workers to practices – the development of primary care teams. The health centre concept, initiated by the opening of health centres at Sighthill, Edinburgh (1953) and Stranraer (1955), provided the physical locus for the coming together of those concerned in child health, and integration of the child health services thus became a reality. A well integrated pre-school child health service, a prominent feature of the Livingstone experiment launched in 1966[19], demonstrated the successful bridging of the gap between curative and preventive medicine. It pointed the way, and revealed the pitfalls, towards full integration of all individuals, medical, nursing, social, educational and voluntary concerned in child health, a goal towards which strides are being taken with steadily increasing success.

Maternity Services

To realise the aims and objects of the Notification of Births (Extension) Act local authorities vigorously undertook their duties as local supervising authorities under the Midwives Act, to ensure as high a standard as possible among midwives. Arrangements were made for medical assistance called in by midwives in emergencies being readily available, the fees incurred being paid initially by the authority which also helped to repay any loss of income sustained by a midwife having to refer a pregnant woman to an authority ante-natal clinic. Sharing of patient care by doctor and midwife was encouraged.

Ante-natal clinics medically staffed with health visitors in attendance were set up by the authorities particularly in more populous areas, and there such facilities as dental care, health talks and cookery demonstrations might be provided. But attendance was slow to develop, as was the whole concept of ante-natal care, and only some 8.7 *per cent* of pregnant women attended authority clinics in 1925, reaching 51 *per cent* by 1946. A weakness in many clinics was the employment of full-time authority medical officers who did not have continuing full obstetric work.

Maternity hospital accommodation was meagre, only about 250 beds being available, almost entirely in the voluntary maternity hospitals of the four cities, supplemented by an unknown number of private and charitable lying-in institutions. One of the consequences of the National Health Insurance Act was the increased demand for hospital confinement[20], and local authorities were encouraged by the central authority to establish, individually or by joint action, small maternity hospitals and homes. Private maternity homes became registrable with local authorities in 1928[21]. Hospital accommodation improved after the local government reorganisation in 1930, and by 1936 over 1,000 beds were available in voluntary and municipal hospitals. At this time too, increased hospital provision became official policy both centrally and locally.

Efficient maternity services for women at all stages of pregnancy, labour and puerperium, suitable to the circumstances and requirements of an area were stressed[22,23] and led to the Maternity Services (Scotland) Act 1937 being passed. This required local authorities to provide services of midwives, general practitioners, obstetricians and, where necessary, anaesthetists, for women applying for home confinement. An inclusive charge was authorised, the amount varying with capacity to pay. The objective was a co-ordinated service designed to relieve pressure on hospital beds.

The outbreak of World War II impeded implementation of the Act somewhat, but by 1941 schemes had been sanctioned for 47 out of 55 local authorities and where the scheme operated, even during wartime conditions, it proved popular and valuable to both local and evacuated women. Emergency maternity homes were opened in reception areas on the outbreak of war, and the seven used provided 200 beds. Obstetric specialists were appointed to the three strategic centres of Inverness, Perth and Dumfries.

The scheme, by its wide application of ante-natal care, revealed many conditions requiring hospital investigation and treatment and, while as many of these women as possible were admitted to hospital, some necessarily had to be treated at home. This emphasised the need for more hospital beds, especially ante-natal ones. With the service under predominant local authority control, partnership of doctor, midwife, obstetrician and hospital was amply provided for and achieved, only to break down with the advent of the National Health Service, in 1948, with its tripartite administrative machinery. It was the difficulties encountered as a result of this that led to a review of the service[24]. The policy of hospital boards was towards centralisation of obstetric care in specialist maternity units and there was, simultaneously, increasing demand for hospital confinement. In 1948, 56 *per cent* of all births took place in hospital, whereas in 1975 it was 99 *per cent* when there were 3,838 obstetric beds available. It was recognised that the movement towards centralisation in specialist units created problems for the development of an integrated maternity service in the reorganised health service after 1974, and a report[25] outlined methods of increasing co-ordination. Various schemes of shared care by general practitioners, community midwives and obstetricians have consequently been evolved[26,27].

Maternity Mortality

Maternal mortality during the present century shows three distinct phases. The first phase, up to the mid-1930s, was characterised by the struggle to get the rate lower than 6 per 1,000 live births, the sepsis component being the primary obstacle. It seemed that the maternity services of local authorities and of maternity hospitals were proving of little avail. Following the recommendation of a committee[28] the central department called for a report by the medical officers of health on every death in their area occurring during pregnancy, parturition, and the first four weeks of the puerperium[29]. A subsequent important report[30] was published with an analysis of 2,500 of these schedules.

The second phase from 1936–39 showed the beneficial effects of the sulphonamides in the control of sepsis and by the outbreak of war the maternal mortality rate was reduced to just under 5 per 1,000 births. During 1940–45 the rate of decline rapidly increased, the mortality rate falling from 4.4 to 2.8. The third phase, initiated by the availability of penicillin and other antibiotics and continued by the striking advances in obstetrics, in medical and sociological attitudes, showed a reduction of the rate to almost nil. In 1982, for example, there were only 6 maternal deaths in all, a rate of 0.1 per 1,000 total (live and still) births. The perinatal mortality rate is now used as an index of the quality of maternity care, as good care during pregnancy, childbirth and subsequently safeguards both mother and child.

Health Visiting

The function of health visiting is quite old but only relatively recently was known under that name. For a long time it was an activity of dispensaries and some hospital outdoor departments, and so could be undertaken by nurses, midwives, and later, women doctors. It became more systematised when medical officers of health, in their efforts to improve health conditions of families smitten with infection, required details of the health of family members and of home conditions. Women sanitary inspectors were often employed in this work, the earliest apparently being in Glasgow in 1870. Leith (1902), and Aberdeen and Dundee (1903) employed them, and when the Notification of Births Act was adopted many local authorities appointed them as official health visitors.

This variety of worker led to a confused situation regarding training. Two colleges, Heriot-Watt, Edinburgh, and Aberdeen Technical, offered courses leading to a Health Visitor's Certificate granted by the Royal Sanitary Institute, London, and the Edinburgh School of Social Study and Training granted a certificate of its own, but neither certificate was officially recognised. In 1919 the Nurses (Scotland) Act provided for the first time for the regulation of nurse training, and Scottish medical officers of health then unanimously insisted on trained nurses as health visitors for maternity and child welfare work. When official conditions of training were issued in 1922, specifying two courses, one for nurses, the other for those without such training[31] the latter was promptly abandoned, and the Edinburgh and Glasgow Schools for Social Study and Training became the officially recognised training centres for health visitor students, certificates being issued by the Scottish Board of Health. In 1932 the Royal Sanitary Association of Scotland was appointed the responsible body for conducting examinations and issuing certificates and in 1948, Aberdeen, Edinburgh and Glasgow health departments became training centres instead of the two Social Study Schools.

In 1962 the Council for the Training of Health Visitors, a United Kingdom body advised by a Scottish Committee, was formed following the recommendation of a working party[32]. It became responsible for all aspects of training and certification and soon introduced radical changes including the transfer of theoretical teaching to six educational establishments, although the former and other health departments provided fieldwork facilities. Aberdeen Health Department in the early sixties pioneered the training of male health visitors whose activities were especially successful with the male adolescent and the elderly man. In 1980 the United Kingdom Central Council for Nursing, Midwifery and Health Visiting was formed, and by 1983 its associated National Board for Scotland had assumed the functions of the former Training Council here.

The health visitor proved her worth in her educative work in maternal and child welfare and her training was progressively extended to cover school health, tuberculosis, family health and welfare, and venereal diseases; and from the 1930s local authorities began to employ her in these services. The National Health Service Act recognised this extension and defined, for the first time, her functions as (a) the care of young children, of persons suffering from illness, including injury or disability requiring medical or dental treatment or nursing, and of expectant and nursing mothers, and (b) the measures necessary to promote health and prevent the spread of infection. From 1965 only qualified health visitors could be employed by local authorities, although there were exceptions[33].

The health visitor is particularly well placed to initiate measures to prevent family breakdown, to perform simple screening tests, supervise children on the 'at risk' and handicapped registers, and with the family doctor can do much to help and encourage the parents of children with defects or disabilities. Close association with voluntary and other bodies, and liaison officers concerned with the health and welfare of immigrant families, is essential.

Maternity and Child Welfare Centres

These were so-called since ante-natal and post-natal care were provided at many of the larger centres, but since a goodly number of the early ones were in rented or adapted premises, conditions were by no means ideal. The opening of the Carnegie and Russell model centres at Motherwell and Paisley, respectively, in the early 1920s, ushered in the advent of the purpose-built centre which usually offered additional facilities for dental care, health talks and cookery demonstrations and school medical service work. Inclusion of the latter was a feature of new centres built following local government reorganisation in 1930. After 1948, the centres became entirely supervisory, diagnostic and educative, with, of course, continued facilities for various vaccinations. From 165 centres in 1920 the number increased to over 600 by the 1970s.

Attendances of infants under one year were generally good, some 60 *per cent* being brought, but numbers fell off dramatically thereafter. Numerous methods have been tried to improve this situation such as mobile clinics, appointment systems calling for birthday and other special examinations, inoculations and other devices. But the hard core remains of those unwilling, for many reasons, to take advantage of the services provided.

Health Services for Pre-School Children

The importance of systematic health supervision of the pre-school child has never been questioned, but measures to achieve this have been slow to develop. Health visitors, after their early concentration on infants, extended their supervision to the 1–5 year olds. Voluntary agencies provided some facilities such as day nurseries, child gardens and toddlers' play centres, and received willing help and financial support from local authorities; but the numbers dealt with were small in comparison to the 1–5 year old population, while official provision has been largely hindered for economic reasons.

Day Nurseries

Early nurseries were opened in Edinburgh, Glasgow and Paisley for working mothers. In 1883 Edinburgh and Glasgow Voluntary Day Nursery Associations provided nurseries later absorbed into the local official schemes. Over 30 were in operation mainly at factories, during World War I, while in the mid-1920s some 24 operated in the cities and industrial areas, usually with a few cots for overnight stays where necessary. During the height of the government sponsored wartime nursery scheme in World War II there were 143 accommodating 6,400 children. Many nurseries were closed after the war in spite of the demand still existing and private nurseries and daily minding of infants and preschool children took the place of official provision. These private concerns became registrable with local authorities under the Nurseries and Child Minders Regulation Act, 1948, as did many of the other private groups of pre-school children which went under a bewildering series of names.

Nursery Schools, Classes and Toddlers' Playcentres

Nursery schools and classes, both official and voluntary, numbered only 19 in 1932. While the Education Act, 1945, made it a duty for education authorities to establish nursery schools and classes, economic considerations constantly precluded any worthwhile expansion but by applying the shift system to those existing a compromise was reached.

Toddlers' Playcentres were pioneered by the voluntary Edinburgh Toddlers' Playcentres Association[34] which opened the first playcentre in 1915. By the 1970s there were 33, including one in a children's hospital.

Welfare Food

From the inception of maternal and child welfare schemes local authorities provided, at cost price or free, milk and dinners for needy, expectant and nursing mothers, and milk and cod liver oil for children. To safeguard the health of these members of the population during World War

II the national welfare foods scheme came into being in 1940 with milk, then vitamin supplements the following year, assuming its present name in 1946 when these became associated with family allowances. Local authorities assumed distribution functions in 1954. Numerous changes have since taken place in the scheme, the most noteworthy being the withdrawal of the two varieties of national dried milk (1977) in favour of proprietary modified dried milks, as recommended by a working party[35].

Home Helps

The untrained midwife or handywoman was generally prepared to do housekeeping duties as well as 'nurse' mother and baby. With her disappearance simple schemes employing neighbours and others for domestic duties in households where the mother was confined, ill or removed to hospital, were adopted. Following the recommendation of the Orr Report (1943) women so employed were officially recognised as doing work of national importance. Later a home help service, at first permissive under the National Health Service, later obligatory (1968), came into being, its administration being assumed by Social Work Departments on their formation. An important development in the 1950s was the provision of long-term assistance, through the service, to problem families and other families with difficulties.

Family Planning

The first Scottish family planning clinic was opened in Glasgow in 1925 as a voluntary administered birth control or 'mothers' welfare centre', as family planning was then called. Other voluntary centres followed elsewhere but progress generally was slow. By the 1950s many local authorities were making a service available by supporting voluntary agencies, and in 1966 they were urged to review and develop the service. In 1970 they were given powers to make provision for advice and services on social as well as medical grounds. In 1974 family planning was recognised as an integral part of health care and became part of the national health service, Area Health Boards gradually assuming control of the centres provided by the Family Planning Association which retained responsibility for arranging conferences, etc. Developments have included a domiciliary service for socially deprived families and arrangements for family doctors to provide free contraceptive advice and supplies on prescription.

Abortion Act, 1967

This Act laid down certain criteria which required to be met for the termination of a pregnancy in national health service hospitals and in certain approved centres.

School Health (Medical) Service

The object of the Royal Commission of Physical Training (Scotland) was not to enquire into the health of children but to enquire into their physical education and that of other students, and to advise on its application in these establishments. With only one medical member, the Commission was not intended to be medically orientated[36]. It was the alarming extent of ill-health among scholars revealed by the Commission's own investigations, and the concurrent disquiet among the public, occasioned by the high rejection rate of army recruits for the Boer War, that led the Commission to make its important and far-reaching recommendations for the provision of medical inspection of scholars and of food and clothing for necessitous pupils.

The Report received a lukewarm reception from the Scottish press. 'The Report... strikes one as... hardly worth the pains spent in concocting it', was one comment[37]. The following year (1904) the Commission's Report was reinforced by that of the Inter-Departmental Committee on Physical Deterioration which, *inter alia*, re-emphasised the need for medical inspections of scholars. Two subsequent Scottish education bills incorporating these recommendations failed to pass but eventually the Education (Scotland) Act, 1908, secured powers to enable, and if necessary require, a school board to provide for the medical inspection and supervision of school children, to employ medical officers or nurses, and to provide the necessary appliances or other requisites. The Scotch (sic) Education Department issued a detailed memorandum of guidance on medical inspection for school boards,[38] all of which, save one, had schemes in operation by 1912. All employed medical officers, full or part-time, but only some provided nurses. The following year the first conference of Scottish school medical officers was held[39].

Earlier in the century proposals for medical inspection of scholars had been made in Paisley[40] and Aberdeen[41], but both foundered on financial grounds. The Carnegie Trust, however, financed an inspection scheme in Dunfermline from 1906 and treatment from 1910.

From its very commencement, medical inspection revealed an overwhelming amount of ill-health and disease, but the treatment facilities available to the general public were unable to cope with the additional burden from school children. So urgent was the situation that a special grant was made available for two successive years towards provision of treatment facilities for necessitous pupils before the Education (Scotland) Act, 1913, made provision for treatment, including surgical and dental, a duty of education authorities. There was little time to implement these provisions, before World War I broke out, which subsequently had a general paralysing effect on the school medical service.

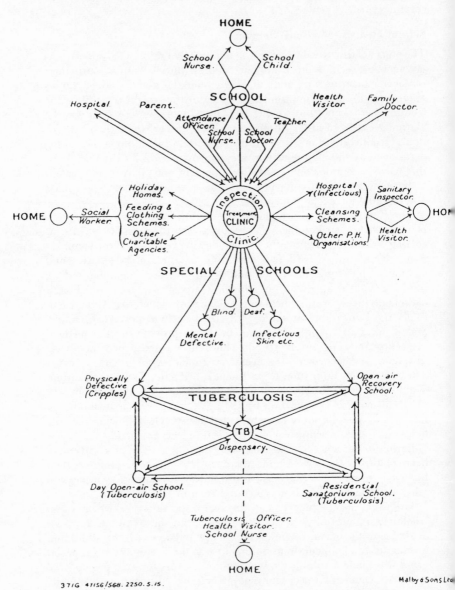

Malby & Sons Ltd.

Figure 1

Schematic Representation of School Medical Service
(From Third Report on the Medical Inspection of School Children in
Scotland, by Lewis D. Cruickshank, 1915, Scotch Education
Department.)

Reform of administration of the educational system including medical inspection and treatment took place in 1919. The school medical service became the responsibility of elected *ad hoc* education authorities for the four cities and the counties, central control of the service being vested in the newly formed Scottish Board of Health. By 1920, 33 authorities out of 38 had submitted schemes to the Board for approval.

Generally schemes covered medical examination of routine and special cases, re-examination of those previously found to need treatment, with provision made for a follow-up by school medical officers or nurses. Measures were also taken for, *inter alia*, cleansing and disinfection of schools, medical supervision of physical education and practical instruction in personal hygiene. The larger authorities made some special provision for the education of physically and mentally handicapped children, a provision made by means of special schools or classes, or of open-air schools, while advantage was taken of convalescent and holiday homes under voluntary management. Medical treatment facilities included clinic provision for nutritional disorders, minor ailments especially of the skin, eyes, ears and nose and throat, visual and hearing disorders, orthopaedic conditions, rheumatism and associated heart conditions, and dental care. (Fig. 1.)

A quiet spirit of optimism prevailed at this time with expansive prosperity which, alas, was soon to end. The country went into a period of economic decline, industrial unrest, and the short-lived enthusiasm for progress and reform waned. The need for national economy prevailed.

Progress

When school medical inspections were first introduced, an effort was made by the central departments concerned to link up the new service with the existing public health service by the appointment of the medical officer of health as chief school medical inspector, and of the medical assistants, required for school work as assistant medical officers of health. This attempt, however, was generally unsuccessful and in some areas the two services were, or became, independent. The re-organisation of 1919 led to a revival of the earlier concept, but again with little success.

The introduction of Dick and Schick testing and immunisation procedures against scarlet fever and diphtheria in the mid-1920s, however, led to closer relationships between the two services since the public health service was responsible for both infectious disease procedures. This was a prelude to the fuller linkage following the reorganisation of local government in 1930 when the two services came under the same local administration, *viz.*, the councils of the four cities and of the counties. By later regulations[42] the medical officer of health was appointed chief administrative school medical officer with a chief executive school medical officer for day to day administration.

A fairly extensive scheme was adopted for the feeding of school children during the coal mining dispute of 1926. In Midlothian, for example, the food was prepared at suitably equipped centres and transported to the schools by motor van. There the children had breakfast, dinner and tea, while meat pies were supplied at weekends. The success of nutritional studies on school children with milk supplements by Orr[43] and others in the later 1920s, was soon put to practical use through the effects of the depression of the early 1930s, by the introduction of the milk-in-schools scheme and of the increased provision of free meals and, incidentally, also of clothing. In 1933, for example, 35,000 children received free dinners, and some 110,000 clothing.

Progress had been slow in the provision of special schools and classes for the handicapped. By the mid-1930s about two-thirds of education authorities had made no provision for the education in special schools or classes of physically handicapped children and nearly one-third of education areas were without local provision for mentally handicapped. Several authorities had made arrangements for such facilities in adjacent areas but little surplus accommodation was available in any area. In 1936 authorities were required to make such provision[44].

This decade also saw some advance in the better regulation of employment of school children; the better recording of defects found at medical inspections enabling a clearer distinction being drawn between major and minor maladies and disabilities in statistical returns (1938). In 1968–69 a further medical record card was introduced from which results could be extracted and analysed by computer.

The serious situation created by the revelations of widespread infestation with vermin, infection with scabies and impetigo and other manifestations of uncleanliness, with the troublesome problem of enuresis among the first evacuees in 1939 was wholly unforeseen by both sending and receiving authorities. The latter were compelled to establish cleansing and treatment centres in addition to the arrangements they had already made for domiciliary treatment, provision of special clinics, hospital care and sick bays in hostels and elsewhere. Consequently, for the months following the initial mass evacuation of September 1939, the scheme for supplementary evacuation which followed required parents to register their children, almost all school children, so that a prior medical examination and any necessary disinfection and/or treatment could be carried out in the sending areas before evacuation. Response to this supplementary scheme was meagre, however, and only some 6,000 children and 123 teachers and helpers were evacuated by March 1940.

In February, 1940, a radically changed scheme was evolved, confined to school children and designed to operate only in the event of actual air attack on an area. Prior registration, medical examination and any necessary disinfection and/or treatment were carried out. Five school camps also became available for evacuees, but once again the response was poor. Only after the severe air attacks on Clydeside did any large scale movement take place, when 12,000 school children were evacuated.

The provision of milk and meals was much extended during the 1940s with the free issue of milk in 1940, and the provision of clothing was also facilitated at this time. In 1946[45] education authorities were required: to provide for medical inspection for free treatment, both medical and dental, for school children and those at junior colleges; to insist on medical inspection when necessary; to provide 'education by special methods' suitable for pupils with 'disability of mind or body'. Increased powers were given to ensure cleanliness; to prohibit or restrict employment of pupils. School medical officers had to report on the hygiene of school premises, and power was given to education authorities to provide child guidance clinics. The service was also concerned with certain remand home duties[46] and its name was changed to School Health Service.

The National Health Service (1948) did not affect the status of the School Health Service which remained a responsibility of the local authority, including the provision of treatment facilities. Nonetheless, there was a decline in the calls on the treatment centres, as an alternative was now provided by the general practitioner and hospital. Many clinics therefore ceased to operate but some specialist ones continued, notably those for ear, nose and throat, ophthalmic and orthopaedic. The Service was, as a consequence, able to participate more fully in preventive measures such as vaccination programmes, the early ascertainment of handicap and ensuring their treatment and management, health education, and fostering closer relationships with other professionals e.g. teachers, educational psychologists, and parents. The discipline became more and more comparable in purpose and scope with industrial medicine and could justifiably assume the name Educational Medicine.

The increasing need for early ascertainment of handicap inevitably led to closer collaboration with the pre-school child health service, family doctor and hospital. The establishment, in 1966, of registers of both handicapped and 'at-risk' pre-school children was a step towards integration of the two local authority child health services. To ensure the best possible use of these registers, regular consultation between responsible medical officers in the two services and in the mental health service became not only desirable but essential. The signpost was now pointing clearly to a unification of the two local authority child health services, an aim which was pursued vigorously by some of the larger authorities.

On implementation of the National Health Service (Scotland) Act, 1972 in April 1974 the School Health Service as a local authority activity came to an end. Thus closed a period of some sixty-five years of honest endeavour to promote the health and well-being of Scottish school children. Henceforth the service became part and parcel of a restructured health service for children.

Three reports dealing with aspects of the health service for school children were issued between 1968–1975[47,48,49] while the Brotherston Report[50], complemented by the Court Report[51] set out the objectives of, and guidelines for, an integrated child health service, which was one of the aims of reorganisation.

Since 1974 steady progress has been made, in spite of numerous difficulties, towards achieving integration of the several branches of the child health service, and several reports[52,53,54,55] have been issued, with observations and recommendations on different aspects of the service.

Medical Inspection, Supervision and Treatment

The original scheme of inspection at 5, 9 and 13 years, and the later one at 16 years for secondary pupils was doubtless the best procedure in the earlier years of school medical inspection. But medical, social and educational conditions have greatly changed since then and the scheme was consequently severely criticised. Modifications of the scheme were therefore sanctioned and encouraged by the central departments since 1962. An earlier modification had been operated in Edinburgh since 1932 with official sanction, whereby the 9 year old inspection was omitted and an annual classroom inspection of *all* children adopted instead, which proved most successful until World War II intervened.

Hearing tests by voice and observation were performed at 7 years, but as methods of testing and techniques improved and earlier management of deafness proved successful, audiometric sweep tests were adopted in 1960 for all entrants. Vision was originally examined at 9 years, later at 7, and finally in 1957 at school entry. From 1962 colour vision testing was introduced and now is practised early after school entry.

Several of the earlier schemes made no provision for the employment of nurses. Effective supervision and follow-up in the home was therefore impossible. After World War I, however, authorities unanimously employed nurses, either full time, or made arrangements with nursing associations for the part-time services of their nurses.

No special qualifications for school nurses were insisted upon but from the 1930s the larger authorities in particular increasingly employed certificated health visitors. In many county areas, however, it was sometimes difficult to attract holders of this additional certificate, although most had district nurse training. Recent years have seen the school health visitor assisted by registered nurses who undertake duties at inspections, clinics and nursing duties at special schools. Welfare assistants undertake clerical and similar duties.

The main function of the school clinic was for treatment of minor ailments, with dental care and specialist sessions for ear, nose, throat and eye conditions, including the issue of spectacles, until the advent of the

National Health Service, occasionally for orthopaedic, rheumatic and cardiac disorders. Changes in the health of school children over the years have produced striking improvements. Ringworm and favus (for which special schools were sometimes opened), impetigo and septic sores are no longer the menace of former years, enlarged glands, anaemia, rickets, rheumatism, rheumatic heart disorders and tuberculous conditions have all but vanished. Infections of the eye and otorrhoea are things of the past. Most ophthalmic, ear, nose and throat work is now concerned with investigation of visual and hearing defects respectively.

Cleanliness clinics for vermin disinfestation and treatment of scabies, formerly part of the school health service facilities, have been provided by local authority environmental health departments since 1974.

Handicapped Children

Legislation in 1890 required school boards to provide for the education and training of blind and deaf-mute children, and this was done by placing them in specific voluntary institutions for such children. In 1906 they were empowered to provide education, medical inspection and conveyance for epileptic, crippled and defective children. The introduction of medical inspection brought into prominence considerable numbers of children whose physical or mental condition rendered them unsuitable for ordinary schools, and some of the larger boards made provision for the modified instruction of these children by opening special schools and classes. Many of the former were constructed on the open-air system. Glasgow appointed two medical officers for special school supervision only, a measure of the attention given to these children. In 1913 school boards were required to ascertain mentally defective children in their areas who were capable of benefiting from special schools or classes but were not obliged to make such provision. Only in 1936 did provision of special schools and classes become obligatory by which time about two-thirds of the authorities had made no provision in their areas for physically handicapped pupils, and nearly one-third were without provision for mentally defective children. Some of these authorities had, however, met the situation, in part at least, by utilising facilities in other areas.

Before 1946 ascertainment was the responsibility of the school medical officer. Once he had signed a certificate of defect it was the duty of the education authority to place the child in a special school or class without consideration of any other opinion, a heavy responsibility for medical officers thus involved, and for which there was no required qualification other than recognition by the Scottish Education Department. In 1946[56] an education authority was called on to consider not only the medical advice but also any reports or information obtained from others e.g. teachers and educational psychologists, before forming a judgement on any child. It was also the duty of an authority, having ascertained the children in its area, to make appropriate provision for them.

In 1969[57] it became mandatory for authorities to obtain an educational psychologists' report *as well as* a medical one and any other views before arriving at its decision on any particular child. They were also obliged to provide a child guidance service, an option open since 1946, and were empowered to ascertain handicapped children under 5 years. In 1981[58] some of the recommendations of the Warnock Committee[59] were incorporated in legislation.

The categories of handicapped children were defined in regulations[60] and comprised pupils who were: deaf; partially deaf; blind; partially sighted; mentally handicapped; epileptic; suffering from speech defects; maladjusted; and physically handicapped. Blind and deaf pupils were required to be educated in special schools for those disabilities. All others were to be educated at ordinary or special schools; hospital classes or at home as the case might be. Whenever possible any pupil with a disability should remain in an ordinary school with such special help as may be necessary e.g. hearing aid, exemption from certain games and exercises, or occupying some particular seat in the classroom.

Prevention of Infectious Disease

The hopeful confidence prevalent at the beginning of the century that school closure or exclusion would effectively control outbreaks of infectious disease is no longer held and school closure is now but rarely practised. Exclusion of individual cases of infectious disease is, however, still operated.

From the 1930s the service became increasingly involved in immunisation procedures and from 1948 this was increasingly shared with general practitioners. Immunisations now current include diphtheria toxoid (national campaign, 1941), combined with tetanus toxoid (late 1950s); B.C.G. vaccine for tuberculin – negative children aged 10–14 years (1950); poliomyelitis vaccine (dead virus, Salk, 1956; live virus, Sabin, 1962); rubella vaccine for 11–14 year old girls (1970).

Environmental Activities

From the very beginning school medical officers were concerned with environmental factors influencing the health of pupils and were expected to report any breaches of the directions on school hygiene issued by central department (1907). In 1946 medical officers became obliged to inspect and report annually on the hygiene of school premises, especially on heating, lighting, ventilation, sanitary arrangements, and equipment, including safety precautions.

Environmental conditions within schools have, from between the two World Wars and subsequently, been very much improved by the construction of new buildings, provision of more ample recreational facilities, better sanitary arrangements with facilities for handwashing, sanitary towel disposal, etc. These improvements in schools and educational advances made for a greater variety of indoor and outdoor exercises, games, and whole-body activities becoming available with abandonment of former formal semi-military 'drill'. Advice as to fitness of any pupil for general physical activities, swimming and other exercises and recreations both indoor and outdoor may be sought from the school medical officers. Adequate guarding of machinery in technical workshops, and prevention of burns and scalds in laboratories and domestic science rooms, are other medical responsibilities.

Health Education

'Every school ought to be a school of hygiene'[61] gave an indication of the desirability of teachers giving instruction to pupils on simple hygienic principles, assisted if required by school doctors and nurses. Much of this early teaching was formal and sufficiently often in schools that were far from ideal hygienically. As environmental conditions improved so health education has become more appropriate. From a general approach to health education there has been a progressive transition to instruction by precept and example and inculcation of good personal standards of hygiene in nursery and primary schools, with the teaching of human biology, accident prevention, dangers of smoking and similar topics in junior departments, and a more deliberate preparation for adult life in secondary school by discussion groups on the social scene, alcohol and drug abuse, sex education and related topics. Films and demonstration material readily available are freely used[62,63].

A Brief Retrospect

Considerable satisfaction can be derived from the much improved health of Scottish children since the beginning of the century. The principal reasons for this improvement may, very broadly, be traced to higher standards of living and education, better housing and environmental sanitation, specific and curative therapy. Problems still remain and present stern challenges to present services.

The following table shows the changes in mortality among infants under one year since 1915, when the maternity and child welfare schemes of local authorities began to take shape.

Year	Infant Mortality Rate (per 1,000 live births)	Neonatal Mortality Rate (per 1,000 live births)	Stillbirth Rate (per 1,000 total births)	Perinatal Mortality Rate (per 1,000 total births)
1911–15	113	43	—	—
1916–20	99	41	—	—
1950	39	23	27	45
1960	26	18	22	37
1970	20	13	14	25
1980	12	8	7	13

From 1900 increasing reference was made to infant mortality in annual reports of the Local Government Board for Scotland, and in its report for 1912 an analysis was given for the first time of the causes of death in infants under one year. Chalmers [64] and Ballantyne [65] repeatedly called attention to the neonatal component of the infant mortality rate (i.e. deaths of infants under 28 days) before it appeared as a rate in 1911. Ballantyne also foreshadowed the perinatal rate (stillbirths and deaths under 1 week per 1,000 total births) which became a regular statistical feature from the 1950s and to which attention is currently being paid [66].

The fall in infant mortality has been most dramatic in the period of 1–12 months while the neonatal mortality rate has fallen less spectacularly, a hard core of deaths during the first day being a major obstacle. The infant mortality rate is highest in the central industrial belt, while illegitimacy and social class gradients act adversely throughout and present considerable challenges today.

Mackenzie [67] wrote that the concentration on infantile death rates had led to the danger of the 1–5 year old being forgotten. He drew attention to the 9,120 deaths of children of this age-group in 1915, giving a related death rate of 21.4 per 1,000. Compare this with 372 deaths of 1–5 year olds in 1956 and a rate of 1.1 [68]. It was the plight of the ex-baby revealed by home visitation by voluntary health visitors in Edinburgh in 1915 which led to the toddlers' playcentre movements.

In 1915 the main causes of death were from the three most deadly infections of pre-school life – measles, whooping cough and tuberculosis. Today the main causes are respiratory infection and accidents with the trend from home to outdoor accidents including drowning. Both these causes are eminently capable of improvement by health education and higher standards of child care.

A measure of morbidity among children of all ages may be obtained from hospital statistics relating to admissions and out-patient attendances. In 1973, for example, there were 57,927 admissions to paediatric beds, both medical and surgical, and total attendances at out-patient departments were 125,978 of which 28,547 were first attendances.

Bassett [69] showed that at Livingston New Town, some 27 *per cent* of the work done by doctors in 5 practices operating from the health centre, concerned children aged from birth up to 14 years. The major contribution made by children to the total number of consultations were for respiratory infections, infectious diseases, skin disorders, and ill-defined and symptomatic maladies.

The fall in mortality among school children (5–14 years) has also been quite striking as have been the changes in the causes of death which have, in the main, been similar to those among pre-school children. In the quinquennium 1926–1930 there was an average annual death rate of 4.4 per 1,000 group population; in 1946, a rate of 2.2, and in 1980 one of 0.3. Active measures are taken in schools for instruction in safety measures in general, on road safety, and in swimming and life-saving in particular.

Since its inception the School Health Service has kept a record of defects and maladies revealed at routine medical inspections and these have been published in annual reports. In session 1967–68 a new medical record card was introduced which made comparisons of the results so obtained with those of the past only of limited value. For example, in 1968 under the new system the percentage among school entrants found with defects was, for boys 51, for girls 47, and for both sexes among leavers 41 *per cent*. During the previous ten years the percentage of children with defects, taking all groups examined together, varied between 24 and 37. This did not imply that there was any increase in unhealthiness of pupils in 1968, but rather that conditions were recorded under the new system which had previously been ignored as having no bearing on the health of the child.

Nevertheless a broad indication of the general improvement throughout the country in heights and weights of scholars may be gathered from Edinburgh figures for 1913–14 and 1971–72.

Entrants (5 years)		*1913–14*	*1971–72*
Boys	Height	41.5 ins	42.9 ins
	Weight	40.6 lbs	42.5 lbs
Girls	Height	41.2 ins	42.6 ins
	Weight	39.6 lbs	41.6 lbs
Leavers		14 years	15 years
Boys	Height	56 ins	61.0 ins
	Weight	78.9 lbs	98.9 lbs
Girls	Height	59 ins	61.2 ins
	Weight	84.3 lbs	104.4 lbs

During World War II the physical condition of pupils, including their nutritional state, was well maintained. Of 205,001 children routinely examined during session 1945–46, 4.54 *per cent* were classed as nutritionally 'slightly defective', while a further 0.4 *per cent* showed evidence of 'bad nutrition'[70].

Among changes in other defects may be mentioned chronic bronchitis which occurred in about 2 *per cent* of pupils examined during the twenties and thirties, in 1945–46 it was 0.6 *per cent* and currently the incidence is around 0.34 *per cent*. Otorrhoea, a chronic, distressing and troublesome complaint occurred in some 1 *per cent* of pupils in the twenties and thirties with an incidence now of 0.2 *per cent*. Verminous heads during the earlier period varied between 2 and 6 *per cent*, and, even after the experiences of evacuation in 1939, some 6–7 *per cent* had nits or verminous heads in 1945–46. Presently the incidence is about 2 *per cent*. Fluctuations occur with changing trends in hair styles in both sexes.

The number of physically handicapped children ascertained by education authorities as requiring special education has progressively declined from 6,637 in 1935 to 1,087 in 1974 due largely to a reduction in the numbers suffering from the effects of rickets, poliomyelitis, tuberculosis of bones and joints, and rheumatism and accidents. To some extent spina bifida and cerebral diplegia have taken their place.

Following the thalidomide episode in the early 60s, an annual survey has been conducted by the central authority since 1964. In 1971 when all victims were at school, 72 attended ordinary schools, 24 were at schools for physically handicapped, 7 were in schools for the deaf or partially deaf, and 2 were in hospital.

Not sharing in the decline in numbers with the physically handicapped were the maladjusted group. Indications are that more behavioural and emotional problems are being brought to light by the introduction of questionnaires to parents. Late in 1970 certain incidents highlighted the problem of drug-taking in school children[71]. The natural curiosity of the young and the urge to experiment lead to trials with alcohol, barbiturates, cannabis, glue sniffing, and other legal and illegal substances which may pose problems[72].

Much has been accomplished since 1900 in improving the prospects and health of children but much remains to be done to constitute the challenges to the new integrated service. Among the problems awaiting solution are the socio-medical ones of: helping families in underprivileged areas to avail themselves of the services available to them; prematurity and congenital malformations; sudden death in infants (S.I.D.S.); and of non-accidental injury in the young child.

Appendix A

A Crowded Two Decades

1901   First ante-natal bed in U.K. Royal Maternity Hospital, Edinburgh.

1902   Royal Commission on Physical Training (Scotland) appointed.

1903 Report of Royal Commission issued. Inter-Departmental Committee on Physical Deterioration, appointed.

1904 Report of Inter-Departmental Committee issued.

1905 First International Congress of Infant Milk Depots, Paris.

1906 First National Conference on Infantile Mortality, U.K. London.

1907 Notification of Births Act. Vaccination Act, authorising conscientious objection to vaccination. Second International Congress of Infant Milk Depots, Brussels.

1908 Second National Conference on Infantile Mortality, U.K. London. Education (Scotland) Act. School Medical Service founded. Children Act.

1909 Education (Scotland) Act operative (1 January).

1911 Third International Congress of Infant Milk Depots (Berlin). Maternity benefits introduced under National Health Insurance Act.

1912 Special Grant of £7,500 distributed among school authorities for urgent treatment of necessitous cases.

1913 Education (Scotland) Act, enabling provision of treatment for school children. Mental Deficiency and Lunacy (Scotland) Act. First Conference of Scottish School Medical Officers, Edinburgh. First English-speaking Conference on Infant Mortality, London.

1914 Milk and Dairies (Scotland) Act, not operative till 1920s. Third National Conference on Infant Mortality, U.K. Liverpool. Outbreak of World War I.

1915 Notification of Births (Extension) Act. Midwives (Scotland) Act. Operative 1 January 1916. First ante-natal clinic in U.K. opened, Royal Maternity Hospital, Edinburgh (July).

1917 Conference on Maternity and Child Welfare, Glasgow. (Mainly Scottish topics discussed e.g. Midwives (Scot.) Act.) Report on Physical Welfare of Mothers and Children. 4 vols., vol.3 on Scotland. Carnegie U.K. Trust.

1918 Education (Scotland) Act, reorganising administration including School Medical Service. Ophthalmia Neonatorum (Scotland) Regulations.

1919 Nurses (Scotland) Act establishing General Nursing Council for Scotland. Scottish Board of Health Act establishing Scottish Board of Health in place of Local Government Board.

References

(1)   Royal Commission on Physical Training (Scotland) Cd.1507 (Edinburgh, 1903).

(2)   Maurice, Sir F., 'National Health: A Soldier's Study'. *Contemporary Review*, (1903) pp.41–56. Lecture given to Civic Society of Glasgow, 1902.

(3)   Inter-Departmental Committee on Physical Deterioration. Cd.2175. (London, 1904).

(4)   Russell, J.B. 'Report upon Uncertified Deaths in Glasgow'. (Glasgow, 1876) p.11. Report to Sub-committee of Committee of Health, Board of Police, Glasgow.

(5)   Local Government Board for Scotland, Eleventh Annual Report. 1905. Cd.2989. (Glasgow, 1906) pp.247–265.

(6)   Chalmers, A.K. 'The Health of Glasgow, 1818–1925'. (Glasgow, 1930), p.203.

(7)   Sturrock, John. 'The Edinburgh Royal Maternity and Simpson Memorial Hospital'. *J. Roy. Coll. Surg. Edin.* 25, (1980) pp.173–187.

(8)   *Lancet*, (1903) 2, 1493.

(9)   Chalmers, A.K., *op.cit.*, p.262.

(10)   Notification of Births (Extension) Act, 1915.

(11)   Carnegie United Kingdom Trust, 'Report on the Physical Welfare of Mothers and Children' vol.3, Scotland, by W. Leslie Mackenzie, (Dunfermline, 1917). A rich source of early historical material.

(12)   Department of Health for Scotland, N.M. & C. Memo No.34/1931.

(13)   Department of Health for Scotland, Annual Report, 1926. Cmd.2881, p.125.

(14)   *Ibid*, pp.128–153.

(15)   Committee on Scottish Health Services (Cathcart Report) Cmd.5204, (Edinburgh, 1936), p.182.

(16)   Department of Health for Scotland. Summary Report, 1 January 1939–30 June, 1941, Cmd.6038, pp.6–7.

(17)   Department of Health for Scotland. 'Infant Mortality in Scotland', a Report of Sub-Committee of Scientific Advisory Committee (Orr Report). (Edinburgh, 1943).

(18)   Scottish Home and Health Department, Circular H. & W.S. 29/1967.

(19)   Scottish Home and Health Department, 'The Livingstone Project – The First Five Years', Scottish Health Services Studies, No.29. Edited by Duncan, A.H. (Edinburgh, 1973).

(20)   Ref. 11. supra. p.616–617.

(21)   Midwives and Maternity Homes (Scot.) Act, 1927.

(22)   Cathcart Report (ref.15 supra) p.178.

(23)   Department of Health for Scotland. 'Maternity Morbidity and Mortality in Scotland', a Report by Douglas, C.A. and McKinlay, P.L. (Edinburgh, 1935).

(24)   Scottish Health Services Council. 'Maternity Services in Scotland'. Report by Committee appointed by Council (Montgomery Report). (Edinburgh, 1959).

(25)   Scottish Home and Health Department, 'Maternity Services: Integration of Maternity Work'. (Edinburgh, 1973).

(26)   Macnaughton, M.C. 'Epilogue' in Dow, Derek, *The Rottenrow: The History of the Glasgow Royal Maternity Hospital, 1834–1984.* (Carnforth, 1984) pp.175–176.

(27)   Boddy, K., Parboosingh, I.J.T., Shepherd, W.C., 'A Schematic Approach to Prenatal Care' (Edinburgh, undated).

(28)   'Puerperal: Morbidity and Mortality'. Report of the Scottish Departmental Committee. (Edinburgh, 1927). p.30.

(29)   Department of Health for Scotland. N.M. & C. Circular No.23/1929 and accompanying explanatory memorandum.

(30)   See Ref. 23. *supra*.

(31)   Scottish Board of Health, 'Conditions for the Certification and Registration of Health Visitors'. (Edinburgh, 1922).

(32)   'An Inquiry into Health Visiting'. Report of working party on field of work, training and recruitment of health visitors. (Jameson Report) (London, 1956).

(33)   National Health Service (Qualifications of Health Visitors) (Scotland) Regulations, 1965. S.I. 1965, No.1490. (S80).

(34) Cuthbertson, E.A. 'The Toddlers' Playground Movement in Edinburgh'. *Nursery Journal* (1962).

(35) Department of Health and Social Security, 'Present-Day Practice in Infant Feeding'. Report of Working Party of panel on child nutrition, committee on medical aspects of food policy. (London, 1975).

(36) Scotch Education Department. First Report on the Medical Inspection of School Children in Scotland, by W. Leslie Mackenzie. London, 1913, pp.3–6.

(37) *Glasgow Herald*, 18 March, 1903.

(38) Scotch Education Department. Memorandum on the Medical Examination and Supervision of School Children. March, 1909.

(39) Mackenzie, W. Leslie and Cruikshank, Lewis D. Editors, 'Problems of School Hygiene'. Report of First Conference of Scottish School Medical Officers. (Edinburgh, 1914).

(40) Robertson, Wm. Letter to *Scotsman*, 21 March, 1903.

(41) Hay, Matthew. Quoted in Local Government Board for Scotland, Eleventh Annual Report, 1905. Cd. 2989 (Glasgow, 1906). pp.209–211.

(42) School Health Service (Scotland) Regulations, 1947 S.R. and O., 1947, No.415/S.13.

(43) Orr, John Boyd, 'Food, Health and Income'. (London, 1936). pp.47–48.

(44) Education (Scotland) Act, 1936.

(45) Education (Scotland) Act, 1946.

(46) Remand Home (Scotland) Rules. 1946. S.R. and O., 1946. No.693/S.25.

(47) Scottish Home and Health Department. Report of Study Group set up by Secretary of State for Scotland on 'The School Health Service'. 1968.

(48) Scottish Home and Health Department. Report of Sub-Committee of Consultative Committee of Medical Officers of Health on 'Routine Medical Examination of School Children'. 1973.

(49) Scottish Home and Health Department. Report of Sub-Committee of Consultative Committee of Medical Officers of Health on 'Re-organisation and the School Health Service'. 1975.

(50) Scottish Home and Health Department. 'Towards an Integrated Child Health Service'. (Brotherston Report). 1973.

(51) Department of Health and Social Security. 'Fit for the Future'. (Court Report) 1976. Cmd.6684.

(52) Scottish Home and Health Department, Scottish Education Department. 'Towards Better Health Care for School Children in Scotland'. Report of Child Health Programme Planning Group of Scottish Health Service Planning Council. 1980.

(53) As for 52. 'Vulnerable Families'. 1980.

(54) As for 52. 'Dental Services for Children at School'. 1980.

(55) As for 52. 'Crossing the Boundaries'. Report of Working Group of Mental Disorder Programme Planning Group of Scottish Advisory Council on Social Work and Scottish Health Service Planning Council. 1980.

(56) Education (Scotland) Act, 1946.

(57) Education (Scotland) Act, 1969.

(58) Education (Scotland) Act, 1981.

(59) Department of Education and Science, Scottish Office and Welsh Office. 'Special Educational Needs'. Report of Committee of Enquiry into Education of Handicapped Children and Young People. (Warnock Report). 1978. Cmd.7212.

(60) Special Educational Treatment (Scotland) Regulation, 1954. S1. No.1239 (S.114).

(61) Scotch Education Department. Memorandum on the Medical Examination and Supervision of School Children, March 1909. Para. 5, xi.

(62) Scottish Council for Health Education. Report of Committee on Health Education in Schools. (Edinburgh, 1950).

(63) Scottish Education Department. 'Health Education in Primary, Secondary and Special Schools in Scotland'. Report by H.M. Inspectors of Schools. (Edinburgh, H.M.S.O., 1979.)

(64)   Chalmers, A.K. 'Infant Mortality'. *Public Health*, 18, (1906). pp.409–438.

(65)   Ballantyne, J.W. 'Antenatal and Neonatal Factors in Infantile Mortality – Analytical Aspect'. *Maternity and Child Welfare*, (1918) No.10, pp.333–339.

(66)   McIlwaine, G.M. *et al.* 'Scotland 1977 Perinatal Mortality Survey'. (University of Glasgow, 1979).

(67)   Mackenzie, W. Leslie. 'Report on Physical Welfare of Mothers and Children, Scotland'. (Dunfermline, 1917) p.270.

(68)   Department of Health for Scotland, Report for 1956. Cmnd.140. p.116.

(69)   Scottish Home and Health Department. 'The Livingston Project – The First Five Years'. Scottish Health Service Studies No.29. (Edinburgh, 1973) pp.34–43. Section Child Health Services by Bassett, W.J.

(70)   Department of Health for Scotland. Annual Report for July 1945 – December 1946. (Edinburgh, 1947) Cmnd.7188, p.29.

(71)   Scottish Home and Health Department, Scottish Health Service Council. 'Health Services in Scotland', Reports for 1971. (Edinburgh, 1972) Cmnd.4970. pp.29–30.

(72)   Scottish Health Education Unit. 'Drugs and Young People in Scotland', by Ritson, A.B. and Plant, M.A. (Edinburgh, 1977).

5. *Public Health Microbiology Services*

Sir James Howie

CONTENTS

About the Author

SIR JAMES HOWIE LLD., MD., FRCP., FRC.Path.

After graduating from Aberdeen University, Sir James held University lectureships in pathology and bacteriology at Glasgow and Aberdeen 1934–1946. After the Second World War, when he served in the RAMC, he was Deputy Director of the Rowett Research Institute 1946–1951, and the Professor of Bacteriology at the University of Glasgow, 1951–1963. He became Medical Director of Public Health Laboratory Service of England and Wales in 1963 and retired in 1973. He has been President of the BMA, the Royal College of Pathologists and the Association of Clinical Pathologists.

Author's Note

In writing the 'history' I am conscious that I have now been retired from laboratory work for ten years, and that my selection is coloured by my personal experiences. Another writer might present different examples of Scottish problems and of the efforts made to solve them. Within the resources available, good work has been done and continues to be done with increasing effectiveness. There have been successes and failures. Scottish microbiology has attracted good recruits, both medical and non-medical, and their contributions have been valued at home and abroad, particularly by the World Health Organisation. The co-operation established between the Scottish Home and Health Department, the Area Health Authorities, the Public Health Authorities and the Universities has been good and fruitful. Even PHLS of England and Wales has enjoyed cordial relationships with individual Scottish workers and departments. May it long continue to do so; and – a last hope – may Scotland's aspect as a national epidemiological entity of great interest increase substantially without regional and local enthusiasm in any way declining as a result.

That this article was written at all is a testimony to the respect and affection which I and many others had for John Brotherston. When he asked me to write for his 'history', I protested that I was not a historian, and that the collection and assessment of reliable information about so wide a topic, over so long a period, would be a task well beyond my resources of time and opportunity. He then persuaded me, nevertheless, to supply whatever I could recollect, and collect, with the help of colleagues; and this I have done with the valued co-operation of those named in the section headed, 'Miscellaneous Significant Items and Events'. John Brotherston himself always listened sympathetically to my arguments that Scotland had mistakenly declined the opportunity to do even more than it had in this field by not having a national public health microbiology service like that of England and Wales, both because Scotland had unique epidemiological situations which would never be fully explored except on a national basis; and because the absence of such a service caused university microbiology departments to be over-burdened with commitments which necessarily made it difficult for them to do as much as they ought to do and could do in the way of teaching and research. John's argument was that Scotland had regional loyalties and rivalries, which made it difficult to picture a nationally-directed service, and that the university departments gained by having to keep their feet securely on the ground!

No doubt this debate could continue, but it is right that I should claim for John Brotherston that he recognised the problems and did most valuable work in helping, so far as was possible, to get the best of both worlds.

Public Health Microbiology Services

From 1900 to 1939

Even before 1900, the discoveries of Pasteur and his followers were being taken up in Scotland. In 1882 Dr David Hamilton, an assistant in the University of Edinburgh department of pathology, was appointed to the Regius Chair of Pathology in the University of Aberdeen. His main research interest was bacteriology and in 1894 the public health department of Aberdeen entered into an agreement with him to provide bacteriological diagnostic services. In Edinburgh, in 1894, Professor Greenfield's assistant in the University Department of Pathology, Dr Robert Muir, was appointed to a lectureship in pathological bacteriology. When Muir was later appointed professor of pathology, first in St Andrews and later (1899) in Glasgow, his duties widened but he retained an active interest in bacteriology, which he regarded as a growing point of pathology. The municipality in Glasgow set up a laboratory to deal with the bacteriology of epidemics, cholera being a principal cause of concern.

These examples do not record all that was going ahead in this field, now referred to as microbiology, but they illustrate that the epidemiological aspects of it, from the beginning, involved an element of co-operation between the universities and the municipal public health authorities.

Up to about 1945 the principal role of microbiology laboratories in Scotland was epidemiological. In this their function was to assist the medical officer of health (MOH) by supplying him with such information about infections caused by the classical bacterial pathogens as would be helpful to him in their control, by such measures as isolation of patients, supervision of carriers and contacts, discovery of sources, tracing pathways of spread, and interrupting these by whatever means were available. In the university departments' relationships with the hospitals, during the period up to 1945, the hospital bacteriological diagnostic services were the poor relations of those for public health. The voluntary hospitals could not afford to fund them adequately, and before the advent of chemotherapy, bacteriological findings sometimes assisted diagnosis, but had little or no influence on treatment. Sulphonamides and antibiotics changed the picture completely, but even their main impact came only from the later 1940s onwards and coincided with the establishment of the National Health Service (NHS) in 1948. Treasury funds then made possible a policy of upgrading the periphery; and the need to know the antibiotic sensitivities of bacteria isolated from hospital patients made this a major element of laboratory work. In the 25 years after 1948 the staffs and numbers of specimens examined multiplied three to four-fold and cost considerably more. Medical Laboratory Scientific Officers (MLSO's) multiplied up to five-fold, but graduate staff much less and auxiliary staffs (clerical, washer-up, and cleaners) only about two-fold. Laboratories able to do this work were set up in places which previously relied on postal services. Meantime the decline in the incidence of some of the major communicable diseases reduced the ratio of the amount of work related to public health, although not its actual volume. The NHS assumed responsibility for providing bacteriological services to the MOH and general practitioners; and this responsibility, to a large extent, devolved on the university departments, which gave a laboratory service to hospitals on behalf of and funded by the NHS. In different places the University-NHS associations eventually came to range from the provision of a complete diagnostic service for the hospital to a looser consultative supervisory role. It varied from place to place and from time to time. In Aberdeen, for example, a Chair of Bacteriology was founded in 1926 under Professor John Cruikshank, who provided a service for the Royal Hospital for Sick Children and the Maternity Hospital but not, until 1938, for the Royal Infirmary. In 1920, the then Deputy Medical Officer of Health, Dr J. Parlane Kinloch, encouraged a young physician at the City (fever) Hospital, Dr John Smith, to teach himself bacteriology and take charge of the laboratory. Its remit was to provide bacteriological services for the City of Aberdeen and for the Counties of Banff, Kincardine, Nairn, Elgin and Moray. From 1934 the County of Aberdeen came into the scheme. Smith's was a part-time appointment until 1924, when it was made a full-time one and he was designated Director of the laboratory. It is no exaggeration to say that Dr John Smith, an excellent physician, discharged his new bacteriological duty with such efficiency and enterprise that he became one of the leading and most effective epidemiological microbiologists that Scotland has produced. His work on the epidemiology of streptococcal puerperal infection, on leptospirosis, on brucellosis and on neonatal and infantile enteritis was and is of fundamental significance and opened up many new lines of thought. His postal service for outlying areas of the north-east was as good as any postal service can ever be. He was essentially a clinician-microbiologist and his laboratory was visited regularly and frequently by medical men of many kinds seeking, and finding, valuable help and advice. Personally, I owe a great deal to this excellent man.

The University Department in Aberdeen under Professor John Cruikshank's successors, Professor Alexander Macdonald and Professor

T.H. Pennington, later made valuable advances in virology and in staphylococcal epidemiology; and it is now collaborating with the Central Public Health Laboratory at Colindale, London, on rotavirus epidemiology and fifth disease.

Inverness lay within Aberdeen's area of service, in the beginning, but in June 1929 a pathology-bacteriology laboratory was set up in the Royal Northern Infirmary under Dr R.G. Bannerman. He was succeeded in 1935 by Dr H.J. Kirkpatrick and at the present time the bacteriology service flourishes under Dr H. Williams, Dr A.B. White, and Dr (Mrs) Williams. The laboratory has a special interest in toxoplasmosis and is now situated (since 1949) in Raigmore Hospital, and in new purpose-built accommodation since 1970.

In Glasgow, a flourishing municipal laboratory was set up in 1899 under Dr Robert McNeil Buchanan, succeeded in turn by Drs Wiseman (1930), Carter (1948) and Elias-Jones (1961). Dr John Brownlee (1868–1927) in Glasgow was one of the first to apply sound statistical methods to epidemiology and the work done in his various laboratories (Belvidere, Ruchill and Medical Research Council) has a classic quality. At Stobhill Hospital there was a large laboratory first set up under Dr Francis Reynolds. In the 1950s Dr John Stevenson established there the Scottish Salmonella Reference Laboratory.

In Dundee, from 1921, Professor W.J. Tulloch made epidemiological microbiology his main interest. He served local authorities willingly, and left the Royal Infirmary largely to its own devices. He gave exciting practical demonstration classes on any microbe, cholera being a special favourite. His set lectures were not so highly rated but his personal and stimulating improvised talks aroused lifelong interest among many who are now well established and much respected microbiologists. Tulloch pioneered the use of microscopy in smallpox diagnosis. From 1963 the present department under Professor James Duguid, an Edinburgh graduate, enjoys a high reputation for the development of basic studies on bacterial fimbriae, on the classification and detailed biotyping of enterobacteria for epidemiological tracing purposes, and for providing a highly effective service in the excellent surroundings of Ninewells Hospital. Professor Duguid retired in 1984. Virology was developed during the mid-1960s and the service to the Royal Infirmary was fully developed.

In Edinburgh, in 1912, the Robert Irvine Chair of Bacteriology was founded and it was occupied by such distinguished microbiologists as James Ritchie, (1913–23), T.J. Mackie (1923–55), Robert Cruikshank (1959–66), Barrie Marmion (1968–78) and Dr Gerald Collee, the present holder. Mackie introduced science teaching in microbiology and was, in every way, a dynamic figure, of whom many stood in great awe. 'He never walked anywhere; he always ran' said one of his oldest friends. A younger friend confirmed: 'I used to see him running part of the way up the stairs to his department on the fifth floor'.

He was honorary consultant adviser to the Department of Health for Scotland, an appointment which began at some point in the 1930s, when he traced some cases of surgical tetanus to the use of imperfectly sterilised catgut, and advised on methods of sterilisation and its control. He played a major part in setting up, equipping, and staffing the pathology laboratories in the Emergency Medical Service (EMS) hospitals during the 1939–45 war. Mackie was not designated as Director of the EMS Laboratories, but he visited the laboratories regularly and dealt with problems of staffing, equipment, and supplies, always tactfully referring professional problems to the professors of bacteriology in the areas outside south-east Scotland. Edinburgh looked after the problems of the Lothians and Borders, including especially Peel Hospital at Galashiels, as well as providing support for Dumfries, which enjoyed cross-border collaboration, in both directions, with Carlisle. Virology was developed by Van Rooyen and Rhodes, pioneers in the subject, and carried on by Richard Swain from 1948 until he retired in 1975.

In Glasgow the Gardiner Chair of Bacteriology was established at the Western Infirmary in 1919 under Carl Browning, within Muir's department of pathology. With very limited accommodation, Browning, with Ernest Dunlop and later W.B. Kyles, provided a service for the Western Infirmary; and Browning was active in the search for new chemotherapeutic agents, following the methods of Ehrlich, with whom he had studied. When war came in 1939, Browning's son, Dr Paul Browning, established an Area Bacteriology Service at the Western Infirmary, with postal arrangements for the widespread Western region and a second base at the Ross Hospital in Paisley. In 1951, Browning was succeeded by the present writer (J.W. Howie 1951–1963), who was followed by Robert White (1963–1981), and he in turn by Professor Delphine M.V. Parrott, the present holder. At the Royal Infirmary (where in the previous century, Lister did his historic work on the use of antiseptics in surgery) a small but active section of microbiology was run within the pathology department by Dr Robert Cruikshank, (1929–36), followed by Dr R.D. Stuart (1936–44), followed by Dr John Dick (1945–47), Dr R.D. Stuart (again) (1947–9) and then by Dr J.C.J. Ives (1950–1980). Dr Ives was succeeded in 1980 by Professor Morag Timbury, whose work on the genetics of herpes simplex virus was a significant contribution. In the early days excellent work was done on infantile pneumonia and leptospirosis; and collaboration between the clinicians and the laboratory has always been carried to a truly effective level with lasting benefit to the work of the hospital. A notable contribution was Stuart's transport medium for the postal transmission of swabs for the culture of gonococci.

Virology in Glasgow was started in 1949 at Knightswood Hospital by Norman Grist (later Professor of Infectious Diseases) at the instigation of Dr Tom Anderson, an infectious disease physician of great driving force, who later became Professor of Infectious Diseases and then of Public Health.

This brief outline indicates the main structure of microbiology up to the coming of the war in 1939. Many details are left out but the main structure may be seen as of a variable collaboration between university departments, hospital laboratories, municipal and fever hospital laboratories, and limited services to general practitioners. With the relatively limited resources made available, a remarkable amount of good work was done; but there were serious gaps, and not nearly enough was done at that time to provide a reliable picture of Scotland's microbiological problems.

Since 1939

With the coming of the war in September 1939 major epidemiological questions faced the Scottish Office and the Ministry of Health in England. First, would the enemy use bacteriological warfare? Second, could we detect its presence if it was used against us? Third, what could we do to prevent the spread of epidemic disease, whether caused by the enemy or arising naturally, especially from large-scale evacuations of people (mainly children) from large towns into the country where, it could be supposed, there might be little naturally acquired immunity to some of the infections all too prevalent in slum areas? Different responses came from England and Scotland. In England, the Emergency Public Health Laboratory Service (EPHLS) was set up. This was a nucleus of three central and sixteen subsidiary laboratories, with the addition of ten emergency hospital laboratories and six existing university laboratories. A scheme of integrated laboratories was devised to cover England and Wales, especially the vulnerable southern area of England, where air raids and invasion risks were likely to be most serious. Staff were recruited from laboratories of the Ministry of Health and from Universities, especially from those in evacuation areas whose activity would be reduced in any case. The whole was run by the Medical Research Council (MRC) for the Ministry of Health. The MRC's name and reputation ensured a good quality of staff recruitment and a non-rigid type of central administration, sufficiently removed from day-to-day ministerial control to ensure that instant answers could be given to questions as they arose, and would be based upon expert technical direction.

Further, regular weekly collection and analysis of laboratory findings from many parts of the country would quickly disclose abnormal patterns of infection in single areas such as might be expected if bacteriological warfare agents were used. Expertise in typing and sub-typing bacteria was developed and made available to all laboratories, whether in the EPHLS or not. The quality of the bacteriological service thus made available by the expertise of the academic bacteriologists, turned loose upon the day-to-day problems of Medical Officers of Health, was a unique contribution to medical epidemiology, and it owed everything to such distinguished men as W.W.C. Topley, Wilson Jameson, Landsbrough Thomson, W.M. Scott, Fred Griffith and Graham Wilson. A stray German bomb eliminated Scott and Griffith together, Topley had transferred to agriculture, but Wilson filled the gap as Director of the service from 1940 to 1963. Microbiologists all over the world look with admiration and envy upon the work of this unique service. The present writer was its Medical Director from 1963 to 1973.

In Scotland, the answers to the wartime problems were, perhaps not surprisingly, quite different. The Scottish Officer sought advice from the four Professors of Bacteriology: T.J. Mackie (Edinburgh); C.H. Browning (Glasgow); John Cruikshank (Aberdeen); and W.J. Tulloch (Dundee – St Andrews). They advised against Scotland's joining the EPHLS of England and Wales or of setting up an identical structure within Scotland. The four universities, they decided, could keep a watchful eye on the situation, which was obviously less likely to be so serious in the less densely populated areas of most of Scotland as it would be in many parts of England and Wales. This was obviously true for Dundee, Edinburgh and Aberdeen, but it was certainly not true for Glasgow and the South West and central areas. There, however, the experienced Glasgow municipal laboratory and the area postal service were judged to be able to carry out the tasks likely to arise. In fact, bacteriological warfare was not used, and alarming epidemics did not follow evacuation. Immunisation against diphtheria was a great success, and the sulphonamides, although restricted in their effectiveness by developing bacterial resistances, helped to keep away modern plagues. Good wartime diet and good advice on elementary hygiene also played their part. What was missed at this stage, however, was the opportunity to ascertain and systematically chart the epidemiology of infectious diseases in Scotland. With its many closed or nearly closed communities, Scotland offers a rich field of microbial epidemiology which began to be properly cultivated only during the 1960s. Since 1967 it has grown rapidly and effectively and is much used and highly valued by the World Health Organisation (WHO) for information and instruction. Right from its beginning the EPHLS of England and Wales was very conscious of the potential value of what Scotland could offer if it were properly organised and indeed – so far as it was allowed – did all that it could to promote collaboration by providing specialised typing services, reagents, and exchanges of information. One name deserves particular mention: Dr Fred O. MacCallum, who joined the PHLS after the war as head of the Virus Reference Laboratory at Colindale. He trained many notable Scottish virologists including Marmion and Grist. Macrae and Pereira, also of

Scottish origin, later succeeded MacCallum as heads of the Virus Reference Laboratory of the PHLS. Indeed, especially since 1963, personal collaboration among bacteriologists has led to many Scottish microbiologists contributing their ideas and efforts to Working Parties of the England and Wales PHLS, now run by its own Board, which does its best to maintain the standards inherited from the Medical Research Council.

The limitations of the earlier Scottish arrangements for epidemiology became apparent in 1964 on the occasion of the typhoid outbreak in Aberdeen; and later when a paratyphoid outbreak in central Scotland was in progress for over two weeks before it was brought to the notice of the Scottish Home and Health Department (SHHD) – oddly enough as the result of a request for further information by the Enteric Reference Laboratory of the PHLS in Colindale, London, which had been receiving specimens from the start of the outbreak for bacteriophage typing. Clearly the arrangements for surveillance of communicable diseases and the communication of information about them to interested parties required to be upgraded.

Dr (later Professor Sir John) Brotherston, Chief Medical Officer (CMO) of the SHHD, advised by Professor Robert Cruikshank, set up an epidemiological sub-committee within the Standing Advisory Committee on Laboratory Services of the Scottish Health Services Council. Its remit was to advise on measures for the surveillance and control of communicable diseases. Its admirably constituted membership included microbiologists, epidemiologists, public health officers, infectious disease physicians, and general practitioners. Its first chairman was Professor Robert Cruikshank, who was succeeded in turn by Professors J.P. Duguid, Tom Anderson and Norman Grist. In 1974 it was reconstituted as the Advisory Group on the Epidemiology of Infection under the aegis of the Scottish Health Services Planning Council and is currently chaired by Dr Dan Reid, consultant in epidemiology and at present Director of the Communicable Diseases Scotland (CDS) Unit at Ruchill Hospital, Glasgow.

The new committee's first task was to organise a weekly collection and publication of all Scottish laboratory identifications of micro-organisms causing communicable infections. For this purpose it sponsored the establishment, in 1967, of the CDS Unit, at first under the joint direction of Professor Grist and Dr Elias-Jones. In 1969 Dr Dan Reid, who had trained in epidemiology at Colindale, was appointed consultant in epidemiology and took over the running of the CDS Unit. The first weekly report was published on 4 February 1967. The weekly reports were achieved by amalgamating the Glasgow information sheets of positive results of virology and other significant infections with the Edinburgh weekly reports plus other invited contributions. Information is currently submitted by 71 laboratories, 11 of these being veterinary laboratories, a most valuable addition. At intervals, summaries are given along with commentaries on the significance of particular data. Information on meningococcal typing and on legionnaires' disease contributed by Dr Ron Fallon, consultant in laboratory medicine at Ruchill Hospital, are worthy of particular mention; but many other topics are received including influenza infections, hepatitis, the unfolding story of polioenteroviruses over the years, whooping cough, measles, venereal diseases, tuberculosis, rubella, food poisoning, travellers' diseases, diseases of deprived groups, and immunisation generally. Communication between members of the different specialities concerned with communicable diseases was fostered by frequent – at least yearly – parochial visits by the Advisory Group to different centres in Scotland. Meetings were arranged with local physicians, microbiologists, veterinarians, and public health officers. Around 1970, Regional Medical/Veterinary Committees were set up in the different health board areas to meet at intervals with a consultant from the CDS. The Unit, in collaboration with the University of Glasgow, has now held 17 very successful annual seminars on communicable diseases which are regularly over-subscribed by applicants from many parts of the world. Many other highly successful courses for various categories of health workers have been run jointly by the CDS Unit and the University Department of Infectious Diseases.

Attempts were also made by a group, under the chairmanship of Professor J.P. Duguid, to improve communication and co-operation between microbiologists in the different Scottish hospital, university, and city laboratories. The idea was to make good the lack of a co-ordinating organisation like that enjoyed by laboratories of the Public Health Laboratory Service (PHLS) in England and Wales. The Directors of Scottish laboratories, however, remained unconvinced of the benefits that would accrue and were resolute in their antagonism to any idea of central co-ordination, even if it amounted only to advice stopping well short of direction.

Two causes of regret seem to me still to continue to make the Scottish arrangement less effective than it could be. First, there are no regular meetings of senior Scottish microbiologists such as there are in the PHLS in England, where there are five such gatherings each year. Out of these come, quite often unexpectedly, very valuable suggestions for new inquiries and working parties. Working parties are set up, if there is sufficient support, to investigate epidemiological, diagnostic and technical problems. These projects arise from relaxed discussions; and as all who get together in the working parties are volunteers, genuine volunteers, the results are good and morale is high. Second, the PHLS is also able to set up, to fund, and maintain, a suitable range of reference laboratories and a surveillance centre to support the investigations approved. In Scotland, it is a cause for regret that far too heavy a commitment may come to lie upon University academic departments which take, or try to take, their epidemiological and diagnostic duties seriously – to the detriment of their duties as leaders of academic research, without which they are not able to fulfil their proper role. Because of the distribution of population this problem was far more serious in Glasgow than in Edinburgh, Dundee, or Aberdeen. But it worried me in the period 1951–63 when, as Browning's successor in Glasgow, I found myself supporting, on an informal basis, what was virtually a regional public health laboratory service, incorporating university and peripheral hospital laboratories as well as my own. So much was this so, that I was invited in 1963 to succeed Sir Graham Wilson as Director of the England and Wales Public Health Laboratory Service. The PLHS Board and the Ministry of Health had decided to promote joint hospital – epidemiological laboratories of the kind which we were in fact running in the South West of Scotland. I appreciated the honour, accepted the post, and found the work all that I had known it could be. In terms of my Glasgow post, which I left with much regret, it had meant that others in my academic department had to do the kind of work which I thought I had been appointed to do! I have no regrets or complaints. It was certainly a Glasgow University doctrine, enunciated by Sir Hector Hetherington in 1951, that Scottish Professors have to 'combine citizenship with their scholarship'. The trouble comes when the former consumes the latter.

Miscellaneous Significant Items and Events

Inevitably the account so far presented is scarcely worthy of being described as a 'history'. It is a summary of events recorded or personally recalled and regarded as significant by myself and others who have generously assisted my memory. These are Professors J.G. Collee, J.P. Duguid, T.H. Pennington, Morag Timbury, and Norman Grist; Drs Peter McKenzie, Dan Reid, Ian Porter, and H. Williams. Without their help this account would be much less well informed; but these generous helpers are in no way responsible for any errors or omissions. The selection of what should be included is my responsibility alone. This applies particularly to what follows. It is a series of brief notes of some items and events, some of which are already mentioned in the foregoing text, and others which did not easily fit into the sequence chosen to give the 'history', in a semi-chronological fashion. Together they may help to fill gaps and to point the reader to relevant references. They are not arranged in any particular order.

Notes

(A) Notable Books

1) Author R. Muir, Professor of Pathology, University of Glasgow. **Textbook of Pathology.** First published in 1924. Now in 11th edition. (1980).
Present Editor – Professor John Russell Anderson.
The first edition was heavy going to some but was nevertheless an eye opener to others, who found in it their first clear insight into pathology as a living science.

2) Authors R. Muir and J. Ritchie. **Manual of Bacteriology.** First published in 1892. Ran to 11 editions, the last in 1949, edited by C.H. Browning and T.J. Mackie. Notable for its remarkable condensation of a fast growing subject and for the directness of its original language and interesting changes in later editions. For example, in early editions tetanus was described as a complication of wounds 'fouled by dirt or dung'. In later editions the wounds were 'contaminated by manured soil or exretal matter'.

3) Mackie and McCartney's famous **Handbook of Practical Bacteriology** (1925) now in its 13th edition retitled 'Medical Microbiology' (present editors J.P. Duguid, B. Marmion, and R.H.A. Swain for Volume 1. Volume 2, editors are J.P. Duguid, B.P. Marmion, and J.G. Collee. A book that is valued throughout Europe and Asia. McCartney became very well known for producing prepared media on a large scale, supplying laboratories of every kind with reliable material and intelligently designed containers.

4) Van Rooyen C.E. and Rhodes A.J. (1940). **Virus Diseases of Man** (second edition 1948 and three more since then). A pioneering work of great significance and value. The first substantial textbook devoted exclusively to medical virology.

(B) Other Matters

5) John Brownlee (1868–1927) an M.D. graduate of Glasgow University, a pioneer in the epidemiology of infectious diseases, was appointed the first Director of the Statistical Department of the Medical Research Council.

6) A masterly report by R.M. Buchanan on plague in Glasgow (1900–1901).

7) **Smallpox**
   (i) *The Tuscania* episode (April 1929) was limited very quickly.
   (ii) *1942:* Passengers of a ship from Bombay to Glasgow caused a spread of smallpox to the population. Over 500,000 people were vaccinated in less than a month. The outbreak was limited to 25 cases.
   (iii) *1950:* The first patient had a few facial spots and atypical pneumonia, and was only slightly ill. He was not diagnosed as a smallpox case with any certainty until staff and patient contacts developed smallpox. Norman Grist had only in 1949 assembled the requisites for the beginning of virology in Glasgow; so he had a rapid and fruitful initiation into what was a tragic outbreak. For details see *Glasgow Medicine* 1984, vol.1, no.5, pages 10–11.

8) A diagnostic virology course, run by Professor Norman Grist in Glasgow, trained 207 postgraduates from all parts of the world between 1965 and 1978.

9) The outbreak of typhoid in Aberdeen in 1964, when over 500 patients were admitted to hospital. The source of the infection was a can of corned beef. For full details of how the infection spread see the report of the Milne Committee (Scotland: Home and Health Department, HMSO, Edinburgh, 1964 Cmnd. 2542).

10) In 1955 a paper of fundamental importance on surgical autoclaves was published by Dr John Bowie of the Edinburgh department of bacteriology (1955, Bowie J.H. *Pharm. J.* vol.174, p.473). This paper stimulated further work (Howie J.W. and Timbury Morag C. 1956, *Lancet*, vol.ii, 669) which in turn led to the setting up of the Medical Research Council's Working Party on pressure steam sterilizers. Chairman J.W. Howie. The three reports of this working party effectively launched the revolution in sterilising procedures. (See *The Lancet* 1959, i, 425; 1960, ii, 193, see also Foreword to 'A Training Handbook for Sterile Supply Staff' edition published in October 1984 by Institute of Sterile Services Management).

11) John Smith's work on leptospirosis among fish workers (Smith J., Davidson L.S.P. 1956, *J. Hyg. Camb.* vol.36, 438) was preceded in 1927 by Buchanan's important work on leptospirosis in wet coal mines (MRC Special Report Series London, No.113). In 1979 Joyce Coghlan found that farmers are now the occupational group with the highest case incidence in the British Isles (*Brit. Med. J.* 1979, vol.ii. p.872). The difficult technology required for successful laboratory work on leptospirosis is worthy of emphasis. Both Buchanan and Coghlan learned their methods in the Edinburgh University department of bacteriology.

12) In 1958 the first university chair of virology in the United Kingdom was established in the University of Glasgow with help from the funds of the Hospital Endowments Research Trust and the support of the Medical Research Council, which established an Experimental Virus Research Unit in the new department. The first Professor was Dr (later Sir) Michael Stoker who was succeeded in 1968 by Dr John Subak-Sharpe. With this fundamental work in virology and its two laboratories devoted to epidemiological and clinical virology, under Professor Norman Grist at Ruchill Hospital (now retired) and Dr Robert Sommerville at Belvidere Hospital (now at the Royal Infirmary), Glasgow is unusually well equipped in this important discipline and the basic and applied aspects are happily balanced and co-operative.

13) What should be included in the list of significant work could well become a matter of unending debate. New additions come thick and fast; not all are quickly assessed. Reference could reasonably be made, however, to the fundamental early work of Duguid in Edinburgh of the mode of action of penicillin. There was also Marmion's work on hepatitis arising from the Edinburgh outbreak among hospital and laboratory staff. Murray and Burrell did significant work on cloning hepatitis B. Fallon's work at Ruchill on meningitis, category-A safety developments, and legionella is of outstanding value. In Edinburgh, Crofton, Wallace, and their colleagues did pioneering work on tuberculosis, and Gillies and Govan collaborated in pyocin and colicin typing. Gould and Bowie made valuable

contributions to antibiotic-sensitivity testing, and Gould's and Arbuthnott's work on staphylococci both have an honoured place. Collee and Watt of Edinburgh are leading authorities on anaerobic microbiology – an exciting variety of work only recently taking its rightful place in British contributions. In Edinburgh, during Robert Cruikshank's time, great progress was made in developing laboratory services to general practitioners and in collaborating with the veterinary profession on all kinds of problems affecting man and animals, notably the prevention of salmonellosis. In this connection Norval's contribution was outstanding.

14) The group comprised Professor J.P. Duguid, chairman, Professor Norman Grist, Dr Ron Fallon, and Dr Frank Elias-Jones. The original object was to set up a communicable Diseases Laboratory Centre at Ruchill. The idea was officially supported but plans were later changed and the laboratory centre has still not been built at Ruchill or Stobhill.

6. *Nursing*

Nursing, Midwifery and Health Visiting

Jessie Main

CONTENTS

About the Author

JESSIE G. M. MAIN O.B.E., S.S.SEJ., R.F.N., R.G.N., R.N.T., S.C.M.(P + I), O.H.Cant.

Miss Main was educated at Kings Cross Hospital, Dundee, The Royal College of Nursing in London, and the University of Edinburgh. She is the former Registrar of the General Nursing Council for Scotland.

Author's Note

This essay is a short history of the work of nurses, midwives and health visitors in Scotland since the beginning of this century. It outlines their achievements, but mainly shows their determination to move forward and develop their professional skills. Without the support of many medical colleagues and other social reformers, however, these changes could not have been possible. Perhaps the greatest developments which affect our lives to date took place in the 1960s and 1970s, during the period when Sir John H.F. Brotherston was the Chief Medical Officer of the Scottish Home and Health Department. He gave advice when needed – for training and education – knowing that in other countries where medical science has developed, and where there has been no change in the education of health workers, the health of the population has not improved. On one occasion he told the writer that these professions undervalued their contributions to the health and welfare of this country.

The present and future generations of these men and women must meet future needs of society. There will be more people living longer, more services will be needed for the mentally ill and mentally handicapped. Community Services will require to be expanded to meet future demands as changes in the lifestyle of young people will make for an increase in the resources of the health services. It is hoped, therefore, that present and future generations of these professionals will meet the challenge when the need arises, and continue to promote the highest professional standards in their work.

Nursing

Nursing, Midwifery & Health Visiting

1900 to 1919

In 1900 in Scotland medical and nursing care of the sick was predominantly hospital based. The hospitals had been built out of voluntary subscriptions from private benefactors, by local authorities, or by religious orders, to meet the needs of the physically ill, the mentally ill and the mentally defective. Due to the high infant mortality rate and the prevalence of infectious diseases (often of epidemic proportions) local authorities were moved toward the provision of specialist institutions for maternity care and the treatment of infectious diseases. Children were usually looked after in designated wards of general hospitals; but in Glasgow and in Edinburgh hospitals had been built wholly for the care of children. The overall responsibility for all or most of these institutions lay with Boards of Management, who were the employing authorities.

There were relatively few trained nurses in these hospitals and they were assisted by partly trained assistants, nurses, and by untrained ward assistants who did the cleaning and scrubbing. The training of student nurses (probationers) was locally organised and of very uneven quality; there was little competition from other sources of employment for the female recruits and nursing, although considered as an independent profession by nurses themselves, was not recognised as such by all doctors. The practitioners were not registered on a professional register. Even in a major teaching hospital the ratio of patients to nurses was low; in the Royal Infirmary of Edinburgh, for instance, there were five patients to one nurse. Hours of work were very long, a day shift could last from 7am to 8.30pm, and wages were low (for a trained nurse £35–£40 *per annum*). The nurse was first and foremost the helper and handmaiden of the doctor. In the Royal Infirmary, Glasgow, in 1893, Mrs Rebecca Strong, the matron, when she addressed the probationers on their entry into the wards of the hospital said, 'In your relation to the medical man remember that the whole object of your technical education is to fit you to become his auxiliary, the least deviation from this is productive of the greatest evil'. The nursing services of the hospital were directed by a lady superintendent or matron, who was responsible not only for the nursing staff in all respects, but also for the catering, domestic and laundry arrangements. Whilst in the hospitals there was skilled nursing for many of those who most needed it. The villages and rural areas depended largely on the 'handy wife', schooled by life experiences, but untrained in any nursing institution, who gave the sick poor the only nursing they could normally obtain in their homes.

Poor Law Nursing

The Scottish poorhouses were the responsibility of the local authorities and were administered by a superintendent. These institutions admitted destitute people who were unable to support themselves or were suffering from chronic illness and who could not be looked after in their homes. The arrangements for nursing the sick and bed-ridden inmates were very inadequate. The wards were mainly dormitory designed wards which were poorly equipped. The beds were low so that if the patients fell out of them the extent of their injury would be minimal. The wards in the poorhouses were not staffed with trained nurses. These pauper nurses were paid for the work they carried out, which might be their only source of income. The authorities were aware of the unsatisfactory situation and made efforts to improve it. A superintendent nurse was appointed who was responsible to the medical officer of health, not to the matron of the adjacent hospital, and she carried out his instructions regarding the care of patients. Gradually the pauper nurses were replaced by trained nurses from the local authorities' training hospitals. The respectable poor had a horror of being sent to these institutions, and it was not until after the establishment of the National Health Service in 1948 that a massive programme of upgrading and reorganisation took place.

Hospital Nursing

By 1900 there was already a considerable specialisation of nursing functions; in addition to the general hospital nurses there were mental, mental deficiency, sick children and fever nurses. These specialisations had arisen out of clinical needs. The prevalence of the different kinds of illness varied widely from those of the present: infectious fevers were common and often life-threatening, and hospital beds for sick children were fully occupied.

Training for these specialisations arose neither out of clinical needs nor educational requirements, but resulted from the fact that the general hospitals did not accept probationer nurses for training until they were 25 years of age. In order to bridge the employment gap between leaving school and commencing general nurse training, many young women started their nursing experience in specialist training schools. For example in 1901 the age of admission of probationers to the Royal Edinburgh Hospital for Sick Children was reduced from 21 to 20 years, 'in order to enable the three years training in children's nursing to be completed before the probationer nurse was eligible for an adult hospital'. In 1913 the age of admission was reduced further to 18 years, partly because the general hospitals had to lower their age requirement and partly on account of competition from recruits from new fields of employment. In this pre-first world war period in the large general hospitals, probationers were given courses of lectures by doctors and senior nursing staff. Medical and surgical aspects of nursing, hygiene and bedside care formed the core of the curriculum, which also included invalid cookery. In the majority of the training schools the practical skills of nursing were developed by instruction mainly in the wards. The nurses received their formal education during their off duty hours. The working day of the probationer nurse might therefore be of 10 or 11 hours, 8 hours on the wards and 2–3 hours' instruction. Probationer nurses underwent a trial period of six months, before being accepted for the remainder of the three years training. Increasingly widely also, nurses at the onset of their training passed through a period of classroom instruction in a preliminary training school. This had been pioneered by Mrs Rebecca Strong, matron of the Royal Infirmary, Glasgow, in 1894, and was later adopted by other large general hospitals throughout the United Kingdom.

In hospitals for the mentally ill and mentally handicapped (known as 'mentally defective' during this period) the nursing staff included a matron, assistant matron, ward sisters, probationer nurses and attendants. Both the male and female wards were staffed by female nurses, with the exception of a few male wards. The majority of these hospitals were divided into a private and public sector.

Many of the assistant matrons and ward sisters had completed their general training, and were appointed on the understanding that they would study and take the examinations of the Royal Medico-Psychological Association. Candidates for training were recruited at a younger age than for the general hospitals. The records from the year 1900 show that the age of entry was usually 19 years of age. Lectures were given by the medical superintendent and other doctors, together with an assistant matron who acted in the capacity of a sister tutor. Most of the probationer nurses who successfully passed the RMPA examinations left to take their general training, but others remained in the staff houses for the rest of their working careers. Many men and women devoted a lifetime of service to the hospitals and encouraged their families to do likewise.

At this time there were very few hospitals built specifically for the mentally handicapped, so the nurses had experience of caring both for the mentally ill and mentally handicapped.

The trained nurses and trainee nurses were involved with many forms of occupational therapy – knitting, sewing, gardening. Patients worked in the public wards, the laundries and the kitchens. The staff and patients formed a close community.

Classrooms in Training Schools

In the voluntary hospitals the nurse training schools consisted of one classroom and a tutor's office. Some of the classrooms had a laboratory bench for demonstrations or urine testing. Glass-fronted cupboards contained items of equipment used in the wards, which the sister tutor made use of when demonstrating nursing procedures. As the recruitment of probationer nurses increased another classroom might be added, but when the classes were large the medical students' lecture rooms could be made available. It was not until the preliminary training schools were established that a fully equipped demonstration room was added. This gave the students an opportunity to practise bedmaking, bandaging, poultice making and other simple procedures which were carried out in the wards at that time. Many of these departments were well equipped, but often the surgical instruments and the equipment had been acquired when they became surplus in the operating theatres. There was no library, but textbooks for reference were held and the collection was enhanced when members of the medical staff had published textbooks and gave a copy to the nurses' classroom. It was not until after the introduction of the National Health Service that major improvements took place.

Midwives

Prior to World War I many women had their children delivered in their own homes, attended by local practising midwives or by pupil midwives attached to the training schools of maternity hospitals, who were prepared to attend a confinement on request. The competence of the midwives was assessed by the chief medical officers of the medical and child welfare departments of the local authorities. But in the cities standards of midwifery practice were often unsatisfactory. Practice was not regulated and training was often inadequate.

The Midwives (Scotland) Act 1915 (which came into operation in 1916) was designed specifically to deal with these deficiencies. In Edinburgh a Central Midwives Board for Scotland was established with wide powers to issue regulations for the training of midwives, to conduct examinations leading to the award of a CMB Certificate, to prescribe rules to be followed by the midwife in the conduct of her practice and to regulate admission to the Roll of Midwives. Under the Act the title 'midwife' was restricted to women who had completed their training and had been 'certified' under its provisions. The local authorities were constituted as the supervising authorities in their own areas.

District Nursing

In 1889 the Queen's Institute of District Nursing (founded in 1887) had been granted a Royal Charter, and most of the district nursing associations already in existence became affiliated to it. It was supported by affiliation fees, donations, subscriptions and a small income from endowments. Its objective was to provide a nationwide home nursing service, as well as the teaching of health promotion and disease prevention to the families visited. Long before the registration of nurses it set up its own syllabus of training in approved training centres and conducted its own qualifying examinations. The successful candidates were admitted to the Roll of Queen's Nurses. The Queen's Jubilee Nurses (as they were called) attended 'the sick poor free of charge, and the working classes at a moderate fee'. Invaluable, however as their work undoubtedly was, the coverage of the country was very far from being comprehensive, and as late as 1936 only 900–1,000 district nurses were employed by the Institute of Scotland. The local authorities discharged their responsibilities for the nursing of the sick poor through arrangements with voluntary nursing associations, the most important of these being the Queen's Institute.

Public Health Nursing

The medical officers of health and other social reformers recognised that it was not enough to build hospitals and staff them with doctors and nurses: the health of the community had to be promoted and maintained. In 1906 antenatal care was pioneered by Dr Ballantyne in Edinburgh, and was spread throughout the country by the opening of clinics staffed by doctors and nurses. The infant mortality rate was very high and the medical profession was convinced that some of the causes of this were preventable; many mothers failed to attend the clinics and it was thought that a system of home visiting of the mother and infants was required.

Health visiting originated in Manchester and Salford in 1892, and Florence Nightingale set up the first course for health visitors in Buckinghamshire in 1892. Gradually health visitors became employed throughout the United Kingdom. In Scotland five 'female sanitary inspectors' were appointed in Glasgow in the late nineteenth century. In 1902 Aberdeen appointed a 'sanitary inspectress' and in 1903 Dundee appointed two 'health visitors'. Glasgow, in 1906, appointed its first health visitor to carry the message of healthy living to homes, schools and factories. Early 'health visitors' were mainly sanitary inspectors, but others were nurses or midwives, and courses for their specialised education were developed by the universities and local authorities in Edinburgh and Glasgow. In 1919 the Scottish Board of Health issued conditions for the certification and registration of health visitors providing two types of training, one for trained nurses and one for persons without previous nursing experience. In 1925 there was a revision of the health visitor training, and this time all health visitors were required to be qualified midwives; additional health visiting courses for trained nurses now extended over six months and for those with only six months experience in nursing, two years. It was not, however, until more than twenty years later that it was made mandatory for all health visitors to hold the Certificate of the Royal Sanitary Institute.

Highlands and Islands Services

Under the National Insurance Act of 1911 arrangements were made for the provision of nursing services in the Highlands and Islands, and there, as in other parts of Scotland, the Queen's Institute of District Nurses contributed greatly to welfare of the people. Small hospitals were built on the islands by the local authorities or benefactors or religious orders. These nurses carried a great responsibility for the care of the patients as many lived in rural areas and outwith the close reach of medical aid. In the early days the practice of midwifery was paramount, but as the islanders moved to the Scottish mainland and worked in large cities many contracted tuberculosis, and on their return to the islands tuberculosis became one of the prevalent infectious diseases. Provision was made for the treatment of the patients in an isolation hospital by the authorities. However, it took another decade before major changes in the nursing service were implemented.

Registration

In 1904 the House of Commons set up a Select Committee to discuss the registration of nurses, and this committee reported in the following year in favour of registration. Not all nurses at that time wanted Registration and many were said to be apathetic. There was ambivalence in the medical profession, with some doctors opposed to the recognition of nursing as an independent profession; this ambivalence was cynically expressed in an editorial in the *Edinburgh Medical Journal* in 1905: 'Now that plumbers and inspectors of nuisances and midwives are all under supervision of one sort or another, there would seem to be nothing whatever to be against the placing of nurses, the handmaidens of medicine, on the same honourable plane'.

The next significant development was the introduction in the House of Lords in 1908 of a Bill whose main feature was the establishment of a National Council for the Registration of Nurses. It passed a third reading in the Lords, but failed to get consideration in the Commons. It was opposed by some of the major teaching hospitals in England, and also had a critical reception from senior nurses and medical administrators in Scotland. Although the proposed Registration Council was to control the teaching, practice and status of nurses in Scotland, Scotland was to have only two representatives (a nurse and a doctor) out of its 16 members. Objection was taken also to the proposal to make examination by the Registration Council an essential qualification for registration. It was thought that in Scotland examinations should be left in the hands of the training schools. An association of the nursing and medical professions was formed and it drafted a Registration Bill exclusively applicable to Scotland in 1909. The nurses in Scotland wanted registration but they also wanted an autonomous Scottish Nursing Council.

It was not until 1919 that a Nurses Registration (Scotland) Act was passed by Parliament. Under its provisions a General Nursing Council for Scotland was constituted. The primary functions of the Council were to protect the public by laying down conditions of training for nurses, and to maintain a register of suitably qualified persons. Nurses paid an annual retention fee to have their names included each year in the Register, and failure to pay this fee led to the exclusion of their names from the Register. The name of a nurse could also be removed from the Register for disciplinary reasons, arising out of professional misconduct. This Act of 1919 was itself repealed by the Nurses (Scotland) Act of 1951.

1920 to 1948

Prior to 1919 nursing in Scotland had grown in numerical strength, diversified its functions and improved training. But progress had been unco-ordinated and not well planned. The large voluntary general hospitals supported skills and staffing levels which were not matched elsewhere. A great deal depended on the individual lady superintendents or matrons. After 1919 nursing had a new professional focus in the General Nursing Council for Scotland, a central body whose main function was to protect the patients, lay down conditions of training for nurses and maintain a Register of Nurses.

The General Nursing Council

The first meeting of the General Council was held in May 1920. The Act of 1919 empowered the Council to maintain a Register of Nurses in several parts, including a general part and supplementary parts for male nurses, nurses trained in the care of sick children and nurses trained in the care of the mentally ill, mental defective and fever patients. Legislation was framed under the Act (which differed slightly from the rest of the United Kingdom as Scotland has its own legal system) in respect of its work, appertaining to the maintenance of the Register, examinations, discipline, meeting of Council and committees and in respect of uniform and badges. Under these regulations admission to the Register could be granted to existing nurses by virtue of experience if they fulfilled the requirements of the Rules. Registration was also granted to nurses trained outwith the United Kingdom, if they satisfied the regulations in respect of registration on the appropriate part of the Register. Other matters such as the employment of staff and finance were included in the Rules.

Soon after taking up office the Council drew up criteria and guidance to enable training schools to be approved, as there were many applications from institutions which were totally unsuitable. An examination system for the whole country was laid down. The examinations were held three times per year in Aberdeen, Dundee, Edinburgh and Glasgow. All candidates were required to present themselves before three approved examiners (two doctors and a nurse) at an oral examination held in a hospital in one of the University cities.

It was apparently the intention of the legislators responsible for the Act of 1919 that men and women who wished to take up nursing as a career would qualify for registration initially on the General Part of the Register and thereafter specialise if they so desired. This, however, did not occur, but the passing of the Nurses Registration (Scotland) Act 1919 stirred both the doctors and nurses working in the hospitals to look closely at the training and education given to the nurses.

In general, sick children's and fever hospitals had a pattern of training and courses of lectures which had already been introduced. However, in the hospitals for the mentally ill and mentally handicapped change took place more slowly. It was not until 1921, that Dr D.K. Henderson (later to become Professor Sir David Henderson), medical superintendent of Glasgow Royal Asylum, wrote in his annual report on the nursing staff, 'It is possible for almost anyone to become a good general hospital nurse, but a good mental nurse has in addition to be endowed with special qualities of heart and mind.' He went on to suggest reciprocity between general and mental hospitals, for three to six months of the training period, and added that he saw no reason why mental nurses should be allowed a year off the regular course of training in a general hospital.

Shortening of the general training for nurses already registered as mental nurses was contained in the General Nursing Council (GNC) Rules framed under the Nurses Registration (Scotland) Act 1919.

Miss Elizabeth Brodie, who had served in HM Forces during World War I in France, and had been appointed matron of the Glasgow Royal Asylum in 1922, was the first nurse to become chairwoman of the GNC for Scotland, following a distinguished nursing career.

The conditions of accommodation and practice in the municipal hospitals generally compared very unfavourably with those in the large voluntary hospitals; and it was not until the end of the 1920s that some of the municipal hospitals were approved as training schools by the GNC. Approval was often given, initially only, to selected wards and departments, pending upgrading of the hospital provision.

Over the decades development in the Highlands and Islands Service had been maintained. Major changes have taken place, and there is a good district nurse service combined with a midwifery service between the islands which contributes to health teaching in these remote places.

Just over 40 years ago, on the tiny island of Islay just off the West Coast of Scotland, the local doctor found that he had a patient requiring urgent hospital treatment. As the sea journey to the mainland was out of the question in view of the urgency and hardship to the patient, the doctor approached a pilot of the Midland Scottish Air Ferries taking passengers from the island, and it was this isolated incident in 1933 which led to the commencement of the Air Ambulance Service in Scotland as it is known today. The Department of Health for Scotland co-operated with the local authorities until 1948 and the cost of the flight was borne by both the patient and the local authorities. Today it is the National Health Service which covers the financial outlay. The service is on a 24 hour day, 7 days a week basis; and specialised volunteer pilots are assigned by BEA to the Ambulance Service. Members of the nursing staff from the Southern General Hospital, Glasgow, volunteer to hold themselves in readiness for these flights in their off duty time. These volunteers attend a course of lectures in preparation for this work, as the aircraft is specially fitted with life saving equipment. On completion of 10 flights a set of miniature silver wings is presented by BEA.

In May 1939 the Department of Health founded the Civil Nursing Reserve (CNR), a special body of volunteers constituting three groups – trained nurses, assistant nurses and nursing auxiliaries. These nurses were recruited to staff the emergency (EMS) hospitals which were newly built, or the wards in already existing hospitals set aside for the reception of casualties. The nursing auxiliaries of the CNR were a new grade of nurse. They were recruited mostly through the St Andrew's Ambulance Association and the British Red Cross Society. They were trained in first aid and the elements of nursing in special courses in hospital before taking up their duties in hospitals or first aid posts. They grew quickly into a considerable and valuable corps. After the war many of them trained to qualify for the Roll of Assistant Nurses, and this was granted if they had fulfilled certain conditions. But the inheritance of a grade of auxiliary, a member of the ward staff to whom the prefix 'nursing' had been applied, despite her lack of training, has proved to be one that nursing administrators have continued to find difficult to accept, manage and control.

Before the outbreak of World War II the introduction in medical practice of the sulphonamide group of drugs followed during the war by penicillin and latterly streptomycin, changed nursing practice in the hospitals. The GNC updated its requirements for registration by revising the syllabuses of training.

Under the provision of the Nurses (Scotland) Act 1943 a Roll of Assistant Nurses was opened. The initiative for this had come from England and Wales, and initially many nurses in Scotland were opposed to it, fearing that it would result in a lowering of professional standards. Moreover, Scotland at this time was training more nurses for the Register than the country itself could employ. Recruitment to the Roll in Scotland was very slow. Some smaller training schools were approved by the GNC for training for the Roll, but overall, until after World War II, very few schools were approved to conduct this training.

The Nurses (Scotland) Act 1943 also enabled the GNC to grant to teachers of nurses Registration as Sister Tutors; and this led to a much better standard of nurses' education and training in the hospitals. Subsequently, in 1946, the Scottish Board of the Royal College of Nursing introduced an educational course for nurse tutors leading to a certificate awarded by the University of Edinburgh.

In 1939 the Royal Medico-Psychological Association (RMPA), which had conducted examinations for their own Certificates in psychiatric nursing for many years, requested the GNC for Scotland to conduct these examinations as a temporary measure, and in 1948 it became a permanent transfer of responsibilities from medicine to nursing. The mental and mental deficiency parts of the Register were opened to all suitable nurses holding the RMPA's Certificate. Perhaps, at least in part as a result of these arrangements, the numbers entering training for the mental part of the Register then showed a significant increase.

During World War II the pay and conditions of nurses were considerably improved. The Scottish Nurses Salaries (Taylor) Committee recommended national salary scales and terms of employment, and most importantly, government aid was forthcoming to provide the employing authorities with the necessary finance for education and training of nurses and midwives.

Midwives

By 1922 the Central Midwives Board (CMB) had prevented any unqualified persons being admitted to the Roll of Midwives. By 1939 the CMB had made it compulsory for all practising midwives to attend a refresher course every seven years of practice.

In the 1920s nursing homes began to add a maternity side and to employ trained nurses with the CMB Certificate to look after admissions to these beds. In order to ensure that reasonable standards were maintained in homes admitting maternity cases, the Maternity Homes Registration (Scotland) Act 1927 was introduced.

Under the Maternity Services (Scotland) Act 1937 it became the duty of the local authorities to make the services of a certified midwife available to any woman 'by whom or on whose behalf application is made.' Recruits to this local authority service were trained nurses with the CMB certificate; and by the 1940s a full time domiciliary midwifery service was well on the way to being satisfactorily established. This Act brought the education syllabus up-to-date and extended the practical training period to one year in the belief that giving the pupil midwife better experience in the community would lead to an improvement in the quality of home confinements.

Health Visitors

By 1928 the health departments decreed that health visitors should hold the Certificate of the Royal Sanitary Institute (in Scotland, the Royal Sanitary Association). The training was to be six months in length for trained nurses and midwives and two years for all others.

The requirement of a qualification and prescribed course of study were set out in the statutory rules and orders of the Local Government Act 1929. After 1932 all health visitor students in Scotland were registered nurses and midwives. Midwifery was to remain an essential prerequisite for health visitor practice until 1931, when changes were made in the training of midwives and Part I only of this training was required for health visiting.

The health visitor's role was defined as prevention and education, advising and assisting in the home in all matters of health. Each health visitor was allocated a certain local area of activity. New births were notified to her, and she was responsible primarily for infant care and, more generally, for domestic hygiene and household management. Women defaulters from antenatal clinics were to be visited by her and persuaded to attend. Although the provision of a home visiting service was required by statute, health visitors had no statutory right to enter homes. At the time of the Cathcart Report (1936) about 100 health visitors were employed by the local authorities, mainly in the large urban areas: elsewhere district nurses undertook statutory duties which had to be fulfilled.

In 1945 the work of the health visitor was extended into the school health service, under the School Health Service (Handicapped Pupils) Regulations. Although authorities were encouraged to employ qualified staff and to arrange for nurses employed in health visiting to acquire the Health Visitor's Certificate, Scotland did not find it practicable to issue Regulations concerning all health visitors until 1965.

Section 24 of the National Health Service (Scotland) Act 1947, in its emphasis of the preventive and social aspects of care, seemed to underline the importance of health visiting, as did the Children's Act and the National Assistance Act, both of 1948. But paradoxically about this time there developed an increasing uncertainty about the respective role of the health visitor and the social worker, and a loss of confidence amongst the health visitors themselves.

Since 1948

In the decade prior to the inception of the National Health Service, the nursing profession had responded by developing its professional skills and responsibilities and changing its curricula, to take full advantage of the great advances in medicine in the 1930s and 1940s. Early in the 1950s there was a radical change in the treatment of the mentally ill which altered the nursing care of mentally ill patients. This was due mainly to the advances in drug therapy, similar to the breakthrough in other fields at an earlier date. Research into the use of drugs in the treatment of mental illness had been going on for some time prior to the 1950s, and in 1952 the tranquilliser group brought about great changes in the treatment of mental illness. This heralded the introduction of others such as the anti-depressants of the tricyclic group four years later, and before the end of the 1950s the mono-amine oxides inhibitors and a range of minor tranquillisers. The introduction of these drugs in the treatment of mental illness very quickly revolutionised the nursing approach to mentally ill patients. In due course the training requirements for the Mental Part of the Register were revised.

The National Health Service, in the organisational changes it has effected and in the enhanced financial support it has given to medical and nursing service across the United Kingdom, has made it possible for nursing to expand and develop its professionalism in the setting of health service teams in hospitals and in the community.

Nurse Training

The Nurses (Scotland) Act 1949 made provision for the establishment of Regional Nurse Training Committees, to supervise the training of nurses in accordance with the training Rules of the General Nursing Council and to report to the Council on matters affecting nurse training in their regions. An inspector of Training Schools (later a second) was appointed by the Council to scrutinise and report upon the local facilities for the training of nurses.

Preliminary training schools and block systems of study were established in the approved training schools. Some of the specialised hospitals found it difficult to attract sufficient candidates to justify the establishment of a preliminary training school, and the GNC approved a joint preliminary training school to serve a group of hospitals. This was the start of a very constructive development, the grouping of student and pupil nurses in joint teaching departments.

In 1961 the lowering of the age of entry to all parts of the Register in Scotland to 17.5 years led to a considerable drop in the number of nurses training for parts of the Register.

The GNC prescribed training in respect of the minimum amount of practical experience and the number of lectures which should be given during the three year period of training for all parts of the Register (the fever nurses were an exception to this, with a minimum two year training period for this part of the Register).

By 1958 the Council had decided that the time had come to introduce a wider basic training, and this became mandatory in 1964. Student nurses were required to have experience in general and psychiatric hospitals, in obstetrics and in community care. At the same time programmes for the mental and mental deficiency parts of the Register introduced elements of care of the physically ill. Since these new programmes involved considerable periods of secondment for student nurses, resulting in staff shortage in the parent hospitals, the management had to be supported by an increased financial allocation from the government to meet the expense of employing replacement staff.

It was appreciated by the GNC that if student and pupil nurses were to gain maximum benefit from their revised training, much of the instruction would require to be given in the wards, and the learners would need to be supported during these periods. The Scottish Board of the Royal College of Nursing agreed and instituted an educational course which prepared suitably qualified nurses to become clinical instructors (later renamed clinical teachers), to complement the teaching of nursing skills in the wards and departments of the hospitals. The GNC amended its legislation in order to grant registration to this new category of teacher.

Candidates for nurse training had traditionally been accepted by the individual training schools which laid down their own educational requirements for entry to training. In 1962 the GNC for Scotland introduced a minimum education requirement. For a long time it was criticised as being too low; but in the intervening years the Schools (now the Colleges) of Nursing had been able to raise markedly the standard for entry to training for candidates both for the Register and for the Roll.

Having widened the basic training, the GNC for Scotland began to evaluate educational change in a more critical way. It encouraged experiments which laid the foundations for future programmes. A combined general and sick children's programme taken over a 4–4½ year period failed, as many student nurses discontinued training during the course. But two other experimental courses succeeded: a one year training for previously registered nurses for entry to the Mental Part of the Register, which led to an appropriate amendment of the Rules to make this the prescribed period of training; and (at Glasgow Royal Infirmary) a two year training for student nurses. It was concluded that the latter was feasible, given that the learner had full student status and the course was followed by one year in hospital practice to acquire clinical judgement. In this use of experimental programmes of training, Scotland generally took a lead in the United Kingdom.

The GNC for Scotland initiative did not end here. By the middle 1960s the Council had carried out a review of the programmes of training for the various parts of the Register and found that there was a great deal of duplication in their content. It proceeded to look at the concept of a comprehensive training for all nurses. It seemed that experience could be given in all major disciplines in a basic programme, followed by post-registration instruction and experience in special fields of nursing. Preparation of the nurse in such a manner seemed desirable on educational grounds, since a general training should precede a specialised one. It would also enable the student to make a more informed choice of the area in which she wished eventually to practise, and it would allow nurses to move freely in areas of employment in the NHS. A discussion document was therefore issued by the Council in 1968 to the nursing profession, suggesting that there might be a comprehensive form of training which would prepare nurses for registration on more than one part of the Register, or for registration on a Register from which all divisions had been removed.

The GNC then decided to move towards a comprehensive training for nurses in stages, introducing phase one in 1972; and at the same time it gave approval for five experimental schemes of training, three in Colleges of Nursing, two in colleges of Higher Education. On assessment it was found that student nurses following these experimental programmes were as satisfied with their training as students for the General Part of the Register, while their teachers generally thought that the breadth of instruction provided a better preparation for the students. The Council therefore decided in 1977 that the future pattern of training should be semi-comprehensive, that is, training should be in two approximately equal parts, the first widely ranging (the comprehensive element) and the second directed specifically towards a qualification leading to registration on a particular part of the Register. This was broadly in accord with the recommendations of the Committee on Nursing in 1972 and it was compatible with the directives on nursing of the European Economic Community which came into force in June 1979. The Council, however, contrary to the recommendations of the Committee on Nursing, agreed to retain the separate parts of the Register rather than have a single Register with endorsements. Other members of the nursing profession would have preferred to accept in full the recommendations of the Committee on Nursing and have one Register without separate parts.

Schemes of training for preparation to qualify for registration on one of four parts of the Register was issued in September 1978. Theoretical and practical objectives were brought closer together in a modular organisational structure, but it proved difficult to ensure that the relevant theory always preceded the related clinical experience.

In the 1970s there were requests from training schools in Scotland for a shortened training for candidates holding a university degree; it was believed that such students could assimilate the theory of nursing in a briefer period. Experimental schemes of training were approved which extended over a period of two years (instead of three) before registration. The first integrated degree was established in the Nursing Studies Unit of the University of Edinburgh in 1959. Its first Director was Miss Elsie Stephenson, who was succeeded in October 1968 by Dr (later Professor) Margaret Scott Wright. In 1973 Europe's first Professor of Nursing was established in the University of Edinburgh, and following this appointment the University established a Nursing Research Unit, its first Director being Dr Lisbeth Hockey, O.B.E. In October 1960 the first group of students was accepted for M.A. or B.Sc. with nursing qualifications. These university departments have contributed a great deal to the development of nurse education in Scotland and the Research Unit is widely known internationally, its publications are circulated in many other countries.

In Scotland in 1978 the University of Glasgow founded a Department of Nursing Studies with Miss (now Professor) Agnes Jarvis as its head, and the first student nurses graduated in 1982. This department has continued to expand; other postgraduate courses have been approved and research into nursing practice continues.

Methods of examination were changed in parallel with alterations in the curricula. In the 1960s practical examinations were held in the clinical areas instead of in the training school. In 1971 continuous assessment of the students' performance was introduced; and for registration the student nurses were required to complete the prescribed training, pass two nationally controlled written examinations and obtain a certificate of proficiency from the training school. These arrangements have stood the test of time.

In the 1960s in Scotland the grouping together of Schools of Nursing progressed, and by the 1970s several new Colleges of Nursing had been built adjacent to the major hospitals and clinical areas.

Enrolled Nurses

The number of enrolled nurses in Scotland whose names had been entered in the Roll of Nurses by virtue of examination was only 76 in 1956, but the employers gradually became more aware of the valuable contribution of this grade of nurse and recruitment steadily improved. In 1962 the Roll was opened to former nursing assistants employed in the mental and mental deficiency hospitals, and legislation made it possible to approve these hospitals as suitable areas for training for the Roll. Scotland differed from England and Wales in that there was only one Roll of Nurses, no reference being made to the field of nursing in which training was undertaken.

In the 1970s the general opinion was that the practical experience of the pupil nurse, being heavily biased towards chronic sick and geriatric nursing, was too narrow, and the syllabus of training was broadened. Subsequent experience suggested that, given good supervision, the length of training could be shortened. Experiments were conducted on schemes of training lasting one year and 18 months, and assessment confirms the adequacy of the latter.

The legislation was amended in 1980 to enable successful candidates to be accepted for enrolment on successful completion of a course, the duration of which could be prescribed from time to time by the National Board for Nursing, Midwifery and Health Visiting for Scotland.

In 1983 the legislation was again amended to permit pupil nurses to register following successful completion of an approved course, of not less than eighteen months, on Part 7 of the Register kept by the United Kingdom Central Council for Nursing, Midwifery and Health Visiting.

District Nurses

When the National Health Service came into being a nationwide district nursing service was already established. The large majority of local authorities provided their own service; they had become members of the Queen's Institute of District Nursing and paid a capitation fee for the Queen's Nurses on their staff. The National Health Service (Scotland) Act 1947 (section 25) made local health authorities statutorily responsible for ensuring that a district nursing service was provided, either by the direct employment of district nurses or by using the existing nursing association on an agency basis; it made no provision for district nurse training and this prevailing system of training remained unchanged.

In 1953 the Ministry of Health and the Secretary of State for Scotland appointed a working party to consider training for nursing in the community. It recommended a norm of four months training in the district for the nurse, registered or enrolled, to add to her hospital nursing skills techniques of nursing in the home, to familiarise her with illnesses she might have met infrequently in hospital, and to acquaint her with the social services.

The next step was to achieve a nationally recognised standard of training. From 1960 all successful candidates were awarded a National Certificate of District Nursing, as well as a Queen's Certificate and a badge for those training under the auspices of the Queen's Institute, which relinquished its own certificate in 1968.

In 1959 training of district nurses in Scotland became the responsibility of the Panel of Assessors for District Nurses' Training and following advice from them circulars were issued to training authorities in 1973, announcing the introduction of a new staff grade of district nurse tutor to be responsible for conducting courses of training leading to the award of the National Certificate. In the following year similar arrangements for practical work teachers was announced.

In Scotland the courses for district nurse training are approved by the National Board, and the qualifications recorded in the professional register held by the UK Central Council.

Midwives

Having earlier in the century achieved satisfactory control over its own training and standards of practice, midwifery has, in the period under review, undergone less organisational change than nursing. In 1981, in Scotland, the course was extended from one year to eighteen months for all registered general nurses. The EEC requirements for the training of midwives has influenced the regulations for training in the United Kingdom, and the Sex Discrimination Act requires that men be accepted for training. Courses in midwifery are now conducted in the Colleges of Nursing and Midwifery which are approved by the National Board.

Health Visitors

A working party report (the Jamieson Report 1956) was instrumental in confirming that the health visitors' central function was 'health education and social advice' in the setting of the family, and the concept of the all purpose family visitor, dealing with the young and the old, emerged. This report prepared the way for the Health Visiting and Social Work (Training) Act 1962. Under its provisions joint councils for health visiting and social work training were set up under a single chairman. It was an arrangement which lasted less than a decade. In 1970, legislation changed the arrangement and created a separate Council for the Education and Training of Health Visitors. The function of this new Council remained as laid down in the 1962 Act: to 'promote the training of health visitors by seeking to secure suitable facilities for the training of persons intending to become health visitors, by approving such courses as suitable to be attended by such persons, and by seeking to attract persons to such courses', and to 'provide or secure the provision of courses for the further training of health visitors' and to 'conduct or make arrangements for the conduct of examinations' and to 'carry out or assist other persons in carrying out research into matters relevant to the training of health visitors'. It was the policy of Council to move the health visitor courses into educational establishments which could provide the resources required for the conduct of the courses. The Council's policy coincided with the growth of resources in further and higher education generally.

National Reviews and Reports

Anyone contemplating the progress of nursing in the first half of this century must be aware that its developments have tended to be fragmented and *ad hoc*. In the past quarter century nursing has been both more self critical and often scrutinised from outside. One major factor promoting this has been the size of the nursing work force and the cost to the National Health Service; another, the nurses' awareness of themselves as an evolving profession with a degree of independence from the medical profession.

Two of the most widely influential of the reviews of nursing have been the Report of the Committee on Senior Nursing Structure (Salmon

Report 1966) and the Report of the Committee on Nursing (Briggs Report 1972).

The Committee, appointed under the chairmanship of Mr Brian Salmon, was given the following terms of reference:— 'To advise on the senior nursing staff structure in the hospital service (ward sister and above), the administrative functions of the respective grades and the method of preparing staff to occupy them'. Its report completely changed the management and administration of nursing in hospitals. Job descriptions were given of posts from the top Grade 10 to Grade 6 (ward sister or charge nurse) in the general field of nursing, and similar gradings were identified for posts in specialised hospitals. An experiment in the new staffing structure was carried out at Glasgow Royal Infirmary; but the structure as a whole was implemented before more widespread testing of its applicability could be completed and before the nursing profession had been trained for its new responsibilities. To meet this need, first-line, middle and top management courses were arranged by the Regional Hospital Boards and the Scottish Board of the RCN and in further education colleges throughout the country. Later the Report of the Mayston Committee (DHSS 1969) led to similar arrangements for nurses working in the community.

On the whole the standardised line management structure has worked reasonably well; but the National Health Service is not a uniform organisation and there have been difficulties in the middle grades with a lack of clarity about responsibilities, and particular problems with grade 7, immediately above that of ward sister.

The appointment of the Committee on Nursing and its Report (Briggs Report 1972) were stimulated by the innovatory approach to nursing education of the GNC for Scotland, and an awareness that reciprocal arrangements across the Scottish/English border were coming under strain. The Report was the most comprehensive and radical review of the nursing profession ever made in this country. It recommended a new structure for nursing in the United Kingdom, and a new approach to nursing education.

The structural recommendations of the Briggs Committee have been carried out. Under the provisions of the Nurses, Midwives and Health Visitors Act 1979, five new statutory bodies, a United Kingdom Central Council, and four National Boards, one for each country, have been established. The educational changes recommended by the Briggs Committee have not generally been carried out; it is doubtful if they have been properly investigated and critically discussed by the Central Council. Nursing in the United Kingdom is currently characterised by the divisions evident between its constituent parts and specialities and there is a strong drive amongst many of its senior members to establish one level of nurse. There are other members of the profession however who wish to retain the enrolled nurse and no longer employ such a high proportion of the nursing auxiliaries and nursing assistants.

The United Kingdom Central Council for Nursing, Midwifery and Health Visiting accept four registration qualifications approved by the four National Boards. At present, at both the UKCC and the National Boards, committees have been set up to plan for the future development of nursing, midwifery and health visiting, and to formulate curricula which will be required for each country.

Continuing Education

A Committee on Clinical Nursing Studies was set up in Scotland in 1974 based on the suitable pattern of the Joint Board of Clinical Nursing Studies in England and Wales. Its remit was 'to consider and advise on the needs of nurses and midwives for post-certificate clinical training in specialised departments of the National Health Service and to co-ordinate and supervise the courses provided as a result of such advice'.

As more and more specialised clinical areas have been established in hospitals, for example in intensive care, renal dialysis, child and adolescent psychiatry, so there has been a national and increasing demand for further training for nurses working in these units. A large number of post-basic courses are now provided, their provision co-ordinated by the National Board to include courses for all branches of the nursing profession and advance courses for midwives and health visitors.

The Nursing Division of the Scottish Home and Health Department has published plans for the future for the continuing education of the profession in Scotland. The National Board for Nursing, Midwifery and Health Visiting for Scotland has given careful consideration to the report and has agreed to base its plans for continuing education for nurses, midwives and health visitors on the recommendations contained in the Report.

The pace of change in medicine and nursing in the National Health Service is bound to reinforce the demand for further professional education during the careers of its professional staff, and they will have to ensure it is provided.

Acknowledgements

The author wishes to thank the nursing, midwifery and health visiting staffs in the hospitals, colleges of nursing and in the community for their help in making available old records and other documents during her research into the early part of this century; to Dr Derek A. Dow, M.A., Dip.Ed., Ph.D. Archivist, Great Glasgow Health Board, for his information regarding the storage of previous records of former statutory organisations.

For much material help I am greatly indebted to Professor Sir Ivor R.C. Batchelor, C.B.E., M.B., Ch.B., F.R.C.P.Ed., D.P.M., F.R.S.E. who encouraged me to write this account and read the scripts, in addition giving me helpful suggestions for the text; my former colleague Miss Margaret W. Thomson, O.B.E., R.G.N., R.S.C.N., S.C.M., R.N.T., for her research into the records of the former General Nursing Council for Scotland and also for reading and checking the script and advising me on recent professional advances.

Bibliography

Agnes E. Pavey	The Story and Growth of Nursing, Faber and Faber Ltd. 1947. p.373.,
Grace M. Owen	Health Visiting, Bailliere. 1977.
Sir Alexander Macgregor	Public Health in Glasgow 1905–1946. E. & S. Livingstone Ltd. 1967. pp.121–4.
Nursing in the Community	The Queens Nursing Institute, White-friars Press. 1970.
Thomas Ferguson	Scottish Social Welfare 1864–1914. E. & S. Livingstone Ltd. 1958, p.8, pp.303–5.

Acts of Parliament

Midwives (Scotland) Act 1915
Nurses Registration (Scotland) Act 1919
The Maternity Homes Registration (Scotland) Act 1927
Maternity Services (Scotland) Act 1937
The Nursing Homes Registration Act 1938
The Nurses (Scotland) Act 1943
National Health Act 1946
The Nurses (Scotland) Act 1949
The Nurses (Scotland) Act 1951
The Nurses (Amendment) Act 1961
Health Visiting and Social Work (Training) Act 1962
The Nurses Act 1964
Teaching of Nursing Act 1967
Nurses Act 1969
Nurses, Midwives and Health Visitors Act 1979

7. *The Highlands and Islands Medical Services*

David Hamilton

CONTENTS

About the Author

DAVID HAMILTON, PhD, FRCS

David Hamilton, PhD, FRCS, is Director of the Wellcome Unit for the History of Medicine at the University of Glasgow. He is author of "The Healers: a History of Medicine in Scotland", Edinburgh 1981.

Author's Note

The Highlands and Islands Medical Service grew out of a radical social policy experiment concerned with providing a sector of the population, living in a large and relatively wild part of Scotland with poor communications, with medical care services. In doing this it was well ahead of the N.H.S. in arranging for a comprehensive health service in which general practitioners worked closely with consultants, hospitals and nurses as well as having an important financial back-up for housing, telephones and transport.

The Highlands and Islands Medical Services

In a small compact State of homogeneous districts, the problem (of public administration) hardly exists; in a large State, without Federal institutions and with one system of public administration throughout, the problem may become more acute if the marginal areas are different in physical character, economic interests, or racial sentiment. The Highlands and Islands have, therefore, become something of a laboratory for administrative and legislative experiments, and this makes them a particularly interesting field of study in so much as experiments thought to be successful, tend to be followed by an extension of the operation to wider areas[1].

Radical social policy experiments have been notable in the north of Scotland, and the Highlands and Islands Medical Scheme was one of them. The sparseness of the population, and the lack of the usual inducements to doctors to settle there, resulted in increasing concern over the medical services towards the end of the nineteenth century, and a bold new initiative resulted in 1912. Though the Highlands and Islands Medical Scheme which resulted was hampered by the financial stringency after World War One, it can be said to have anticipated the features of the National Health Service later, in particular by removing the cash nexus between patient and doctor and by the comprehensiveness of its aims. The reasons for concern for health and the medical services in much of the Highlands and Islands[2] from the mid-nineteenth century onwards are numerous. Perhaps the shift of population from the Highlands to the Lowlands made it difficult to support a desirable number of doctors, and perhaps the landowners, who had traditionally subsidised the doctor, became increasingly absent and occasionally impoverished. Perhaps the new sophistication of the Lowland hospitals made a career in the country less attractive, and towards the end of the century a Highland doctor, more than others, required expert support services and aids such as the telephone and a car, these were most required by those who could least afford them. A similar change occurred in the provision of nurses. In earlier times nursing care was expected only from the family or neighbours, but as standards rose in the voluntary hospitals of the

Lowlands, the Highlands were at a relative disadvantage. This concern led to an increasing number of investigations into medical practice and the health of the Highlands from the mid-nineteenth century onwards. It should be noted that the Highlands were not unknown to the leaders of the profession and to politicians: it was to become increasingly the habit for such men to holiday in the areas, and many claimed to be experts in the local conditions. At any rate, from the mid-century onwards there was a series of investigations. The first of these was by the Royal College of Physicians of Edinburgh, who conducted a postal enquiry, and on the basis of the returns made some proposals involving a subsidy of medical men to practise in the North[3]. Other enquiries were made but little was done[4]. This was perhaps because the mode of operation of the new Poor Law from 1845 in these remote areas had given a public service of a kind. The Poor Law meant that a parish could employ a doctor to look after its poor, and give him a modest salary to tend a few paupers. The Poor Law (Amendment) Act of 1845 allowed for proper medical attendance on the poor and encouraged the appointment of a qualified medical officer. But the local parish had to raise part of the salary from their own poor rate before the Board of Supervision would add their matching grant. The extreme example, well known at the time, was that the parish of Westray in Orkney paid its doctor £70 a year[5], ostensibly to look after their one official pauper, the understanding being that the doctor would do much other work gratis: he would also be in residence and available for those who could afford the normal fees. The availability of this Poor Law money made it possible to have a resident doctor where otherwise none could have been supported. The pressure for a resident doctor was often a major local issue and 'probably animated our grandparents more than any other issue of the day...'[6].

On the nursing side there had been a similar evolution, although the voluntary principle succeeded more prominently in maintaining the nursing service in the Highlands than it did elsewhere. The fund-raising voluntary movement was known as the Nursing Association, which raised money to pay and even train nurses, sending them for training in the Lowlands. These Associations were successful, since the work and object of the Association appealed to the wives of the gentry, and it became a fashionable charity. Its status was confirmed when, in 1897, Queen Victoria allocated part of her jubilee fund to the training of nurses for district work, with special attention to medical care far from the improving facilities of the town's hospitals. The great Scottish Local Government Act of 1889 made possible further development of the district nursing services. The nursing services in the Highlands were probably better supported locally than were the medical men.

By the turn of the century, however, a change in the distribution of the Poor Law medical grant to the Highlands and Islands occurred and resulted in a fall in the amount of State spending on health care in the Highlands. In 1885, the Board of Supervision made the training of nurses in the poorhouses a first charge against the Medical Relief Grant. Immediately a large part of the grant was taken up in the necessary and worthy work of improving nursing in the large poorhouses of the Lowlands. The Highlands had almost no poorhouses: small poorhouses had been experimented with in the area but proved to be relatively costly. The effect of this shift of priorities was that by 1912 the State medical grant to the Highlands had been halved. Further concern for the medical services in the area was expressed by two reports. In 1909 the Royal Commission on the Poor Laws became aware of the need for change and recommended that the number of Parochial Medical Officers should be increased. The Minority Report went further, listing the seriousness of some diseases in the Highlands – such as tuberculosis – and the clear evidence of delay in treatment, or even no attendance by a doctor in the area, during a last illness. In 1912 another event occurred which adversely affected the already serious situation. The National Health Insurance Scheme was emerging, and it covered those in regular employment; it was obvious that the irregular income and bartering economy of the crofters would exclude most of the inhabitants in this area from the benefits of the Scheme[7]. Moreover, for those few to be included in the Scheme by reason of their conventional income there was only a patchy health service available. Separate proposals would have to be made, and the Chairman of the Scottish National Insurance Commissioners expressed his concern over the matter to the General Assembly of the Church of Scotland in May 1912[8]. Political unrest might have resulted; the heavy poor rate, but bad services, in the area had already provoked protest by the governed and the governors. The Highland landlords had a grievance about the rates. In 1906 there had even been a mass resignation of elected local councillors in the Long Island.

The speed at which a bold State plan emerged to meet the problem suggests that the case for a special plan for the Highlands was clear to many sections of opinion. Unusually, the Highland landowners were probably in favour of such a radical experiment, since they were no longer prepared to subsidise the Poor Law medical services through their heavy rates bill, and hence were not prepared to raise ideological objections to a State medical service. J.P. Day has pointed out that in the Highlands new initiatives 'where proprietary rights and the interests of the community are opposed, are likely to bring up in an acute and practical form the question of the proper limits of State action'[9]. In the case of the medical services, the landowners, the administrators, the politicians and the poor were now on the same side.

The enquiry was chaired by Sir John Dewar, MP for Inverness, and after taking evidence in Edinburgh, they moved round the Highlands investigating local conditions there[10]. Their travels and the evidence given were followed attentively by the Scottish newspapers. The Dewar Report which resulted[11] gave a gloomy picture of the health of the area, as judged by infant mortality rates and tuberculosis, and it echoed much of the findings of earlier reports[12]. The housing and nutrition of people were poor, and they noted much reliance on patent medicines and even the survival of witchcraft. Nor were they pleased with the conditions of general medical practice as revealed by their investigations. The figures for uncertified deaths – deaths which could not be certified because a doctor did not attend the last illness – again caught the attention of the Committee, as it had the investigators. This figure could reach 90 *per cent* in some of the remote parishes on the Ardnamurchan peninsula. The description of the quality of the doctors in the Report is carefully drawn up, but it suggests that at worst the area was affected by a constant turnover of doctors, and that many of the older men had problems of some sort. They considered that the nursing services in the area were unimpressive compared with the new sophistication of the town's voluntary hospitals and district services.

The Committee seem to have quickly agreed on their conclusions and the remedies, and their proposals were novel and imaginative[13]. Though some heritors had given the Committee stern warnings that a State scheme would switch off local philanthropy, the proposals were for a major State subsidy for the medical services and the nursing services. The doctors were to have a minimum salary, and the cost of their travel to remote patients was to be reimbursed. They were free to obtain a small fee from those who could afford it, about a quarter of the usual visit fee[14]. By 1915 70 *per cent* of their visits were under the Scheme. In return for this secure employment the doctors were to undertake to visit all those requesting visits, to assist with public health and school work, personally to attend midwifery cases, and to provide themselves with transport[15]. The nursing services were to be expanded by providing new salaries. But the Report went much further, and recognised that a broad service, with State-supported hospitals and salaried specialists, would be required. Hospices combined with nurses houses were planned, ambulances were to be purchased, and grants to be made for telephone installation.

The proposals were put to Parliament, and with remarkable speed and absence of debate, the Report was accepted. The Act appeared eight months after the Report. A new nominated Board was set up in 1913, as the Highlands and Islands (Medical Services) Board, to administer the Scheme under Sir John Dewar. The Board was to have not more than nine members, and not less than five, and one member had to be a woman, an early example of a now familiar condition. The Board sent out enquiries to the local government authorities asking for a statement of their needs under the remarkable number of categories of medical care dealt with in the Report. The enthusiastic responses to this open-ended invitation were studied and modified by the Board, and the Board then visited parts of their area to study conditions for themselves. Their estimates were that fifteen new doctors would be needed to add to the 170 already in post, and that no less than 100 new nurses were required. Their request for an annual grant of £42,000 was made to the Treasury. This sum was agreed, and was to be the annual budget of the Highlands and Islands Medical Scheme.

But the Scheme was in trouble from the start. They had a slow start in early 1914, but they did manage a start with the travel support scheme, a support of the salaries of some existing doctors, and to send a resident nurse for the first time to St. Kilda. There the McLeod of McLeod provided a cottage for her, furnished by the Board. The Board also appointed a relief doctor who was available to do locum duties in the area: he was probably the first salaried State practitioner in Britain.

But the start of the war caused a curb on all but vital expenditure, and wartime inflation eroded the value of the once-generous fund. The grant could not be spent in full each year, and money was only released for doctors' salaries and expenses. This subvention was even more welcome during the war than before, since the new seriousness of the nation had reduced the influx of summer shooting tenants and other paying patients, who had been important in the economy of the Highland doctor. Little else was allowed as expenditure, although a sum of £400 was allowed in 1916 to the Belford Hospital in Fort William to prevent its closure. Even then, the scheme which had hoped to attract young men into the area now found that the young men were instead away at war work. Though the budget of the Board was shackled in this way, they were allowed to keep the unspent surplus and, paradoxically, a healthy balance built up. But the end of the war brought no relief as tough government spending cuts were once more introduced, after a short period of optimism in 1919. None of the imaginative aspects of the Scheme could be introduced. The funds were now entirely devoted to the doctors' salaries, and travel. But the verdict on this limited scheme was favourable. It was commented at the time that this had been a notable success in bringing good medical men and women into the Highlands, and that they stayed in the area longer than before. This can be judged from the staffing of the area[16].

In 1919 the Board was put under the new larger Scottish Board of Health. The First Annual Report of the Scottish Board of Health in 1919 was still optimistic. It felt that the limited scheme had undoubtedly fulfilled the purpose for which it was designed, namely to bring an adequate medical service within the reach of persons of limited means, and at the same time to provide reasonable remuneration for the medical practitioners[17]. To their surprise, the civil servants were also obtaining statistics on the doctors' work load and journeys, since each visit had to be itemised for reimbursement, and the Annual Report commented that this sort of information was not available in any other part of the country[18]. By 1920 the Second Report of the Scottish Board of Health was preoccupied with 'the grave financial position of the country over-shadowing all present endeavours at social betterment'. The Scheme still had a healthy reserve to spend from all the previous years of limitation, but was not allowed to use it, in spite of what the Annual Reports of the Scottish Board of Health in succeeding years called 'claims for sickness benefit... genuinely attributable to lowered vitality as a result of un-employment'. Small sums were allowed to be granted for worthy projects: the payment of locums, the maintenance of the wartime emergency telephone circuits, essential repairs to hospitals and doctors' houses, and to help the tuberculosis work.

By 1930, the Treasury could relax their limits on spending and the allocation to the Highlands and Islands Medical Service was doubled, but only on the Treasury's terms. A heavy hint was given to the Board to release their budget to the local authorities, thus removing the central control of the fund and perhaps weakening the Board's political power[19]. The support for the doctors continued as before but at last some other parts of the original scheme were implemented, and there were improvements to many hospitals in the north. The first consultant to be appointed was the surgeon at Stornoway in 1924. Other surgical appointments followed, and an Ear, Nose and Throat specialist and physician were appointed at Inverness in 1929 and 1938. The first laboratory in the north was opened in Inverness, which provided a postal service. X-ray services were also set up. More newsworthy was the provision of the air ambulance service to the Western Isles starting in 1936, linking them with Glasgow hospitals. Even lifeboat journeys for medical emergencies to remote places were paid for from the Highlands and Islands Medical Service.

In 1936 the Cathcart Report[20] planned a national health service for Scotland, and in its review of health services it acknowledged the success of the Highlands and Islands Medical Service: the Highlands, for the first time in centuries, were no longer a problem[21]. It was the only area of the country in which the health services were aiming to be administered as a whole, in which general practitioners, consultants, hospitals and nurses were seen as part of a comprehensive service, and where money was available for houses, telephones and transport. The central adminis-tration was admired for its simplicity and directness and the central staff of civil servants were familiar with the area served. The doctors were contented and relieved to deal directly with Edinburgh rather than work with their ancient fear of local political control[22,23]. Even the British Medical Association seemed happy with the arrangements[24], and being State employees was habit forming; this led the Highlands and Islands Medical Service doctors, in 1928, to seek a superannuation scheme.

In the end the Highlands and Islands Medical Service was merged without fuss into the new National Health Service, many of whose features it had anticipated.

Acknowledgement

The careful work of Dr John Brims is gratefully acknowledged.

Sources

The Highlands and Islands Medical Service papers are held in the SRO File HH65: these are disappointing, having been heavily culled at some time. No minutes of the Board meetings remain, nor any detailed accounts of finances. The private papers of Katherine, Duchess of Atholl, Marchioness of Tullibardine have been preserved as NRA(S) 980 but have little on the Highlands and Islands Medical Service, nor do her memoires *Working Partnership*. The relevant Treasury files are TI/11703/726910, TI/11836/24638 and TI/11908/5814 for the years 1913 to 1916. The Highlands and Islands Medical Services Board published an Annual Report from 1914 onwards (first Report Cd 7977), which later merged with the Annual Reports of the Scottish Board of Health from 1919 (Cmd 825) which have a section devoted to the work of the Highlands and Islands Medical Service.

References

(1) From the perceptive and neglected work by John P. Day *Public Administration in the Highlands and Islands of Scotland* London 1918, p.6.

(2) The area covered in this paper and covered by the Highlands and Islands Medical Service, is known as the crofting counties, namely Argyll, Caithness, Inverness (excluding the burgh of Inverness), Ross and Cromarty, Sutherland, Orkney, Shetland and the Highland District of the County of Perthshire. The area was about half the land surface of Scotland and at that time had one-fifteenth of Scotland's population. At the committee stage of the Commons debate on the Dewar Report, the Highland District of Perth was taken out of the proposals, but at the Report stage, it was back in again. This led to requests from adjacent areas, notably Perthshire, Forfarshire, Moray and Nairn to be included as did all the Border counties.

(3) The Royal College of Physicians of Edinburgh holds the original returns of this simple survey of workload and travel: they have not yet been analysed fully.

(4) Other reports on medical services in the Highlands and Islands are the *Select Committee on Scottish Poor Law 1869*, the *Royal Commission on the Poor Laws and Relief of Distress (Scottish Report) 1909*.

(5) The announcement of this salary in 1897 brought a sharp letter from the Marquis of Zetland to the Local Government Board protesting at the burden it would place on the rates paid by the local landowners.

(6) Rex Taylor 'Doctors, paupers and landowners: the evolution of primary medical care in Orkney.' *Northern Scotland*, 4, p.98, 113–120.

(7) This was confirmed later, when in some parishes only the minister and the teacher were eligible for National Health Insurance.

(8) *The Scotsman* May 31st 1912.

(9) Day, J.P., *op.cit.*, p.6.

(10) This included a visit to the island of Foula and the news that several medical men were on the island led to several cases being brought to them for consultation and advice. '*First Annual Report of the Highlands and Islands Medical Services Board*'.

(11) The Dewar Report is Cmd 6559. The printed volume of evidence contains submissions by public bodies and the verbatim evidence from 258 witnesses.

(12) Some of the language of the Dewar Report owes much to the earlier Minority Report on the Poor Laws: eg. the Minority Report complained of 'intolerable conditions within twenty-four hours' journey from Edinburgh', while the Dewar Report deplored 'such conditions within twenty-four hours of Westminster'.

(13) For some comments on members of the committee see David Hamilton 'The Early History of the Highlands and Islands Medical Scheme'. *Scottish Medical Journal* 19/9 24, pp. 64–68.

(14) The fee was to be 5/- for a first visit, and 2/6 for a return visit, and £1 for midwifery. The guaranteed minimum salary was £300, which rose to £800 by 1948. A similar scheme of inducement payments was a natural outcome after the National Health Service was started. The salary of the nurses was hoped to be £120/year, but in the end little support was given.

(15) The doctors had other benefits notably to allow them to travel to postgraduate meetings and to pay for locums.

(16) Data from *The Medical Directory* and *Annual Report of the Registrar General for Scotland*.

(17) *First Annual Report of the Scottish Board of Health* 1919 Cmd 825.

(18) No trace of these itemised claims can be found in the relevant files; they were perhaps destroyed to preserve confidentiality.

(19) 'my Lords certain considerable doubts as to whether the highly centralised administration of the scheme by your Board may not be a serious obstacle to obtaining satisfactory contributions from local sources. My Lords would press your Board to consider whether the time has not arrived for placing the administration of the Schemes in the hands of the public health authorities...' 1920.

(20) 'The service (HIMS) revolutionised the whole standard of medicine in an area where, without assistance, comparable improvement would have been unobtainable, and set a pattern for similar services in other parts of the world presenting kindred geographical problems'. Thomas Ferguson, *Scottish Social Welfare 1864–1914* Edinburgh 1958. Though this verdict was widely repeated there are no accounts of where the Scheme was copied.
For other laudatory references see R.D. Martin 'The Highlands and Islands Medical Scheme', DHSS Reports 1956, pp.47–50 and A. Shearer (1938) 'The Highlands and Islands Medical Services' *Transactions of the Medico-Chirurgical Society of Edinburgh* 1937–38, pp.85–89. Shearer was for a time from 1922 an itinerant locum for the then central liaison officer in Edinburgh.

(21) The Cathcart Report is *Committee on Scottish Health Services* (1936 Cmd 5204).

(22) The Birsay Report of 1967 (Cmnd 3257) had no serious criticisms of the medical services in Highlands and Islands.

(23) The island of Papa Westray had fifteen resident doctors in the eighteen years prior to the scheme, but only four in the thirty-two years after it – Taylor, *op.cit.*, p.120.

(24) The Scheme was also unique in having the political support of the British Medical Association. The only dispute was the ritual threat not to join the early scheme, a threat which astonished the chairman of the Board – they do not lack courage – he commented (HH 65/7; letter from Lord Forteviot). In 1920 there were only 29 doctors in the area who were not part of the scheme.

PART IV:
Other Significant Factors in Development

CONTENTS

1. *The Scottish Medical Schools*

David Hamilton

CONTENTS

About the Author

DAVID HAMILTON, PhD, FRCS

David Hamilton, PhD, FRCS, is Director of the Wellcome Unit for the
History of Medicine at the University of Glasgow. He is author of "The
Healers: a History of Medicine in Scotland", Edinburgh 1981.

Author's Note

The reputation of the Scottish medical schools arose in the eighteenth century when the high quality and breadth of medical education available attracted students from afar. This resulted in a high output of medical students in the nineteenth century. In Scotland the extramural medical schools were a feature and in the twentieth century the Scottish medical schools still attracted students from other countries. The relations between the medical schools, universities and doctors' corporations in Scotland are different from England and explain some of the unique features of Scotland's medical schools.

The Scottish Medical Schools

A Unique Evolution

The Scottish medical schools (more accurately known as the Medical Faculties of the universities) have always had a distinctive place in British medical education, and at some periods in their history the eminence and individuality of Scottish medicine has attracted analysis, and many factors found to have been at work[1]. In Scotland, the relationships between the medical corporations, the health boards and medical schools are different from England and these have always and still make a Scottish medical training distinctive. As Sir Edward Wayne pointed out, the English student is more like an apprentice with a continuing system of clinical attachments, but the Scottish medical student is more like a student in any other faculty in the university[2]. The ability of poorer students to reach university has always been a feature in Scotland and the relative absence of private practice has perhaps influenced students in their career goals.

In the mid-eighteenth century the first Scottish medical school or faculty (i.e. a *group* of teachers) appeared in Edinburgh in 1726. Earlier, in mediaeval times, the Scottish universities usually had one teacher of medicine who taught the few students who might appear for instruction from time to time (e.g. Aberdeen's 'mediciner'). Shortly after the Reformation there was a proposal for a five year course to be set up at St Andrews University. What was new in Edinburgh was the collective effort by a group of teachers. The inititative was a civic one by a town in need of a new role after the Union of Parliaments. A medical school

495

might attract students from afar to the Town: Scottish medicine (unlike
the Church or Law) was international. In this experiment Edinburgh
succeeded beyond any reasonable expectation. Building on this fame, the
universities in Glasgow and Aberdeen also started teaching medicine in
an organised way in the late eighteenth century and there followed a long
period of dominance by Scottish universities of medical education in
Britain, attracting many students from overseas, and supplying huge
numbers of doctors to the rest of the world. It is known that of those who
graduated in medicine in Scotland (not all were required to or wished
to do so) in the period 1800–1850, no less than 95 *per cent* were Scottish
graduates, many coming from furth of Scotland to study[3]. The reasons
for success in Scottish teaching at that time were that the Scottish universities gave short economical and practical courses of use to the young
students and medical men who in mid-career returned to study. The
university teaching was closely linked to the teaching hospitals, and the
Scottish teaching broke with tradition since medicine, surgery and midwifery were included, whereas in England the two ancient universities at
Oxford and Cambridge, remote from the London hospitals (where there
were individual teachers of skill) taught theoretical physic only. Surgery
and midwifery were not suitable subjects for gentlemen. In London,
clinical instruction was good: the Scottish teaching was hampered by a
relative lack of patients compared with the numbers taught. The same
sort of problem vexed the Scottish anatomists. The eclectic Scottish
medical curriculum served to produce competent general practitioners
and practical medical men for the armed services. Thus useful medical
education harmonised with the teaching of the Scottish philosophers of
the day[4].

It was Glasgow and Edinburgh that attracted the students. St Andrews teaching never became regular, but the university made a steady
income from awarding the M.D. degree by examination, and even in
absentia on the basis of testimonials. This period of dominance of British
medicine by the Scottish medical schools lasted until the 1850s, when
English medical education changed. The first medical school in London
was based on the Scottish model, and the new University College Hospital Medical School was staffed from the start by Scottish graduates.
However, the earlier dominance by Scotland led to a natural self-
confidence in matters medical which persisted into the late nineteenth
century, even when it was obvious that the English medical schools were
now much improved and were fostering excellent research. But it was
Germany which now rivalled the British teaching, and by the early
twentieth century there was a mood of critical self-examination by the
Scottish medical schools: the old ways were not good enough. True, there
had been occasional signs of radicalism: Edinburgh had been liberal in
being first to admit female medical students, but in other ways there was
much stagnation. The teaching methods and the hierarchical structure

of the universities were under question[5]. The system of paying the professor directly by the fees from the students attracted to the class, though defended by traditional 'free enterprise' lobby, was no longer tenable. This ancient system had worked well in the eighteenth century, but now discouraged the appearance of new specialties and discouraged the ageing professoriate to put money towards purchase of the necessary equipment. Moreover the clinical professors were also absent at their private practices, and hence had little time for study or research. Reluctantly, the German system of salaried teachers had to be considered in Scotland. But it was the English medical schools, now much improved, which were ready to experiment. The chance came when the pre-First World War Haldane Commission on the London medical schools, to which Flexner gave evidence, proposed the setting up of new posts for full-time teachers in the London medical schools where it was obvious that teaching and research did not flourish because of the attractions of private practice[6]. After the First World War the new University Grants Commission funded full-time clinical chairs in clinical subjects in the London teaching hospitals: the new Medical Research Council (MRC) also added money for junior staff, and grants for laboratory equipment came from the Rockefeller and Sir William Dunn trusts. These London clinical units were not a success and the MRC withdrew their support ten years later[7]. It was to be in Scotland that the full-time principle for clinical teachers was to be established and succeed for the first time in Britain. Aberdeen University appointed their first full-time clinical professors in 1930. The habit spread from North to South and when the post-graduate hospital at Hammersmith opened a few years later. Scottish graduates were prominent in the new full-time staff in London who were to make such an impact on clinical research.

In the inter-war years, central control of medical education increased. The General Medical Council continued to regulate the medical curriculum. The new University Grants Committee (UGC) and its funds became an increasingly important factor in the universities finances, and the MRC funds meant that research was no longer dependent on local philanthropy. The MRC were not generous to Scotland, though a short-lived grant to Edinburgh was made, and some Rockefeller money also reached Edinburgh in the late 1930s. In pre-World War II Scotland, the academic clinical units were hardly different from others. Only in the period after World War II in Scotland was the full-time principle to have such profound effects.

During this time there was continual lengthening of the medical course. It increased in Scotland from the three year course of 1861 to four years in 1877 and in 1892 it was extended to five years. Later, in 1949 a six year course was set up, though this was later reduced to five. In Scotland poor students had two advantages when seeking a medical education. The first was that grants were available from the trust set up by Andrew Carnegie, the Scots-born American steel millionaire. The second was the economical education provided by the Scottish medical schools.

Extra-mural Teaching

Extra-mural medical teaching[8] (i.e. non-university teaching) had arisen early in Scotland. Because of the numbers seeking tuition in Edinburgh and Glasgow in the late eighteenth century, and since graduation was not mandatory until the Medical Act of 1858, rival teachers appeared outside the universities in both Edinburgh and Glasgow. These thrived in the competitive spirit of the times, and made good the deficiencies of the university teachers. The local Edinburgh and Glasgow medical corporations (the Royal Colleges and Faculty) recognised these teachers and courses, and the corporations, often in rivalry with the university, gave their own diplomas to the students taught extra-murally. These extra-mural schools and individual teachers added to the academic communities in the two cities: teaching was often a way of earning a living for a young man before promotion within the university or gaining private practice. It also meant that there were closer links in Scotland between the corporations and the universities. The education at the extra-mural schools was cheaper than at the university and poor students (the most distinguished being David Livingstone who studied at Anderson's College, Glasgow) could become doctors. It was estimated in 1894 that a London medical education might cost £587 in total whereas a Scottish extra-mural school education might need only £350 for the same time of study. The diplomas of the extra-mural medical schools were recognised by the 1858 Act. Initially the two Edinburgh Colleges joined together to hold a 'conjoint' examination: the Glasgow Faculty joined them in 1884 to make a 'triple' examination and qualification.

In the inter-war period in the twentieth century, as scientific technology increased and practical classes became necessary to teach these skills, the university medical schools were increasingly supported by the University Grants Committee. By contrast, the extra-mural teaching by 'chalk and blackboard' became less favoured and looked increasingly deficient. The Goodenough Report of 1944 reported on these extramural schools and the report caught the mood of the times. Because of their 'unscientific' structure they were shut down[9]. As part of these changes the laboratory of the College of Physicians in Edinburgh was transferred to the university. In their last years before the Second World War, the extra-mural schools were educating about 15 *per cent* of the Scottish medical students, including many, such as Jewish students, who could not obtain a medical education elsewhere[10]. There was one final unorthodox school in Scotland: the Polish Medical school set up in

Edinburgh in the Second World War taught many Poles intending to return home[11].

Women in Medicine

Though the battle for the admission of women medical students had been won in Scotland by the 1890s, women medical students were not immediately made welcome in large numbers. In the 1930s the proportion of women in the intake was 15 *per cent* and by the 1970s this had reached about 40 *per cent* in Scotland. By then, too, in some universities the number of female students had almost risen to parity with the male students.

Post-World War Two

Though there were initial shortages of money and equipment in the universities and hospitals after the Second World War[12] the medical schools thereafter showed a remarkable vitality and in this Glasgow perhaps surpassed Edinburgh. The medical schools in Scotland had two great advantages at this time. One organisational factor was important. A major difference between the 1947 National Health Service Acts for Scotland and for England and Wales was that in Scotland the Teaching Hospitals were administered by the Regional Hospital Boards and not, as in England, by separate Boards of Governors. The reason for this difference was that in Scotland the Teaching Hospitals were such an important component of hospital provision that had they been separated off the Regional Hospital Boards would not have been viable. For this reason the relationship in Scotland between the Health Service and Universities has been much closer and more important. It is to bring out certain points in this relationship rather than to attempt any history of the medical schools that these paragraphs are included. Whereas before the War all major hospitals had the facilities for treating and teaching on all types of case, the post-war growth of specialties meant that smaller hospitals now often housed a specialist regional referral centre such as paediatrics, chest surgery or brain surgery. In Scotland these hospitals were all within one administrative group, and this centred on a university; hence students and postgraduates were more easily taught. The second advantage in post-war Scotland was that of the new arrangements under the National Health Service which allowed those consultants not wishing to do private practice to have an adequate salary. In Scotland this was enough to encourage many to set out on an academic or specialist hospital career without private practice. Added to this, men discharged from the Forces were given a salary for a time to attach themselves where ever they wished in order to restart their careers. These factors allowed the teaching hospitals and academic units in Scotland to encourage talented and ambitious men, and in Glasgow Sir Charles Illingworth used all these dispensations to create a notable school of surgery[13].

Emigration and the Medical Schools

Emigration from Britain and Scotland has always been a feature of medical education, and because of the large output from the Scottish medical schools, the Scottish doctor abroad has always been a familiar figure. In 1982–83 the number of medical students in the United Kingdom was 19,940 and of these 3,372 were in Scottish Medical Schools. The much greater number of medical students in relation to the population has been a feature for many years and many more doctors have been trained in Scotland than have been needed for the local population. Study of Aberdeen graduates had shown that there was always a marked exodus of medical graduates at all times, and over 70 *per cent* of graduates left Scotland for abroad even in the inter-war period[14]. This loss became a political issue in the 1960s, though the numbers leaving were, as politicians found, difficult to count. The reasons for the loss were not only poor career prospects in Britain (mostly through too many hospital doctors being trained at a junior level) but also the lure of large salaries, particularly in North America. The exodus to Canada and America, which gave a new reputation to the Scottish medical schools, stopped before questions of regulation, control or repayment of fees could become a reality. North American jobs became fewer and tougher entry regulations were enforced: these doctors who had gone to Canada in the pioneer days now found themselves to be not only prosperous but also respectable. The same sequence of events and attitudes may be evolving in the current expansion of medical care in the Middle East.

The Decade of Optimism

The 1960s were a time of growth in public expenditure and optimism in the medical schools and universities. The growth of public sector expenditure seemed unlimited and every reasonable project seemed to be reachable: new staff posts were easily funded. Labour governments announced major rebuilding programmes for the hospitals, many of which were ageing rapidly, having been built in Victorian times. The editor of the *Scottish Medical Journal* could say of Scotland in 1963 that 'we look forward to a decade of new hospitals and new research institutes.'

This time of expansion also seems to have been remarkable for a concern with the medical curriculum, which diverted the attention of many university teachers for some time. Medical teaching had always been controlled by the General Medical Council, and the signal for experiment came from them in 1957. Its policy had fluctuated, but in that year the GMC proposed that the universities should 'educate more and instruct less.' Many medical schools hastened to experiment with their own interpretation of this philosophy and international comparisons were endlessly made: the Western Reserve Medical School teaching in America was particularly admired. As a result Glasgow introduced their 'integrated year' and Edinburgh their basic science degree. These innovations were seldom followed by an audit of the results and even the aims were often unclear[15]. In 1975, the Merrison Committee had reported redefining the responsibilities of the General Medical Council, but left the deficiencies of the pre-registration year unchanged. Much valuable information about the medical schools in the British Isles, their curricula and profiles, are contained in "Basic Medical Education in the British Isles" published by the Nuffield Provincial Hospitals Trust in 1977 and presenting the result of a survey conducted by the General Medical Council. "Medical Education and Medical Care" (NPHT 1977) also contains useful reviews of relationships between medical education, specialisation, government and resource allocation. The outcome of the debate on the student curriculum seemed to sharpen awareness that much of the real training was done after graduation. Sir Charles Illingworth commented that the medical course had traditionally met the needs of a former time when a young doctor who 'on the morrow of graduation might sail for Patagonia to undertake full medical responsibilities, perform major operations and perhaps supervise the control of public health.'[2] Another traditional view was that the medical course aimed at producing 'safe GPs'. But many commented that by the 1960s the aim seemed instead to be to turn out research-minded specialists and those who did not care for this career or who 'fell off the ladder' became general practitioners instead. To deal with this, expansion of postgraduate education was emphasised. In particular, the general practitioners were better organised, better paid and politically stronger. The 'safe GP' could only emerge after more years of in-service training.

The entry of Britain into the European Economic Community in 1976 allowed for free movement of specialists between the member nations, but in the end little change resulted.

The statutory provision in the Scottish Act of 1947 for liaison with the universities through Medical Education Committees did not prove to be a very successful provision and some, at least, of the Medical Education Committees ceased to meet. Much more important were the *ad hoc* arrangements, many of which were initiated and fostered by Brotherston.

For example, he started regular meetings at St. Andrew's House between himself and his senior staff and the Deans of Medical Schools. At these meetings many mutual problems were ventilated and goodwill created. For mutual benefit the Scottish Health Service has funded a number of new University Departments in subjects of special concern in health care but in which a university might be better able to attract first rate staff.

The University Clinical Departments, and especially the laboratory-based departments, have provided a high proportion of the routine care for the population. There have, of course, been arguments as to costings, but, in general, the close relationship between the two services ensured that these were fairly resolved.

Certain university departments merit special mention. The first professorial appointment in General Practice was made in Edinburgh in 1963 and the Departments in the medical schools have played an important part in the improved status and training of general practitioners. The changes in the names of the Departments of Community Medicine have mirrored the changes in health care. In Edinburgh, for example, the Chair of Public Health was instituted in 1898. In 1946, it became the Chair of Social Medicine, and in 1974 the Chair of Community Medicine. The department's role in training formerly for the Diploma in Public Health and more recently for the MSc in Community Medicine has been a very important one for the Scottish Health Service.

Retrenchment

In the 1970s, it was David Owen who first said that money for health care had to be rationed: the first alarm had sounded as Britain's economic base weakened and borrowing was brought under control. Existing hospitals plans were phased: then the unbuilt phases were postponed. The new formulae for calculating allocation of resources (RAWP and Scotland's SHARE) directed money away from the heavy spending city hospitals to the new District General Hospitals at the edge of the cities where the population had now settled. These cuts increasingly hit the medical schools of the city centre who started to make economies[16]. By the early 1980s hard times made the medical schools look for funds from novel sources, sources other than government or grant-giving bodies. Fund-raising methods familiar in other countries, namely from the local community, or from the business community or from the forgotten Scottish alumni were introduced. High fees were charged to students from other countries: laudatory accounts of the Scottish universities were printed in Arabic. A further blow to the old style of the Scottish schools was the extension of private practice by the Conservative governments of the early 1980s. This meant that all consultants could indulge in private practice: recruitment into academic medicine became less likely.

Whereas in 1976 for instance only 40 *per cent* of Scottish surgeons did private practice (compared with 80 *per cent* of English surgeons) the new regulations meant that all Scottish surgeons could do private practice if they wished, and usually without detriment to their NHS income. The great Scottish advantages of the 1950s were lost. It was also a time when, almost without notice being taken, the number of students at the Scottish medical schools had lowered to reach the proportion expected for the population of Scotland.

By the middle of the 1980s many of the essential features of Scottish education had gone, and the medical schools faced instead a retreat from the collectivism of the post-war period and a new pluralism of funding. Perhaps it was not really a new situation: perhaps it was a return to the entrepreneurial medical schools of the eighteenth century. At any rate, Adam Smith's textbooks were now back in favour.

References

(1) For general accounts of the Scottish Medical schools see Comrie, J.D., *History of Scottish Medicine*, London 1932, and Hamilton, D., *The Healers: a History of Scottish Medicine*, Edinburgh 1981. More detailed information is found in *Fortuna Domus: A series of Lectures delivered in the University of Glasgow in commemoration of the Fifth Centenary of its Foundation*, The University of Glasgow 1952, Horn, D.B., *A Short History of the University of Edinburgh 1556–1889*, The University Press Edinburgh, 1967, and Mackie, J.D., *The University of Glasgow 1451–1951: a Short History*, University of Glasgow 1954. See also *Royal Commission on Medical Education 1965–68* Cmnd 3569, 1968, and the *Royal Commission on Scottish Universities 1826–30*. British medical education is described in Poynter, F.N.L. (ed), *The Evolution of Medical Education in Britain*, London 1966, and McLachlan, G. (ed), *Medical Education and Medical Care: a Scottish-American Symposium*, London 1977 gives the comparison and links between Scotland and America.

(2) Wayne, E.J. in *The Future of Medical Education in Scotland*. Published by Scottish Medical Journal, Glasgow 1963, p.40.

(3) Hamilton (ref. 1), p.151.

(4) Holloway, S.W.F., "The Apothecaries Act 1815: a reinterpretation." *Medical History* (1966), *10*, pp.107–29 and 221–36.

(5) *Scottish Review*, January 1894, p.1.

(6) For Scottish concern over the German lead, see Patrick Geddes, *Closing Address for 1889–90*, Leng and Co, Dundee 1890.

(7) Landsborough Thomson, A., *Half a Century of Medical Research*, London 1973, vol. 2, pp.13–23.

(8) Guthrie, D., *Extra-mural Medical Education in Edinburgh*, Edinburgh 1965.

(9) *Report on the Interdepartmental Committee on Medical Schools*, HMSO, London 1944.

(10) See Collins, K., "Asher Asher MD (1837–1889)". *Glasgow Medicine*, March/April 1984, pp.12–14.

(11) The Universities of Edinburgh and Poland. ed. Wiktor Tomaszewski, Edinburgh 1968 (privately published but printed by the Aberdeen University Press). Other numerous books on the Edinburgh Polish School of Medicine are listed in Hamilton (ref. 1), p.304.

(12) See Robert Campbell Garry, *Physiology in the University of Glasgow to 1970*, University of Glasgow 1980.

(13) Sir C Illingworth, "Founding a school of Surgery". *Review of Surgery* (1966), 23, pp.77–83. See also *British Medical Journal*, 6th November 1976.

(14) See MacKay, D., *Geographical mobility and the Brain Drain*. London 1966.

(15) Note that the Association for the Study of Medical Education was founded in 1957 and has its headquarters in Dundee.

(16) The recent economies have given rise to suggestions that some classes formerly heavily dependent on experimental work e.g. physiology, might be given without practical instruction. Anti-vivisection sentiment adds to this re-examination.

2. *The Impact of Technology*

Derek Dow and John Lenihan

CONTENTS

About the Authors

Dr DEREK DOW, Ph.D.

Derek Dow graduated in history from Edinburgh University in 1973. Four years later he was awarded a Ph.D. for a thesis on nineteenth century Scottish Churches' foreign missions. He has been archivist to the Greater Glasgow Health Board since 1979, and is currently Joint Honorary Secretary of the Scottish Society of the History of Medicine.

PROFESSOR JOHN LENIHAN, O.B.E., M.Sc., Ph.D., F.Inst.P., F.I.E.E., F.I.Biol., F.R.S.E.

John Lenihan is Senior Research Fellow in the Department of Nursing Studies at Glasgow University, where he was formerly Professor of Clinical Physics.

Authors' Note

Scotland has made a large and distinctive contribution to the impact of technology on health care. Recognition, during the nineteenth century, of the importance of physical science in medical education and practice provided a favourable environment for the combination of scientific, industrial and clinical interests which gave the country a prominent role in the early achievements of radiology. This pattern of innovation was repeated, half a century later, in the development of ultrasonic diagnosis.

The study of these two episodes illuminates matters of wider significance – in particular the historical, administrative and financial influences relevant to Scotland's leadership in many aspects of the technological revolution, which began, fortuitously, just after the inception of the National Health Service.

The Impact of Technology
Part 1

Pointing the Way: Technology Prior to 1948

Charles Newman's 1954 Fitzpatrick lectures on medical history[1] contain a number of sweeping generalisations about the technology of medicine at the beginning of the nineteenth century. Newman's definition, in which 'technology' gradually replaced the 'wisdom' and 'long experience' of the clinician by means of advances in 'medical science'[2], is clearly too broad for a chapter of this length. A detailed analysis of the impact of technology on Scottish health care in the present century awaits a book of its own. The framework required in such an undertaking can be gauged from the range and complexity of themes identified by Paul Durbin and his collaborators in 1980[3]. Many of the origins of twentieth century developments may be discerned in Reiser's recent work on medicine and technology in the nineteenth century[4]. The focus for this study of the period prior to 1948 is of necessity a much narrower one.

In the introduction to his 1890 guide to young doctors entering private practice Jules de Styrap claimed that medical education was regarded as 'that worst of all educations – a technical one'[5]. Less than twenty years later this attitude, if it had ever existed, was largely extinguished. In July 1908 the British Medical Association held its annual meeting at Sheffield where the section of physiology conducted a spirited 'Discussion on the Scientific Education of the Medical Student'[6]. Sir Felix Semon's suggestion for a six-month compulsory postgraduate course in methods of physical diagnosis was warmly applauded. The range of techniques advocated by Semon was an impressive one – auscultation and percussion, urinary analysis, ophthalmoscopy, laryngoscopy, otoscopy, rhinology, Roëntgen rays, staining, electrical reaction and medical uses of electricity.

Dr Dawson Turner, medical electrician to the Royal Infirmary of Edinburgh and lecturer in natural philosophy at the extra-academical medical school[7], made an even more radical demand. His proposal that medical or biological physics should be taught by medically qualified men was given cautious support by Dr R.C. Buist, gynaecologist to Dundee Royal Infirmary. This idea was opposed by Dr Wells of Greenwich, and the Chairman of the Section later drew attention to the fact that Turner was the only one of the speakers who had not advocated putting pressure on the public schools to improve science teaching. Leaving aside the apparent differences between the favoured school science curriculum north and south of the border the debate contained three elements which may be used to illustrate the effects of technology on Scottish medicine, namely electricity, diagnostic equipment and the bonding agent provided by the physicist *cum* clinician.

The potential use of electricity for therapeutic purposes was recognised in the eighteenth century. On drawing up regulations for the new Glasgow Royal Infirmary in 1794 the Managers decreed that the Surgeon's Clerk was 'to electrify those patients for whom electricity is ordered'[8]. Ten years later the Managers agreed to purchase a galvanic battery[9], in the wake of the visit to this country in 1803 of John Aldini, nephew of Professor Galvini. The most dramatic exploitation of this new technology occurred in 1818 when James Jeffray, Professor of Anatomy at Glasgow University, conducted a number of experiments on the body of Matthew Clydesdale after his execution for murder[10]. The alarm which attended this apparent revival of the dead almost certainly put paid to further research in the immediate future[11].

The contemporary introduction by Laënnec of the stethoscope (1816) saw the introduction of technology as a diagnostic rather than a therapeutic aid to medicine. Subsequent developments, such as the microscope and the ophthalmoscope, resulted in more sophisticated methods of viewing the human body. A feature of many of these advances was the role of the individual, working independently of other researchers and frequently providing his own funding. Within Scotland this trend continued throughout the nineteenth and well into the twentieth century. The earliest recorded venture into print by John Macintyre, who later played a leading part in the development of radiology, was an 1885 article on the use of the electric light in medicine[12]. Dissatisfied with existing lamps, Macintyre commissioned a local optician to manufacture a lamp to his own specification. A leading firm of Glasgow instrument makers gave Macintyre access to all their electrical apparatus and informed him of the existence of a French lamp, designed by M. Laverne and similar to his own[13]. Macintyre concluded his article with the prediction that electric light was still in the experimental stage but would certainly be used extensively as doctors became more familiar with it.

A further example of personal initiative was provided in 1898 when Dr Samuel Sloan, best known as an obstetrician, demonstrated his faradimeter to members of the Philosophical Society of Glasgow[14]. Sloan's project was prompted by the inability of instrument makers in the UK or on the Continent to supply a suitably sensitive instrument to measure the very small currents used in electro-therapeutic practice. The apparatus which Sloan devised, apparently without commercial backing, was constructed by another local firm, Baird and Tatlock.

Some of these projects were doubtless born of frustration. One of the major drawbacks to the spread of technology in the hospitals at this period was a lack of funding. Voluntary hospital managers were in some cases reluctant or dilatory in approving expenditure; in April 1884 the directors of the Glasgow Maternity Hospital agreed to buy a microscope for clinical use but the purchase was not completed until February 1886, almost two years later. In such circumstances it was common for individual members of the medical staff, despairing of action, to present equipment to the hospital as a gift or extended loan[15]. As an alternative to this the medical staff might attract individual sponsors, either from the management committees or from their own circle of friends. Of the four microscopes purchased by Glasgow Royal Infirmary in 1914–15 for use in the wards, two were paid for from Infirmary funds while the cost of the others was met by the Chairman and one of the other managers[16].

The problems of introducing and accepting new technology are perhaps seen most clearly in the case of radiology. Electrical knowledge and diagnostic theories could now be combined in a manner not previously possible. Within a relatively short span of time considerable use was being made of the new X-rays for therapeutic purposes although enthusiasm sometimes outstripped caution and knowledge in these pioneer days, with disastrous results. The emergence of radiology as a distinct specialty, which later sub-divided itself even further, provides a model from which to study the more general fragmentation of medicine as new technologies become more widespread or invasive. The history of radiology in Scotland provides an early embodiment of factors which became even more critical in the post-1948 era, namely the increasing dependence of medicine upon non-clinical personnel and resources, the growing trend towards an institutionalisation and centralisation of services and the rapid upward spiralling of costs.

On the announcement in November 1895 of Roëntgen's discovery of X-rays Glasgow was particularly well-placed to take advantage of this exciting news. Glasgow Royal Infirmary already possessed a medical electrical department, supervised by Dr John Macintyre since his appointment a decade previously. Thanks primarily to Macintyre's growing reputation the department had been enlarged in 1894 with the assistance of Henry Mavor and a number of anonymous donors[17]. More importantly, Macintyre was a protégé of the 72-year-old Lord Kelvin, the most distinguished physicist of his generation, and Archibald Campbell, Lord Blythswood, an extremely talented 'amateur' with a well-equipped private laboratory[18]. The establishment at the GRI in 1896 of what is arguably the first hospital radiological department in the world owed much to the technical and moral support of these two great figures.

The capabilities of the 'new photography' as it was swiftly dubbed were almost immediately apparent. In 1865, barely thirty years earlier, Dr John Taylor had devised an electric probe to detect bullets remaining lodged in the body[19]. The invention seemingly aroused little interest although the problem remained. In 1896 Macintyre located a bullet in the body of an officer stationed at Maryhill Barracks in Glasgow[20]. *The Bailie*, a local satirical weekly, reported the occurrence in rather less awed tones than the medical press.

"An Inkerman bullet in the brain of an old soldier in the Royal Infirmary has been spotted by the Roëntgen rays. The anxiety for a 'howk' by the surgeons is considerable. Seeing that the old man has had quiet possession of the Russian lead for forty-two years, why disturb him now?"[21]

Although *The Bailie* questioned the utility of acting upon this information, the fact that it was now available paved the way for the modern advances in operative possibilities and techniques.

Spurred on by this example the Glasgow Western Infirmary and the Royal Infirmary of Edinburgh installed electricity in 1896–97 and appointed medical electricians to set up X-ray departments[22]. The ease and speed with which this was accomplished was an indication of the low capital costs and the relatively simple technology required at this time[23].

Not surprisingly, in view of its priority, the GRI was able to raise funds to erect and equip a new electrical pavilion in 1903[24]. The Infirmary was fortunate – or foresighted – enough to attract sufficient funds to run and maintain its X-ray department. In 1919 this commitment was extended to pay for a full-time technician to service the electrical apparatus[25]. Other hospitals were less well-endowed. In both Keith

(1913) and Huntly (1919) the use of donated X-ray equipment was hampered by the lack of an adequate power supply. In the latter case the X-ray department at Huntly Jubilee Hospital was indebted until 1936 to the local woollen factory for its power, permission being required prior to each use of the equipment because of the resultant surge which interfered with the factory's own equipment.

By the mid 1920s X-ray apparatus was becoming more sophisticated and, inevitably, more expensive. In the pioneering days the required components could be assembled relatively cheaply by individual doctors, aided by manufacturers such as Henry W. Cox who advertised Cox's Record Portable Coil in the 1904 *Medical Directory* as, 'The most suitable apparatus for General Practitioners'. By 1926, when the Edinburgh Royal erected a new radiological department, the cost had risen one hundred-fold from the £500 required to establish the department thirty years earlier[26]. In addressing the GRI annual meeting on 8 February 1926, James Macfarlane LLD, chairman of the Board, drew attention to the average cost per bed which had risen two and a half times since 1899. Although the effects of World War I were traditionally blamed for this steep rise Macfarlane refuted this explanation:

"The real reason was the growing complexity and cost of medical diagnosis which had been steadily going on during the last twenty years, and which entailed expenses in connection with departments of the Infirmary unheard of or only in their infancy 20 or 25 years ago"[27].

Prominent in the list which followed were X-rays.

Later that year the Glasgow Western Infirmary managers authorised the expenditure of £420 on a new X-ray outfit, purchased from a local firm of X-Ray and Electro-Medical Engineers. This was only the prelude to a much greater outlay. After preparing the ground in their annual reports for 1924 and 1925, drawing attention to the need for regular replacement of X-ray equipment due to wear and tear and to technological advances, the Western Infirmary managers launched an appeal for £20,000 to rebuild the radiological department. With the aid of three individual donations of £5,000 this was accomplished by 1928 and the new department was completed in 1930.

X-ray equipment, whether for diagnosis or treatment, was thus becoming more sophisticated and, in the case of smaller hospitals, prohibitively expensive. The same was true to an even greater extent in the related field of radium therapy. Although radium had been discovered by the Curies in 1898, it was not used successfully in the treatment of carcinoma until 1903[28] and it never gained the widespread adoption of X-rays. In 1909–10 Dr John Levack, Medical Electrician to Aberdeen Royal Infirmary, requested the sum of £88 to purchase a supply of radium. Before ultimately refusing this request the Directors obtained information on the use of radium in other Scottish hospitals. The results of this survey are illuminating. The RIE claimed to have been purchasing radium for the past eight years, paid for from Infirmary funds; the GRI had access to radium but did not pay for it; both the Western and Victoria Infirmaries in Glasgow were marking time in the hope that generous donors might provide sufficient quantities of radium to be useful[29].

The cost of radium was such that centralised co-ordination of its distribution was seen as the optimum approach from an early stage. In May 1914, a committee was formed under the chairmanship of Sir John Stirling Maxwell to obtain a supply of radium for Glasgow and the West of Scotland[30]. This committee comprised representatives of the three city infirmaries, the Royal Cancer Hospital and the Royal Samaritan Hospital for Women, together with 'certain experts' including Frederick Soddy[31] and J.T. Bottomley[32]. The five institutions received an equal share of the radium available and were subject to strict controls requiring the appointment of a recognised radiologist and the provision of clinical and pathological evidence on cases treated[33]. In 1929, a National Radium Trust and Commission was established as the result of a nationwide appeal for funds[34]. The establishment of this new body was intended to maximise the efficiency of what was recognised to be an increasingly specialised and costly field. The Glasgow Committee already possessed some 700 mg of radium, purchased at a cost of £9,000. In 1928, however, the Cancer Hospital received a donation of £10,000 from Lady Burrell to purchase additional radium[35]. At around the same time Sir Henry Mechan, vice-chairman of the Western Infirmary, gave £5,000 to his own hospital for a similar purpose. Allied to the opening of the new radiological department this led to the designation of the Infirmary as the National Radium Centre for the West of Scotland[36]. In a parallel development the Royal Infirmary of Edinburgh, which in 1929 received an anonymous donation of £5,000 for the purchase of radium, was selected as the Centre for south-east Scotland[37]. This concentration of effort and resources set a pattern which was copied in many future instances.

During the 1930s those hospitals which could afford it were obliged to spend heavily on updating or installing X-ray equipment. Between November 1931 and March 1935 the Glasgow Royal Maternity Hospital directors debated this subject on numerous occasions, delaying on each occasion through anxiety about the availability of accommodation and the capital and recurring costs of such a commitment. The decision to proceed was finally approved on 17 April 1935 when the Walker Trustees agreed to bear the capital costs (c. £2,500) and the Hospital Ladies' Committee offered to meet the first year's running costs[38]. Similar hesitations were experienced by other voluntary hospitals in this period.

In 1933 a Committee was appointed by the Department of Health for Scotland:

"To review the existing health services of Scotland in the light of modern conditions and knowledge, and to make recommendations on any changes in policy and organisation that may be considered necessary for the promotion of efficiency and economy"[39].

While reasserting its belief that the family doctor should continue to be the lynchpin of the health system[40] the Cathcart Committee recognised the need for a national policy to avoid overlap and duplication, especially between the voluntary and local authority sectors[41]. The implications for advanced technology were clearly seen in the recommendation that a single deep X-ray therapy plant might serve several different kinds of hospital. Although it was not stated explicitly in the report, such requirements would contribute to the move towards a nationalised and centralised hospital system[42].

In 1938 a detailed survey of hospital buildings and facilities in Scotland was undertaken on behalf of the Department of Health for Scotland[43]. The reports of the surveyors, all medical men experienced in hospital work and administration, were published for each of the five Scottish regions in 1946[44]. The report on hospitals in the Western Region revealed wide discrepancies in the quality of X-ray equipment and in the level of expertise available to operate it. Some hospitals possessed no electricity or gas supplies; Bute Cottage Hospital at Old Cumnock had an X-ray room which was not used; at Kirkcudbright and District Cottage Hospital the X-ray work was 'done by matron'[45]. Ayrshire fared rather better than some of the other sub-regions in that 'the equipment is better than the buildings would suggest, like new wine in old bottles'[46]. In reporting on the needs of a Cancer Service the surveyors highlighted the need for centralised facilities in order to effectively meet the cost of modern equipment and to gather 'a large staff of experts including physicists and trained technicians'. In recommending that the posts of radiotherapist and radiologist (previously separated) should be combined the surveyors also accepted that technological requirements had a part to play in shaping medical as well as ancillary staffing structures[47]. Although it would be erroneous to claim that technological requirements, particularly in the field of radiology, shaped the National Health Service which came into being in 1948, it is fair to say that the location, cost and increasingly specialised nature of medical technology had a significant impact on decision making in the new system.

The *ad hoc* developments revealed by the 1938 Survey were clearly inappropriate given the Cathcart Committee's assertion that priority should be given to the integration of separate services into a national health policy. Five regional committees had been established after the Local Government (Scotland) Act of 1929 to co-ordinate the efforts of the voluntary hospitals. Based on the four teaching schools (Edinburgh,

Glasgow, Dundee and Aberdeen) and Inverness these bodies were still inactive when Cathcart reported[48]. Sir William Beveridge's insistence on the creation of 'a comprehensive medical service for every citizen ... under the supervision of the Health Department'[49] gave further weight to the view that increased co-ordination of services would be required in future. The implications for technology were spelled out in the 1949 reports of the Department of Health for Scotland and of the Scottish Health Services Council. It was intended that X-ray and other electro-medical equipment should be purchased centrally and installed by the Ministries of Health and of Works. In the particular case of Cancer and Radiotherapy a sub-committee was established under that heading in March 1949 to control developments in these related spheres[50]. The second half of this chapter examines some of the factors which determined the practical application of this theoretical framework.

The Impact of Technology
Part 2

Technology in Health Care: 1948–1985

The growth and management of technology in health care in Scotland after 1948 was influenced by a number of earlier developments. In addition to those recommended (or foreshadowed) by the Cathcart Report of 1936, three others were significant:

(1) The Highlands and Islands Medical Service, established just before the first world war, demonstrated the feasibility of a system providing both primary and specialist health care under the direct control of central government.

(2) The Emergency Medical Service, established during the second world war, made good conspicuous deficiencies in the country's hospital provision, enhanced the opportunities for research and practice in several specialties (including radiology, neurosurgery, anaesthetics, orthopaedics, pathology, plastic surgery and the treatment of burns), and showed how the activities of local authority hospitals, voluntary hospitals and State-run hospitals could be integrated.

(3) The National Health Service (Scotland) Act of 1947 placed all

hospitals under the control of Regional Hospital Boards. This arrangement (though viewed with some displeasure by the Conservative opposition, and with some anxiety by the Minister of Health) was to prove advantageous, since it facilitated the integration of teaching hospitals (and other voluntary hospitals) with local authority hospitals in the strategic planning and management of specialist services. These tasks were more difficult in England, where teaching hospitals were committed to the care of separately-financed Boards of Governors.

The environment characterised by these distinctive features was favourable to the growth of technology in health care, as new opportunities arose in rapid succession after 1948. The first twenty-five years of the new service saw the emergence of major new clinical specialties (including cardiac surgery, renal medicine and nuclear medicine) and the growth, from modest beginnings, of others, including anaesthetics and radiotherapy; all were heavily dependent on technology. Many established specialties (including radiology, obstetrics, neurology, neurosurgery, ophthalmology and ear, nose and throat surgery) were considerably influenced by new technical developments contributing to investigation and treatment. Experience (gained during the second world war) of the benefit of specialised post-operative care encouraged the transformation of recovery rooms into intensive care units. The increasing complexity (and, later, the automation) of biochemical investigations necessitated great expansion of hospital facilities for clinical chemistry.

These developments required the recruitment and training of large numbers of staff in various new and existing paramedical and technical occupations. Managerial responsibility for some groups (including radiographers and electrocardiography technicians) remained in clinical hands. As laboratory medicine became less attractive to doctors, who now had many other opportunities for salaried work, graduate biochemists, seldom employed in clinical laboratories before 1948, were recruited in considerable numbers and attained parity of status with medical graduates similarly occupied. Medical laboratory technicians (later designated medical laboratory scientific officers) aspired, without success, to managerial control of clinical laboratories.

A wide range of scientific and technical services was provided by the departments of medical physics established by the five Regional Hospital Boards. Each was based on the concept, initiated in Glasgow in 1953, of an organisation independent of any clinical specialty, but staffed and equipped to provide advice and assistance to hospitals, community health agencies and university clinical departments. This support took several forms:

(a) design and construction of equipment;
(b) collaboration of complex diagnostic and therapeutic facilities;
(c) guidance in the choice of commercially-available equipment (to supplement the Home and Health Department's central pur-

chasing schemes for radiological, electromedical and sterilising equipment);

(d) teaching and training;
(e) participation in the formulation of managerial policies related to the impact of technology.

Administrative and financial arrangements varied among the regions. In Aberdeen and Edinburgh, the Universities accepted the substantial administrative commitments and shared the costs in agreed proportions. In Dundee and Inverness, the departments were managed and funded by the Regional Hospital Boards. In Glasgow the University made a nominal financial contribution.

The importance of physics in medical education and practice had long been advocated by Scottish physicians[51]. The concept of medical physics as a service organised on a regional basis, but providing expert staff and specialised resources in the front line of the clinical realm, was a Scottish invention. In England, small (sometimes one-man) physics departments survived for many years in association with individual clinical specialties; some hospitals had three or four such departments. The Scottish pattern was better able to support, in an economical way, the technological revolution in health care which began in the mid 1950s.

The Scottish experience had a significant influence on the recommendations of the Hospital Scientific and Technical Services Committee, appointed in 1967 by the Minister of Health and the Secretary of State for Scotland. In 1970, the chairman of the committee (Sir Solly – later Lord – Zuckerman) said, in opening the new building of the Glasgow department of Clinical Physics and Bio-Engineering:

"The growth of the scientific and technical services... has been fragmented, with little units of a few isolated people working in particular specialties and individual hospitals... The guidelines which were set by the Committee in its deliberations were to bring about concentration in place of multi-fragmentation, teamwork in place of isolation and to build multi-disciplinary groups of physicists, electronic specialists, mechanical engineers, biochemists, all working together in a group, focusing their attention on the same problems... Several of our recommendations added up to what I have seen here today... I am quite sure that the evidence my committee was given about the desirability of bringing about a concentration of scientific power – which we see represented here – came because there already was the knowledge that you had done this in Glasgow."

The recommendations[52] of the Zuckerman Committee, based on the integration of pathology and biological sciences with medical physics, bio-engineering, nuclear medicine and applied physiology in a Hospital Scientific Service, were not fully implemented, but Regional Departments of Medical Physics were established cautiously in the English provinces during the 1970s and early 1980s.

Before 1948, hospital managers had developed a variety of stratagems to solve (or to circumvent) financial problems created by the growth of technology. Substantial innovations, such as new radiology departments (which, until the 1940s, provided both diagnostic and thereapeutic services) were often financed by benefactions or public appeals. In teaching hospitals, university departments provided resources for practice and research in major clinical specialties, as well as in pathology and bacteriology.

After 1948 the financial management of technology became more difficult. Hospital Boards operated under an accounting system based on annual allocations for revenue expenditure and for capital expenditure on new buildings, including their equipment. They had no power to set aside adequate sums to build up funds for the purchase or replacement of costly items in future years. In effect, equipment was written down to zero value on the day of acquisition. This unsophisticated accounting system was not altogether appropriate, in a period when the demand for technical resources was increasing rapidly for several reasons:

(1)   As private practice fell to a very low level in Scotland, full-time senior and junior medical staff in hospitals generated increased demand for laboratory, radiological and other investigations.

(2)   Research became an essential activity for those aspiring to consultant status or to academic appointments.

(3)   Manufacturers exerted themselves to meet the specialised needs of the increased number of research workers. Sensitive to the availability of increased funds, disbursed in a less frugal way than before, they also exerted themselves to stimulate demand by producing equipment in greater variety and of greater complexity for routine clinical use.

(4)   Scientific advances, sometimes in disciplines, such as electronics and nuclear physics, not directly related to health care, were adapted to produce new (and often costly) devices and techniques for investigation or treatment.

(5)   Equipment which was expensive to buy was usually expensive to maintain, and sometimes became obsolete before it was worn out.

Despite these considerations, the technological revolution proceeded without undue difficulty. Financial control by the Department ensured that high-technology specialties, such as radiotherapy, neurosurgery, cardiac surgery and some components of nuclear medicine, were concentrated in a small number of centres with adequate equipment and staff.

Support for Research

The impact of technology on health care was enhanced by the advantageous arrangements enjoyed in Scotland for the support of research.

The existence of four medical schools – two of them very large – ensured a generous share of the funds disbursed by the University Grants Committee, the Medical Research Council, and other grant-giving bodies with responsibilities covering the United Kingdom. These resources were substantially augmented by a number of organisations with an exclusively Scottish remit.

The Secretary of State for Scotland, (who is effectively the Minister for health, education, local government, agriculture and much else) has considerable powers if he chooses to use them. Holders of the office since 1948 have given vigorous support to the health service in general and to medical research in particular. The Advisory Committee on Medical Research, appointed in 1950, considered applications from medical and scientific research workers in hospitals and universities. The Secretary of State provided support from public funds for projects approved by the Committee.

An imaginative venture was initiated in 1949, with the appointment of the Hospital Endowments Commission, constituted under the National Health Service (Scotland) Act of 1947. The endowments held by hospitals before 5 July 1948, were not immediately transferred to the State, as were buildings and equipment. Instead, they were, after some deductions for 'liabilities inherited by the State from voluntary hospitals generally', transferred to the new Boards of Management constituted to operate the hospitals. At that stage, the endowments were very unevenly distributed. Some of the voluntary hospitals had been well provided with endowments from which the income met a significant part of their running costs; but these costs were now to be taken over by the State. Local authority hospitals, and others less attractive to private benefactors, had little or no endowment income.

Charged with the task of preparing a scheme for the redistribution of endowments, the Commission recommended that most of the available funds should be allocated to Boards of Management and Regional Hospital Boards, to be used for the provision of additional amenities for patients and staff, or for research. The remaining funds, producing an annual income of about £100,000, were to be administered centrally by a body of independent trustees. This body was constituted in 1953 as the Scottish Hospital Endowments Research Trust. During its first 30 years, the Trust, with scientific advice from the Advisory Committee on Medical Research (until its dissolution in 1975, and thereafter from the Biomedical Research Committee) supported almost 400 projects at a cost of more than £5 million. Many of these projects required advanced technology, in the form of specialised equipment and scientific or technical staff.

The Chief Scientist Organisation, established by the Scottish Home and Health Department in 1973 (in response to the recommendations of the Rothschild Report and the subsquent White Paper *Framework for*

Government Research and Development, Cmnd 5046, 1972) appointed committees to advise on the allocation of government funds for research relevant to the needs of the health service. By 1985, the committees with a significant interest in technology were those responsible for advising on:

(a)   bio-medical research;
(b)   equipment research, development and evaluation;
(c)   research on equipment for the disabled.

In 1985 the expenditure under these headings was more than £2 million. Regional Hospital Boards, Boards of Management and, later, Health Boards generally took a responsible view of their obligations and opportunities in relation to research. Small projects were funded locally. Novel experimental or investigative facilities provided by one Board but available to all were jointly funded by a simple administrative procedure, which was used also to maintain support for innovative work which had passed beyond the research stage but had not yet been assimilated into the clinical repertoire.

The informal but close contacts among the organisations supporting research was exemplified in the financial arrangements for the costly nuclear magnetic resonance imaging system installed at the Southern General Hospital, Glasgow in 1985. A sum of nearly £1 million, needed for building conversion, equipment and start-up costs was met by contributions from the Scottish Home and Health Department, the Scottish Hospital Endowments Research Trust, the University of Glasgow, the Greater Glasgow Health Board and the Medical Research Council.

The cost of providing this one machine exemplifies the rapid rise in the real cost of medical imaging resources. In 1896, George Watson of Keighley (afterwards Professor of Medicine in Leeds) expressed the view that Roëntgen's discovery could hardly come into practical use in medicine because of the cost of the apparatus; his equipment cost £5. In the same year the cost of providing an X-ray department in the Royal Infirmary of Edinburgh was £500; the new department established in 1926 cost £50,000.

Ultrasonic Diagnosis

The story of the development in Scotland of ultrasonic diagnosis illuminates many features of the impact of technology on health care.

When, in 1954, Mr Ian Donald came to Scotland as Regius Professor of Midwifery in the University of Glasgow, he brought with him an imaginative plan for clinical and scientific research.

His aims were:

(1)   To continue and extend his work begun in London, on the study and treatment of respiratory distress in the newborn (then the major cause of neonatal mortality) using novel electronic instruments and techniques.

(2)   To develop non-invasive techniques for continuous measurement and recording of blood pressure.

(3)   To study the reflection of ultrasonic radiation at tissue interfaces as a means of localising tumours and cysts.

(4)   To study the possibility of selective destruction of cells by ultrasonic radiation.

Early in 1955 the Regional Hospital Board provided a technician (on the staff of the Regional Physics Department) who worked on the development and construction of electronic equipment for respiratory physiology. Later in the year an application to the Scottish Hospital Endowments Research Trust, based on the four projects already mentioned, was well received and funds were provided for the employment of a post-doctoral physicist to augment the experimental resources already deployed.

The respiratory physiology programme, supported also by the British Oxygen Company, led to the commercial production of an ingenious servo-respirator, but was later overtaken by the emergence of other methods for the management of respiratory distress in the newborn. The development of the servo-respirator was impeded for a time by the lack of reliable equipment for the measurement of low pressures and flow rates. The device, invented by the physicist in the project (Dr J.R. Greer), was suitable for a number of scientific and industrial uses and attracted much attention. Dr Greer was even less successful than Dr Sloan (p.509) in arousing commercial enthusiasm. After several manufacturers expressed lack of interest, he founded his own company (Mercury Electronics) which went on to make a range of successful products.

Before long, a major project in ultrasonic imaging took shape. The objective was to obtain useful diagnostic information by exploiting a distinctive property of ultrasonic radiation – reflection at a tissue boundary. The radiologist, relying on differences in the absorption of X-rays by different tissues, can readily distinguish air and bone from soft tissues but (in the days before computerised axial tomography) all soft tissues looked much the same to an X-ray beam and could be distinguished only with difficulty, or by specialised techniques using contrast media. An ultrasonic beam is partially reflected whenever it reaches a tissue boundary. If an ultrasonic beam is sent into the body, the reflected signals should, in principle, be capable of delineating any circumscribed mass, such as a cyst or a foetus.

This theoretical possibility was applied to the detection of submarines during the First World War – and, more successfully, during the Second World War. Clinical applications were attempted during the early 1950s by several teams in the United States, but with limited success. The Glasgow group were late arrivals, but they soon took the lead. A decisive factor was the intervention of Kelvin Hughes, a Glasgow-based company (forming part of the Smith's Industries group) who were already well known for the manufacture of equipment using ultrasonics for the detection of flaws in metal welds and castings. This company made a considerable investment in the development of ultrasonic equipment for medical diagnosis. Their collaboration with Professor Donald and his team achieved great success, both commercially and clinically, despite early scepticism in many quarters. The pioneers themselves were cautious; in their first publication[53], in 1958, they recorded surprise that meaningful signals had been obtained in the ultrasonic examination of abdominal masses, and concluded that their findings were of more academic interest than practical importance.

The team's unusual combination of scientific insight, technical skill and clinical virtuosity soon dispelled these misgivings. The Diasonograph (as the scanner made by Kelvin Hughes was known) was shown to be valuable in the diagnosis of abdominal masses (such as tumours) and in the study of normal and abnormal foetal growth. It became particularly attractive in obstetrics, since it avoided the hazards (to the mother and, more particularly, the foetus) associated with X-ray examinations during pregnancy. Later developments extended its use to many other parts of the body.

Imaginative collaboration of University, Hospital Board and industry had a decisive influence on the spectacular growth of medical ultrasonics throughout the world. It was nevertheless appraised in some quarters with the scepticism accorded in earlier times to the stethoscope, the sphygmomanometer, and other technological innovations. In 1977, Professor Donald recalled[54] the judgement of a clinician from Edinburgh who returned from a demonstration 'only to announce to a hilarious group of students that in Glasgow we needed a machine, then costing about £10,000 to diagnose an ovarian cyst which he with God-given clinical acumen could diagnose with a twopenny glove.'

His words were echoed in the comment of another gynecologist, who wrote[55] in 1980: '... this is a field in which the capability of the techniques may be far greater than their clinical relevance. The ability to say that there is a mass the size of a grapefruit present in the pelvis is something which any self-respecting clinician can do without the need or assistance of expensive machinery'.

In 1963, Smith's Industries reduced their commitment to industrial electronics in a reorganisation which led to the closure of the Kelvin Hughes factory. With financial assistance from government funds, the ultrasonic manufacturing and marketing operations were taken over (together with unsold or unfinished equipment, workshop and laboratory apparatus and commercial goodwill) by Nuclear Enterprises, an Edinburgh company which had been founded several years earlier by two Scottish physicists. In 1982 this company's ultrasonic interests were acquired by the Fisher Corporation, an American company seeking an outlet in Europe for their own equipment.

This was not the end of the story. By 1985, former employees of Nuclear Enterprises, and others, had established four companies in Scotland, which were the only manufacturers of all-British equipment for medical ultrasonic imaging.

The growth of this technique illustrates many important aspects of the relationship between technology and health care. The basic scientific and technical knowledge was available in the 1940s, but it was not exploited with appreciable success, clinically or industrially. In Professor Donald's original research programme, the major effort was in respiratory physiology, with the possibility of ultrasonic imaging in gynaecology as a subsidiary development. The support given to this programme by the Scottish Hospital Endowments Research Trust, the University, and the Regional Hospital Board provided a secure base for the later development of ultrasonic imaging in obstetrics, the achievement which stimulated such massive clinical and industrial activity. Scotland provided the decisive factors which emerged, not from the deliberations of a clinical think-tank, but from the spontaneous support of many people and organisations, dominated by the charismatic leadership of Professor Donald. He may be compared to that earlier Glasgow pioneer, John Macintyre; indeed, history will probably judge his achievement to be the greater. When Macintyre, an ear, nose and throat surgeon, began his work with X-rays, there were no radiologists. But Donald, the gynaecologist, outshone the multitude of radiologists in breaking their monopoly of imaging technique, which had been unchallenged for more than half a century.

Scottish industry, as so often in the past, lost its early advantage, not through failings in design or marketing, but in the face of inexorable commercial and financial forces which, since the beginning of the technological revolution in the mid-1950s, have concentrated the production of sophisticated medical equipment in the hands of English and foreign manufacturers.

Industrial Participation

The decline of the heavy industries in which Scotland held a dominant position during much of the 19th Century stimulated many efforts to develop new foundations for economic prosperity. The Bio-engineering Study Group, appointed by the Secretary of State in 1971, considered ways of encouraging the growth of the medical equipment industry in Scotland. They reported[56] that Britain's share of the world market was only about 2.5 *per cent* and had been falling sharply during the 1960s; Scotland's output was less than 10 *per cent* of the modest UK total.

They considered that Scotland's tradition of technical ingenuity, wealth of skilled manufacturing capacity, long-standing reputation in medical practice and rapidly-growing resources in medical physics, offered good scope for commercial success in medical engineering. An eightfold increase in manufacturing output over a period of seven years was suggested as a realistic target.

The Study Group advised that, in pursuit of this goal, two new organisations should be established to improve communication and collaboration between clinical users and manufacturers:

(1) An Advisory Council on Medical Engineering, which would forecast the equipment needs of the health service and identify areas of technical innovation appropriate for support on the basis of clinical need, of country-wide priority and, in general, of commercial viability. This support would be provided by the Scottish Home and Health Department, in the form of development contracts and the underwriting of initial production expenses. Where social needs were judged to be more important than commercial viability, additional subsidies would be recommended.

(2) An Evaluation Agency, which would commission studies in approved laboratories (such as medical physics departments) and provide a seal of approval for equipment which reached prescribed standards of design and performance.

The cost to public funds of implementing these and other policies was estimated at £6m during the first seven years.

The report was received politely, but its major recommendations were not accepted. It is doubtful whether they would have succeeded in their aims. The outcome of enterprise in medical equipment manufacture does not depend wholly on what expert committees think the health service needs. To a much greater extent it depends on an accurate prediction of what the service will buy if a manufacturer makes it available. The early development in Britain of ultrasonic diagnosis (p.519) was determined by the enthusiasm and insight of one clinician and one unsubsidised manufacturer. At that stage there was no clearly-expressed clinical need.

Conversely, as the later history of ultrasonics showed, the provision of support from public funds, after clinical need has been clearly established, does not guarantee commercial success.

What Has Technology Achieved?

The period since 1948 has been characterised by three significant changes in the health care systems:
(a) the inception of the National Health Service;
(b) the rapid spread of technology;
(c) the increasing ascendancy of the hospitals in relation to other agencies providing health care.

These changes were inter-related in various ways. In the 1950s it became apparent that the long-cherished concept of general practice as the keystone of the system could not be maintained. General practitioners, whether working single-handed or in groups, could not command the financial and other resources needed to embrace the new technology. Consequently their patients were more often referred to hospitals for investigation or treatment. There was no corresponding reduction of doctors' work loads, because the existence of a service which was (at the point of delivery) free of cost to the consumer encouraged more frequent consultation.

For the hospitals, the availability of funds to meet the increased demand allowed investment in specialised equipment, staff and buildings. The transfer of financial responsibility from private and corporate charity to the state was, however, not the decisive factor in this change. The technological invasion proceeded as briskly – sometimes more so – in other countries, whether health care was supported by taxes, insurance or patients' fees. In Britain, the foundation of the National Health Service, with ultimate control of expenditure by the Exchequer, helped to avoid the excessive enthusiasm for technology seen in some sectors of the American health care system.

Health Care as an Industry: Limitations and Prospects

The health care system has two of the characteristics of a consumer-oriented industry: it delivers a product shaped by technology; and its output is based on demand rather than on need.

Technology influences demand in many ways. In the public perception, diagnosis is more attractive than treatment or prevention, particularly if it depends on high technology. When official policy does not match this perception, large sums are readily found, by public collections and donations, to provide sophisticated diagnostic devices (such as body scanners), though not always in places where they are most needed.

Sometimes (as in other industries) technology has a negative impact on progress. Investment in technology has continued to grow even though it has for many years been apparent that the major problems facing the health service during the rest of the century, and beyond, will require the role of technology to be reassessed in a radical way. Technology has contributed (though by how much is a matter of debate) to the spectacular improvement in the public health during the present century. Through this success, the pattern of morbidity has greatly changed. Many of the acute diseases of early and middle life have been reduced in importance – some almost to insignificance – with the result that more people survive long enough to suffer the chronic degenerative disorders of later life (such as cancer, rheumatic diseases, mental illness and stroke) which require long-term care rather than short-term intervention. The National Health Service, as it has developed since 1948, is not well-adapted to dealing with built-in obsolescence, expressed in creeping morbidity which progressively impairs the quality of life.

The scope for technology in tackling this challenge has not yet been adequately evaluated, but useful work on aids for the physically disabled has been done with the help of the Bio-engineering Unit of Strathclyde University and the associated National Centre for Training and Education in Prosthetics and Orthotics. Some of the medical physics departments have also been active in this work, as well as in collaborative research and development on the management of deafness and of incontinence. Much more remains to be done in harnessing technology (often in relatively simple ways) to the service of the increasing number of patients who are not sufficiently ill or disabled to be in hospital, yet not sufficiently fit to enjoy the quality of life that they expect the health service to provide.

References

(1)   Newman, C. *The Evolution of Medical Education in the Ninteenth Century* (Oxford, 1957).
(2)   *Ibid*, p.6.
(3)   Durbin, P.T., (Gen. Ed.), *A Guide to the Culture of Science, Technology and Medicine* (New York, 1980).
(4)   Reiser, S.J., *Medicine and the Reign of Technology* (Cambridge, 1978).
(5)   de Styrap, J., *The Young Practitioner: With Practical Hints and Instructive Suggestions...for his Guidance on Entering into Private Practice* (London, 1890), p.xi, quoted in Peterson, M.J., *The Medical Profession in Mid Victorian London* (London, 1978).
(6)   *British Medical Journal*, 1908, II, pp.374–87.
(7)   Comrie J.D., *History of Scottish Medicine* (London, 1932), pp.710, 713; *Edinburgh Medical Journal* XXXVI, 1929, p.127.
(8)   Glasgow Royal Infirmary minutes, 25 November 1794, (Greater Glasgow Health Board Archives).
(9)   *Ibid*, 6 August 1804.
(10) The episode of the Clydesdale chair continues to arouse interest and controversy. *Vide* the correspondence columns of the *Glasgow Herald*, 7, 14, 22, 27 and 30 June, 6, 12, 15, 20, 21 and 26 July, 1983.
(11) The publication in 1818 of Mary Shelley's *Frankenstein* could have done little to assuage public anxiety.
(12) Macintyre, J., 'Some Notes on the Use of the Electric Light in Medicine', *Glasgow Medical Journal*, January 1885, pp.17–24.
(13) The firm in question was W.B. Hilliard & Son. William Macewen, a leading surgeon of this era, apparently had difficulty obtaining good quality surgical instruments in this country and was forced to look to Germany. *Vide* Bowman, A.K., *The Life and Teaching of Sir William Macewen* (London, 1942), p.12. It would be interesting to trace the role of firms such as Hilliard. In 1886 Hilliard agreed to purchase an incubator from Paris for the Glasgow Maternity Hospital. There followed a disagreement about the level of commission which was appropriate and the hospital eventually acquired a cheaper incubator in London. *Vide* Glasgow Maternity Hospital minutes, 8 November and 13 December 1886, 10 January and 14 February 1887, (GGHB Archives). This Continental influence deserves fuller study. In 1915 the Royal Hospital for Sick Children in Glasgow agreed to the purchase of equipment from Mayer & Meltzer only if it was proved that this was not a German company. RHSC minutes, 10 August 1915 (GGHB Archives).
(14) *Proceedings of the Philosophical Society of Glasgow*, Vol.29 (1897–8), pp.230–7.

(15) This practice was doubtless encouraged by the fact that doctors at this time received the bulk of their income from private practice and few voluntary hospitals paid honoraria to their medical staff. The rising cost of equipment and the introduction of full-time salaried doctors ended this trend.

(16) GRI minutes, 30 September and 25 November 1914, 27 January and 24 February 1915. The cost of equipment took on a much larger significance with the provision of another 36 microscopes for teaching purposes in 1918–19. Six of these were paid for by the Infirmary and the remainder by Glasgow University. GRI minutes, 9 January and 27 February 1918, 19 March 1919. It is not yet known whether the teaching hospitals accurately reflect attitudes in local authority or non-teaching hospitals.

(17) Scott, J., 'The Birth of Radiology in Scotland', *Radiology, 17*, 1951, pp.46–9; Goodall, A.L., 'John Macintyre, Pioneer Radiologist', 1857–1828', *Surgo*, Whitsun 1958, pp.120–1. Henry Mavor, an electrical engineer and father of the playwright 'James Bridie' possibly had a vested interest in encouraging the installation of an electrical system. When the Western Infirmary of Glasgow followed suit in 1896 his firm, Mavor & Coulson, was awarded the contract, worth almost £6,000. Another early X-ray pioneer, A.A.C. Swinton, was commissioned in 1906 to draw up specifications for electric lighting at one of Scotland's premier asylums. Easterbrook, C.G., *The Chronicle of Crichton Royal 1833–1936* (Dumfries, 1940), p.298.

(18) The early impact of Glasgow on the history of radiology is admirably described in Christopher Smith, *Medical Radiology: its practical application 1895–1914*, Checkland, O., and Lamb, M., *Health Care as Social History: The Glasgow Case* (Aberdeen, 1982), pp.100–16.

(19) Taylor, J., 'On an Electric Apparatus for Detecting the Presence of Pieces of Metal, such as Musket Balls, etc., in Gunshot Wounds', *Proceedings of the Philosophical Society of Glasgow*, Vol.6, 1865–8, pp.9–12.

(20) Goodall, *op.cit.*, p.122.

(21) *The Bailie*, 15 April 1896.

(22) Turner, A.L., *Story of a Great Hospital: The Royal Infirmary of Edinburgh 1729–1929* (Edinburgh, 1937), pp.289–92; Glasgow Western Infirmary annual report 1897–8.

(23) Aberdeen Royal Infirmary already possessed a medical electrician when the Directors agreed on 8 July 1896 to spend not more than £75 to 'furnish the apparatus necessary for the Roëntgen Skiagraphy'. For this and other developments in the Grampian region I am indebted to Mrs Kirsteen Macpherson, formerly archivist to Grampian Health Board. The information quoted on Radiography in the North-East is taken from the unpublished text of her lecture to the Aberdeen Branch of the Society of Radiographers on 23 February 1982.

(24) *Vide* Macintyre, J., 'The new Electrical Pavilion of the Glasgow Royal Infirmary', *Glasgow Medical Journal*, Vol.58, 1902, p.161. The new department was visited by Princess Beatrice in November 1903 when she was in Glasgow as a guest of Lord and Lady Blythswood. *Vide Glasgow Herald*, 19 November 1903.

(25) GRI minutes, 13 February 1919. John Scott, who was invited to accept the post, first met Macintyre in 1914. Scott was then an apprentice electrical and scientific instrument maker in Kelvin's laboratory. Scott, *op.cit.*, p.48.

(26) Turner, *op.cit.*, p.293; Catford, E.F., *The Royal Infirmary of Edinburgh 1929–1979* (Edinburgh, 1984), p.40. The problem of cost was exacerbated by the growing awareness of the necessarily expensive protective measures which were essential.

(27) GRI annual report, 1926.

(28) Mould, R.F., *A History of X-Rays and Radium* (London, 1980), p.7.

(29) The Western Infirmary annual report for 1908–9 claimed that if funds could be obtained for a supply of radium this would lead to greater efficiency in the treatment of locally malignant affections.

(30) The minutes of the Glasgow and West of Scotland Radium Committee, 1914–34, are held in Glasgow University Archives, at GUA 35904. This new technology

prompted the creation of a radium extraction plant, housed in a disused sawmill at Balloch, near Loch Lomond. *Vide Glasgow Herald*, 12 February 1915.

(31) Lecturer in physical chemistry at Glasgow University, 1909–14, then Professor of Chemistry at Aberdeen, 1914–19, and Oxford, 1919–36. Soddy received the Nobel Prize for Chemistry in 1921.

(32) Nephew of Lord Kelvin and a distinguished physicist in his own right, Bottomley had been involved with X-ray work in Glasgow from the outset.

(33) Glasgow and West of Scotland Radium Committee minutes, 4 June 1914.

(34) The Trust was responsible for the purchase of radium while the Commission dealt with its custody, distribution and use.

(35) This trebled the supply available to the hospital. Dr P.R. Peacock, appointed Director of Research in 1928, was sent to the Middlesex Hospital and to Paris to evaluate how this might be utilised since the existing supply was used at less than 20% of its capacity. (Unpublished transcript of tape-recording provided by Dr Peacock for Dr John Paul's address to the Scottish Society of the History of Medicine on 19 April 1980.)

(36) *British Medical Journal*, 1930, II, p.117. The new scheme posed problems for those hospitals not selected. Addressing the annual meeting of the GRI on 8 February 1932 the Chairman, Dr James Macfarlane, explained that the GRI quota from the Commission would be small. This would mean relatively high administrative costs unless 'some generously disposed friend or friends' presented an additional supply. The GRI became a designated Radium Centre in 1933.

(37) Catford *op.cit.*, pp.41–3. The RIE was the first hospital in Scotland to draw up plans for a Radium Institute for Scotland, in December 1928. *Vide British Journal of Radiography*, 1929, p.43. Glasgow was the first Scottish city to inaugurate such an Institute, opened in 1930. *ibid.*, 1930, p.154.

(38) These included salaries of £250 p.a. for a radiologist and £182 for a radiographer. Glasgow Royal Maternity Hospital minute, 20 March 1935.

(39) *Report of Committee on Scottish Health Services*, Cmd 5204 (1936), p.9.

(40) *Ibid.*, p.151.

(41) *Ibid.*, pp.84–7, 236–7. It is beyond the scope of this paper to examine the relative speed of adoption of new technology in the voluntary and local authority sectors. Opinions differ as to the level of commitment and funding in each and this is a question worthy of detailed consideration.

(42) The argument that specialised services should be concentrated in a number of key hospitals serving a peripheral ring was not new. Sir Napier Burnett proposed such a scheme in his evidence to the Voluntary Hospitals Committee, Cmd 1335 (1921), pp.14–15. Burnett argued that money should be withheld from any smaller units which refused to enter what he termed 'this spider-web arrangement'.

(43) The original survey sheets are retained in the Scottish Record Office, at HH65/150–1.

(44) *Scottish Hospitals Survey*, HMSO 1946.

(45) *Ibid.*, paras.217, 233, 280.

(46) *Ibid.*, para.268.

(47) *Ibid.*, paras.39–56.

(48) *Ibid.*, para.677.

(49) Sir W. Beveridge, *Social Insurance and Allied Services*, Cmnd 6404 (1942), para.105.

(50) *Report of the Department of Health for Scotland and of the Scottish Health Services Council* (1949), pp.34, 110.

(51) For example, Neil Arnott (1788–1874: MD Aberdeen, 1814) in his Elements of *Physics or Natural Philosophy*. London, 1827, p.xxviii:

> Physics is also an important foundation of the healing art. The medical man, indeed, is the engineer pre-eminently; for it is in the animal body that the true perfection and the greatest variety of mechanism are found ... Yet will it be believed, that there are medical men who neither understand mechanics, not

hydraulics, nor pneumatics, nor optics, nor acoustics, beyond the merest routine; and that systems of medical education are put forth at this day which do not even mention the department of Physics!

In the sixth edition (1864, p.xxiv) he added, rather optimistically:

And the day is probably arrived, when members of the medical profession generally will understand how very much the correct knowledge of animal structure and function, and of remedial means, depends on precise acquaintance with Physics.

Also Sir William Gairdner (1824–1907: Regius Professor of Practice of Medicine in the University of Glasgow) in *The Physician as Naturalist*, Maclehose, Glasgow, 1889, p.28:

... most of the great advances in medical diagnosis in the present day, through the stethoscope, microscope, laryngoscope, ophthalmoscope, sphygmograph, electricity as applied to muscle and nerve, etc, involve applications of pure physics which are neither remote from practice nor yet very easily mastered by the beginner ... I am persuaded that in a very few years the physical laboratory will become an absolutely essential preliminary step in the education of the physician of the future, and that those who have not undergone this training will be hopelessly distanced in the race.

(52)   Hospital Scientific and Technical Services: *Report of the Committee, 1967–68*. HMSO 1968.

(53)   Donald, I., MacVicar, J., and Brown, T.G. Investigation of abdominal masses by pulsed ultrasound. *Lancet*, i, 1188, 1958.

(54)   Donald, I. The ultrasonic boom. *J. Clin. Ultrasound*, 4, 323, 1976.

(55)   Scott, J.S. The impact of technology on obstetrics and gynaecology 1955–1980. *J. Med Eng. Tech.*, 4, 275, 1980.

(56)   Medical Engineering: *Report of the Bio-Engineering Study Group (Scotland)*. HMSO 1972.

3. *The Population and Vital Statistics of Scotland: 1900–1983*

Stanley Sklaroff

CONTENTS

About the Author

STANLEY SKLAROFF. B.A.

After studying and teaching at the London School of Economics, Stanley Sklaroff worked in the Social Medicine Research Council before joining the Department of Public Health of the University of Edinburgh, now the Department of Community Medicine, in which he is currently Senior Lecturer in Population and Health Statistics.

He served on the Medical Research Council's Committee for Research and General Practice, and has been particularly involved in socio-medical studies of common diseases, e.g. tuberculosis and family staphylococcal infection. More recently, he has undertaken studies of disability in and outside of hospital.

Author's Note

This essay explores the trends in population and vital statistics which shaped the problems faced by the Scottish Health Services between 1900–1983. The divergent demographic experiences of Scotland and England and Wales are used to focus particular attention on Scotland's continuously higher mortality, and its temporarily different pattern of fertility.

The specific links between Scotland's vital statistics and its health service problems are illustrated with reference to the dominance of the Clydeside conurbation on Scottish statistics and also to the variations within Scotland of the problems identified by Dr Peter McKinlay in his analysis of Scotland's population and health statistics in the 1930s – and also in his detailed studies of infant and maternal mortality, and of the ill-health of the insured population. The continuing importance of these links was illustrated by John Brotherston himself in his 1975 paper on 'Inequality: is it inevitable?'

A review of the trends in the numbers in the population, the death rates and the expectation of life at different ages, reveals not only a Scottish population with increased numbers of elderly women, but one in which these women now have a lower expectation of life than women of the same generation in England and Wales.

Scotland's relatively lower infant mortality at the start of the period was followed by a higher adult mortality than most European countries and may indicate a particularly heavy burden of chronic disease for those reaching old age at the end of the period.

With the disappearance of the unmarried daughters whose high prevalence once provided a source of home care, the demographic impact of Scotland's ageing population is inevitably heavy on the community health services of today. The ability to see how the demographic trends of the past shaped the health service problems of the present and future was an essential element in John Brotherston's unique understanding of how the health of the Scottish people could be improved.

The Population and Vital Statistics of Scotland: 1900–1983

Demographic Trends

Between 1900 and 1983, Scotland experienced the same slowing down of population growth, the decline in its mortality and in its fertility and the ageing of its population as did England and Wales and most other European countries[1,2]. There are nevertheless distinctive features of Scotland's demographic experience which are associated with an environment and history different from those of England and Wales[3,4,5]. Apart from an apparently lower infant death rate at the beginning of the period, Scotland has had, and continues to have, higher death rates than England and Wales[6]. Until recently, the fertility levels in Scotland were also higher than in England and Wales[7]. From the 1860s, up to the outbreak of the Second World War, the number of emigrants from Scotland exceeded the number of immigrants[4]. Within Scotland, regional variations in population increase were dominated by migration from the rural Highlands and Islands into the industrial and commercial areas of the central Lowlands particularly in the west[4,5].

From 1920 onwards, Scotland's vital statistics have been increasingly dominated by the concentration of its population in this central industrial belt[5,7]. Only since 1961 has there been any significant outward movement from this and other central areas, and a rise in the population of the Highlands and Islands after several decades of decline or little growth[7].

Vital Statistics and Health Administration

Between 1900 and 1983, the system of preparing and publishing Scottish vital statistics has been twice reorganised. The first reorganisation, in 1911, involved the adoption of Public Health Districts – burghs and county districts – as the geographical units, as defined by the Public Health Act of 1897. It also introduced the practice of correcting all local birth and death statistics for those events occurring and registered in public health districts different from those of usual residence. This was intended to eliminate the effect on local statistics of the presence of large institutions and of the residents of one public health district moving to another. The new districts meant the loss of the pre-existing grouping of registration districts into urban districts of different population sizes which had been in operation since 1855. This grouping had been valuable in demonstrating differences in the mortality of town and country districts. A new grouping of public health districts still allowed some urban/rural distinctions to be made, but the large burghs which constituted the most urban group were dominated by the urban areas centred on Glasgow.

It had become recognised that large cities extended beyond their administrative boundaries and often were closely associated with industrial towns and villages to form conurbations. In 1951, in Scotland, such a combination of burghs and county districts formed the statistical entity of the Central Clydeside Conurbation centred on Glasgow. In that year it included more than one third of the population of Scotland. It had a higher birth rate and a much higher death rate than the rest of Scotland, especially for tuberculosis and other chronic chest diseases.

The introduction of the National Health Service in 1948, did not involve a major restructuring of Scotland's vital statistics. As the five Regional Hospital Board areas were composed of combinations of the 57 existing Public Health Districts, the new Hospital Board Regions reflected the differences in the vital statistics of their constituent public health districts. In 1965, the vital statistics of the Western Regional Board, which included the County City of Glasgow, still reflected the relatively poor environment and health of its population, although the high levels of its mortality and morbidity were not reflected in its hospital discharge rates[9]. Even outside the conurbation, the health of the population in the inter-war period was still poor[10].

The reorganisation of the existing local authorities under the 1973 Local Government (Scotland) Act created 9 regions, plus the island areas. The establishment of the new Health Board areas in place of the Regional Hospital Board areas in 1974 provided another set of geographical divisions deliberately designed to combine the urban centres with their less urban hinterlands. Today, the computer and the use of postal codes have created the opportunity for combining small area units in many different combinations, thus freeing vital statistics from outgrown administrative boundaries[7].

When, in 1933, the Secretary of State for Scotland appointed a committee to review existing health services, the opportunity was taken to review Scotland's vital statistics from the point of view of health service provision. The report of this (Cathcart) committee identified many of the features of Scotland's population situation which still exist today. Among its conclusions were:

(1)   that the population would not expand much further,

(2)   that future numbers would not be affected by changes in death rates,

(3)   that the low birth rates were due to the deliberate prevention of births and could be assumed to continue,

(4)   that migration would not now be a substantial factor modifying the numbers of Scotland's population,

(5)   that there would be an older population with 'the diseases of later life tending to represent a larger, and those of earlier life a smaller proportion of the sum total of the diseases of the whole population'.

Much of the analysis of Scotland's vital statistics for the Cathcart Committee was the work of Dr Peter McKinlay, the unsung William Farr of Scottish health statistics. Between 1930 and 1960 he acted as the medical link between the Scottish Registrar General and the Department of Health for Scotland. He was instrumental in analysing and displaying the geographical and social dimensions of maternal and infant mortality in association with Dr Charlotte Douglas. He was also responsible for epidemiological analyses of the statistics of incapacity for work among the insured (more than one third of the entire) population of Scotland, which appeared in the Annual Reports of the Department of Health for Scotland in the 1930s[12]. In providing information on the causes that rarely appeared in death records, Peter McKinlay anticipated the analysis of sickness and injury benefits statistics of the Department of Health and Social Security, and of the Studies of Morbidity in General Practice – sadly only carried out in England and Wales.

Trends in Birth Rates

In the decades following the introduction of the national system of vital registration in the 1850s, the birth rates of Scotland, England and Wales shared the same level and the same trend. They had fallen from the high plateau of 35 live births per 1,000 population, which ended in the late 1870s. From 1900 onwards, however, although the Scottish birth rate continued to show the same fluctuations as the birth rate in England and Wales, it remained at a higher level until 1977. By the time of the economic recession years of the 1920s and 1930s, the Scottish birth rate was 3 per 1,000 above the rate for England and Wales. Only in 1977, when the birth rates of both countries reached their lowest point since birth registration began, did the rates of Scotland, England and Wales again converge. Since 1977, the Scottish birth rate has dropped below that of England and Wales. Its lower birth rate is not due to differences in the size, or age composition, of the child bearing population of women in the two countries.

Only after the Population (Statistics) Act, which came into operation in July 1938, did birth registration information become available for calculating birth rates by age of mother. It was then possible to see that, just before the Second World War, Scottish women not only had a higher birth rate than women in England and Wales but the rates were particularly high in those under 20 years, and in those over 30 years – more than 25 *per cent* higher than in England and Wales. The child-bearing of Scottish women was thus spread more widely over the child-bearing ages than in England and Wales. The convergent fall in the level of fertility in the two countries was, by the 1980s, accompanied by a convergence in the age patterns of fertility as well. As Scotland and England and Wales began to share a common fertility pattern, the differences in fertility between the regions within Scotland also narrowed.

It has been suggested that three tendencies have combined to create, at a low level, the convergence of area differences in Scottish fertility. These are:

(1)   the narrowing of socio-economic marital fertility differentials in so far as they are measured by the Registrar General's social class classification of husband's occupation,

(2)   the decline of fertility in the Catholic areas of West Central Scotland, and

(3)   perhaps most significantly, and not unrelated to the first two causes, the rise in the proportion of married women at work.

It is possible to detect a rising trend in this proportion from approximately 6 *per cent* at the 1911 census to more than 50 *per cent* at the 1981 census, the major acceleration having taken place between the censuses of 1931 and 1951[7].

Trends in the Expectation of Life in Scotland, England and Wales

As a summary measure of current death rates, the expectation of life at birth, or at other ages, provides a simple indicator of the overall level of death rates unaffected by changes and differences in the age distribution of the population. Between 1900 and 1982, the expectation of life at birth increased by 50 *per cent* for males and females. The expectation of life at 15 years and at 45 years also increased, although not to the same extent. At 15 years and at 45 years they increased by 25 *per cent* for males and by 32 *per cent* for females.

The expectation of life at birth was lower in Scotland than in England and Wales at each census year between 1901 and 1980, an average difference of 1 to 2 years, with a maximum of 2.5–3.5 years at the 1931 census. In 1981, the expectation of life at birth in Scotland was still 2 years lower than in England and Wales.

Until 1960, the expectation of life at birth increased at the same rate for males and females. After 1960, the expectation of life at birth increased more rapidly for females than males. At later ages also, at 45 and at 65 years, the life expectancy of women increased to a greater extent than that of men. The expectation of life at age 65 rose, however, only to a little extent for men from 10.34 years to 12.2 years between 1901 and 1981, an increase of 18 *per cent*. Whereas for women aged 65 years it had increased by 41 *per cent* from 11.3 years to 16 years.

In 1900 there was little difference between Scotland, England and Wales in the expectation of life of men or women aged 65. After 1950 a difference in the expectation of life of the elderly population of the two countries became apparent, particularly for women. There is a difference of one year in the expectation of life of women aged 65 years in the two countries at each census year from 1951 to 1981, Scotland having the lower figure.

Trends in Death Rates in Age Groups

Infant Mortality

Infant and maternal mortality are dealt with more fully in the essay on child and maternal health services. Infant mortality is mentioned here partly because, at least in the early years of the period, its level had a considerable influence on the expectations of life at birth. It also has relevance as the source of a paradox, *viz.* that although for much of the period infant mortality was higher in Scotland than in England and Wales, at the beginning, Scotland's infant mortality rate was less than that of England and Wales. Infant mortality also has relevance as a socio-economic indicator. In 1936 the Scottish Registrar General first analysed infant mortality (including neonatal) by legitimacy, and demonstrated an excess infant mortality of 50 *per cent* among illegitimate births. This difference has now disappeared.

The grouping of fathers' occupation into social classes for the analysis of infant mortality was introduced into the Scottish Registrar General's Annual Report for 1943, although the first figures to be analysed were for the year 1939, on the grounds that any later year would have been affected by the large numbers of fathers in the services. This analysis showed that the mortality rate was higher for the infants of fathers in unskilled occupations than for infants of fathers in other occupations but that the effect of father's occupation was altered by urban status. Overall, infant mortality was higher in the large burghs than in other areas. The social dimensions of infant mortality that were revealed were not simple. The infants of fathers in social class 1 occupations who lived in the counties (excluding the large burghs) had a higher mortality than those whose father's occupation was also classified to social class 1, but who lived in the large burghs.

Mortality Trends in Children 1–14 Years

By 1921, death rates at ages 1–4, 5–9 and 10–14 years had fallen by a third from their levels in 1901. The death rate in children aged 1–4 years fell more steeply, particularly during the war years 1940–45, to reach a fifth of its 1901 level. The death rates of children aged 5–9 years, and of children 10–14 years, declined more slowly, but had nearly reached their 1981 level by 1951.

Mortality Trends in Adults 15–34 Years

The mortality rate of young adults had also fallen by 1921 to a third of the 1901 level in each of the three age groups of 15–19, 20–29 and 30–34 years. A further, but less marked, decline occurred in these rates by 1931. The 1939–1945 war halted the decline in mortality of these young adult age groups. In the 15–19 year age group no marked decline of civilian mortality occurred and civilian mortality rose in the age group 20–24. Total mortality in 1940–1944, including war deaths, amounting to twice the level of mortality for men aged 20–24 in 1901, left a permanent mark on the sex-ratio and on the life of the survivors. By 1951, death rates in all three young adult age groups and for each sex had fallen to levels which were a quarter to one fifth of those in 1901. From 1961 onwards, death rates in these age groups changed very little with two exceptions: a rise in the death rate for men aged 15–19 years associated with road accidents and a marked fall in the death rate for women aged 25–34 years.

Mortality Trends in Adults 35–64 Years

In the age groups 35–44, 45–54 and 55–64 years, death rates had fallen to two thirds of their 1901 level by 1921. By 1941 the decline in death rates at these years was greater for women than for men. This sex difference in the extent of the decline in mortality continued to the end of the period in 1981. Two other features are to be noted. In 1971 women aged 45–54 had a higher death rate than in 1961, although the rate was slightly lower again by 1981. For both sexes, the decline in death rates had slowed by 1951 and slowed down again by 1981.

Mortality Trends in Persons Aged 65 Years or More

Death rates for men and women declined in both the younger (65–74 years) and older (75–84 years) elderly age groups but the decline was much less than that of age groups under 65 years. The decline was less marked in the older than in the younger of these two age groups and the decline was steeper for women than for men, the death rate for men aged 65–74 years having increased between 1951 and 1971.

By the 1950s the Scottish male death rates at 50 years and over were among the highest in Europe and the rates for women were high at all ages[13]. By the time the Scottish children, who, surviving infant death rates lower than those of England and Wales at the beginning of the period, had reached their old age, their death rates had become among the highest reported in 30 developed countries (WHO, 1982).

The combination of a declining birth rate with improved survival has given Scotland, as other countries, an ageing population. The population of Scotland grew by 13 *per cent* between 1901 and 1981, (an annual rate of 1.5 per thousand). The ageing of the Scottish population took place from the beginning of the period, the numbers of the population aged 65 years or more rising with each decade until their numbers had been tripled by 1981. Up to the second world war, the age distribution of the population aged 65 and over remained stable but from 1951 onwards, it became increasingly more elderly. The number aged over 80 years rose from 66 to 124 thousand by 1981.

The population of working age (15–64 years) grew continuously up to the first world war, and fell slightly thereafter. The ratio of dependents, children under 15 years plus adults 65 years and more, to the population aged 15–64 years, fell in each decade until 1931; the ratio regained its 1901 value in 1971 but fell again in 1981.

It is relevant to the tasks of the Scottish Health Service of today that the modern service was launched in 1948, just when an accelerated ageing was taking place within Scotland's elderly population. In this chapter only a brief sketch has been given of some of the main features of Scotland's vital statistics between 1900 and 1983. These end points are arbitrary. Scotland's history before 1900 casts its shadow upon the period reviewed. For example, the Scottish women whose child-bearing years coincided with the beginning of the twentieth century included a high proportion – one fifth – who had not married by the end of their child-bearing years. In contrast to their experience, the majority (92 *per cent*) of the generation of Scottish women who entered their child-bearing years after the second world war had been married by the end of those years. The disappearance of a generation of maiden aunts has contributed to the change in the nature and dimensions of the care of the elderly who have survived until today.

References

(1)   *Demographic Trends in the European Region.* WHO Regional Publications, European Services No.17. (World Health Organisation, 1984.)
(2)   Mitchell, B.R. and Deane P., *Abstract of European Historical Statistics* (Abridged Edition), (MacMillan), 1978.

(3)   Kellas, James G. *Modern Scotland*. (2nd Edition.) (Allen & Unwin, 1980.)

(4)   Tranter, N.L., *Population and Society 1750–1940 (Themes in British Social History. Contrasts in Population Growth)*. Longman, 1985.

(5)   Flinn, M. (Ed.). *Scottish Population History*. (Cambridge University Press, 1977), p.5.

(6)   *Annual Reports of the Registrars General for Scotland and England and Wales.*

(7)   Jones, H. (Ed.), *Population Change in Contemporary Scotland*. Royal Scottish Geographical Society. (Geo Books, Norwich, 1984.)

(8)   Ferguson, Thomas, *Scottish Social Welfare, 1864–1944*. (E. & S. Livingstone Ltd. Edinburgh and London, 1958.)

(9)   Sklaroff, S.A., *Hospital Use and Population Needs: Implications of Recent Vital Statistics for the Scottish Hospital Board Regions*. (Health Bulletin, XXVI, *3*, 1968.)

(10) Stein, L. and Sklaroff, S.A., *The Health of an Urban Community*. (British Journal of Medicine, 6, S.A., 1952), pp.119–151.

(11) Douglas, C.A. and McKinlay, P.L., *Maternal and Infant Mortality in Scotland*. (Health Bulletin of the Departments of Health of Scotland, XVII, *2*, 1959), pp.17–44.

(12) *Second Annual Report of the Department of Health for Scotland, 1930*. (Cmd.3860, HMSO, 1931.)

(13) Gwilt, R.L., *Mortality in the past 100 years*. Transactions of the Faculty of Actuaries in Scotland, 24, 1956. (Faculty of Actuaries, Edinburgh, 1956), pp.40–176.

(14) Lopez, A.D. and Hanada, *Mortality Patterns and Trends among the Elderly in Developed Countries*. (World Health Statistics Quarterly, WHO vol.35, Nos.3/4, 1982.)

4. *The Evolution of Health Information Services*

John Womersley

CONTENTS

About the Author

Dr JOHN WOMERSLEY

John Womersley is the Community Medicine Specialist in the Greater Glasgow Health Board, with responsibility for Information Services and particularly information relating to the public health. He has a particular interest in investigating differences in health between communities, and in considering inequalities. This type of analysis has been undertaken for over 150 years in Glasgow – which includes inner city and suburban populations of very different types – a city which represents in microcosm the full spectrum of social circumstances found in the United Kingdom.

Author's Note

From about 1820 throughout the nineteenth century, health statistics were used in Scotland to promote radical sanitary and environmental changes, and so to improve the public health. The statistical techniques used, particularly by the first medical officers of health of Glasgow and Edinburgh, were as sophisticated as any in use today. In contrast, during the first two-thirds of the twentieth century, there was little advance either in the use of statistical methods, or in the routine use of information – for monitoring purposes and to effect change – notable exceptions being in the fields of obstetrics and infant and maternal mortality.

In 1967, a Working Party chaired by Professor John Brotherston, made a series of far-sighted recommendations concerning the uses of information in the hospital service including the encouragement of self-audit by clinicians, the evaluation of different clinical and diagnostic practices, and participation in operational research, both centrally and at hospital level (including junior medical staff as well as consultants). It was envisaged that operational research would eventually be extended to a study of the total medical needs of communities, and of the efficiency of all services – general practitioner, local authority and hospital – designated to meet them. Unfortunately, little progress has been made towards these important objectives during the subsequent two decades: although computer technology has made data processing immeasureably more efficient, corresponding advances have not been made in converting data into an effective tool for stimulating change. As a result, clinical audit, the allocation of resources according to measures of need, health service planning and routine epidemiological analysis remain, in the mid 1980s, relatively unexploited activities. Now, however, there are signs that financial constraints, the appointment of general managers to health authorities, and recommendations on management budgeting, may provide the necessary stimuli to realise something like the full potential of the powerful basic framework of health information, which has existed in Scotland for many years.

The Evolution of Health Information Services

The history of the development of information systems in Scotland is interesting in that in many ways more effective use was made of statistics in earlier days than has been the case more recently. In the 1860s, for example, relatively sophisticated techniques – which were later discarded for almost a century – were used to focus down on localised areas of ill health. Information was then collected for the specific purpose of effecting change usually by individuals who were directly responsible for the public health. These pioneers were also more expert than many of their counterparts today in projecting their message through whatever media were available – from statistical reports to eloquent prose, and from talks to influential societies to direct action through the local authority. The following pages trace the development of health and related information systems from the mere documentation of events prior to the nineteenth century through the period of active use of data to effect change during the nineteenth century, to systems in the twentieth century which are more complex, but which have often lapsed into passive recording mechanisms. In the final years of the twentieth century, however, there is a renewed interest in the public health, in fitness, and in the effective and efficient use of services; inevitably information services will require to reach their own full potential if this interest is going to be put to maximum effect.

I. The situation prior to 1800

The best source of information for this period is the work *Scottish Population History* by Flinn and his colleagues[1].

Parish registers

The documentation of health events appears to have begun with a Synodal Decree in the 14th century which required clergy to keep lists of those who died in each parish. In 1552 the General Provincial Council of the Church required all parishes to keep a register of baptisms and proclamations of Banns, and in 1565 the Reformed Church recommended that every minister should keep a register of burials. In 1616 the General Assembly decreed that each parish should establish and keep a register of baptisms, marriages and burials. Unfortunately these stipulations were often not put into effect, and an attempt to enforce the keeping of an adequate register by Act of Parliament in 1703 failed. The situation was worsened by the many secession movements from the main Church of Scotland during the eighteenth century, by the stamp duty imposed on registrations during the years 1783 to 1794, and by the secession of the Free Church in 1843. In a survey by local enumerators during the first national census of 1801, only 99 of 850 parishes in Scotland which made census returns were found to keep regular registers (most of these being parishes on the East coast), and fewer still kept adequate records of burials. Not surprisingly, therefore, relatively few old parish registers exist in Scotland, and there are almost none for the sixteenth century, although considerably more have survived in England and Wales.

Bills of mortality

The publication, at regular intervals, of deaths, subdivided by age group and cause, was begun in several towns towards the end of the seventeenth century. These were often published in newspapers when they became established during the mid eighteenth century, although this practice was continued only until the early 1800s. The bills of mortality were derived from records of interments in burial grounds, which – in towns – became the responsibility of a paid official (e.g. in Edinburgh from 1658, and in Glasgow from 1670).

Webster's census

Dr Alexander Webster established a fund for ministers' widows in 1743, and possibly as a result of this took an interest in population matters which led him to publish an *Account of the number of people in Scotland in 1755*. This was conducted through church presbyteries, failing which through individual ministers. The total population of Scotland was found to be 1,265,000.

Other sources of information

Kirk Session records sometimes provide information about disease and social conditions at times of crises. The Old Statistical Account of Scotland, produced beteen 1791 and 1799, also includes information about social conditions and, for a number of parishes, about the sex and age distribution of the population, which was of particular interest in some areas because of the effect of emigration. Burgh records provide information about action taken with respect to the poor, and describe visitations of the 'plague' (but rarely of other epidemics). The register of the Privy Council (which ceased to exist during 1708) also provides some information about poor relief, food supplies, and epidemics of the plague. Some information about occupied households, about householders and their wives and servants, may be obtained from records relating to hearth taxes and to poll taxes respectively: taxes which were imposed to finance the armed forces during the period 1690–98. Poor people, however, were excluded from these taxes, and there were problems collecting them in some of the more remote parishes.

In addition to sources covering the whole of Scotland there are data for particular groups of people in different localities, such as listings of individuals for ecclesiastical purposes (these were rarely complete listings of inhabitants), and private censuses (usually of individuals who were liable for particular taxes). Information about emigrants from Scotland is also available from a special survey of Highland parishes for the years 1772 and 1773, and by returns collected for the period 1772 to 1782 for the Treasury by local customs officers. These returns ceased after the American War of Independence; were resumed with the Passenger Act 1803; but were collated only after 1825 since when they provide a continuous series of records for emigration from Scotland.

From these various sources of information, it is possible to follow the disastrous effects on mortality of famines during the sixteenth and seventeenth centuries, and to show how harvest failures in the eighteenth century had less devastating effects as trade and transport improved, as mechanisms for poor relief became more effective, and as central and local government took emergency control over food supplies. Vivid descriptions are also provided of the progress of plague during the sixteenth and seventeenth centuries, culminating with the last catastrophic epidemic of 1644–49. It is also possible from these records to identify some epidemics of other diseases (e.g. smallpox, typhus, diphtheria and influenza), although it is not always possible to determine the particular disease; also, some diseases – such as smallpox – were so much accepted as normal events that outbreaks were probably frequently not recorded.

Hospital information

Among the earliest infirmaries established in Scotland were those in Edinburgh (1729), Aberdeen (1742) and Glasgow (1794). The first voluntary hospital in England (the Westminster Hospital, London) opened in 1720, and shortly afterwards (1732) Dr Francis Clifton[2] published a book on *The State of Physick* in which he made the following suggestion:

"I humbly propose, first of all, that three or four persons should be employed in the hospitals (and that without any ways interfering with the gentlemen now concerned), to set down the cases of the patients there from day to day, candidly and judiciously, without any regard to private opinions or public systems, and at the year's end publish these facts, just as they are, leaving every one to make the best use he can for himself. Would not some such method as this let us more into the nature of diseases in a few years than all the books of theories, or even the books of observations, hitherto published? Certainly it would; and yet if proper encouragement were given, it is not at all unlikely but that persons would soon be found every way qualified for such an undertaking; and even if good salaries were allowed them, and everything made as easy and agreeable to them as they could desire, the benefit the public would receive from them would vastly more than balance the expense".

Clifton proposed a tabular form for documenting cases, which included the following headings: sex; age; occupation; date of onset and duration of illness; signs and symptoms; treatment; and outcome.

Some type of annual report was probably produced by most of the voluntary infirmaries in Scotland and England. Their original purpose was to show the work of the hospital – preferably successful and increasing – in order to attract funding. From time to time, comparisons would be drawn with other institutions around the country, if the analysis was favourable to the issuing hospital. In Glasgow Royal Infirmary the responsibility for keeping patient statistics was delegated to the Apothecary, and from these the annual report was compiled. Unfortuantely the reports at this time were mainly narrative with relatively little statistical information apart from the numbers of cases admitted and discharged, and the numbers of deaths.

II. Health Information in the Nineteenth Century

Censuses

The first government census was conducted for the whole of the United Kingdom in 1801 under the supervision of John Rickman, Speaker of the House of Commons. Local responsibility for the census was delegated in Scotland to the Sheriff Depute in each county and to the (Lord) Provost in each town. Schoolmasters were appointed as enumerators, and enumeration was conducted between 10th March and the end of April, 1801; it was not until 1841 that the census was conducted on a single day. No age breakdown was provided until 1821, and then not until 1841; from 1851 onwards progressively more information (e.g. occupation, country of birth, civil status) was included on the census until 1881 when information about Gaelic speaking was requested for the first time.

Because the first government censuses in 1801 and 1811 were mere counts of the numbers of men and women in the various parishes, James Cleland (1770–1840) persuaded the magistrates of the City of Glasgow to conduct what he called a 'voluntary enumeration' of the inhabitants in 1820. This included not only numbers and sexes, but also the ages, country of origin, duration of residence, occupation, religion and status (as householders, lodgers, servants, married etc.), and represents probably the first classified enumeration of any large town in Great Britain. The detailed census results were published for each of the nine parishes 'within the Royalty', for the five districts of the Barony parish, and for Gorbals parish[3]. The population of the City of Glasgow and its suburbs (the same area as that from which the bills of mortality were drawn) was enumerated by sex and for the age groups 0 to 11 years, 12 to 17 years and 18 years and over.

Deaths and births prior to civil registration, 1855

Early analyses and interpretation of data:

Because of improvement and standardisation of documentation relating to burials, instituted by the Lord Provost in 1783, Glasgow has undoubtedly the best records of deaths in Scotland for the period prior to the introduction of civil registration. The first attempt to collate and interpret mortality records on a diagnostic basis appears to be that of Robert Watt in 1813[4] who in an appendix to his book *A treatise on chincough* made a detailed analysis of the causes of deaths of children under the age of ten years, for whom diagnostic information was likely to be more reliable. Watt was able to demonstrate a dramatic reduction in the number of deaths from smallpox after the provision, by the Faculty of Physicians and Surgeons of Glasgow, of free vaccination for infants in 1801: during the period 1783 to 1800, smallpox accounted for about one third of all deaths in children aged 0 to 9 years, whereas over the period 1807–1812 the proportion was only 7 *per cent*. Despite this, however, and due to an unexplained increase in deaths from measles, whooping cough and other conditions, there appeared to be no decline in overall mortality. Watt also noted an increase in the proportion of stillbirths, attributing this to 'the introduction of particular manufactures, by which immense numbers of women are employed in public works or confined to sedentary employment', the children being more likely to be born 'puny', and being less likely to be well cared for.

In 1819, in order to improve the collection of burial dues, James Cleland persuaded the City Fathers to establish a register of deaths to be kept by wardens of each of the burial grounds in the city, and he took great care to try and obtain information about all burials including the age and sex of each of the deceased. As a result, he was able to publish annual totals of burials by sex and age grouping from 1821 onwards. He made several attempts to try and obtain some diagnostic information, but abandoned them on the grounds that any information he could obtain was likely to be extremely inaccurate. Cleland also attempted to determine the true numbers of births during the years 1821 and 1830 by writing to individual pastors and others within the city: about 50 *per cent* of births had not been registered.

In 1835 T.R. Edmonds[5] analysed Cleland's mortality bills for the period 1821–35, commenting that 'there are two points in which (these bills) excel all others – in supplying an authenticated list of all the deaths with their ages, whilst in England we have only the deaths entered in the parish registers . . . and in a second (voluntary) enumeration of the living *and their ages* made in the year 1830, [whilst] in England we have only one such enumeration made in the year 1821'. Edmonds calculated age-specific mortality rates for three five-year periods, and was able to show a very marked increase in mortality in all adult age groups between 20 and 60 years for both men and women (about 20 *per cent* between each five year period even after excluding the effects of the cholera epidemic in 1832). Edmonds emphasised the need to analyse mortality in relatively small age groups (decades), demonstrating that crude mortality changed little over the period 1821–30 because the increasing mortality of adults was counterbalanced by a declining mortality in children.

Cleland was undoubtedly a pioneer in understanding the necessity for detailed and accurate denominator data; and in processing information about the age structure of the population, he presumably understood the need to take this into account – when considering death rates – as Edmonds subsequently so ably demonstrated. The unique quality and interest in Glasgow, in population data and burial statistics, provided precisely the baseline information required to mount compelling arguments for public health measures to overcome the recurrent devastating tides of epidemic disease. These arguments were taken up principally by four individuals.

Information as a tool for social reform:
Dr Andrew Buchanan (1798–1882) produced in 1830 what appears to be the first quantitative statement of the variability in disease between different parts of a city, stating that among the six 'districts' (each being the responsibility of a single district surgeon), the proportion of fever cases among all those treated varied between 3 *per cent* and 10 *per cent*[6]. Buchanan observed that fever was most prevalent where overcrowding was greatest, and that its spread was most rapid in circumstances of bad ventilation, poor nutrition and inadequate clothing; and he believed that many of the poor died of undernutrition – resulting in a disability which caused them to succumb to illness which better fed individuals would

readily have recovered from. Buchanan wrote vivid accounts of the circumstances in which he found many citizens to be living, and argued that it would be a saving even in financial terms to allow the 'sick-poor' clothing and certain articles of diet, as well as medical aid.

Dr Robert Cowan (1796–1841) attributed the worsening mortality in Glasgow to excessive immigration without any corresponding increase in housing[7]. He also observed that the increase in mortality and in still-births was associated with the steady decline in the proportion in the population of the wealthy middle class. He noted that the increase in mortality, particularly from fever, had occurred at a time of unparalleled prosperity and full employment, and concluded that the reasons for this were lack of cleanliness, ventilation and sanitation; overcrowding; strikes; fluctuation in prices; and 'the recklessness and addictions to the use of ardent spirits'. He also produced a map which showed that fever was most prevalent in the most densely crowded districts. Cowan appears to have been among the first in Glasgow to urge the establishment of a 'medical police' to help resolve these problems, and he urged the pro-vision of more adequate permanent hospital provision so that epidemics could be prevented rather than being dealt with only once they had become established. He also proposed the unification of municipal local government to overcome the inequalities and increase efficiency; that the children of the poor should have the right to treatment by the district surgeons; and 'that a uniform system of co-operation be established among the guardians of the poors' funds, the managers of our hospitals, lunatic asylums, houses of refuge and other charitable establishments'.

Robert Perry (1783–1848) showed six-fold differences between parts of Glasgow in the proportions of the population attended by the district surgeons for fever, and demonstrated the extent and progress of the 1843 typhus epidemic on a map on which affected households were individu-ally identified[8]. It was, however, the fascinating but horrifying reports which he collected from the district surgeons which he used as his main argument for change. He lamented the refusal to provide hospital beds at the time of epidemics until they commenced their 'ravages among the upper classes, when fears for their own safety compel them to take measures, when it is too late, to check the progress of the pestilence'. He also advocated a tax for the support of the poor in hospitals, the estab-lishment of a board of health in every town and city to help prevent the onset and spread of infectious disease, and improvement in poor relief for rural areas.

John Strang (1795–1863), as Glasgow City Chamberlain, took on the task of collating and reporting to the Council the vital, social and com-mercial statistics of the city, and his meticulous tables and commentary were published annually from 1847 until his death. Strang demonstrated marked diversity between the mortality of different quarters of the city[9]. He was aware of the complication introduced in small area analyses by the presence of hospitals, but concluded that even after 'making a due deduction for these disturbing elements, there is enough left to show that there exists, within certain registration districts, causes more destructive to life than in other portions of the city'. Strang emphasised the danger of collecting information merely for its own sake as distinct from using information to determine aetiology and to effect change. He was very much aware of the association between health and socio-economic circumstances, observing 'no idea can be justly formed as the real sanitary condition of towns or districts from looking merely at the death-rate figures, or without taking into account the birth-rate and the ages of the inhabitants to which those figures relate. The poverty or riches of a people also is absolutely needful to be known before we can truly determine the ratio of death to any population'.

Comparative statistics for the mid nineteenth century:
Not all data for this period, however, related to Glasgow. For example, in 1840 the General Committee of the British Association resolved to set up a comparative investigation of the vital statistics for six large towns in Scotland[10]. The membership of the Committee included Dr W.P. Alison and Edwin Chadwick, but the statistical data was collated by Mr Alexander Watt, who was responsible for maintaining the bills of mortality for Glasgow. The towns selected were Edinburgh with Leith, Glasgow, Aberdeen, Perth and Dundee. It was demonstrated that whereas there were 3.2 births registered per 100 total population in England and Wales, the corresponding ratio was only 0.99 for Edinburgh and Leith, 1.31 for Aberdeen, 1.16 for Glasgow, 1.50 for Dundee and 1.70 for Perth. It was concluded that recording of baptisms or births in Scotland was so deficient and variable that no use could be made of the data.

The Committee also found that no uniform or systematic method of recording the causes of death had been adopted in Scotland, except in the parish of South Leith where a system recommended by the Royal College of Physicians of Edinburgh had been introduced. However, it was possible to make certain comparisons, for example the proportion of deaths under the age of five years to the total deaths was in the range 29 *per cent* to 34 *per cent* in Aberdeen, Perth and Edinburgh, but was 45 *per cent* to 47 *per cent* in Glasgow and Dundee. The crude death rates in 1841 were 3.1 *per cent* for Glasgow, 1.6 *per cent* for Aberdeen, and in the range 2.2 to 2.5 *per cent* for the other four towns. The Committee observed a relationship between mortality and factors such as climate, free circulation of air, drainage, cleanliness, temperance, the absence of wholesome food, clothing, fuel, and the occupations of the people. Differences in the means of affording medical relief however were not considered to be important since the various hospitals and dispensaries exhibited 'the same high character of efficiency'. The recorded causes of deaths were available for certain towns only, but it was noted that the greatest excess of deaths in Dundee over those in Edinburgh was caused by asthma, bowel complaints, catarrh, croup, dropsy, whooping cough, measles, nervous diseases, scarlet fever and smallpox.

In 1851 James Stark, later to become the first statistician to the Registrar General in Scotland, published a review of vital statistics for Scotland[11] in which he argued that their quality was among the poorest in Europe – due to failure of the Church to improve its system of registration, and to obstruction by the Church to the Bills brought before Parliament for a national registration system. Much of his data was derived from the second Statistical Account for Scotland (1845). Stark's review began with a detailed account of the prevalence of insanity and idiocy in various parts of Scotland, England and Wales, Ireland and elsewhere in Europe, and he concluded that the apparently greater prevalence in Scotland and England was associated with a greater frequency of intermarriage of near blood relatives. Estimates of the numbers and proportions of deaf and dumb, blind, paupers and orphans were also given for the various counties of Scotland. Stark estimated that even in Edinburgh, Glasgow and Dundee, 'where registration is conducted with some care', less than one third of births is entered in the registers, although he was able to use the existing figures to calculate that 7.6 *per cent* of births in Scotland were illegitimate, compared with only 2.1 *per cent* in Sardinia and 20.6 *per cent* in Bavaria. The statistics relating to marriages were more accurate, although possibly of little practical value. For mortality data, Stark used the Second Statistical Account and other sources to show that the mortality in towns was considerably higher than in the country (26.7 per thousand v. 20.3 per thousand). He observed that Glasgow was 'out of all proportion the most unfavourable to childhood', whereas Dundee was 'the most favoured town in Scotland to the aged'.

Deaths and births after civil registration, 1855 to 1899

Although civil registration of births, deaths and marriages was introduced in England and Wales in 1837, and despite the fact that ecclesiastical registration was considerably less adequate in Scotland, opposition by the Church, the burghs and lairds, and lack of co-ordinated effective pressure by bodies such as the British Association for the Advancement of Science, the London Statistical Society and the Royal College of Physicians, led to the delay of civil registration in Scotland until 1855[11].

The Act in Scotland was compulsory, whereas that in England and Wales was still merely permissive for death registration (and remained so until 1874), and so the quality of the vital statistics for this period is likely to be superior in Scotland. The range of information collected at registration was initially considerably greater than that required in England and Wales, with the result that it was six years before the first Detailed Annual Report could be published; from 1856, therefore, the data collected was much reduced. Detailed annual reports were published until 1910, thereafter being re-named Annual Reports, which have been published ever since. Decennial supplements, surveying trends in mortality, fertility etc., were produced for the ten year periods 1861–70, 1881–90 and 1891–1900. No further decennial supplement was published until 1932 (for the years 1920–29). Since that time decennial supplements have not been published, but occasional supplements have been produced on topics such as occupational mortality and life tables. There was a medically qualified person in charge of vital statistics since the appointment of Dr James Stark in July 1855. His post was equivalent to that of William Farr, Compiler of Abstracts to the Registrar General for England and Wales, who was responsible for the scientific content of the reports and was probably the most outspoken interpreter of the official mortality statistics.

Stark produced the reports from 1855 until 1870, when Dr William Robertson took over. The 1879 to 1901 reports were compiled by Dr R.J. Blair Cunynghame, and those from 1902 to 1919 by Dr James Crawford Dunlop, whose title became Superintendent of the Statistical Branch of the Department. Crawford Dunlop became Registrar General himself within three years and – perhaps because of his own statistical background – no Superintendent of Statistics appears to have been appointed. On his retirement in 1931 Dr Peter McKinlay was appointed to superintend statistics until his retiral in 1960. During this long period McKinlay wrote a large number of papers on a wide variety of topics[12], most of which were published in the *Health Bulletin*, and he contributed to the reports of several departmental committees (see later).

In 1960, Dr (later Professor) Alwyn Smith was appointed as 'medical statistician' giving professional guidance to the Registrar General for Scotland, and he was succeeded in an advisory capacity in 1966 by Dr Michael Heasman, who had been Principal Medical Officer of the Health Services Research and Development Unit.

Small area statistics during the nineteenth century

As we have seen, medical statisticians in Glasgow had compared mortality in different parts of the city, and had related this to differences in living conditions, for 20 or 30 years prior to the introduction of civil registration. This tradition was continued after 1855 by John Strang, who became responsible for producing the vital statistics of Glasgow; using subdivisions of registration districts he was able to demonstrate a range in infant mortality from 19.6 to 213 per thousand, and in the crude death rate from 5.3 to 34.4 per thousand (although much of the latter was due to a marked difference in age structure).

The first medical officers of health in both Edinburgh (Dr Littlejohn, appointed 1862) and Glasgow (Dr Gairdner, appointed 1863) were both much concerned with the variability in death rates within their respective cities, and conducted analyses for smaller spatial units than the registration districts which were the basis of the report of the Registrar General. In the words of Gairdner 'A registration district contains so vast a sum of lives (population usually 30,000 to 40,000) that the causes of mortality, as affecting individuals and small groups of persons, are completely lost in the consideration of such enormous aggregates'[13]. For census purposes, the City of Glasgow had been subdivided in 1861 into 960 enumeration districts, each comprising some 70 to 120 families. Gairdner proposed that these be used as the basic units for epidemiological measurement – each being 'a little town within a town'. He further suggested that the Registrar tabulate his returns for each enumeration district weekly, in order to 'afford instant information of the rise of the death rate in any particular locality, and to enable precautions to be specially directed to that quarter'. He envisaged that such returns would also be useful for identifying the causes 'of that permanent excess of mortality which we know to exist' and to discover to what extent this was dependent 'on faults in the arrangements of families, the construction of houses, overcrowding, deficient comforts, poverty, and so forth'.

Not surprisingly, this ambitious scheme proved unworkable, and Gairdner was compelled to reduce the number of subdivisions of Glasgow to 54 'sanitary districts', each being reasonably homogeneous 'in the social position and sanitary circumstances of their population'. He felt certain, however, that a systematic examination of deaths, by cause, for five or six years – arranged according to sanitary districts – would lead to results of great importance as regards prevention. In Gairdner's view his subdivision of the population for sanitary purposes was much more complete than that attempted for any population of equal magnitude. But he was careful to emphasise that death rates for individual sanitary districts could only be calculated with certainty for census years, and condemned the press and others for publishing rates based on a census several years earlier, at a time when dramatic population changes were taking place.

Unfortunately, Gairdner's warnings went unheeded, and the publication of 'utterly absurd and erroneous conclusions from the incorrect figures upon which they had operated so unwisely'[14] forced Gairdner to abandon his system. The result was that his report for 1871 was described as the most unsatisfactory, simply because he could supply only masses of figures, 'from which no pressure could extract a drop of juice, and which no human ingenuity could prove to any reasonable conclusion'[15]. Dr J.T. MacFadyen, in an address to the Glasgow Philosophical Society[16], therefore urged a return to a 'minute subdivision' of Glasgow in order to ascertain whether local death rates in the vicinity of clearances had fallen, and to find out whether the clearances had resulted in 'huddling together elsewhere, so as to create a mortality counter-balancing the good effect'. For each subdivision he indicated the need for the population, the occupations, ages, birth and death rates and 'all those particulars that students of the public health so much desiderate, but very seldom obtain'.

As a result of the support for the return of small area statistics the Glasgow Committee of Health agreed to create 20 subdivisions within the 10 registration districts, although it was realised that these sub-districts were likely to be much less homogeneous than the 54 aggregates of enumeration districts previously defined by Dr Gairdner. These new subdivisions, like the former, were called sanitary districts. Death rates were published each year from 1871 for all ages (all causes, for consumption and for certain other causes) and for children under the age of five years. The population density for each enumeration district was also given. As time went on information about average numbers of rooms per house, birth rate, infant mortality and illegitimate birth rates were included in the statistics, and crude death rates for some 20 causes of death were published for each of 22 sanitary districts. In 1903, however, the sanitary districts were replaced by municipal wards as statistical subdivisions of the city and these were considerably less homogeneous entities than even the subdivisions of registration districts; the wards remained in use for this purpose until 1973, although from 1911 onwards very little information about specific causes of death (apart from tuber-culosis) was provided.

In 1865 Dr Littlejohn published an extremely detailed report on the sanitary condition of the City of Edinburgh[17] in which the character-istics of each of 19 'sanitary districts' (population range 1,886 to 18,307, each being defined subjectively as having a reasonably homogeneous population) were described. Included in the data for each sanitary district were the number of legitimate and illegitimate births, the birth rate, the number of deaths (for 17 causes), the death rates for those under and over the age of five years, the number of fever cases (for the years 1847/48 and 1857/58), and the cases of cholera (for 1848); also given were the percentage of paupers, and the numbers of untrapped cesspools, lodging houses, wells, drinking fountains, urinals, other public conveniences, public houses, byres and alehouses (and their state of cleanliness and ventilation), and the number and distribution of manu-factures and trades. Almost as comprehensive a range of data was provided in addition for certain individual streets and even for particular tenements where overcrowding was severe. Detailed analyses of death rates were also given for individual causes of death, age groups and occupations. Undoubtedly this book must rank as the most comprehen-sive and detailed report of the health and related circumstances of any town in Scotland, and possibly even in Great Britain. It is a model report, and one which has been approached in excellence at no time since.

Hospital statistics

By the early 1920s hospital managers began to keep more formal registers of admissions and discharges with the aims of establishing how long individuals remained in the hospital and of identifying cases which were incurable, or inappropriate for treatment in the hospital. The registers were also used to ensure that subscribers sent only the number of patients for which they had paid. In 1823, in reference to an enquiry about increased death rates by James Ewing of Strathleven, one of the directors of Glasgow Royal Infirmary, the hospital minute book included a lengthy statistical account by the hospital medical committee for the period since the opening of the hospital. Mortality in the hospital had increased from one death per 17.1 cases for the period 1795–1801, to one death per 11.5 cases for 1816–22. This increase was, however, very adequately explained by the facts that the population of Glasgow had doubled over this period – almost entirely due to an influx of 'the lower orders', and that in 1816 district surgeons had been appointed to attend the sick poor in their own homes – the result being that only the more serious cases were transferred to the infirmary. The hospital medical committee made the very pertinent observation that hospital deaths could not be looked at in isolation from those occurring in the districts, and from the proportion of cases treated by the district surgeons; but the committee did concede that increasing overcrowding in the hospital may have contributed to the increasing mortality.

Early performance analysis:

In this 1823 report, tables were presented in which death rates in some 20 hospitals in England, Scotland and France (Paris) were compared. The only Scottish hospitals represented were the Aberdeen and Glasgow Infirmaries, and this may indicate that these were the only two which published statistics; indeed it was specifically stated that no annual reports were available for Edinburgh Infirmary. The committee warned of the dangers of making such comparisons, quoting 'the comparative mortality of different hospitals is a most fallacious test of successful practice unless the nature and intensity of the several diseases are taken into account'. It was suggested that many statistical reports from other hospitals were produced 'rather for the purpose of pleasing than instructing the public,' and that some hospitals dismissed patients 'at a time well chosen as to free the hospital from as many dying patients as possible'. The committee observed that the statistics suggested that the diseased poor of Nottingham were 'healthier than the inhabitants of the most salubrious spot which can be found elsewhere on the surface of the whole world', and accused Edinburgh Infirmary of admitting none who are incurable, and selecting only those who were 'suitable subjects for clinical discussion'. The committee concluded that it was preferable to review trends in a single hospital than to try to compare hospitals which may have radically different practices of admission and discharge.

Growing comparisons:

Until 1812, Glasgow Infirmary published only the numbers of patients who were admitted and who died; subsequently lists of diseases treated, operations, and the number of cases in each category were published. Proposals to compile medical and statistical tables to throw light on the nature, progress and termination of diseases in the infirmary were put forward by Dr Richard Millar at at a meeting of managers in 1827, and thereafter the annual reports give the results of treatment (separately for medical and surgical cases) in terms of 'relieved', 'dismissed' ('with advice', 'irregular', 'improper', 'incurable' or 'own desire'), 'remitted', 'cured' or 'dead'. Regulations for the infirmary, published in 1830, show that the responsibility for recording each case was the responsibility of the Physicians' Clerks:

> "They shall make up the Register Book of Admissions, Dismissions etc, and at the end of the year the Senior Physicians' Clerk shall make out a list of the number of Patients in the House at the end of the preceding year; stating the number admitted since – distinguishing the males, females – how many medical, surgical, how dismissed ... and showing the number of Patients remaining at date of list".

In 1832 Dr Moses Buchanan published a *History of the Glasgow Royal Infirmary* which included a review of financial and medical statistics[18]; in this he urged further investigation 'of the laws which regulate the course of population and mortality in the city', and while recognising the contribution made by Dr Cleland, regretted that this had not been matched by similar efforts from the medical profession.

Buchanan praised the efforts made by the Editors of the Glasgow Medical Journal who, since its inception in 1828, had procured from the district surgeons quarterly lists of the diseases treated by them, together with the mortality and the number of cases transferred to the Royal Infirmary. In this journal, Dr John McFarlane published in 1828 a paper on 'the diseases of the poor' in which he described the work of the six district surgeons and tabulated the cases visited by them during August to October 1827[19]. He calculated that the average cost per patient treated at home by the district surgeons amounted to only eleven pence three-farthings, whereas in the Infirmary the average cost of each patient 'for medicine and medical attendance, including wine and spirits', amounted to 10s 1d. The average length of stay in the Infirmary at that time was calculated to be 33 days, compared with 43 days during the first 20 years of its existence.

Increasing sophistication:

By 1838 the annual report for Glasgow Royal Infirmary had been extended to tabulate the causes of death of each patient and the average length of stay for medical and surgical cases separately. In that year a summary of all cases treated since the opening of the hospital was given: 13,275 dismissed, 7,379 died, 59,313 cured and 255 still 'in house'. Unfortunately an earlier attempt (1834) to publish a yearly account of interesting cases was thwarted by opposition from senior clinical staff who were unwilling to accept these additional duties. By 1843 the number 'cured', 'relieved' or 'died' was given for individual diseases and operations, together with the diagnoses for all fevers admitted to the annexed fever house. In 1844 the statistics were given for each month, and the location of residence of the patients was also documented in some detail. In that year statistics for all other medical institutions in Glasgow were also provided in the report.

Not all hospitals in Britain, however, produced such detailed reports, and many probably produced no annual or other statistics at all. Thus Charles Cowan, Physician to the Royal Berkshire Hospital and Reading Dispensary, wrote (1840), that 'were 100 practitioners annually to publish the results of their experience on any uniform or comprehensive plan, much valuable information, as to the locality and treatment of disease, would be obtained, and many points on the natural history of particular complaints, now uncertain or contested, might be satisfactorily demonstrated and for ever set at rest'[20]. He urged the provision of synopses of cases – 'by a few brief words more real essential points might be secured than are often included in pages of unmethodised description'. He was also fully aware of the influence of social and environmental factors and of variations in the quality of practitioners, and recognised that problems in the classification of disease and in diagnosis often made the correct interpretation of health statistics difficult.

An editorial[21] in *The Lancet* in 1841 attacked practitioners for 'failing to lay down a general plan of hospital registration – an obvious duty when it is universally admitted that medicine is a science of facts, and the results of experience'. For this it blamed undue attention being paid to 'curious, strange, uncommon, miraculous cases, instead of generalising the phenomena of most frequent occurrence', and suggested that only an Act of the Legislature could now put matters right.

The editorial cited among various examples of good statistical reports Dr Cowan's statistics of fever in Glasgow, Dr Balmanno's statistics of Glasgow Infirmary, Dr Craigie's reports in the *Edinburgh Medical and Surgical Journal*, and the Reports of the Clinical Clerks to the Edinburgh and other infirmaries. It gave a detailed list of the various factors which should be entered in a register, and warned of the dangers of attempting 'to seize everything, which invariably ends in grasping nothing'. It was suggested that special detailed reports should be made from time to time on particular diseases, and that the registers and reports should be the responsibility of 'reporters with good salaries, who had nothing to do with the treatment'. The editorial concluded that in view of the many advantages of introducing an adequate recording and analytical system ('to progress the knowledge and treatment of disease; to differentiate quackery from science; to reduce the uncertainty of medicine by demonstrating that death and recovery were regulated by determinate physical laws and influenced by physical agents') it was impossible to understand the objections to the proposal.

In the eighth annual report of the Royal Statistical Society (1842) it was stated that the 'Committee for prosecuting inquiries relating to vital statistics' had issued a form to 11 London hospitals for the 'registration and annual collection of their experience'[22]. The Committee considered that without some standard of comparison it would be impossible to determine the relative value of different methods of treatment; consequently there was a danger that 'medicine will be open to charges of inutility, and the public health will be the sport of fashion, the perilous innovation of empirics and superficial theorists'. The need for a control group was clearly recognised, as also was the difficulty of withholding what might be effective treatment. It was suggested that London hospitals should collaborate in the completion of a simple but uniform statistical return, and once this had proved itself it was expected that it would be extended elsewhere.

In 1861 a meeting of physicians and surgeons from eight of the General Hospitals of London resolved that the metropolitan hospitals should adopt one uniform system for the registration of patients (very similar to that proposed 130 years earlier by Dr Clifton) using the nomenclature employed by the Registrar General, with additions suggested by Miss Nightingale to the International Statistics Congress[23]. It was suggested that annual summaries should be submitted for publication in the *Journal of the Statistical Society*, with a full annual report produced for each hospital, and that in every hospital there should be an officer charged specifically with the duty of attending to the registration of patients.

Little action appears to have been taken on these recommendations, and it was over 50 years before any further advance was made in the collection of statistics for general hospitals. The Lunacy (Scotland) Act of 1857, however, provided for the establishment of a mechanism for registering patients with mental disorders, and these data have been analysed by Cameron (1954)[24]. He estimated that about 1,240 patients had been admitted to mental hospitals in Scotland over the period 1850–54 (0.43 patients per 1,000 population). From 1857 the annual admission rate rose to 0.48 per thousand plus 0.09 per thousand insane residents in private dwellings who were also included on the register. From 1862 a small but steadily growing number of voluntary patients was also admitted to mental hospitals. After 1875 the number of admissions increased considerably (to 0.70 per thousand population during the period 1880–89) as a result of central government funds being provided towards the upkeep of pauper lunatics. A special report, published as a supplement to the 36th Annual Report (1894) of the Board of Lunacy noted considerable differences in the proportion of the population in the various types of establishment – from 29 per 100,000 in Shetland to 177 per 100,000 in Edinburgh; it was emphasised that this difference, and the increasing admission rate, was due to differences in hospital provision and not to differences in, or an increasing level of lunacy in Scotland. An interesting comparison was made in 1871, 1881 and 1891, between the census returns for the number of insane in the population and the numbers registered by the Commissioners; the census figures were in excess by 18 *per cent*, 14 *per cent* and 11 *per cent* respectively.

III. Health Information in the Twentieth Century

General practitioner records

National developments:

Until the 1911 Insurance Act general practitioners were under no obligation – apart from that of good medical practice – to record details of any consultation with or procedures carried out on patients, although most practitioners presumably did record, in a day or medicines book, attendances and any medicines given.

Under the terms of the 1911 Insurance Act general practitioners were awarded an Exchequer grant as a supplement to their remuneration from the Insurance Fund, provided that various conditions, including an obligation to keep certain prescribed records, were complied with. The form adopted, which had been approved by the British Medical Association, was based on the day book or prescription book previously used by many doctors (and which continued to be used for non-insured persons).

This form was unsatisfactory, and in 1913 a two-part record card was introduced to be used for individual insured patients. At the end of each year the part of the record containing identifying details and attendances was sent to the Insurance Committee, and the part containing the particulars of illness and summary of attendances was sent to the Insurance Commissioners. In order to preserve confidentiality, no mechanism was provided to enable the two parts to be linked subsequently: an arrangement which was obviously inadequate both for clinical and for statistical purposes since it was impossible, even for the doctor, to bring together the particulars of illness of the same patient in successive years.

In 1917 the Insurance Commissioners decided, as a temporary measure, to suspend the enforcement of the obligation to keep records because of the strain on the general practitioner service occasioned by the withdrawal of so many for military service.

In the new Medical Benefit Regulations (Scotland) 1920, it was stated – with the support of the Conferences of the Local Medical and Panel Committees – that 'a practitioner is required to furnish records of the diseases of his patients and of his treatment of them in such form as the Board may from time to time determine'. In order 'to consider and advise the Minister of Health and the Scottish Board of Health as to the form of Medical Record to be presented, having due regard to the clinical purposes as well as to the administrative and the statistical purposes which such records may serve' an Inter-Departmental Committee on Insurance Medical Records was set up in 1920[25]. The Committee observed that the prime purpose of the medical record is to contribute to the more efficient treatment of patients, both by the doctor who makes the record, and by other doctors, under whose care the same patient may subsequently come. A continuous record, kept by the general practitioner at all times, was therefore necessary. This meant that the record would not be readily available for statistical and administrative purposes. In order to overcome this difficulty it was suggested that doctors might submit returns – possibly on a detachable portion of the record card – summarising certain particulars relating to certain categories of patients. Alternatively, a routine extraction of the requisite particulars could be made by officers of the Departments concerned.

The Committee attached great importance to the possibilities of the Departments (in England and Scotland) promoting *ad hoc* enquiries such as enumeration of the sickness experience of persons of a particular age or ages, or engaged in a particular occupation, through several years; or investigation of the prognostic significance of various symptoms in the aetiology of serious disease; or assessment of selected portions of the record of insured persons who are certified as incapable of work. It was also suggested that routine tabulation from the records of insured persons who have died, or gone out of benefit, might be made on their eventual return to the Central Department. The Scottish representatives of the Committee, unlike their English counterparts, considered that the best method of providing summary information would be for the doctors themselves to produce this on a summary card without identifying information – provided that they were then freed from the need to record attendances and visits.

The Committee was very much aware of the need to minimise the clerical work of the doctor, and made several recommendations to this effect. However, it was also very aware of the enormous potential value of the general practitioner record for medical research purposes, for clinical work, as a means of effective communication with other professionals and of assessing a doctor's own clinical performance, and as an important link with other medical records such as school medical records, institutional records and the medical records of the Ministry of Pensions. Unfortunately, although the recommendations of the 1920 Report were accepted, only the design of the medical record envelope and of the continuation card appear to have been implemented. None of the proposals for statistical work, epidemiological research, or improved training in the observation and recording of clinical details appear to have been acted upon.

With the implementation of the 1946 National Health Service Acts, use of the 1920 medical record envelope was extended to cover all patients registered under the NHS, and this is still the official mechanism for registering, transferring and de-registering patients today. In 1963 a sub-committee of the Standing Medical Advisory Committee (Chairman Anne Gillie) emphasised the value of almost everyone having a medical record which was maintained throughout life despite changes in the general practitioner[26]. The committee reported that 'continuing easy survey of the data recorded opens the way for the doctor's check on his diagnosis and on trends (epidemiological, environmental and other) exhibited among his patients'. Participation in research by the general practitioner was encouraged – 'research through planned observation should be a normal activity for the family doctor'. It was suggested that cross-referencing and the maintenance of an age–sex register were desirable and even necessary. No suggestion was made that Departmental representatives might make occasional *ad hoc* studies of certain aspects of general practitioner records, but it was stressed that means must be found to co-ordinate and finance research projects involving family doctors.

The 1963 committee was 'far from satisfied' with the format and size of general practitioner records and urged a trial of new sizes, including the use of report summaries in order to reduce bulk and facilitate reference. Two years later the Tunbridge Report (1965) in England reiterated a dissatisfaction with the general practitioner record and expressed the hope that 'general practitioner organisations will continue to give serious study to the purpose and best use of the existing records as well as to their improvement'[27], although in Scotland the corresponding Walker Committee (1963) made reference only to general practitioner referral letters[28]; both reports recommended standardisation of hospital records to A4 size.

In 1971 a report was published of a survey commissioned by the Scottish Home and Health Department – *The General Practitioner's Use of Medical Records*[29]. This survey was answered by 167 Scottish general practitioners, 49 *per cent* of whom said that they would welcome a radical change in the general practitioner record (although 20 *per cent* felt that the medical record system was, in fact, ideal). It was concluded that after an era of half a century of unprecedented change in the practice of medicine and of improvements in public health due to environmental and therapeutic advances, reform of the virtually unchanged general practitioner records was long overdue, and that a working party should be set up to look at the whole field of medical records in general practice, and to recommend changes. In 1971 such a working party was set up – the Joint Working Party on Re-design of Medical Records in General Practice – with representatives from Scotland as well as England and Wales. Its report (1972) recommended that Health Departments should take steps to replace, as soon as practicable, the medical record envelope by an A4 size record system with a suitable folder and a specified range of insert sheets printed in distinctive colours[30]. These included a summary sheet (unstructured), an immunisation and screening investigations record, a maternity record, a paediatric development chart, a mount sheet and a nurses' and health visitors' record.

In 1978 the Royal College of General Practitioners published its own report *Medical Records in General Practice*[31]. The authors found that there was increasing evidence from general practice and the hospital service that present records were inadequate, both for service purposes and for planning medical care. This was considered likely to decrease the effectiveness of the management of patients' care, to prevent satisfactory medical audit and to make the appropriate allocation of resources within the health care system more difficult. The lack of any routine information on a local or national scale about general practice where the vast majority of health service consultations take place (about 250,000 annually), and the lack of integration with hospital and community records, were also considered to be serious deficiencies.

Local initiatives and microcomputer developments:

In 1959 the Research Committee of the Royal College of General Practitioners produced a comprehensive classification related to the International Classification of Diseases and Causes of Death (ICD)[32], and this was replaced in 1963 by a shorter list selected according to frequency of occurrence and severity. This classification opened up the possibility of individual general practitioners setting up their own disease indices, for example the 'E-book' of Dr T.S. Eimerl and the 'W-book' of Dr Walford[33]. Again, in the early 1970s, experimentation was begun with the Problem Orientated Medical Record (POMR) introduced from the United States. This structured record is intended to contribute to better patient care by encouraging a systematic approach to the resolution of problems. The problem-orientated medical record provides a very effective mechanism for the transfer of information between general practitioner and hospital doctors (both for in-patient and out-patient care), it improves the continuity of care by clearly recording each active problem and its current status, and it interfaces well with structured hospital discharge summaries; current and past therapy is also recorded, as is an indication of what the patient has been told about his illness. The problem-orientated medical record enables the reader to assimilate key information at a glance, guards against wasteful duplicate investigations, improves follow-up, assists in monitoring the process and outcome of care, optimises the use of resources and has an important educative influence on both doctor and patient.

In 1974 Dr R.McG. Harden described a feature card system, each card representing a particular feature (eg diagnosis, occupation, age group) and each being divided into numbered squares which refer to individual patients[34]. Using the system it is possible within minutes to relate any one feature to another or to any combination of features. This system was extended in Howden Health Centre, Livingstone, to provide readily available information for analysing the age-sex distribution of the practice population, for monitoring the elderly and patients on long-term therapy, for monitoring immunisation and other programmes for children, for identifying other groups for whom preventive measures were thought desirable (eg the administration of influenza vaccine to chronic bronchitis), and for epidemiological and other research activities[35].

General Practitioners are obviously in the best position for measuring morbidity among their patients. Three national studies of morbidity statistics from general practice have been conducted in England and Wales jointly by the Royal College of General Practitioners (RCGP), the Office of Population Censuses and Surveys (OPCS) and the Department of Health and Social Security (DHSS): the first in 1955/56 (53 practices), the second in 1970/71 and subsequent years to 1975/76, and a third in 1981/82 (43 practices – 36 being the same as in 1955/56). Practitioners who agreed to take part in the studies recorded details about patients, consultations, diagnoses and referrals. OPCS analysed the data received and was thus able to estimate the national incidence and prevalence rate for each condition. The national morbidity studies have been used for estimating national morbidity treated in general practice, for investigating trends, and in studies on adverse reactions to pertussis vaccine, raised blood pressure, the prevalence of diabetes and malignant hypertension, and virus infections in pregnancy. Despite the unique information generated by these three morbidity surveys, no similar investigations have been conducted in Scotland and none is planned. The pattern of morbidity and workload in each practice can also be determined, summarised statistical information being produced as Practice Statistical Reports (PSRs).

A very ambitious computer-based system became operational in Exeter in 1975[36]. This was an experimental project funded by DHSS, one of the main aims of which was the integration of information so that all relevant data would be quickly and easily available at any of the points at which a patient makes contact with the health service. Real time computing was used for most functions so that recall and updating could be almost immediate, both in the health centres and hospital. The system included clinical and administrative functions in both the health centre and in the hospital nursing and service departments; it also included the administrative practices of the outpatient and inpatient departments of the hospital. The aim was to create a single 'integrated patient record' which would be available at each patient contact to all authorised users. Each general practitioner surgery at the health centre is provided with a visual display unit (VDU) which is used by the doctor to review the previous history of each patient who attended, and then to key in details of the attendance. The record is structured, clear and concise. The system is able to print prescriptions, summary records for hospital referral, and the entire record for patients who transfer to other practitioners. It can also be used to identify patients due for screening or in particular age, sex or diagnostic categories.

This is obviously a system with enormous potential, but also one of extremely high cost. It is likely that most of the benefits of the system can be achieved more simply and much more cheaply by a modular approach – whereby general practitioners have their own micro-computers which can exchange information with larger computers in hospitals and elsewhere. This information exchange would take place in 'batch' mode (ie not on-line) which is much less expensive and of little or no disadvantage for most applications.

In 1982 a 'Micros for GPs' scheme was announced to promote aware-ness of information technology in General Medical Practice. The Department of Trade and Industry offered to meet half the cost of purchasing and installing a micro-computer system of appropriate size in up to 150 British general practices. The offer also covered the cost of training and maintenance for the first three years, and a grant of up to 20 pence per record was made available towards the cost of record conversion during the first year. The systems were designed for the registration of patients, the issue of repeat prescriptions and the screening and recall of patients, and 17 of these were installed in Scotland. A report on experiences over the first year[37] showed that most practices had established computer routines for patient registration and repeat prescriptions, and many had started computer screening and recall programmes. Although significant time savings were not apparent and many organisational difficulties had to be overcome as the computers were introduced, the vast majority of doctors and staff thought their computer systems worthwhile and wished to maintain or expand their use. The report identified a growing awareness that the main benefits of computers do not lie in the mimicry of manual procedures for the day-to-day routine of General Practice administration, but rather in the aggregation and analysis of information: practices had started to use these techniques to assess what they were doing, to plan and review their activities and to introduce change. The report also emphasised the importance of linking health authority and general practice computing systems in order to promote the effective co-ordination and targeting of health care.

The microcomputer systems available under the 'micros for GPs' scheme were restricted to the products of two companies, and perhaps the most serious limitation of the scheme was the inability of the system to link with any of the information systems run by health authorities. Dr David Ferguson, however, a general practitioner in Glasgow, had by this time developed his own general practitioner microcomputer system – primarily for repeat prescribing. In 1984 funds were obtained from the Scottish Home and Health Department to extend this system to include morbidity recording and the development of linkages to health authority information systems, and it is likely, therefore, that exploitation of the full potential of general practice computing in Scotland will be achieved through this system (known as GPASS or general practitioner adminis-tration system, Scotland). By early 1986 about 80 practices had adopted GPASS, and plans were being made for developing direct commu-nication between individual general practices and patient indices held by the health authority. In Glasgow the health board was providing the GPASS system on loan to general practitioners who were willing to participate in its campaign for the reduction of cardiovascular disease by introducing screening procedures for their patients.

Information relating to community health

The introduction of legislation for the notification of infectious disease (1889) extended the very limited information systems of the time to assist in initiating measures for the control of the spread of disease and to provide early intelligence of the onset of epidemics. A further extension took place as a result of the Notification of Births Act (1907) which was probably the first public health measure taken not exclusively for protec-ting the community against the spread of disease or for humanitarian purposes, but for protecting the next and succeeding generations. Infor-mation on tuberculosis was collected from 1912 when the illness was made compulsorily notifiable and a State grant of 50 *per cent* was made available towards the cost of treatment, on venereal disease from 1916 when local authorities were required to provide free, efficient, convenient and secret treatment of affected persons, and on diabetes from 1925, when local authorities became authorised to provide medicines and treatment to persons suffering from the disease.

At the beginning of the present century there was a general uneasiness regarding the health of the nation, the immediate reasons for this being the high death rates of infants during their first year of life, the falling birth rate and the unsatisfactory condition of army recruits during the South African War. This concern led to the appointment of the Royal

Commission on Physical Training, Scotland (1903), and of the Inter-Departmental Committee on Physical Deterioration (1904). These enquiries were the most comprehensive ever made into the health of the Scottish people, and their findings and recommendations have influenced the development of the health service ever since; they have also been instrumental in popularising the idea that the State should concern itself not merely with the removal of specific conditions inimical to health, but should also accept responsibility for measures designed to promote the health of the people. The reports recommended routine medical inspection in schools, and emphasised the opportunity provided by schools for taking stock of the physique of the whole population and securing the conditions most favourable to healthy development. They showed that the high rate of infant mortality had varied little over the previous 25 years, and that about half of the mortality occurred in the first three months of life. The Notification of Births Act (1907), and the development of the school medical service (Education (Scotland) Act 1908) and of maternity and child welfare services since 1915 were also direct consequences of these enquiries.

In 1905 the School Board of Glasgow recorded the physical measurements of 72,857 children attending 73 primary and secondary schools – at the time the most extensive assessment of heights and weights ever undertaken in schoolchildren. The subsequent Education Act made it possible for local authorities to provide for medical examination and supervision, and to take appropriate action in cases of child neglect. The subsequent reports of the school medical service provide a dramatic indication of the improvements in child health which have taken place during the 20th century.

Moves to comprehensive measurement:

A detailed statistical account of the various aspects of the health of Glasgow from 1818 to 1925 was produced in 1930 by the former Medical Officer of Health for the City[38]. A very comprehensive review of the health of the whole population of Scotland was published in 1936 in the *Report of the Committee on Scottish Health Services*, under the chairmanship of Professor Edward Provan Cathcart[39]. This included analysis of the growth and distribution of the population of Scotland, of the social and economic conditions, of the state of health of the people, and of the health services. The Report noted that although the public health system had developed to embrace research, the prevention of disease and the promotion of healthy living, the administrative system had not kept pace with this widening conception. Also services were often not adapted to the changes which had taken place in social and economic conditions, in the habits and outlook of the people, in the size and distribution of the population, and in the nature and incidence of ill health. It was the view of the Committee that the general standard of health in Scotland was then far below what could be attained, but that this could be improved by expenditure in the application of established knowledge, with the co-operation of the people themselves. The Committee defined the main objective of policy as the promotion of fitness, and therefore emphasised the importance of health education, improved environmental conditions, and facilities for healthy recreation. It also envisaged increasing dependence being made on the general practitioner for the medical contribution to further progress in public health – bringing him and the official services together in a co-ordinated effort to improve the health of the people. Its proposals included the extension of existing medical services to the general medical care of the dependents of insured persons and others, the recognition of the voluntary hospitals as an integral part of the health service, strengthening the powers of the central department for initiating and securing schemes of co-operation among local authorities 'to provide inspiration for the whole health service and to give a lead and guidance throughout', removing the isolation of the general practitioner, and raising the standard of entrants to general practice. In addition, the Report made some 20 pages of detailed recommendations concerning almost every facet of health care. The Report provided much vital information which was used in formulating the structure of the National Health Service, and the White Paper (1944) which presented these proposals for the United Kingdom, acknowledged that the Cathcart Report was one of the most complete official surveys of the country's health services and health problems yet attempted. No such similar comprehensive survey of the nation's health, or of the changes necessary to improve health, has been published since.

Specific reports:
The Cathcart report is one of a large number of reports produced by expert *ad hoc* committees, appointed by the Scottish Home and Health Department and its equivalent earlier organisations, to make recommendations on topics of current interest or concern. Two other such reports which were based on detailed statistical analyses, and which have had far reaching effects, were those on maternal morbidity and mortality, and on infant mortality.

The *Report on Maternal Morbidity and Mortality in Scotland (1935)* expressed an urgent need for improvement in the standard of midwifery, and recommended a comprehensive and co-ordinated service to adequately cover the whole field of maternity provision in Scotland[40]. Its detailed recommendations were based on analyses conducted by Dr Peter McKinlay, the medical statistician to the Registrar General. These included analyses by cause of maternal death since 1911; detailed cross-tabulations including parity, maternal age, overcrowding and cause of death; and comparisons of maternal mortality in different towns and counties over different time periods.

The *Report on Infant Mortality in Scotland* (Department of Health, 1943; Chairman, John Boyd Orr) was described by the then Secretary of State for Scotland, Thomas Johnston, as 'momentous', and showed that infant mortality in Scotland was 40 *per cent* worse than in England and higher than in the USA or in any nation in Western Europe except Spain and Portugal[41]. The Secretary of State remarked that 'here for the first time all the known comparisons are carefully marshalled and a medical committee of great experience and authority, under the chairmanship of one of the leading nutritional scientists of our time, has diagnosed the causes of the lamentable place Scotland takes among the great nations in the saving of infant life'. He attributed much of the blame to unemployment, overcrowding and to poverty. Dr Peter McKinlay was again responsible for the very detailed analyses which included international comparisons for countries and cities, comparisons of infant and neonatal mortality in the various counties and cities of England, Wales and Scotland, analyses by cause over a number of years (1911–39), and investigations of the incidence and influence of prematurity, of the association between infant mortality, overcrowding and unemployment, and of the relationship between infant mortality and illegitimacy.

Other national reports which have been produced from time to time since 1966 include those of special research studies commissioned by the Scottish Home and Health Department and undertaken by its research and intelligence branch (later the Information Services Division). Some of these are published as 'Scottish Health Service Studies', and a list of these is included as Appendix 1.

Ongoing surveys:

There are three continuous sources of health and demographic information during the twentieth century and the latter part of the nineteenth century. First, there are the annual reports of the Registrar General for Scotland, and occasional surveys and supplements. Secondly, there are the annual government reports of the Board of Supervision for the Relief of the Poor in Scotland (1847–94), of the Local Government Board for Scotland (1895–1918), of the Scottish Board of Health (1919–28), of the Department of Health for Scotland (1929–61) and of the Scottish Home and Health Department (1962–present time). Thirdly, there were the reports of the Medical Officers of Health which the holders of that office were expected to provide on an annual basis. Unfortunately the main problems of the time and the changes which were taking place are documented only in the individual reports, and in no very consistent manner, and so it is impossible to make any detailed analysis without spending considerable time in perusing them one at a time. What commentary there is, tends to be very much more bland than that of the mid-nineteenth century, and there is less attempt to focus on areas which have the greatest degree of ill health, or to campaign for reduction in the more extreme inequalities in health.

An additional source of health information is the annual General Household Survey; this is based on a sample of the general population resident in private (non-institutional) households in Great Britain, and has been running since 1971. The sample of addresses is selected from the Electoral Register and information is collected week by week throughout the year by personal interview. A total of 1,560 addresses was selected for the survey in Scotland for 1982, and contact was made with 1,481 households (95 *per cent*) although 4 *per cent* of these refused to take part.

The survey aims to provide a means of examining relationships between the most significant variables with which social policy is concerned and, in particular, of monitoring changes in these relationships over time. It is thus of particular importance as a source of background information for central government decisions on resource allocation between social programmes. The survey is also a valuable source of data about some particular social groups, though its sample size is such that it is sometimes necessary to aggregate data over a number of years in order to obtain large enough sub-samples. The survey can also supplement administrative statistics in various major policy areas; and, together with the Family Expenditure Survey and Labour Force Survey, it helps to fill some of the information gaps about social changes between censuses.

To meet these aims, the survey covers five main subject areas, namely: population, housing, employment, education, and health. Certain subjects are covered periodically by the GHS, although not every year. For example, questions on smoking, included each year from 1972 to 1976, have been asked every second year since then and, since 1978, questions on drinking have also been asked in alternate years. Analyses include the relationship of cigarette smoking and drinking habits to self-reported chronic and acute sickness, the household circumstances of the elderly, frequency of contact with the health service, and data on pre-marital cohabitation and on fertility patterns among women. Also included is information on the economic activity of married couples, a section on private medical insurance cover (which describes the characteristics of people who are covered by private medical insurance policies, and the relationship between insurance cover and reported ill health), and sections on self medication, sight and hearing loss, and the use of contact lenses. The General Household Survey is currently the only means of examining morbidity levels in the community, including that which does not result in health service contact. There is, however, a need to validate the responses in relation to the actual physical condition of the respondent since there will obviously be much variation between respondents in what they consider to be worth reporting. Also, the survey does not include the population resident in communal establishments and this undoubtedly will distort any measure of the apparent level of illness in the community.

Three further enquiries:

Finally, there are three detailed ongoing enquiries in Scotland into particular causes of death. The first of these is the enquiry into maternal deaths in Scotland; this commenced with an investigation of each death during pregnancy and labour or within one year of delivery or abortion, for the period 1965 to 1971. A similar enquiry in England and Wales has run continuously since 1928, but a system of scrutiny established in Scotland for the period 1927 to 1932 appears to have lapsed until 1965. The first investigation in Scotland of individual maternal deaths was probably that set up in Aberdeen during the 1920s by Professor Matthew Hay, Medical Officer of Health for the city. The enquiry attempts to assess whether factors associated with the deaths were potentially avoidable, and to attribute responsibility for these factors.

The second ongoing enquiry relates to perinatal mortality, and this was initiated in 1977 by Professor M.C. Macnaughton, Dr Gillian McIlwaine, and others in Glasgow, based on a method adopted by Professor Dugald Baird in the City of Aberdeen in 1948. Obstetricians and Paediatricians throughout Scotland provide detailed information on every stillbirth and first week death, and are asked to decide the principal obstetric event that started the sequence that led to the perinatal death, and also to assign a paediatric cause to the first week deaths[42]. The enquiry has now been taken over as a routine national system by the Information Services Division.

Professor Sir Dugald Baird was a pioneer of clinical audit. In a *Lancet* editorial to mark Sir Dugald's 80th birthday his former colleague, Dr Angus Thomson, wrote[43]:

> "Baird almost single-handedly began the task of compiling hand-written summaries onto cards and extracting statistics by laborious manual methods. This work, undertaken in addition to a busy routine of teaching and clinical work, gave him exceptional insight into the realities behind impersonal statistics. In consequence, his department became noted for the liveliness of its ideas and discussions; in due course this grew into a multidisciplinary research team, which not only contributed much to the scientific understanding of human reproduction but also saw the perinatal mortality rate in Aberdeen fall from about the Scottish average to one of the lowest in the United Kingdom".

Almost half a century after this work began, obstetricians in most health authorities in Britain have established methods for monitoring their own maternity services. In Glasgow, the obstetric teams from seven or more local hospitals meet annually to compare and discuss statistics relating to patient management and outcome. Such continuous and careful monitoring, by increasing awareness and inducing critical discussion, has undoubtedly played a major part in reducing perinatal mortality and otherwise improving obstetric outcome. The only regret is that doctors in other disciplines have been so slow to follow this example.

A third ongoing system of monitoring, relating to infant deaths, was established in 1979 by Professor Gavin Arneil of Glasgow. This enquiry is very similar to that of the perinatal survey and aims to monitor the numbers of deaths which are birth-determined, the result of illness or accident, or unknown ('cot deaths'); the post mortem findings of the cot deaths are investigated in particular detail.

Hospital Statistics

The development of Scottish Hospital In-patient Records

For virtually the first half of the twentieth century the only standardised hospital statistics were those for the mental hospitals. These showed little change in the annual registration rate over the period 1900 until 1943, although this concealed a gradual decrease from about 130 to zero in the number of patients in private dwellings and a substantial increase in the numbers of voluntary patients (from just over 100 prior to the First World War to 1,423 in 1943). Between 1944 and 1953 the proportion of the population admitted to mental hospitals each year almost doubled (from 0.85 to 1.43 per thousand), the number of voluntary patients admitted rose to 5,375 *per annum* and the number of certified patients admitted was 2,580. Cameron (1954) attributed the reasons for the dramatic increase in admission to mental hospitals to (*a*) an increase in public confidence in mental hospitals, thus greatly increasing voluntary admissions, (*b*) hospital treatment becoming free under the National Health Service, (*c*) some poorhouse inmates who were certified and transferred to mental hospitals in 1949, (*d*) an increased proportion of readmissions, (*e*) increasing age of the population and (*f*) a reduction in family size so that fewer people were available to look after mentally sick people at home. Cameron noted that the Board of Control records did not include information about the age of admissions or about readmissions, although the former at least could be obtained from individual mental hospitals[24].

Early moves to create information systems:

Until the time of the First World War (1914–18) very little progress had been made in the development of information systems for general hospitals. Some hospitals kept registration and diagnostic details in ledgers, but summary statistics were difficult to produce because of the time-consuming tabulations required and the lack of clerical assistance.

Some doctors and groups of doctors did scrutinise records in order to assess their practice, but at that time there was no obligation even to record clinical details and even less to preserve data for investigation later. It is possible that in some hospitals clerical help of a sort was provided, but training was probably non-existent or minimal even for relatively simple tasks such as filing, and almost certainly was not provided for registration and analytical tasks.

After the war the increasing prominence of chronic disease, in contrast to infectious disease, and the development of a variety of techniques to combat these made it important to keep careful case notes so that the progress of patients could be assessed over a relatively long time-period and the effectiveness of different forms of therapy assessed. More clerical staff to assist with documentation and the filing of records were appointed, but little in the way of training or facilities was provided.

During the Second World War (1939–45) the Emergency Medical Service demanded increased, often standardised, record keeping and many new therapeutic procedures were developed. Cancer registration was introduced in 1945, and shortly afterwards the Nuffield Provincial Hospitals Trust sponsored studies into hospital treated illness in Stirlingshire and Ayrshire. In order to try to bring some structure to the disorganised records function which pertained in most hospitals, a meeting of records officers was held in 1946 at the Christie Hospital, Manchester; a working party was set up as a result, and two years later the Association of Medical Records Officers was formed. This body is responsible for the maintenance of professional standards and for ensuring adequate training.

Medical records in general hospitals:

A report on *Medical Records and Secretarial Services* (1959) made a variety of recommendations relating to medical records practices and needs in hospitals other than those for mental illness and mental handicap[44]. This went into considerable detail regarding filing and clerical functions, and organising appointments and secretarial services. Very little of the report was devoted to the production of hospital statistics, and none at all to emphasising the importance of this aspect of the work. A small section was devoted to the maintenance of diagnostic indices, but there was no mention of annual reports or other summaries of workload. Unfortuntely these guidelines represented a rather narrow view of the work of the hospital records officer, and this may still be reflected in what records officers perceive as their role today.

The Joint Working Party on the Organisation of Medical Work in the Hospital Service in Scotland (1967) observed that setting up medical records departments had not so far resulted in any general increase in the dissemination of clinical statistical information – possibly because of the increasing workloads of the staff, but probably also because clinicians 'do not yet realise the potential usefulness of the information, nor the part they have to play in encouraging accuracy and completeness in its collection'[45]. The Working Party considered that the medical records officer had an important part to play in operational research at hospital level, and that he or she should be encouraged and trained to prepare and analyse data, and to help clinicians in appropriate studies. In order to provide time for such work it was regarded as essential to eliminate any unnecessary duplication of statistical returns.

The National Health Service – A new impetus for systematic information:

Soon after the implementation of the National Health Service Act in 1948 the need became apparent for some detailed information about available facilities and the use made of them. In 1949 an annual return was instituted for all hospitals in England and Wales and this became known as the SH3 return in 1953. The equivalent returns appear to have been introduced rather later in Scotland. These were purely numeric hospital workload summaries including availability of beds, numbers of admissions and discharges, mean length of stay, number of transfers and deaths. This information was of fundamental importance for the planners of the new National Health Service, but it was a crude substitute for the much more ambitious schemes suggested two centuries and again one century before.

The beginnings of modernity:

In 1950 agreement was reached between the Department of Health for Scotland and representatives of the then five Regional Hospital Boards for the introduction of a uniform system for the collection of hospital statistics, including diagnostic information, for the whole country; the scheme was begun in April 1951 in general and maternity hospitals, but because of technical and financial problems this was restricted to the Northern region. The scheme was gradually extended to include hospitals in other regions, but it was not until 1961 that this system of Scottish Hospital In-Patient Statistics (SHIPS) was extended to general hospitals throughout the country under the charge of Dr Willie Robertson; mental and mental handicap hospitals were included in a similar scheme from 1963, and maternity hospitals from 1969. The information was collected on a summary discharge document which included diagnostic and other data relating to individual patients.

One hundred *per cent* coverage was thought necessary in Scotland because facilities such as the provision of diagnostic indices, feedback to consultants about individual cases, and the ability to link episodes of care for individual patients were envisaged from the outset. Dr Heasman, then co-director of the Scottish Home and Health Department Research and Intelligence Unit, gave four reasons for the introduction of SHIPS:

to provide administrators with facts about the most costly hospital element of the National Health Service (including the social and demographic characteristics of patients) in order to make best use of current resources and to plan effectively for the future; as a source of epidemiological information about the most serious end of the disease spectrum; to increase doctors' awareness of some of the problems of the management of groups of patients and the utilisation of hospital resources; and provision of diagnostic indices for research and other purposes[46].

SHIPS: The details:

Data for SHIPS are collected on a general hospital discharge document known as SMR1. This is one of a series of Scottish Morbidity Records (SMRs) which include patient identification and administrative details together with diagnostic and operation codes. The SMR2 maternity hospital discharge document includes considerably more clinical information (e.g. blood group, height, method of induction etc.). The other hospital discharge records are the SMR4 (mental) and SMR11 (neonatal) documents. Scottish In-Patient Statistics for general hospitals have been published annually since 1961, and unpublished tables, and tables requested by administrators and clinicians on an *ad hoc* basis, are also available. Prior to 1967 patients' names were excluded from analysis and identification could be obtained only from the case reference number. Since then, however, in order to assist in data retrieval, in the evaluation of patient care and in research, diagnostic and operation indices are produced for each hospital, and also a national disease index. In 1985 a total of almost 1.2 million SMR documents was completed and processed.

It should be stressed that SHIPS does not give a true indication of the prevalence or incidence of morbidity in the community. Whether or not a patient is admitted to hospital depends on a variety of factors such as the severity of the condition; whether hospital treatment is appropriate; the age and social circumstances of the patient; the attitude of the patient, general practitioner, and possibly also of the hospital doctor; and the availability of general practitioner and hospital services. Hospital discharges will thus include only a proportion of total morbidity except for conditions for which hospitalisation would seem obligatory – for example perforated peptic ulcer or fracture of the femur. Also, it must be remembered that SHIPS data relate to discharges rather than persons; although statistics based on discharges are adequate for most administrative purposes, person-based information is needed when attempting to assess variations in the incidence of individual diseases. For most epidemiological purposes repeated admissions to hospital of the same patient require to be linked, and although this can be done on an *ad hoc* basis a national facility for linkage of a variety of SMR1 and other records relating to the same person (including links to death registrations so that survival studies may be facilitated) is still not available[47].

One of the most consistent criticisms of SHIPS is error. A check is made to ensure that the number of returns received from each hospital corresponds reasonably well with the number of discharges recorded on the statistical summary ISD(S)1 returns, and the unexplained discrepancy between the two totals is usually under 1 *per cent*. Hospital consultants in particular make this criticism, but it should be remembered that the Joint Working Party on the Organisation of Medical Work in the Hospital Service in Scotland, 1967, of which John Brotherston was Chairman, recommended that the consultant in administrative charge should be responsible for ensuring the accuracy and completeness of the discharge summary record[45]. This was re-emphasised in the Scottish Health Services Council Report (1967) on *Hospital Medical Records in Scotland* (Chairman Professor James Walker) which stated 'the consultant in administrative charge of a unit should be responsible for the quality of medical records maintained there and also for ensuring the accuracy and completeness of the Hospital In-Patient Records Summary Sheet and, in co-operation with the medical records officer, for the efficient handling of the records in his unit'[28].

A quick visual check is made of each form prior to data-processing to identify omissions or obvious errors. Automated (computer) data-vet procedures are then used to identify other omissions and some of the other more obvious errors or unlikely occurrences (e.g. impossible dates of birth or diagnostic codes, or events which are unlikely at a particular age or in a particular sex) and these are sifted out for checking prior to any analyses being commenced. A study by Lockwood (1971) of the accuracy of SHIPS data over its first nine years of publication (1961–69) showed that the administrative information collected for the year 1969 was very accurate, and that national data either in published or unpublished form were little affected by errors and omissions in transcription except for the recording of social class[48]. For 1969 the principal diagnosis, which forms the basis of both published and unpublished national statistics, was found to be 95 *per cent* accurate. There was thus no reason to believe that for Scotland as a whole the data were not sufficiently accurate for the various purposes for which it was intended. There is always the possibility, however, that returns for particular hospitals, or particular specialties or consultants within a hospital, may be more incomplete or seriously biased in some way.

The system is extremely flexible in that a wide range of investigations can be undertaken on any chosen variable. For example diagnoses may be investigated on the basis of duration of stay, waiting time, bed usage or geographic variation, and standardisation for age and sex can readily be conducted. Hospital activity may be examined in relation to diagnosis, age, catchment area and a variety of other variables; data are available for medical consultants for research purposes, evaluation of patient care and for assessing workload; and diagnostic indices are available to assist with administrative, research and evaluation functions. All these data are available for general hospitals since 1967, and some of it since 1961, so a great variety of analyses of trends is possible. Spaces are also available on the records for use by consultants for their own purposes, with analyses being undertaken for them on request. And there is strict control over confidentiality so that data relating to individual patients or consultants are only available to the consultant concerned.

The provision of feedback to hospital consultants:

In 1967 the Brotherston Working Party (see above) recommended that data should be provided for individual clinicians in a form which is brief, relevant, and accompanied where necessary by a short commentary on the outstanding findings. Such information would assist clinicians to compare their work with that of colleagues, and to consider the implications of these comparisons; for example, differing practices (including analyses of lengths of stay) and other studies which would 'follow almost automatically once interest has been aroused'. It was realised by the Working Party that routine statistics will often only raise questions which require more detailed studies, and outlines were given of a wide variety of important studies – few of which had in fact been initiated. In order to facilitate such studies it was recommended that staffing resources for operational research should be strengthened both centrally and locally, including encouraging the involvement of both hospital consultants and junior medical staff.

It was suggested that the development of operational research be divided into three main phases. The first phase might consist of the presentation to clinicians of readily intelligible statistical data concerning work done, the development of patient care evaluation based on these data, the initiation of local *ad hoc* studies, and the extension of work study techniques into the clinical field. This would be followed by studies of a more ambitious nature requiring the increased participation of clinical and diagnostic departments in operational research generally. The third phase would involve in-depth study of the total medical needs of a community and of the efficiency of all services – general practitioner, local authority and hospital – designed to meet them. The Committee recognised the need to discuss important issues in such a way as that the information penetrates to the individual doctor or nurse. Use of the Divisional system of clinical specialties, 'house' magazines and the *Health Health Bulletin* were suggested as possibilities, and also the 'Scottish Health Service Studies' series for the dissemination of information about operational research projects conducted by, or on behalf of, the Scottish Home and Health Department.

In response to the recommendations of the Working Party the Scottish

Consultant Review of In-Patient Statistics (SCRIPS) was initiated, in which statistical reports of their work were distributed in confidence to most consultants (or sometimes to groups of consultants) in Scotland between the years 1969 and 1979[49]. The reports comprised a summary of in-patient work together with national norms for comparison, and a diagnostic index of cases, including the number of cases treated, ages, waiting time for admission, duration of stay (total and prior to any operation) and the outcome (in terms of transfer, discharge or death). No interpretation was given, since this would have been impossible without detailed local knowledge. The hope was that the data might be analysed critically by the consultant, leading sometimes to improvements in efficiency and effectiveness. The data showed considerable differences between consultants, between hospitals and between teaching and non-teaching hospitals in variables such as lengths of stay (total, pre- and post-operative), and the proportions of patients with particular diagnoses which were operated upon. This suggested, for example, that there was often considerable scope for reducing lengths of stay with no detriment to the patient.

When this project had reached its sixth year of operation Dr Heasman reported that the main response to this form of feedback had been apathy, with criticism outweighing favourable comments among the more responsive minority[49]. The major criticism was error. Some error is almost inevitable in any health information system, but unfortunately many clinicians considered the whole output to be wrong whenever an error was detected. Other criticisms included irrelevancy, lateness (the data were on average 15 months out of date, although clinical practice would probably not change very much over this time), expense (although this is small, and should readily be able to pay for itself many times over in terms of increased efficiency), and unattractive presentation coupled with difficulty in interpretation. Few clinical divisions or groups of consultants had made use of the SCRIPS system, and Dr Heasman suggested that community medicine specialists, as members of clinical divisions with no particular axe to grind, should adopt the role of interpreters of the data. He also advocated the production of more detailed special reports for particular specialties or even for individual diseases.

The SCRIPS system was abandoned in 1979 in favour of an annual production of 'hospital activity comparison tables', in which for each National Health Service hospital in Scotland a concise resumé of activity is given for the previous year. The tables are subdivided by specialty, and again by hospital type, and by formatting the data on one line per hospital it is possible to make rapid comparisons between hospitals of similar type by eye. Tables are sent to the Chief Administrative Medical Officer and Community Medicine Specialist in each Health Board as intermediaries who should provide interpretation in the light of local circumstances.

Despite the enormous potential of the systems of Scottish Morbidity Records, this has never been exploited to the full. The main reason for this lies in the training and attitudes of doctors and – to some extent – administrators. Doctors are still not trained to critically evaluate their work, and they are not trained to recognise the importance of ensuring that diagnostic and other information is recorded accurately and in such a way that records staff can readily enter this onto summary documents for subsequent data retrieval purposes. As a result most hospital consultants have failed to take responsibility for ensuring the accuracy and completeness of the SMR discharge documents. And those individuals who are usually left with this responsibility – the hospital records officers – rarely receive adequate support or encouragement from the medical staff or from the administrators.

Except for a few examples, such as the shared problem-orientated medical record in Aberdeen and the shared antenatal record used in Sighthill Health Centre in Edinburgh, records are generally unstructured, and summaries rarely available; communication between those responsible for the care of the patient is thus unreliable, and data stored for automatic retrieval are sometimes inaccurate. Until suitable training is provided in medical schools the main hope may be that more Community Medicine Specialists will become appointed to Clinical Divisions, and that with their skills in epidemiology and in the presentation of data they will gradually start to demonstrate to clinicians how hospital in-patient data may be used in an interesting and exciting way for self evaluation and to help make the best use of available resources.

The organisation of health service information systems in Scotland

The Research and Intelligence Unit of the Scottish Home and Health Department was established in 1965 under the directorship of Dr M.A. Heasman to bring together the statistics, in-house research and work study sections of the Department. The statistics and research branches expanded considerably during the subsequent nine years, but the work study branch returned to an administrative division where it was largely involved with pay-productivity schemes. The Unit played a leading part in the development of Health Services Research in Scotland and this became a principal component of the Chief Scientist's Office when this was established in 1974. The Unit also became responsible for the development of the Scottish Health Services computer policy. A special study on medical computer development in Scotland by Scientific Control Systems Ltd (SCICON), was commissioned by the Nuffield Provincial Hospitals Trust in 1969. The report recommended concentration on batch processing systems and central co-ordination of computer development, and these have since formed the main components of the Scottish Health Service computer policy[50].

In 1970 the Scottish Home and Health Department commissioned SCICON to report on the requirements for a health service information system. Its report[51] emphasised that for effective management it was necessary to have access to information which was already collected for administrative, diagnostic, therapeutic and social purposes, and that it was necessary to determine how this could best be achieved whilst safeguarding privacy; for the manager, as for the epidemiologist, information was said to be 'the raw material of his activities'.

The report identified three major functions of an information service:

Research and intelligence:
Three components were described: medical/epidemiological (including research into the working of the National Health Service), operational research (including work study) and scientific intelligence (including the investigation of new techniques and equipment).

Publication and statistics:
These comprised the provision of operational data to doctors, administrators, and functional groups in the CSA; annual provision of statistics for public, parliamentary, and National Health Service comment and question; publication of advice in the form of booklets and pamphlets on health; and advertising, such as that on the dangers of smoking, pep pills, and hazards to children. It was emphasised that routine statistics could form only part of the activity of an information system: it was necessary to support this with an interrogation capability to provide facilities for follow-up inquiries.

Data processing:
This was regarded as the essential supporting activity to all others, involving data capture, data processing, information retrieval techniques, and the use of computers.

The report emphasised the need to strike a correct balance between routine data collection in anticipation of requirements and special collection exercises to answer particular kinds of inquiry. It urged a constant review of activities to ensure that the scope of routine data collection continued to reflect the demands which were being made of the data.

The report also stressed the importance of the establishment of a basic register of the people in each area, to which can be linked such activities as hospital discharges, immunisation programmes, and notifications of special disabilities or risks. Such a development was soon afterwards put into effect in Tayside[52], and then modified as a 'Community Health Index' for use in other health boards. The SCICON report also recommended that existing registers (e.g. for cancer, the blind, handicapped, cytology and other screening systems) and discharge data should be developed into a unified system for use in forward operational scheduling as well as for retrospective analysis and future longer-term planning. Furthermore there was managerial, clinical and epidemiological need to link medical records relating to individual patients – both those originating in different locations and also those generated over a period of time (several years); this would require the introduction of a satisfactory identification number and the commitment to use it, and a trial use of personal identification cards was suggested. The Community Health Index (CHI) provides a mechanism for achieving such linkage. The CHI also provides a unique method for the identification of individuals who fail to receive some prophylactic measure (e.g. immunisation), who escape health surveillance (e.g. young children or the elderly), or who fail to attend for some screening procedure (e.g. cervical cytology or screening for cardiovascular risk factors).

The Common Services Agency: Information Services Division:

Following the reorganisation of the National Health Service on 1 April 1974 the Common Services Agency (CSA) was set up to provide the Scottish Home and Health Department and the new Health Boards with a variety of services which are provided most efficiently by a single agency. One subdivision of the CSA is the Information Service Division (ISD), which has the following functions:

(a)   To develop agreed standards in information collection and processing in Scotland, and to process, analyse and interpret major data sets collated from all the health authorities in Scotland.

(b)   To co-ordinate computer services within Scotland, monitor computer developments and provide advice on computing and information processing in general.

(c)   To publish statistical and research reports, and maintain liaison with the General Register Office, Office of Population Censuses and Surveys, and other departments responsible for health related data.

(d)   To conduct health service research.

ISD is a National Health Service institution and differs from its parent Research and Intelligence Unit in being separated from the civil service, and hence in having a degree of independence in its function and particularly in the way that information is interpreted. ISD is under the control of a medically qualified Director (Dr Heasman until 1986), and this is important since the Division is responsible for handling large volumes of confidential medical data. There is a mixed complement of some 75 medical and other professional and administrative staff. One of the community medicine specialists in the division also acts part-time as medical statistician to GRO.

The research and statistics activities of ISD very closely parallel those of the Statistics and Research Division and the Operational Research section in DHSS. The exceptions are that Social Security Statistics (e.g. sickness and injury benefit claims for people absent from work, statistics on attendance allowances) are collected by DHSS for the whole of Great Britain, and statistics on prescribing in general practice are analysed by DHSS staff on behalf of SHHD, and tables are provided to ISD.

Regular meetings are held between the Division and community medicine specialists, statisticians, and records officers responsible for information services at health boards. The improved liaison has resulted in much greater co-operation between health boards and the Division and a greater understanding of each other's problems.

In 1976 a records officer was appointed to the Information Services Division. She maintains liaison with and fulfils a co-ordinating function for the health board records officers to ensure that they are complying with national policies as far as possible. By this liaison she promotes the standardisation of records and the uniform use of terms used for recording data for statistical purposes at both national and local level, and advises on standard codes of practice and on systems to safeguard against unauthorised access to records. In consultation with the manpower services division of the CSA and other appropriate bodies she provides guidance on suitable training programmes for records staff.

The research branch of ISD may conduct its own projects or respond to requests from the Scottish Home and Health Department. It was closely associated with the SHHD working party on Revenue Resource Allocation which derived a formula (including population, 'cross boundary flow', the availability of 'supra-specialties' and regional specialties, and the standardised mortality ratio for the 0–64 year age group of the population) for determining the annual revenue allocation for each health board. The final report of this working party – *Scottish Health Authorities Revenue Equalisation* (SHARE) – has, since 1975, been applied in the health service in Scotland, and the research branch is now responsible for the on-going statistical calculations which form the basis of revenue allocation to health boards. Further research work is also taking place in an attempt to improve the allocation method. This is particularly concerned with attempts to measure morbidity and the effect of social deprivation on health, and to more accurately assess work relating to out-patients who are treated outside their health board of residence.

Specific data schemes:

ISD collects a very wide range of data relating to the resources in the NHS and their utilisation. Data may be obtained for individual patients or as statistical aggregates. Schemes for which data are collected in respect of individuals include general hospital, maternity and neonatal discharges; mental hospital inpatients (admissions and discharges); abortions and the young chronic sick; cancer and handicapped children registrations; school health examinations; mass miniature radiography; and dental services.

Data on individuals are made available for research purposes only, and strict control is exercised over this. Most requests for individual data are met by omitting the name of the patient but including the hospital record number; the customer must then approach the consultant if he wishes to consult the medical record.

Data which come as statistical aggregates (i.e. counts only) can be grouped into statistics on service use and provision, on manpower, and on morbidity in the community. They include hospital bed use and outpatient statistics; dental statistics; vaccination and immunisation; chiropody; community nursing; community services for children; cervical cytology; family planning; ophthalmic services; laboratory statistics; radiography workload; manpower statistics for all hospital staff, general practitioners and all other health board employees; infectious diseases notifications; food poisoning; and sexually transmitted diseases.

The output from these various schemes is provided in a variety of publications and computer printouts, including disease and operation indices.

Apart from the production of routine statistics the ISD receives between 700 and 800 *ad hoc* requests for information per year. These vary from simple one figure answers to extremely complex requests, some of which may involve record linkage or the collection of considerable additional data. Most requests for detailed analysis come from SHHD and from the Scottish Health Service Planning Council and its supporting groups including the National Consultative Committees: SHHD has no in-house statistical advice and ISD provides its only source of such advice. Requests from research workers and from health boards, however, are more often concerned with the provision of data which they then analyse for themselves.

There are advantages in the existence of a centralised service and in a continuing collection of routine data: paramount is the need of SHHD, ministers, and other central and national bodies to have information available to assist them in administration and planning. A central body of data enables many questions to be answered readily, although data needs which require an *ad hoc* approach clearly arise from time to time. More complex questions on the operation of the NHS will require research projects to be undertaken to examine problem areas in more depth.

One of the main disadvantages of a centralised data system is the delay in production of data which occurs, partly from the sheer volume of data which requires handling, but mainly because the national picture requires records from all sources to be received before analysis can take place, and late returns from one health board can cause delays in the feedback of data to all other boards. Difficulties also arise in producing detailed information for local use from centrally held data, which necessarily are held in summary form, and in ensuring uniformity of standards in records practice.

Deficiencies in current health information systems, and prospects for the future

Some 6 *per cent* of the gross national product is consumed on the National Health Service. In order to secure the optimum use of resources, it is essential that this massive expenditure is managed in the best possible way. At present, information processing and statistical analysis for the entire Scottish Health Service (including those functions in the SHHD) probably consumes less than one *per cent* of the total revenue resources. The scope for increased efficiency and for savings is not great, and further development must rely on greater investment both centrally in ISD and in individual health authorities.

An effective information system should function at all levels of management, from clinicians responsible for patient management (for treatment, legal and research purposes) through administrators of health services, to those responsible for planning, both at a local level and nationally; it should also provide a framework for specific studies by clinicians and research workers. Even the most flexible and detailed systems will not be able to answer all questions, however, and there will therefore also be a facility for conducting special investigations into particular problems. The research branch of ISD can carry out a limited number of such projects but the Chief Scientist organisation exists to identify and sponsor research needs on a larger scale.

The outputs from an information system should enable comparisons to be made over a period of time (i.e. several years), and between units, hospitals, districts and regions. They should include procedures for monitoring the incidence of disease; the demand for services; service bottlenecks (using criteria such as waiting lists and waiting times for various forms of care, services or facilities which are not available, misplacement in acute beds); and all aspects of workload, including costs, related to specific client groups and to individual patients, where possible related to the seriousness of the condition – including community support and investigative procedures as well as hospital treatment. Information, however, should not relate only to the process of care. The outcome of care must be investigated, for example in terms of case fatality rates, complications and recurrence/readmission rates, time lapse before return to work, quality of life and patient satisfaction. Also the effectiveness of existing systems (e.g. for screening) or of innovations must be evaluated.

Information is needed to identify changes quickly and to project future improvements. It should also be possible to develop models in order to determine how changes in resources are likely to influence workload and throughput[53].

The basic framework for establishing a comprehensive information system of this type was developed in Scotland during the period 1961 to 1970, but this has not been exploited to anything approaching its full potential. The central problems – which are probably common to all health information systems – can be assessed as follows:

Lack of interest in evaluation and monitoring among clinicians:
This is a fundamental problem which relates to undergraduate and postgraduate training, and shows little sign of being resolved.

Reluctance by managers to insist on evaluation and a sound information base:
This situation may well now be changing with increased interest in management budgeting, as will be discussed later.

Accuracy:
Ideally information should be collected as a by-product of some other essential activity – either administrative (such as computer based 'hospital patient administration systems') or relating to patient care. Where this is not possible, information should be collected by skilled records staff who are an integral part of the information system and who are provided with regular feedback on the uses to which their data are put; without such feedback records staff lose interest and motivation, with resulting loss in accuracy.

User involvement:
The users of information are frequently not actively involved in the development of information systems, and as a result the data is often not exactly what is required. Worse still, it is often impossible to extract the required data from computer systems, either because of technical problems or else because coding is inadequate or un-standardised. For too long highly organised computer systems have created a gulf between the user and the data which has prevented their lively interaction – an interaction which existed in the public health administration in the latter half of the nineteenth century, and which has existed in the field of obstetrics from the 1940s until the present time.

Making the 'best' the enemy of the good:
There has undoubtedly been too much emphasis on the development of new systems and on exploiting 'leading edge' technology rather than on maximising the use that can be made of existing and well-tried systems. There is little point in adopting sophisticated techniques such as

networking, desirable as these are in the longer term, until more fundamental problems have been resolved.

Interpretation of financial manpower and clinical data:
It has not been possible to integrate data sources in order to enable comparison, in relation to outcome, of the costs of different forms of care. This synthesis of information is needed for different diseases (or diagnosis related groups) and for different client groups, and should include care and services in the community as well as in hospital. The information should be capable of being collated for hospital specialties, units or wards. By costing the product in relation to outcome it should be possible to direct expenditure to where it is likely to be most effective.

Record linkage:
No routine facility exists for linking over a prolonged time period records pertaining to individuals: such a facility is necessary for purposes such as
(i) monitoring the process of care (e.g. the number of laboratory investigations, transfers or readmissions) or for assessing the services used by or required by individuals or groups with special needs;
(ii) monitoring the outcome of care (e.g. long and short term reactions to drugs; the long term sequel of operative procedures);
(iii) determining the family history and pedigree of patients with genetic disease (this would require record linkage for individuals within families).

Inter-professional communication:
Communication between the various professionals concerned with the care of individual patients is often inadequate. It is desirable to develop, as is being achieved in Aberdeen, an integrated medical record which can be shared by the variety of professionals who may be concerned with the care of the patient (general practitioner, health visitor, consultant, midwife, clinical medical officer, paramedicals). Extracts of the record could also be used by professionals from other agencies (e.g. social work, housing). The problem-orientated medical record is ideal for sharing information for the benefit of the patient and the service.

Intra-professional insularity:
Where far-sighted and effective organisational changes have been made, there is often reluctance to adopt these elsewhere; good examples of this are the Sighthill (Edinburgh) system of shared antenatal care, and the Aberdeen problem-orientated medical record. Similarly, recommendations made for improving patient care, such as the reports of departmental subcommittees, are all too often ignored – important

examples being the Warnock report on Special Educational Needs[54] and the Timbury report[55].

General practitioner involvement:

Clinical information originates with the general practitioner, and the primary care team is responsible for the majority of contacts with patients and is the most effective mechanism for preventive care. Health authorities in Scotland are fortunate in that, in contrast to the situation in England and Wales, computing for primary care administration family practitioner committees (FCPs) has not developed as a separate entity. In consequence, the possibility exists for linking primary care and health authority data systems using a computer based index (the community health index, or CHI) of all patients registered with a general practitioner who are resident within a health authority area. This should enable the needs of primary care practice populations to be more accurately assessed, so that resources may be redeployed as appropriate, and so that preventive measures such as screening procedures and health surveillance may more adequately be evaluated.

The need for reliable measures of outcome:

Improved measures are required to permit monitoring of outcome over longer and shorter periods of time. It is important to be able to assess disability in various groups (e.g. the elderly or those with particular handicaps) so that the need for services can be assessed, and changes in disability monitored over time in relation to service provision. Such information would enable norms of good practice to be formulated, against which performance could be measured, and this would permit more effective planning of preventive, primary care, and hospital services for individual client groups. A reliable set of indices is also required for sensitively monitoring the overall health of populations, both for health authorities as a whole and for smaller areas or communities within health authorities.

Extension of information systems:

Information systems and norms of good practice need to be developed to encompass hitherto neglected areas such as the supply of drugs, the preventive maintenance of capital equipment, and health board services such as transport, hotel services, waste disposal, and energy expenditure.

A new stimulus to remedy at least some of these deficiencies has been provided by the appointment of general managers in health authorities throughout the United Kingdom, and more specifically by the recommendations[56] on management budgeting. The response to this in Scotland has been a proposal to link the introduction of management budgeting to the simultaneous improvement of management information systems at hospital level, and includes proposals for testing the feasibility of collecting and disseminating data at ward level. Pilot studies have begun at two Scottish hospitals to test the viability and the cost effectiveness of the proposals. The development of a national information system strategy which incorporates the following elements has also been suggested[57]:

(a) provision for individual Boards to submit to the Department plans for the development of their own information systems within the framework of the national strategy;

(b) proposals for local computer advisory structures to allow top management to mould and influence local plans for the development of information systems;

(c) incentives for the adoption of standard systems to facilitate integration of systems at both Board and national level and to minimise the unnecessary dissipation of scarce skilled computing resources:

(d) plans for increasing the funds available for the acquisition of computer hardware and centrally developed software;

(e) guidelines on the definition and collection of minimum sets of information for national purposes, and on the appropriate technology for given operational systems.

(f) the aim of maximising data integration, beginning with integrated hospital information systems.

It is the view of the Scottish Home and Health Department that greater investment in relevant information systems is likely to be highly cost-effective in improving the quality of management decisions. This is clearly the judgement in the private sector where a much higher proportion of costs is accounted for by information services.

Digest of main conclusions

Since 1732, and particularly during the eighteenth century, attempts have been made to develop information systems in hospitals which would permit evaluation of clinical practices and promote epidemiological enquiry. It was hoped that such systems would lead to more efficient use of resources and provide the basis for more effective planning. These efforts have not succeeded. During the past 30 years a variety of sophisticated information systems have been developed in Scotland, but their very considerable potential has still not begun to be fully realised. The more important reasons for this failure are lack of training and interest in the use of information for management and evaluation purposes among both clinicians and administrators; insufficient attention being paid to training records officers in the need for meticulous data recording and in the uses to which the data for which they are responsible are put; undue emphasis on exploiting new technology with neglect of the needs of users or potenital users of information; the insistence of many health authorities in developing their own systems rather than contributing to the development of standard systems; and insufficient investment being made in developing quick and easy methods for data analysis by users, and in improving methods of presenting data. The appointment of general managers to each health authority, the emphasis by the Scottish Home and Health Department on managing budgeting and greater efficiency in the use of resources may, however, provide the necessary stimulus to overcome at least some of these problems in the late 1980s.

Methods of analysing and presenting data relating to the health of communities have also advanced little since the remarkable efforts of the early Medical Officers of Health and of some of the medical statisticans who preceded them. Also, translating the information into action is now much more difficult with the separation of community health functions from those of the local authority: housing, the environment and social circumstances are fundamental determinants of health. Even within the health service, information systems are often separated from managers at the centre and from clinicians at the periphery, with the result that information is not fully exploited in planning and evaluating services.

Perhaps the most exciting recent development resulting from the new technology is the Community Health Index (CHI). This is a computer held index of all persons resident within the area served by a health authority who are registered with a general practitioner. It enables health services to be targetted on that section of the population which has the worst health or is most at risk, and this is extremely important in a country in which adult health is amongst the poorest in the developed world. The index can also be used to demonstrate variations in health and in the uptake or availability of health services, and to measure health characteristics for general practice populations. Another extremely important feature is the possibility of using the CHI to target health services through primary care teams, and to bring together community health, general practitioner and eventually hospital data sets.

Unfortunately, we are still looking forward to the grand horizon, where information is presented in a compelling way and in the required form to administrators and clinicians who insist on high quality data for effective management, planning, evaluation, resource allocation and epidemiological investigation. Until this goal – which has been sought for over two and half centuries – is reached, the limited resources of the health service will continue to be deployed to considerably less than maximum effectiveness, and the health of the population will remain poorer than it need be.

APPENDIX I
SCOTTISH HEALTH SERVICE STUDIES

1. Patients under Psychiatric Care in Hospital: Scotland 1963 by Dr Alwyn Smith and Vera Carstairs, 1966.

2. Home Nursing in Scotland by Vera Carstairs, 1966.
3. Nurses' Work in Hospitals in the North-Eastern Region, 1967.
4. An Assessment of the Current Status of the "At Risk" Register by Dr R.G. Walker, 1967.
5. Cancer Registration 1959–61.
6. Dietary Study of 4,365 Scottish Infants – 1965 by Dr Gavin C. Arneil, 1967.
7. Student Nurses in Scotland. Characteristics of Success and Failure by Dr Margaret Scott Wright, 1968.
8. Cancer Registration 1962–64.
9. Nursing Workload per Patient as a basis for Staffing, 1969.
10. A study of the work of hospital junior medical staff by Dr. R.G. Walker, W.R. Miller and I.G. McLean, 1969.
11. Channels of communication by Vera Carstairs, 1970.
12. Comparative Survey, Professional Surgical Unit, Aberdeen Royal Infirmary, 1970.
13. A Study of Unmarried Mothers and their Children in Scotland by Sylvia Weir, 1970.
14. Health Education and Alcohol by Dr L Boyd, 1970.
15. The General Practitioner's Use of Medical Records by Dr J. Cormack, 1971.
16. Infant Mortality in Scotland by Dr I.D.G. Richards, 1971.
17. Studies of Illness and Death in the Elderly in Glasgow by Dr B Isaacs, 1971.
18. The Evaluation of a Direct Nursing Attachment in a North Edinburgh Practice by Dr S.W. Macgregor, Dr M.A. Heasman, and Dr E.V. Kuenssberg, 1971.
19. The Elderly in Residential Care by Vera Carstairs and Marion Morrison, 1971.
20. Scottish Hospital Morbidity Data 1961–1968 by Dr E. Lockwood, 1971.
21. The Elderly in Scottish Hospitals 1961–66 by Mr B.N. Downie, 1972.
22. A Study of Long Stay Admissions to the Acute Medical Wards of the Aberdeen Hospitals by Dr Audrey Sutherland, 1972.
23. Outpatient Services in the Scottish Border Counties by Dr Rosamond Gruer, 1972.
24. Health Services in a Population of 250,000 by Vera Carstairs and Vida Howie, 1972.
25. The Sanitary Inspector in Scotland by Dr Geroge Cust and Mr James Pearson, 1973.
26. Cancer Registration 1965–67, 1973.
27. Time Study of Consultations in General Practice by Professor I.M. Richardson and I.C. Buchan, 1973.
28. Scottish Ambulance Service by Mr D. Davidson, 1973.
29. The Livingston Project – The First Five Years by Dr A.H. Duncan, 1973.
30. The Evaluation of an X-Ray Unit in a Health Centre by Vida Howie, 1974.
31. Patient Costing Study by Dr E.M. Russell, 1974.
32. Value of a day-bed unit in a General Hospital Practice by Dr Ian W. Kemp, 1975.
33. Needs of the Elderly in the Scottish Borders by Dr Rosamond Gruer, 1975.
34. The Measurement of Need in Old People by Professor Isaacs and Mrs Y. Neville, 1976.
35. Meals Services for the Elderly in Scotland by Gillian Stanley and W. Lutz, 1976.
36. Survey of Present Health Care Provisions for Staff of Health Boards by James Pearson, William Prentice and Dorothy Radwanski, 1976.
37. Work Study of District Nursing Staff by Mrs Jean B. McIntosh and Professor I.M. Richardson, 1976.
38. Mental Subnormality in North-East Scotland. A Multi-disciplinary Study of Total Population by Dr G. Innes, A.W. Johnston and W.M. Millar, 1978.
39. Detoxification of Habitual Drunken Offenders – Dr J.R. Hamilton, Ann Griffith, Dr B. Ritson and Professor Cairns Aitken, 1978.
40. A Nutrition Survey of Immigrant Children in Glasgow (1974–76) by K.M. Goel *et al*, 1979.
41. The Establishment and Development of Local Health Councils by Dorothy Bochel and Morag MacLaren, 1979.
42. Services for the Elderly, a survey of the characteristics and needs of a population of 5000 old people by John Bond and Vera Carstairs, 1982.

References

(1)   Flinn, M., Gillespie, J., Hill, N., Maxwell, A., Mitchison, R., and Smout, C. *Scottish Population History from the 17th Century to the 1930s*. Cambridge: Cambridge University Press, 1977.

(2)   Clifton, F. *The state of physick, ancient and modern, briefly considered: with a plan for the improvement of it*. London, 1732.

(3)   Cleland, J. *Enumeration of the inhabitants of the City of Glasgow and its connected suburbs*. Glasgow, 1820.

(4)   Watt, R. "Treatise on the history, nature and treatment of chincough to which is adjoined an inquiry into the relative mortality of the principal diseases of children and the numbers who have died under ten years of age, in Glasgow, during the last 30 years". Glasgow: John Smith & Son, 1813.

(5)   Edmonds, T.R. "On the Mortality of Glasgow and on the increasing mortality in England". *Lancet*, 1836, ii, pp.353–59.

(6)   Buchanan, A. "Report of the diseases which prevailed among the poor, during the summer of 1830". *Glasgow Medical Journal*, 1830, 3, pp.435–50.

(7)   Cowan, R. "Vital statistics of Glasgow illustrating the sanitary condition of the population". Paper read before the statistical section of the British Association, 21 September 1840.

(8)   Perry, R.C. "Facts and observations on the sanitary state of Glasgow during the last year showing the connection existing between poverty, disease and crime with appendices containing reports from the district surgeons". Pamphlet dedicated to the Lord Provost of Glasgow.

(9)   Strang, J. *Economic and social statistics of Glasgow and the West of Scotland for various years from 1851 to 1861*. Glasgow, 1862.

(10)   "Report of a committee of the British Association for the Advancement of Science (1843). Vital statistics of large towns in Scotland". *J. Stat. Soc.*, 6, pp.150–66.

(11)   Stark, James. "Contribution to the vital statistics of Scotland". Journal of the Statistical Society, 1851, 14, pp.48–89.

(12)   McKinlay P. Selected papers: private compilation.

(13)   Gairdner, W.T. "Reports by the Medical Officer of Health for the City of Glasgow to the Board of Police". Appendix III. Memorandum in regard to the Preparation of the vital Statistics of Glasgow.

(14)   Gairdner, W.T. *Annual Report on the Health of the City* (of Glasgow) for the year 1870. 1871.

(15)   Sanitary Department Review (1871), Glasgow, p.516.

(16)   MacFadyen, J.R. "The theory of the death rate, with measurements of the comparative force of mortality, in Glasgow and other cities – Proceedings of the Philosophical Society of Glasgow", February 22, 1871, pp.425–42.

(17)   Littlejohn, H.D. *Report on the Sanitary condition of the City of Edinburgh*. Edinburgh, 1865.

(18)   Buchanan, M.S. *History of the Glasgow Royal Infirmary*, Glasgow: Lumsden & Son, 1832.

(19)   McFarlane, J. "Report of the diseases which prevailed among the poor of Glasgow during the autumn of 1827". *Glasgow Medical Journal*, 1828, 1, pp.97–109.

(20)   Cowan, C. (1841) Referred to in *Lancet*, 1841, i, pp.649–52, (ref.21).

(21)   Lancet (1841). 'On the advantages of statistical records of disease in our hospitals, dispensaries and asylums'. Editorial. *Lancet*, 1841, i, pp.649–52.

(22)   Statistical Society. "Report of the Committee on Hospital Statistics". *J. Stat. Soc.*, 1842, 5, pp.168–76.

(23)   Medical Officers of Metropolitan Hospitals. "Statistics of the General Hospitals of London, 1861". *J. Stat. Soc.*, 1862, 25, p.384.

(24)   Cameron, D. "Admissions to Scottish Mental Hospitals in the last 100 years". *Brit. J. Prev. Soc. Med.*, 1954, 8, pp.180–86.

(25) Inter-Departmental Committee on Insurance Medical Records. "The Form of Medical Record to be Prescribed Under the Terms of Service of Insurance Practitioners". London: HMSO, 1920.

(26) Gillie, A. Ministry of Health: Central Health Services Council. Standing Medical Advisory Committee. The field of work of the family doctor, report of the sub-committee. London, HMSO: 1964.

(27) Tunbridge, Prof. R.E. Ministry of Health: Central Health Services Council. Standing Medical Advisory Committee. The standardisation of hospital medical records, report of the sub-committee. London: HMSO, 1965.

(28) Scottish Home and Health Department. Scottish Health Services Council. Hospital medical records in Scotland, development and standardisation, report of a sub-committee of the Standing Medical Advisory Committee (Chmn. Prof. J. Walker). Edinburgh: HMSO, 1967.

(29) Cormack, J.J.C. "The General Practitioner's Use of Medical Records". Scottish Health Service Studies No. 15. Ed: Scottish Home and Health Department. 1971.

(30) Department of Health and Social Security. "Interim Report of the Joint Working Party on Redesign of Medical Records in General Practice". London: HMSO, 1972.

(31) Zander, L.I., Shirley, A.A., Thomas, P. *Medical Records in General Practice*. Occasional paper 5. Royal College of General Practitioners ISBN 85084 062 7, 1978.

(32) College of General Practitioners. "College Classification of Disease". *Journal of the College of General Practitioners*, 1959, 2, pp.140–59.

(33) Walford, P.A. "The art of record keeping in general practice". *Journal of the Royal College of General Practitioners*, 1962, 5, pp.265–69.

(34) Harden, K.A., Harden, R.McG., and Reekie, D. "Use of feature cards in general practice". *British Medical Journal*, 1974, 2, p.162.

(35) Burchell, K, Barclay, R., Ryan, M.P. "The use of the Problem Oriented Medical Record and Feature Cards in Practice Management and Research". *Health Bulletin*, 1975, xxxiii, pp.210–13.

(36) Grummitt, A. "Real-Time Record Management in General Practice". *Int. J. Bio-Medical Computing*, 1977, 8, pp.131–150.

(37) General Practice Computing. "Evaluation of the 'Micros for GPs' Scheme: Final Report". London: HMSO, 1985.

(38) Chalmers, A.K. The Health of Glasgow, 1818–1925, *An outline*. Glasgow, Glasgow Corporation, 1930.

(39) Cathcart, E.D. "Report of the Committee on Scottish Health Services". Edinburgh: Dept. of Health for Scotland (Cmnd.5204). 1936.

(40) Department of Health for Scotland. Maternal Morbidity and Mortality in Scotland. Report of a clinical sub-committee of the Scientific Advisory Committee (Chmn. Professor D.P.D. Wilkie). Edinburgh: HMSO.

(41) Department of Health for Scotland. "Infant Mortality in Scotland". Report of a Sub-committee of the Scientific Advisory Committee (Chmn. Sir John Boyd Orr). Edinburgh: HMSO, 1943.

(42) McIlwaine, G.M., Howat, R.C.L., Dunn, F., and Macnaughton, M.C. Scotland 1977 Perinatal Mortality Survey. Glasgow: University of Glasgow, Department of Obstetrics and Gynaecology, 1979.

(43) Lancet. "Sir Dugald Baird's Birthday Present". Editorial. *Lancet*, 1980, ii, pp.839–40.

(44) Department of Health. "Medical Records and Secretarial Services", (5) Hospital Organisation and Management Service Report No. 2. London: HMSO, 1959.

(45) Scottish Home and Health Department. *Organisation of Medical Work in the Hospital Service in Scotland*. First Report of Joint Working Party (Chmn. John Brotherston). HMSO: Edinburgh, 1967.

(46) Heasman, M.A. Scottish Hospital In-Patient Statistics: Sources and Uses. *Health Bulletin*, 1970, xxvi, No. 4.

(47) Heasman, M.A., and Clarke, J.A. Medical Record Linkage in Scotland. *Health*

Bulletin, May 1979, pp.97–103.

(48) Lockwood, E. Scottish Hospital Morbidity Data 1961–1968. Scottish Health Service Studies No. 20. Edinburgh: Scottish Home and Health Department, 1971.

(49) Heasman, M.A. SCRIPS Success or failure. "A critical study of the Scottish Consultant Review of In-Patient Statistics". Unpublished paper.

(50) Ockenden, J.M., and Bodenham, K.E. *Focus on Medical Computer Development*. A study of the Scottish scene by Scientific Control Systems Ltd. London: Nuffield Provincial Hospitals Trust, 1970.

(51) Bodenham, K.E., and Wellman, F. "Foundations for health service management". A Scicon report for the Scottish Home and Health Department on the requirements for a health service information system. London: Nuffield Provincial Hospitals Trust, 1972.

(52) Tayside Health Board. "The Tayside Master Patient Index". Dundee: Tayside Health Board, 1976.

(53) Alderson, M.R. Health Information – general aspects. In: National Health Survey Systems in the European Economic Community. Proceedings of a conference held in Brussels. Commission of the European Communities, (Ed. P. Armitage). 1974.

(54) Special Educational Needs. Report of the Committee of Enquiry into the Education of Handicapped Children and Young People (Chairman Mrs. H.M. Warnock). London: HMSO, 1978.

(55) Timbury, G.C. Scottish Home and Health Department. Scottish Education Department. Report on services for the elderly with mental disability in Scotland – a report by a Programme Planning Group of the Scottish Health Service Planning Council and the Advisory Council on Social Work. Edinburgh: HMSO, 1979.

(56) Scottish Home and Health Department. "General Management in the Scottish Health Service: Implementation – The First Steps: Circular 1985 (GEN) 4." Edinburgh: SHHD, 1985.

(57) ICSAG. Paper submitted to the Information and Computer Services Advisory Group by SHHD, 1985.

5. *Economic Aspects of Health Care in the Twentieth Century*

Pat Stuart and Gavin Mooney

CONTENTS

About the Authors

GAVIN MOONEY

Gavin Mooney graduated from the University of Edinburgh in 1969. From 1977 he was Director of the Health Economics Research Unit at the Univesrity of Aberdeen and in 1982 he was appointed Professor of Health Economics there. In June 1986, he went to live and work in Denmark where he is Visiting Professor in the Department of Social Medicine, University of Copenhagen.

PAT STUART

Pat Stuart graduated from the University of Aberdeen in 1983. At the time of writing she was a Research Assistant at the Health Economics Research Unit at the University of Aberdeen.

Authors' Note

This essay is a review of the twentieth century development of the health care sector in Scotland from the point of view of political economists.

The first section traces the economic development of selected Scottish hospitals throughout the period. This is followed by a more general outline of the growth of the National Health Service since its inception.

The second section offers an economist's analysis of changing patterns of care throughout the period. Developments in the health services are set in the context of the economic and social circumstances prevailing in the nation, the changing policy objectives are examined to identify shifts in the economic rationale underlying the development of services.

In the final section, it is suggested there is some distance to be travelled in pursuit of the original goals set for the National Health Service in 1948. The economic objectives of efficiency and equity are implicitly present, at least in part, but the history of the health service in Scotland this century suggests a need for more explicit rational planning if these important goals are to be met more effectively in the future than they have been in the past.

Economic Aspects of Health Care in the Twentieth Century

Introduction

In preparing this chapter, we have been aware of two problems. First, we are economists by training, not economic historians. This has meant that while we understand the economic issues underlying the Scottish health service in this century, we are not skilled in presenting that understanding in a proper historical perspective. Second, we were perhaps initially over-ambitious, not appreciating that historical research may be severely constrained because of lack of availability of appropriate data, a lack which often is absolute. The data are not there and now cannot be resurrected, assuming they ever existed at all. Consequently the final product suffers from being designed initially on the assumption that a complete data set would be available. That has proved not to be the case.

Given the lack of data on trends in expenditure, resource use etc, especially in the period up to the formation of the National Health Service in 1948, we have not placed undue emphasis in this chapter on the presentation of economic figures. However, the next section does highlight some changes through time, especially in the post 1948 era when the data are inevitably so much better.

Thereafter we review the changing health care sector in Scotland in this century very much from an economic perspective. In particular we emphasise the changes that have occurred in the underlying economic rationale. Finally we attempt to suggest some lessons from the past which may prove relevant to the economic well being of the health service in Scotland for the rest of this century and perhaps beyond.

Economic Trends

To trace the growth of expenditure on health services over the entire century has proved impossible, due to the complex and unco-ordinated pattern of services before 1948. However, we can gain some impression of the development of the main teaching hospitals from the data we have for five of these.

Table 1 shows for these hospitals, changes in total expenditure from 1900 to 1980.

Table 1   Total Expenditure in January 1974 Prices (£'000)

	Edinburgh Royal Infirmary	Glasgow Royal Infirmary	Glasgow Western Infirmary	Dundee Royal Infirmary	Aberdeen Royal Infirmary
1900	476.7	—	262.4	109.3	104.6
1910	490.0	416.9	345.2	150.6	119.6
1920	360.0	343.4	275.8	132.2	98.6
1930	839.4	612.8	472.2	269.1	193.3
1940	—	795.5	600.3	314.6	379.9
1950	2,197.2	1,846.5	1,256.2	869.1	—
1960	2,591.8	2,360.8	1,833.4	1,125.4	1,465.8
1970	4,665.3	4,194.5	3,507.3	2,741.6	3,238.8
1980	9,783.1	8,471.5	2,951.2	2,951.2	7,852.7

Sources: *Burdett's Hospitals and Charities Annual* (London, various years) and SHHD Scottish Health Service Costs (Edinburgh, various years).

Clearly these figures are difficult to interpret in isolation. Nonetheless for these hospitals – all major hospitals over the whole of the twentieth century – the rate of growth of expenditure is *much* greater in the 40 years after 1940 than in the 40 years before. Whether that is a function solely of growth in expenditure in health care or in hospital care generally or a result of centralisation in these facilities is difficult to judge. However, we can form some view of the changing size of these hospitals by examining the number of available beds through time, as in Table 2. (The figures in brackets are percentage occupancy.)

Table 2   *Numbers of Available Beds* (Percentage Occupancy)

	Edinburgh Royal Infirmary	Glasgow Royal Infirmary	Glasgow Western Infirmary	Dundee Royal Infirmary	Aberdeen Royal Infirmary	Total
1900	780 (89)	582 (94)	420 (97)	300 (74)	240 (87)	2,322
1910	926 (91)	589 (103)	540 (97)	400 (75)	240 (94)	2,695
1920	963 (90)	665 (102)	600 (93)	400 (86)	270 (92)	2,898
1930	1,010 (96)	782 (104)	642 (98)	420 (107)	366 (102)	3,220
1940	—	1,151 (64)	674 (73)	507 (60)	560 (66)	—
1950	1,157 (89)	918 (83)	625 (92)	510 (?)	610 (94)	3,820
1960	1,068 (83)	896 (83)	636 (89)	549 (84)	615 (87)	3,764
1970	985 (85)	849 (82)	658 (84)	585 (83)	699 (82)	3,776
1980	965 (82)	766 (77)	539 (76)	249 (77)	752 (77)	3,271

Sources: as Table 1.

While there has clearly been an increase in beds in these hospitals over the century – approaching 50 *per cent* on average – the more significant change is clearly in the growth of expenditure per bed.

With reference to in-patients for these same hospitals, there is again a marked rise through time.

Table 3   *Number of In-patients*

	Edinburgh Royal Infirmary	Glasgow Royal Infirmary	Glasgow Western Infirmary	Dundee Royal Infirmary	Aberdeen Royal Infirmary
1900	9,569	6,802	4,850	3,335	2,646
1910	12,342	8,311	9,230	4,098	3,140
1920[1]	11,751	9,772	8,718	5,456	3,009
1930[2]	19,626	16,688	12,576	8,967	5,763
1940[2]	n.a.	16,483	10,492	8,174	8,495
1950[3]	23,239	17,821	13,116	13,613	14,238
1960[4]	26,919	20,861	17,185	14,083	18,706
1970[5]	27,730	27,767	20,846	17,642	19,808
1980[5]	31,819	28,116	19,269	6,697	25,128

[1]Figures for 1919; [2]new in-patients; [3]in-patients admitted; [4]average in-patients × 365 average length of stay; [5]in-patients discharged.

Sources: as Table 1.

Combining Table 2 with Table 3 gives a picture of what was happening to average length of stay. This is presented in Table 4.

Table 4   *Average Length of Stay (days)*

	Edinburgh Royal Infirmary	Glasgow Royal Infirmary	Glasgow Western Infirmary	Dundee Royal Infirmary	Aberdeen Royal Infirmary
1900	26.5	29.4	30.7	24.3	28.8
1910	24.9	26.6	20.7	26.7	26.2
1920	26.9	25.3	23.4	23.0	30.1
1930	18.0	17.8	18.3	18.3	23.6
1940	—	41.5	17.1	13.6	15.9
1950	16.2	15.6	16.0	—	—
1960	12.0	13.0	12.0	12.0	10.4
1970	11.0	9.2	9.7	10.0	10.6
1980	9.1	7.7	7.8	10.4	8.4

Sources: as Table 1.

Clearly there are various possible explanations for the very substantial fall in length of stay – greater centralisation in these facilities, greater use of convalescent hospitals, changing case mix as patterns of morbidity changed and so on. It would require a separate research study to determine the extent to which these figures reflect increased productivity in hospital care through time. It is certainly difficult to believe that this is not an important contributor to these large falls in lengths of stay over time.

In Table 5, we illustrate the growth of health service expenditure during the National Health Service period, by relating it both to population growth and to growth of Scottish Gross Domestic Product (GDP).

Table 5   *Expenditures on the National Health Service*

	Total NHS Expenditure (January 1974 = 100) (£000)	NHS Expenditure per Head of Population (£)	NHS Expenditure as % of Scottish GDP
1949–50	142,869	28.04	—
1951–52	133,948	26.28	—
1956–57	153,777	30.03	—
1961–62	186,124	35.94	4.57
1966–67	245,834	47.27	5.32
1971–72	315,567	60.35	6.20
1976–77	390,317	74.99	6.17
1981–82	506,685	97.28	8.24

Sources: *Scottish Health Statistics*, Department of Health for Scotland (later SHHD), (Edinburgh, various years), and A.M. Gray op.cit.

In comparison to England expenditure per capita in Scotland has increased more rapidly so that today Scotland receives about 24 *per cent* more per capita than England. Most of this growth has occurred in the hospital sector. Indeed over the thirty years to 1981 the proportion of total National Health Service expenditure going to hospitals rose from less than 61 *per cent* to over 70 *per cent*.

Table 6 shows some interesting differences in growth rates of labour and non labour costs over time.

Table 6 *Average Annual Rates of Growth of Labour and Non-Labour Hospital Services Expenditure* (excluding capital expenditure)

	Average Annual Growth Rate of Labour Costs (%)	Average Annual Growth Rate of Non-Labour Costs (%)
1951–57	8.3	6.1
1957–63	8.2	4.7
1963–69	9.5	6.3
1969–75	19.9	16.1
1975–81	19.1	23.9
1951–81	12.9	11.2

Source: A.M. Gray, *The Rising Cost of Scottish Hospitals, 1951–81*, Ph.D. Thesis, University of Aberdeen, 1983, Table 5.9. Gray op.cit.

For the whole period, average growth in labour costs was significantly higher, at 12.9 *per cent* compared with 11.2 *per cent*. The figures for sub-periods show growth in labour costs to be higher in every period, except the last i.e. from 1975 to 1981. While a number of explanations are possible, it may well be significant that this last period was one of relatively high unemployment when the bargaining power of National Health Service staff was comparatively weak.

Finally, Tables 7 and 8 show how the major resources in any health service – doctors and nurses – increased during the period of the National Health Service.

Table 7 *Total Qualified Hospital Nursing and Midwifery Staff*

	Whole Time	Index (1948 = 100)	Part Time	Index (1948 = 100)
1948	17,300	100.0	3,250	100.0
1951	18,984	109.7	2,878	88.6
1954	20,427	118.1	2,890	88.9
1957	21,586	124.8	4,150	127.7
1960	22,971	132.8	5,209	160.3
1963	24,212	140.0	7,411	228.0
1966	26,251	151.7	8,853	272.4
1969	27,697	160.1	11,686	359.6
1972	29,805	172.3	16,356	503.3
1975	33,659	194.6	23,620	726.8
1978	34,487	199.3	23,032	708.7
1981	38,051	219.9	23,974	737.7
1983	41,337	238.9	24,115	742.0

Source: Gray, op.cit.

Of course, the increase in numbers indicated has been affected to a considerable extent by shorter working hours and longer holidays. Gray[1], for example, estimates that over this period the reduction in annual hours worked by whole-time and part-time nursing staff of all grades ranged from 20 *per cent* to 35 *per cent*.

Table 8   *Total Numbers of Qualified Doctors in Hospitals and Primary Care*

	Total Hospital WT + PT (excluding honorary)	Index (1948 = 100)	Primary Care[1]	Index (1948 = 100)
1948	1,900	100.0	2,600	100.0
1956	2,678	140.9	2,936	112.9
1965	3,304	173.9	2,771	106.6
1974	5,260	276.8	2,959	113.8
1983	6,305	331.8	3,460	133.1

[1]Includes trainees and assistants.
Source: Scottish Health Statistics, op.cit.

The overall picture appears thus to be one of substantial growth in health care expenditure and resources particularly it would seem in the second half of the eighty year period examined (although the paucity of data prior to 1948 makes this a difficult judgement to make). Certainly the National Health Service period indicates very substantial growth placing us, perhaps surprising for a relatively poor country in West European terms, up among the leaders in terms of the proportion of our national income that we spend on health care.

Economic Views

Beyond the above presentation of data on trends,we move to consider the changing picture through time of health care in Scotland from an economic perspective. As a first step, it is potentially enlightening to consider what the objectives of health care policy have been and how they have changed over time. It is not possible for example to consider the notion of economic efficiency in any empirical way unless we have some idea of what it is that individuals or society are attempting to be efficient about.

In looking back to the early part of the century to get some idea of the standard of living it is worth noting that average civil earnings (in 1984 prices) were running at a level of about £1,700 *per annum*[2]. However this figure masks the fact that there were very wide variations in income across different groups and from year to year, especially as a result of variation in food prices.

Generally in the early twentieth century, the majority of Scots enjoyed a very low standard of living. This was reflected in the housing conditions. Even by the time of the First World War nearly half of the population of Scotland was living in one- or two-roomed houses compared with only 7 *per cent* of the population of England[3]. Mitchison[4] points to the observed association between living conditions and health, the infant mortality rate for one-roomed dwellings being double that for 4-roomed dwellings (not that all of this could be ascribed to housing differences). It is hardly surprising then that the Royal Commission on Scottish Housing reporting in 1917[5] drew a horrifying picture of over-crowded dwellings with pathetically inadequate and insanitary toilet facilities.

It is also to be noted that it was in the first decade of this century that figures for mortality rates, infant mortality rates and expectation of life in Scotland began to compare unfavourably with the equivalent English figures. In the late nineteenth century, Scotland had enjoyed a slight advantage over England by all of these measures.

In looking at the economics of health care policy in twentieth century Scotland various theories can be put forward for health care activity and somewhat more specifically for state intervention in health care – the latter being in effect the central, dominating issue in the provision of health services in twentieth century Scotland.

The earliest state intervention was designed to isolate the infectious and contagious sick in an attempt to limit the spread of disease. This reflected concern over the devastating effects of frequent epidemics, and the essence of such policy was to preserve the health of the uncon-taminated, rather than to treat the victims. By the nineteenth century the connection between dirt and disease was becoming ever more apparent, and an increasing amount of state activity was directed toward inter-vention. By the beginning of the twentieth century in the words of the Cathcart Report[6] '... the sanitary code of Scotland embraced among other things the registration of births and deaths: notification, isolation and treatment of infectious diseases; vaccination against smallpox; pro-vision of water supplies, sewerage and drainage; public cleansing and lighting; removal of nuisances; control of density of buildings and regu-lation of streets and highways; internal sanitation of houses; smoke abate-ment; inspection of food to prevent adulteration and ensure purity; and provision for burial of the dead.'

The nature of the Scottish Poor Law and the economic philosophy it espoused is of particular significance to the history of health care pro-vision in Scotland. It was a central tenet of Scottish Poor Law that relief should only be made available to those who were both poor and disabled (i.e. incapable of work). The eligibility of dependent members of a household was defined solely with reference to the capacity of the bread-winner to work, and thus to provide for care. The 1845 Poor Law Amendment Act, designed to rationalise the Scottish Poor Law system, made clear the responsibility of the Parochial Boards to see that, wher-ever poorhouses were built or expanded, there should be adequate arrangements for the dispensing of medicines to the sick poor and that there should be medical attendance, provided by the Parish, for the inmates. It was in this way that a framework was provided for the development of a Poor Law hospital service.

There was considerable variation in provision, conditions and rates, between Scottish parishes and consequently major locational inequities. In spite of such variation, however, parishes were careful not to provide more than a basic minimum of care. The guiding principle was that pauperism was an avoidable failure on the part of the individual. Benevolence or compassion would only encourage resort to the parish and were, therefore, inappropriate. Poor relief was to be seen as a last resort, when self-help had failed. Provision was spartan. The contrast between care in the voluntary hospitals, and in the Poor Law hospitals, was stark. New techniques were invariably slow to make their appearance in the Poor Law hospitals. This in turn helped ensure that social class inequalities were increased since conditions were not attractive to medical staff, who could work in far better conditions, with access to new technology, in the voluntary hospitals.

In 1904, the Medical Relief Committee recommended that any poor houses erected in the future should have separate hospital buildings[7]. A trend toward such separation had begun in England around 1867, but by the time of the 1909 Poor Law report only three custom-built hospitals had been erected in Scotland for the sick poor, and all of these were in Glasgow. Everywhere else in Scotland, provision for the sick was still made in the general poorhouse[8].

In the 1909 report, the Commissioners observed that 'Attached to a few of the large poorhouses, we found well equipped hospitals or hospital wards and some of those recently erected are excellently planned. But in our opinion, they all suffer from the fact that they form part of the general poorhouse, and are managed under conditions which militate against their success as hospitals for the treatment of the sick'[9]. It was also stated in the report that of the 68 poorhouses in Scotland 26 still had no trained nurses. 'Not only so, but pauper nursing it appears, is permissible in all Scottish poorhouses'[10] (Pauper nursing, that is the use of inmates to provide care for others, had been prohibited in England and Ireland 12 years previously.) As the Poor Law report states:

"the Scottish Sanitary Authorities unlike the English have no power to provide hospitals other than those for the treatment of infectious disease. On the one hand we have the voluntary hospitals struggling to cope with the demands made upon them, and unable to accommodate everyone seeking treatment within their walls; on the other hand, we have the Poor Law Authority gradually providing hospitals which are primarily for pauper cases, but which also receive others whose destitution mainly consists in the fact that they are in need of hospital treatment which they cannot obtain elsewhere"[11].

Terms of admission to the voluntary hospitals varied considerably between towns. In 1909, admission to the Edinburgh Royal Infirmary was free, but in the other major towns, the main means of gaining admission was by subscriber's line. Admission terms for those without a subscriber's line varied also. At Glasgow Royal Infirmary, these were charged £2.4s. to cover residence of no more than a month. There were generally no inquiries into the financial circumstances of people seeking admission, and it was alleged by the Commissioners in 1909 that 'the benefits of the infirmaries are not infrequently taken advantage of by persons well able to pay for treatment'[12]. Furthermore the treatment of the great majority of cases, once admitted, was absolutely free. This contrasted starkly with the situation in the Poor Law hospitals, where patients or their families were liable to be required to refund the cost of treatment, in whole or in part. Some were being charged as much as 15 shillings per week. Besides this financial cost, patients had to bear the stigma of reliance on the Poor Law, and the risk of disenfranchisement. There is thus little to suggest that, even in their own terms, either hospital sector was particularly efficient.

There was no effective or consistent co-operation between the voluntary and the Poor Law hospitals, and no clear distinction between the cases dealt with in the two sectors. However there was a tendency for the voluntary hospitals to concentrate their resources on the treatment of acute, or unusual cases, and to send the residue to the Poor Law hospitals, which consequently had to deal with a high proportion of chronic illness. This imbalance tended to override consideration of the economic status of patients.

The benefits of hospital care, of course, were generally only available to those living in or near cities and large burghs. It was pointed out quite forcefully in the Scottish minority report of the Poor Law Commissioners that for thousands of people, no medical attendance at all was provided. On some of the Hebridean islands, infectious disease was rife, and there was a high incidence of tuberculosis. The proportion of deaths not certified by a doctor could reach 60 or 70 *per cent* on some islands[13]. Change however was on the way. At the beginning of the century, Britain remained very much a colonial power and a major trading nation in international markets. Much of the wealth and income of the country was dependent on that power and trade. It was therefore with some considerable concern, given the need to defend these sources of power, that it was revealed from studies of army recruits that the general health status of the working class was declining at the start of the century. This coincided with growing militarism in other countries, especially Germany, adding weight to the argument of those who called for a re-appraisal of attitudes to social problems.

This was a major shift in political thinking. Health – beyond the immediate concerns of controlling the spread of epidemics rather than the treatment of the sick – had been seen very much as the responsibility of the individual, alleviated only and to a very limited extent by the philanthropy of those to whom the health of others mattered for whatever reasons (an issue we will return to later in the century at the formation of the National Health Service).

Health thus became a matter of public concern – not just environmental health for the benefits it could bring through reduction of epidemics and their carnage but also individual health as a major input to the defence of the realm.

Out of these concerns and – according to Gilbert – a large dose of political realism and of wheeling and dealing, emerged the 1911 National Insurance Act. It had little to do with sound insurance principles. Indeed Gilbert[14] argues that it 'was more clearly the result of the powerful and conflicting political pressures exerted by the three great social institutions most affected by health insurance – the friendly societies, the commercial insurance industry and the British medical profession'. What the Act did in effect was to provide compulsory insurance coverage for all workers over 16 earning less than £160 per annum (the income tax limit) and all manual workers, regardless of income. Contributions were originally set at 7s. per week for men and 6s. for women, Benefits included: medical treatment by a panel doctor of the patients' choice for the insured; sickness benefit of 10s. per week for men and 7s.6d. for women for up to 26 weeks; disability benefit of 5s. per week; admission to sanatoria for certain diseases for the insured and dependants.

By the mid 1930s, the Cathcart report was reflecting a more humanitarian attitude to health care objectives while at the same time still accepting the economic argument that investing in health was good for business. It is stated, for example, that 'health among the workers and industrial efficiency are but two aspects of the same question'[15].

The purpose of the National Health Service (Scotland) Bill was stated to be to provide for '. . . the establishment in Scotland of a comprehensive health service designed to secure improvement in the physical and mental health of the people of Scotland and the prevention, diagnosis and treatment of illness. . .'[16]. The National Health Service, as conceived by Bevan, was to establish a system of health care for all, with as equitable a pattern of access, both social and geographic, as possible. Services were to be provided free of charge, except where special provision should be made for charges.

Certainly the 'cradle to the grave' objective of the National Health Service has not been fulfilled in the way that the founding fathers presumably expected. But they did not foresee the changing needs and expectations of the population nor of the medical profession.

At the same time it has to be recognised that the National Health Service, as Watkin[17] has remarked, 'created no new hospitals, trained no new doctors, brought no new drugs or methods of treatment into being'. However, to suggest, as he adds, that it can only be justified 'from a legal or administrative standpoint' is to sell it short. It represents at least potentially a major shift in the objectives of the health care sector. The ideals on which it is based are truly humanitarian with interests specifically in health as a means of furthering human welfare but at the same time not just the promotion of the health of the individual but the concern for the health of the community as expressed in its equity goals. It is this 'caring externality' or concern for the community (the caring about caring) which was the guiding light by which the National Health Service's original goals were set.

Indeed in terms of the changing economic framework of health care it is worthy of note that the issues of caring and of freedom were crucial. Opposition to the National Health Service stemmed largely from those who saw the economic independence of the medical profession being threatened by the state. Specifically the nationalisation of hospitals was viewed as a major assault on the laudable principle of voluntarism.

The key issue here is not so much voluntarism versus nationalisation but rather the choice of what weights to attach to freedom of choice, to equity and to health. It is not a simple choice but it is clear that as conceived the latter two were intended by the founders to be given much more weight than the first, indeed, if necessary, at the expense of the first.

Against the background of the existing system of health care provision, it is difficult to see how the planning of a national, co-ordinated hospital service could have been contemplated without nationalisation. Furthermore the re-distribution which becomes possible within a nationalised network means that provincial hospitals can better compete for medical staff with the urban hospitals, by offering comparable salaries and conditions.

At the time the National Health Service was set up, it was widely believed that there would be a high initial demand for care, followed by a tailing off, as accumulated 'need' for care was met. This view was expressed in the Beveridge Report[18]. However, although demand for dentures and spectacles did ease off after the first few years, as a backlog was satisfied, throughout the rest of the service, no such thing happened. There is no objective and universally acceptable definition of need. The nature and extent of an individuals' expressed need for health care, indeed for health, depends on the perception of that need by the person involved, by her/his family or friends, and by the health care professionals with whom she/he has contact.

A variety of factors has contributed to shifts in levels of total demand over time: (1) as more life-threatening diseases are brought under control, and more effective means of dealing with acute ailments are found, it is to be expected that less obviously pressing ailments will assume a greater significance. (2) Any success in terms of extended life-span brings added demand from the aged. Indeed, the care of the elderly consumes an ever-increasing volume and proportion of health service resources. (3) The growth of real incomes in the post-war years bred a rise in expectations – a demand for better standards of health along with improved standards in housing, education and nutrition. (4) Rapid technical progress in medicine and surgery also bolstered expectations, particularly among the medical profession. New drug therapies or advances in such areas as transplant surgery offer fresh hopes of survival or recovery. Such new treatments may be more cost-effective than the possible alternatives, but they may not. Whatever the costs, there is a common attitude in our society that it is immoral to withhold treatment on the grounds of cost. Such an attitude implies either a belief that available input resources are infinite, or a refusal to acknowledge the opportunity cost of any particular resource use (that is, the sacrifice which will be required elsewhere in the system).

During the years of relatively rapid growth it seemed possible for those committed to the health service to believe, if not that resources were infinite, at least that provision would continue to be expanded until demand was met. Among those with reservations about the service, there was considerable alarm over the increasing cost to the Exchequer.

The economic recession of recent years has led to a growing acceptance of the reality that the health service cannot expand indefinitely. In an era in which the service is faced with an absence of growth, or even with contraction in real terms, the choices between alternative patterns of provision appear more stark. However, it is important to be clear about the fact that those choices are inescapable, even if they are not made explicit.

It is possible to identify several key economic events in the development of the National Health Service in Scotland since its inception in 1948. First, there was the early concern with the growth in expenditure leading to the imposition of charges and the breaching of the principle of 'free' provision as set out at the start of the service. Spectacles, dentures and prescription charges all came in in 1951 or 1952 and of course have remained ever since (with the exception of prescription charges in the mid sixties.)

Second in 1962 the 'Hospital Plan for Scotland' was published. This represented the most important document in planning terms in the history of the National Health Service in Scotland. Yet it was very limited in terms of its approach to planning, first, in being based on the assumption that there was an existing level of need that it was possible to meet in full and secondly, being wholly capital led in the sense of simply assuming that the revenue consequences of the capital schemes would be met – and indeed did not have to be planned for. It is hardly surprising that concern about the growth of spending on health care grew over the sixties, being reflected in the setting up of the Public Expenditure Survey Committee (PESC) in 1964 whose concern was with *total* spending and not just capital.

Third, the reorganisation of 1974 resulted in the formation of Health Boards and the closer integration of what had previously been three separate entities – the hospitals, the community service and the primary care services (GPs, general dentists, etc). This most certainly represented an important move in terms of economic efficiency – in allowing a greater potential for substitutability of services across these three sectors. A further reorganisation in 1982 shifted the emphasis within health boards more towards functional units, with less emphasis than previously on geographical areas within boards as the locus of management.

Fourth, in 1976 and again in 1980, priorities documents in the form of first, *The Way Ahead*[19] and second, *Scottish Health Authorities Priorities for the Eighties* (SHAPE)[20] appeared from the Scottish Home and Health Department. While in retrospect it is strange to think that the Scottish Health Service could exist for nearly 30 years *without* setting out its priorities it has still to be recognised that the extent to which these documents were anything other than reflections of statements of political policy already enunciated was limited. Certainly, there was little attempt at rational analysis in *The Way Ahead* and little more in Scottish Health Authorities Priorities for the Eighties.

Fifth, in the interests of promoting greater equity across the different health boards, the *Scottish Health Authorities Revenue Equalisation* (SHARE) *Report*[21] formalised a needs-based formula which replaced a hitherto largely supply based approach to allocation. While little more than a copy of its RAWP counterpart south of the border it nonetheless represents the most important – if limited – contribution to the pursuit of equity in the Scottish National Health Service.

Sixth, in 1976 planning by volume was replaced by cash limits. Prior to this time, allocations were made to the boards in terms of last year's spending plus an allowance to meet any inflation and then some small growth monies on top of that. Cash limits mean just that – with no guarantee that such limits will allow the full extent of inflation to be covered. This has led to increased emphasis on financial control in the health care sector and less on service planning.

Lastly, there has been the Griffiths Management Inquiry[22] which has led to the appointment of general managers and increased concern with management efficiency generally. It has also led to more being done by way of experimenting with different budgeting systems to attempt to control and influence expenditure patterns within the service.

It is too early to say what the cumulative effect of all these changes has been. Certainly the awareness of the need for efficiency has increased but there is a long way to go before any real success can be claimed in meeting that goal.

The issue of setting priorities for different client groups remains too closely associated with medical opinion, despite the attempts to change the position through *The Way Ahead* and *Scottish Health Authorities Priorities for the Eighties.* Even the clearest official statement of policy objectives may not in itself be sufficient to ensure the attainment of those objectives. For example, one of the principal themes in both priorities documents was that there should be a shift of emphasis away from general and acute hospital services, and more on provision for the mentally ill, the mentally handicapped and the elderly. However, from 1977 to 1982, the number of beds per 100,000 population aged 65 and over rose by only 7 *per cent*, while the numbers of psychiatric and mental handicap beds fell by 7.3 *per cent* and 3.8 *per cent* respectively. If we use numbers of consultants as an indicator, those in geriatrics rose by only 6 *per cent*, in mental illness by 9 *per cent*, but in acute care by 13 *per cent* (Cole, McGuire and Stuart)[23]. If the reason for setting priorities is (as it should be) that, for a given extra expenditure, the benefits to be gained in a high priority area is greater than in any other, then a failure to pursue agreed objectives effectively is clearly inefficient.

On equity too there has to be some disappointment that so little has been done in the wake of the *Scottish Health Authorities Revenue Equalisation* report. There is scope for improving equity by Health Boards – particularly as the current method of costing of cross boundary flows breeds centralisation and protects the two main Boards, Lothian and Greater Glasgow, at the expense of those around them. But there is even greater scope for beginning to tackle the major inequities that exist across social classes.

The Century in Economic Perspective

Clearly there have been very substantial changes in health care during this century in Scotland. From the inequitable and, even in terms of their own goals we would submit, inefficient Poor Law and voluntary services of the start of the century, major advances have been made. These stem largely from the formation of the National Health Service in 1948 which has led clearly to greater equity and at least created the potential for greater efficiency.

Yet the potential has not been realised on efficiency. Certainly the integration of services in 1974 helped foster efficiency but the efforts at planning since then have been disappointing and based insufficiently on any perceptible economic rationale. There has been a lack of will to grasp the efficiency nettle.

Equity both geographic and social was a major pillar of the National Health Service in Scotland when it was established and there can be little doubt that Scotland enjoys a more equitable health care system than most other countries in Western Europe. Yet advances on equity since 1948, with the exception of *Scottish Health Authorities Revenue Equalisation*, seem small.

Scotland does relatively well for the funding of its National Health

Service compared with England. Increasingly, however, questions have to be asked about whether this additional funding has not meant a growing complacency and acceptance of inefficiencies and inequities. New initiatives in management and policy making are needed and perhaps general managers and new forms of budgeting introduced by Griffiths will help.

To date private medicine, while recently growing, has constituted less of a threat to the National Health Service in Scotland than in England. But unless the right sorts of incentives are devised and actions taken to try to ensure a more efficient National Health Service, it may well be that more and more of the Scots will turn to private medicine – especially the medical profession. We doubt if that would be socially efficient; we are convinced it would not promote equity.

Acknowledgements

We wish to acknowledge financial support from the Scottish Economic Society and to thank Rochelle Coutts for typing the manuscript.

References

(1) Gray, A.M., *The Rising Cost of Scottish Hospitals, 1951–81*. Ph.D. Thesis, University of Aberdeen, 1983.
(2) Feinstein, C.H., *National Income Expenditure and Output of the United Kingdom, 1955–1965*. Calculated from various tables.
(3) Lenman, B., *An Economic History of Modern Scotland. London, 1977*. p.202.
(4) Mitchison, R., *A History of Scotland. London, 1970*. p.402.
(5) *The Housing of the Industrial Population of Scotland, Urban and Rural*. Cmnd 8731. Edinburgh, 1917.
(6) *Committee on Scottish Health Services Report*. Cmnd 5204. Edinburgh, 1936. para. 14.
(7) *Report of Departmental Committee on Poor Law Medical Relief (Scotland)*. Cmnd 2008. London, 1904. para. 54.
(8) *Royal Commission on the Poor Laws and Relief of Distress, (Report on Scotland)*. Cmnd 4922. London, 1909. Part IV, para. 7.
(9) *Ibid.*
(10) *Op. cit.*, Part IV, para. 14.
(11) *Op. cit.*, Part IV, para. 16.
(12) *Op. cit.*, Part IV, para. 17.
(13) *Royal Commission on the Poor Law and Relief of Distress, (Report on Scotland)*. Cmnd 4922, (London 1909), Separate Report by the Very Reverend the Dean of Norwich, Mr F. Chandler, Mr George Lansbury and Mrs Sidney Webb, p.259.
(14) Gilbert, B.B., *The Evolution of National Insurance in Great Britain: The Origins of the Welfare State*. London, 1966. p.290.

(15) *Committee on Scottish Health Services Report, op. cit.,* para. 29.

(16) *National Health Service (Scotland) Bill, (Bill 49).* London, 1947. para. 1.

(17) Watkin, B., *The National Health Service: The First Phase 1948–1974 and After.* London, 1978. p.1.

(18) Beveridge, Sir W., *Social Insurance and Allied Services.* London, 1942.

(19) Scottish Home and Health Department, *The Health Services in Scotland, The Way Ahead.* Edinburgh, 1976.

(20) Scottish Home and Health Department, *Scottish Health Authorities Priorities for the Eighties.* Edinburgh, 1980.

(21) Scottish Home and Health Department, *Scottish Health Authorities Revenue Equalisation.* Edinburgh, 1977.

(22) House of Commons, Social Services Committee, *Griffiths NHS Management Enquiry Report.* London, 1984.

(23) Cole, P., McGuire, A., and Stuart, P., *More money better health care? A comparison of NHS spending and health service provision in Scotland and England.* HERU Discussion Paper, University of Aberdeen, No. 03/85.

EPILOGUE

TRIBUTE TO
SIR JOHN BROTHERSTON

Delivered at the KIRK of the GREYFRIARS,
EDINBURGH, 17th May 1985

by

Professor A. S. Duncan D.S.C., F.R.C.S.E., F.R.C.P.E., F.R.C.O.G.

JOHN HOWIE FLINT BROTHERSTON – the very name has a ring of importance and dignity fitted to the man whose life and achievements we commemorate today. The name 'John' has come to mean one who is specially loved – and more of that presently. The name of a Howie forebear is to be found on the Covenanters Roll in this the Covenanters' Kirk. 'Flint' derives from good farmer and merchant stock in Ayrshire, but suggests to me the spark of fire of enthusiasm. And 'Brotherston' reminds us that John's father was an Edinburgh Writer to the Signet and that his mother was one of the pioneer women doctors in Scotland. She developed Maternity & Child Welfare Services and lived to know the distinction that her son had achieved both in that field and in general.

With such a background and heredity it is not surprising that the man in our thoughts today was determined to achieve his ideals and objectives and that he became one of the foremost Scots of his generation. He was very very proud of Scotland and its people. He lived and worked for them and, in order to remain here, he chose not to accept distinguished posts elsewhere.

Born and educated in Edinburgh, John Brotherston has had an outstanding career both in academic life and in the Health Service. As a student he was Senior President of the Students' Representative Council. Perhaps it was this which led him, when Dean of the Faculty of Medicine from 1958 to 1963, to involve students in Faculty affairs long before such a development in other Faculties. But I think, rather, that this was part of his lifelong policy of involving as many groups as possible in discussion and in decision-making. This was one of his great strengths for it made people think for themselves and be concerned with the issues of the day. He was essentially an ideas man and his enthusiasm was infectious.

Before he started Medicine John graduated Master of Arts with History and Political Economy as special subjects and he has maintained a great feeling for the Scottish tradition both in Medicine and in Society. He was Honorary President of the Campaign of the Scottish Assembly and, at the time of his death, he was in the late stages of editing and writing a history of health care in Scotland from 1900 to the present day. That work will shortly be completed by his fellow contributors, and, when published, will be a further memorial to him.

John Brotherston had two very fruitful spells as head of the University Department at the Usher Institute and led the department from strength to strength. In between he was Chief Medical Officer at the Scottish Home and Health Department and, in both these important posts he has been a great innovator and the pioneer of integration of health care. As Chief Medical Officer he travelled extensively all over Scotland so that he could see problems at first hand and so that individuals got to know him personally.

Although essentially a Scot and indeed an Edinburgh Scot, his influence and interests have been much wider. His early appointments were in the United States and in London and he has since travelled extensively. He played an important part in the work of the World Health Organisation and that led to the establishment in Edinburgh of the first Diploma course in medical service administration and also to Edinburgh's six-year link with the Medical College in Baroda in India. John's international reputation led in 1971 to his being the first Briton to be awarded by the American Public Health Association the prestigious Bronfman Prize in recognition of achievements leading to improvements in Community Health. Many other awards included honorary degrees from Aberdeen and Bristol. He was knighted in 1972 and was Honorary Physician to the Queen from 1965 to 1968.

He did not often speak of his war experiences except in praise of others but he had a distinguished Army record in the Middle East and in Europe. He was wounded in the Sicily landings and carried shrapnel in his body for the rest of his life.

There has been wide publicity recently for the Black Report on Inequalities in Health Care but, as the Black Committee though perhaps not others recognise, John Brotherston in his Galton Lecture in 1974 had said it all and had drawn attention to the special needs of deprived areas.

Sir John was a great champion of general practice. In the University he had set up, based on the Scottish Dispensary system, a General Practice Teaching Unit which later became a full University Department – the first in the United Kingdom. He led the campaign in Scotland for Health Centres and links with hospitals. He initiated the

Livingston experiment where General Practitioners also have hospital appointments. All this work led to the greatly enhanced status of the Family Doctor. At the same time he was a great believer in the responsibility of the public for their own health and, in this connection, he was amongst other things Scottish Chairman of ASH.

As Chief Medical Officer John Brotherston will be mainly remembered for his joint working parties on integration. We tend to forget already that at the beginning of the National Health Service, general practitioners, hospital staff and the Public Health Services were all run by different authorities and collaboration was difficult to say the least. Parallel with change south of the border led by George Godber, John Brotherston's work on integration in Scotland has changed all that and now we have a unified health service. During that work he drove himself and never let up *and* he got others to do likewise – such are the attributes of a great leader. He was greatly concerned with the long stay services, and the Medical Advisory Structure was his brainchild as was the Scottish Health Services Planning Council. He was an innovator; he emphasised clinical integration and saw management as a means to an end. As Chief Medical Officer he introduced regular meetings with the Deans of Medical Schools and these greatly improved relationships between Universities and the NHS.

It was during the Brotherston deanship that the first radical change in the medical curriculum was planned and, during that phase, I know that his home was littered for months with tables and graphs. The new curriculum, like the health service changes, featured close integration. John was for many years a most successful chairman of the Education Committee of the General Medical Council. He instituted the series of national conferences on various educational topics and he mounted the Survey of Medical Education in the British Isles. In this regard and in studies of Quality of Care and many others he worked in close association with the Nuffield Provincial Hospitals Trust which supported him strongly and found him most persuasive.

Two important developments stemmed from the restructure of the Health Service and John was greatly involved in both. The first, the evolution of the specialty of community medicine has not yet had time to reach full fruition but now Medical Officers of Health, Administrative medical officers and academics are finding common ground and the University Department of Community Medicine in Edinburgh under Sir John has played a leading rôle in planning appropriate training for the new breed of specialist. The second related development is now well established. The Faculty of Community Medicine sponsored by the Royal Colleges of Physicians is now the national forum for all the groups I have mentioned. In planning the Faculty John was more involved than anyone else and he filled a missionary rôle, explaining that by integration the functions of the three disparate groups could be unified and enhanced. Despite his stroke, which occurred during his term of office as the Faculty's third President, he travelled the length and breadth of the United Kingdom to link the grass roots membership with the London Headquarters.

Already the Faculty has established a Student Essay Prize in memory of his presidency – he was looking forward to presenting the first prize this summer.

While he was accomplishing all this John's family was a great joy to him. Lady Brotherston, herself a doctor, has been a tremendous support in all he did and his sons and daughters added strength. His nine grandchildren delighted him. He was very proud that one of the grandsons will become a fourth generation medical student in Edinburgh this autumn. On the occasion of his 70th birthday in March of this year John received a card from his daughter Margaret who lives in the United States. The card said 'Hope my present arrives in time'. A few hours later the present was on the doorstep – Margaret herself. She is with us today but knowing of her father's serious illness she came in March without telling anybody and this of course delighted her father. All the family have memories of energetic holidays exploring Scotland, of John's recent interest in cooking and wine-making and of his insistence on taking photographs on every possible family occasion from breakfast onwards.

When illness struck John some years ago and again more recently the support of his wife and family again gave him extra strength. He was also full of praise for all those who looked after him in hospital and at home. He bore his illnesses with great courage as indeed he had done with other illnesses throughout his life about which he didn't speak. After his stroke he and Bunty resumed their yachting and last summer John fulfilled a dream to explore his beloved Scotland in his boat right up the west coast to the Summer Isles. Before the yachting phase he had returned to golf after many years and of course nothing less than the redoubtable Muirfield was for him.

He was much loved by all his friends and we will continue to enjoy happy memories of our association with him. His work will continue in the inspiration which he has instilled in others. John had a great flair for spotting talent and he was kind, loyal and supportive to those whom he had chosen. This is not to say he was not tough for how else could he have achieved so much; but he had great charisma and we will remember him for himself as well as for his tremendous contribution to the integration of health care. What greater memorial could a man have than such a legacy to society as well as to medicine.

Index

Acknowledgements

Because of the circumstances of my taking over the editorship and presentation of this volume, I am grateful for the help afforded me by a large number of people which is testimony to the high regard which Sir John Brotherston's colleagues and friends had for him.

Thus, I must first pay tribute to the authors of the essays in this collation who bore with great patience my many trespasses on their time when I was getting to grips with the magnitude of the problem presented in taking over another's work, while at the same time trying to be faithful to his approach and intention. Coupled with them is Jemima Porter who typed their manuscripts efficaciously.

In connection with the Introduction, Norman Graham and Archie Rennie kindly consented to read the third section 1948–84 and made very useful comments, as did Stuart Morrison from a professional Public Health point of view, which helped me considerably in my task as Editor.

John Brims who was the Research Assistant was a great help in providing me with invaluable information about the course of the study, and responded nobly to the demands I made on him in connection with one or two of the essays and the vast number of prime source references involved. Derek Dow answered magnificently my appeal for help in checking the page proofs, and went far beyond, by drawing attention to a host of discrepancies most of which, I hope I have eliminated.

Mrs Hilary Flenley at very short notice and in difficult circumstances produced the Index which was no mean feat.

My daughter Tessa who was working with me when I assumed the task, gave me immense support at a difficult time when not only was I beginning to realise what I had taken on, but I was also on the point of retiring after 31 years as Secretary of the Trust. Her work in the initial sub-editing when we were getting to know the authors, and her preparation of the manuscripts, kept me and the project going.

Above all however, without the constant encouragement, advice and comments from that Prince and wisest of friends, Archie Duncan, this collation in John Brotherston's honour would never have been completed.

The Editor

Gordon McLachlan C.B.E., B.Com., F.C.A., LLD. (Hon), F.R.C.G.P. (Hon), was born, brought up and educated in Leith and Edinburgh. After war service in the Royal Navy and appointments in Local Government and the NHS he was from 1955 to 1986 Secretary of the Nuffield Provincial Hospitals Trust and General Editor of their Publications List. Since 1974 he has been a Member (by election) of the Institute of Medicine of the National Academy of Sciences, Washington, D.C.

G. McL.